HEALTHCARE TECHNOLOGIES SERIES 61

Artificial Intelligence and Blockchain Technology in Modern Telehealth Systems

IET Book Series on e-Health Technologies

Book Series Editor: Professor Joel J.P.C. Rodrigues, College of Computer Science and Technology, China University of Petroleum (East China), Qingdao, China; Senac Faculty of Ceará, Fortaleza-CE, Brazil and Instituto de Telecomunicações, Portugal

Book Series Advisor: Professor Pranjal Chandra, School of Biochemical Engineering, Indian Institute of Technology (BHU), Varanasi, India

While the demographic shifts in populations display significant socio-economic challenges, they trigger opportunities for innovations in e-Health, m-Health, precision and personalized medicine, robotics, sensing, the Internet of things, cloud computing, big data, software defined networks, and network function virtualization. Their integration is however associated with many technological, ethical, legal, social, and security issues. This book series aims to disseminate recent advances for e-health technologies to improve healthcare and people's wellbeing.

Could you be our next author?

Topics considered include intelligent e-Health systems, electronic health records, ICT-enabled personal health systems, mobile and cloud computing for e-Health, health monitoring, precision and personalized health, robotics for e-Health, security and privacy in e-Health, ambient assisted living, telemedicine, big data and IoT for e-Health, and more.

Proposals for coherently integrated international multi-authored edited or co-authored handbooks and research monographs will be considered for this book series. Each proposal will be reviewed by the book Series Editor with additional external reviews from independent reviewers.

To download our proposal form or find out more information about publishing with us, please visit https://www.theiet.org/publishing/publishing-with-iet-books/.

Please email your completed book proposal for the IET Book Series on e-Health Technologies to: Amber Thomas at athomas@theiet.org or author_support@theiet.org.

The Institution of
Engineering and Technology

Artificial Intelligence and Blockchain Technology in Modern Telehealth Systems

Edited by
Agbotiname Lucky Imoize, Chandrashekhar Meshram, Joseph Bamidele Awotunde and Dinh-Thuan Do

The Institution of Engineering and Technology

Published by The Institution of Engineering and Technology, London, United Kingdom

The Institution of Engineering and Technology is registered as a Charity in England & Wales (no. 211014) and Scotland (no. SC038698).

First published 2023

The Institution of Engineering and Technology
Futures Place
Kings Way, Stevenage
Hertfordshire, SG1 2UA, United Kingdom

www.theiet.org

British Library Cataloguing in Publication Data
A catalogue record for this product is available from the British Library

ISBN 978-1-83953-863-6 (hardback)
ISBN 978-1-83953-864-3 (PDF)

Typeset in India by MPS Limited

Cover Image: Yuichiro Chino/Moment via Getty Images

Contents

About the editors

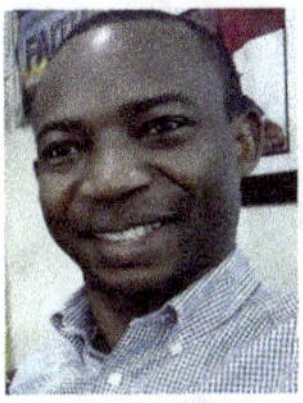

Agbotiname Lucky Imoize (senior member, IEEE) received the B.Eng. degree (Hons.) in Electrical and Electronics Engineering from Ambrose Alli University, Nigeria, in 2008 and the M.Sc. degree in Electrical and Electronics Engineering from the University of Lagos, Nigeria, in 2012. He is a lecturer in the Department of Electrical and Electronics Engineering at the University of Lagos, Nigeria. He was, until recently, a research scholar at the Ruhr University Bochum, Germany, under the sponsorship of the Nigerian Petroleum Technology Development Fund (PTDF) and the German Academic Exchange Service (DAAD) through the Nigerian-German Postgraduate Program. He was awarded the Fulbright fellowship as a visiting research scholar at the Wireless@VT Laboratory, Bradley Department of Electrical and Computer Engineering, Virginia Tech., USA, where he worked under the supervision of Prof. R. Michael Buehrer from 2017 to 2018. Before joining the University of Lagos, he was a Lecturer at Bells University of Technology, Nigeria. He worked as a core network products manager at ZTE, Nigeria, and as a Network Switching Subsystem Engineer at Globacom, Nigeria. His research interests cover the fields of 6G wireless communication, wireless security systems, and artificial intelligence. He has coedited five books and coauthored over 180 papers in peer review journals and conferences. Imoize is an active reviewer and editor for over 50 international journals and conferences. He is the Vice Chair of the IEEE Communication Society, Nigeria chapter, a Registered Engineer with the COREN, and a member of the Nigerian Society of Engineers (NSE).

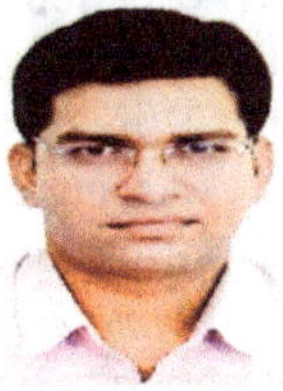

Chandrashekhar Meshram is an assistant professor in the Department of Post Graduate Studies and Research in Mathematics, Jaywanti Haksar Government Post Graduate College, Chhindwara University, Betul, India. His research interests include cryptography and its applications, neural networks, the IoT, WSNs, medical information systems, ad hoc networks, number theory, fuzzy theory, time series analysis, climate change, mathematical modeling, and chaos theory. He has published over 150 scientific articles in international journals and conferences on these research fields. In addition, he is a regular reviewer for over 60 international journals and conferences. He is a member of IAENG, WASET, CSTA, IACSIT, EAI, ILAS, SCIEI, MIR Labs, and a lifetime member of the Indian Mathematical Society and Cryptology Research Society. He received his Ph.D. degree in Mathematics from R.T.M. Nagpur University, Nagpur, India.

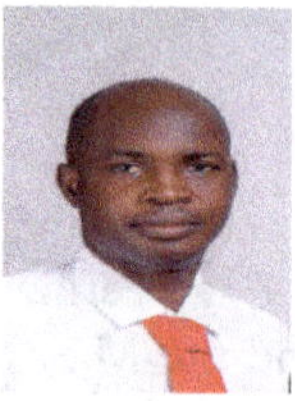

Joseph Bamidele Awotunde received a B.Sc. degree in Mathematics/Computer Science from the Federal University of Technology, Minna, Nigeria, in 2007, M.Sc. and Ph.D. degrees in Computer Science from the University of Ilorin, Ilorin, Nigeria, in 2014 and 2019, respectively. He was formerly a Lecturer with McPherson University, Nigeria. Currently, he is a Lecturer with the Computer Science Department, University of Ilorin, Nigeria. He has authored or coauthored over 100 articles, 50 book chapters, and over 40 conference proceedings. His research interests include Information Security, Cybersecurity, Bioinformatics, Artificial Intelligence, the Internet of Medical Things, Wireless Body Sensor Networks, Telemedicine, m-Health/e-health, Medical Imaging, Software Engineering, and Biometrics. He is a member of the International Association of Engineers and Computer Scientists (IAENG), the Computer Professional Registration Council of Nigeria, and the Nigeria Computer Society.

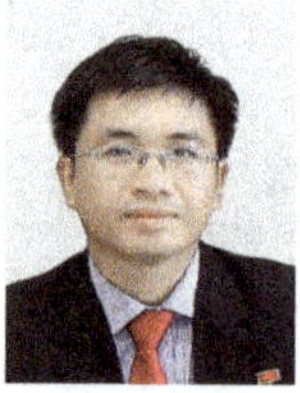

Dinh-Thuan Do is an Assistant Professor in the School of Engineering, University of Mount Union, Alliance, USA. He was a Research Scientist at the Electrical Engineering Department, University of Colorado Denver, Denver, USA. Also, he was formerly a Research Scientist in the Department of Electrical and Computer Engineering at the University of Texas at Austin, USA. Prior to joining The University of Texas at Austin, he was an Assistant Professor at Asia University in Taiwan and a Research Assistant Professor at Ton Duc Thang University in Vietnam. His research interests include signal processing in wireless communications networks, non-orthogonal multiple access, full-duplex transmission, and RIS. He received the Golden Globe Award from the Vietnam Ministry of Science and Technology in 2015 (Top ten excellent scientists nationwide). He is currently serving as an Editor of Computer Communications, Associate Editor of EURASIP Journal on Wireless Communications and Networking, Associate Editor of Electronics, Associate Editor of ICT Express, and Editor of KSII Transactions on Internet and Information Systems. His publications include over 100 SCIE/SCI-indexed journal articles and 40 international conference papers. In addition, he is the author of two textbooks and six book chapters. He is a senior member of the IEEE. He holds a Ph.D. degree in communications engineering from the Vietnam National University (VNU-HCMC), Vietnam.

Preface

Telehealth systems support healthcare professionals to monitor, diagnose, and treat patients remotely at minimal costs. The traditional telehealth systems are centralized and suffer limited service delivery, security, and privacy of user data. However, the security of sensitive user information is critical to effective and efficient healthcare delivery. Artificial intelligence (AI) and blockchain technology are identified as key drivers of emerging telehealth systems, enabling efficient delivery of telehealth services to billions of patients globally. These technological drivers assist in managing limited healthcare resources to satisfy the particular needs of patients in critical health conditions. Specifically, AI facilitates the processing and analysis of complex telehealth data, and blockchain technology offers decentralized, transparent, traceable, reliable, trustful, and robust security to telehealth systems. Blockchain uses a distributed architecture to manage the shared ledger of complex health data seamlessly. In order to gainfully exploit the enormous benefits of AI and blockchain in telehealth systems, there is a need to critically examine their technical design characteristics and how they are integrated into the telehealth system. Besides, the wide adoption of AI and blockchain technology in telehealth systems is still in its infancy, and several research issues need to be addressed to aid the rapid deployment of AI and blockchain in telehealth systems.

In this edited book, we review the proliferating design, application, security, and privacy issues in traditional telehealth systems, and present key promising AI and blockchain technology-based frameworks and efficient architectures to support telehealth systems. The book discusses the critical AI and blockchain-based applications to resolve security and privacy issues that affect all parties in the telehealth ecosystem and provides practical machine learning-based solutions to solve these problems. Specifically, the book beams a laser focus on the technical considerations, potential opportunities, and critical challenges inhibiting the ubiquitous adoption of AI and blockchain in telehealth systems. The book also discusses extensively, the prospects and societal benefits envisioned in AI and blockchain-based models for telehealth systems. Finally, the book presents case studies, highlights critical lessons, and provides valuable recommendations for designing future AI and blockchain-based telehealth systems.

The key features of the book are outlined as follows:

- Brings new insights into real-world scenarios of the deployment, applications, management, and associated benefits of robust, and efficient AI and blockchain techniques in telehealth systems.

- Discusses critical security and privacy issues which affect all parties in the healthcare ecosystem and provide practical AI and blockchain-based solutions to resolve these issues.
- Beams a laser focus on the technical considerations, potential opportunities and critical challenges inhibiting the ubiquitous adoption of AI and blockchain in telehealth systems.
- Proposes solutions to revamp the traditional telehealth architecture to address the emerging security challenges in modern telehealth systems.

Specifically, the book is structured into 21 chapters outlined as follows:

Chapter 1 gives an overview of AI and blockchain technology in telehealth systems, focusing on the background and basic features of a telehealth system that facilitates communication between medical experts and recipients of healthcare services. The chapter highlights the geographical statistics of countries that are effectively adopting AI and blockchain technology in telehealth systems. Chapter 2 presents a taxonomy that explores the integration of AI and blockchain in telehealth systems. The taxonomy aims to categorize, classify, and analyze the various applications, benefits, challenges, and future directions of this integration, providing a comprehensive understanding of the synergistic relationship among AI, blockchain, and telehealth. Chapter 3 torchlights wireless communications channels, models, and protocols used in telehealth systems. The study aims to enable researchers and healthcare providers to decide on the telehealth system that best suits their needs and requirements.

Chapter 4 provides a blockchain-based framework that incorporates AI to streamline the process of compiling the medical history of patients from several sources such as prescriptions (printed or handwritten) and imprinted documents into a single record. In this case, the medical report is kept safely via a decentralized blockchain network and displays just the most important facts in a succinct style for ease of access. Chapter 5 dwells on AI and blockchain enabling data access authorization in telehealth systems. The chapter explores the integration of AI and blockchain and their implications for secure and transparent data access in telehealth systems. Chapter 6 discusses AI and blockchain-enabled synergies for telehealth projects. The chapter revealed the applicable tools and approaches for creating synergies between AI and blockchain technology. Selected AI and blockchain-enabled projects in telehealth comprising MedCredits, MedChain, BlochHeal, and MyHealthMyData were lucidly presented. The findings showed that strengthening the synergies between AI and blockchain technology in telehealth will significantly engender the trust of patients and clinicians.

Chapter 7 provides recent advances in AI and blockchain technology applied to telehealth systems. The chapter beams a laser focus on the deliverables of telehealth and the remarkable enhancement of telehealth systems using AI and blockchain technologies. Last, the chapter highlights the recent advancement in rapidAI, ProvChain, extreme data privacy, and the application layer security for application in modern telehealth systems. Chapter 8 examines architectural design criteria for AI and blockchain technology in telehealth systems. The chapter discusses the implementation of four design criteria, such as the development of secure blockchain networks, the use of smart contracts to automate the processing of transactions, the development of user-friendly interfaces to facilitate control of patient data, and the consideration of ethical and legal issues in the overall system design framework.

Chapter 9 focuses on addressing computational complexity issues in telehealth systems using AI and blockchain technology. The chapter begins by highlighting the increasing utilization of telehealth services, particularly during the COVID-19 pandemic, and the advantages they offer, such as convenience, cost savings, and improved patient insights. Particularly, the study explores the architecture, functionality, and key applications of AI and blockchain in telehealth systems. The chapter also outlines the challenges and research gaps in telehealth systems, including privacy concerns, efficient data processing, regulatory compliance, and the urgency associated with resolving the ensuing computational issues arising from the use of AI and blockchain in telehealth systems. In addition, the chapter discusses the implications of recent research findings in the telehealth care domain, emphasizing the ethical considerations of bias in AI algorithms and the importance of transparency and accountability. Chapter 10 examines the potential issues and risks associated with the integration of AI and blockchain technology in telehealth systems. The authors emphasized that all stakeholders in telehealth systems must collaborate to develop robust technical standards, governance mechanisms, and regulatory frameworks to mitigate the identified issues and risks in modern telehealth systems.

In Chapter 11, various telehealth concerns triggered by cybersecurity from a universal telehealth system perspective, its vulnerability, and what the future could hold for telehealth systems at the facility, patients' level, and other stakeholders in the telehealth ecosystem are highlighted. Identifiable attacks and imperatives for telehealth systems, and global significances for medical data are demonstrated. Chapter 12 presents testing and validation of AI and blockchain-based models for application in telehealth systems. Specifically, AI-inspired algorithms were employed to predict chronic kidney diseases for early detection and prevention. Classifiers such as the Random Forest and eXtreme Gradient Boosting were utilized for the forecast with an accuracy of 97.50% and 96.50%, respectively.

Chapter 13 x-rayed the importance of cybersecurity in healthcare, exploring various cyber threats faced by healthcare systems, including malware attacks, ransomware attacks, and social engineering attacks. The chapter examines the impact of these threats on healthcare, such as patient privacy breaches, financial losses, and reputational damage. Furthermore, the chapter delves into the regulatory and legal requirements that healthcare organizations must adhere to in order to safeguard patient privacy and security. Chapter 14 dissects the regulatory policies for telehealth data protection using AI and blockchain technology. The authors opine that AI can detect and respond to threats in real-time by continuously monitoring telehealth platforms, which lowers the chance of data breaches and illegal access. The study revealed that blockchain technology could be harnessed to establish secure, decentralized data storage and sharing, and telehealth providers can ensure patient confidentiality while improving the efficiency and accessibility of healthcare services. The chapter also reviews current telehealth regulatory frameworks that can foster innovation and ensure patient safety in the rapidly changing telehealth landscape.

Chapter 15 investigates the legal frameworks surrounding the utilization of AI and blockchain in telehealth systems. The chapter examined key aspects such as data privacy, security, liability, consent, and intellectual property rights in the context of these emerging technologies. Chapter 16 explores the technological difficulties in adopting blockchain and AI in telemedicine, including the requirements for interoperability and guidelines to ensure that various systems can effectively communicate seamlessly. The chapter emphasizes the significance of data standardization to guarantee consistency and accuracy in healthcare data management. The chapter concludes with a call to action for government and healthcare professionals to embrace the opportunities of blockchain and AI in telehealth while also being aware of the associated technical and ethical issues involved.

In Chapter 17, a method for location information privacy protection considering human presence probability is discussed elaborately. Specifically, the chapter proposes a method to mitigate service quality loss, which is a quantifiable indicator of user convenience, by considering the probability of human presence. Chapter 18 provides recent case studies on the application of AI and blockchain technology in telehealth systems. The chapter explores the critical case studies with the aim of identifying the gaps inherent in existing works and provides potential solutions to the identified gaps. The work also explores the relevant AI algorithms and architecture for related studies in telehealth systems. The authors conclude that the findings from the case studies have the potential of transforming the telehealth system into a more efficient and effective platform.

Chapter 19 focuses on achieving quality healthcare using blockchain technology for detecting fake drugs. The chapter proposes a private permissioned blockchain as well as IoT technologies for detecting fake drugs. The approach enables pharmaceutical companies to upload information about their drugs, attach unique ID in the form of QR Code or Snaptags and push it to the blockchain network. Chapter 20 projects cybersecurity in centralized healthcare systems, giving an overview, design framework, challenges, and research trends. The chapter gives an in-depth evaluation of the role of cybersecurity in modern healthcare systems and highlights the importance of designing and implementing effective cybersecurity measures, as well as the need for ongoing research to address the ever-evolving threats posed by malicious actors in the healthcare ecosystem. Finally, Chapter 21 focuses on AI and blockchain for healthcare from the perspective of security, privacy, and confidentiality. The chapter concludes by offering recommendations on how to ascertain secure and private use of AI and blockchain in modern healthcare systems.

Gelsenkirchen, North Rhine-Westphalia, Germany
Agbotiname Lucky Imoize

Acknowledgments

I sincerely express my profound gratitude to God for His faithfulness and divine wisdom to edit this book. This book would not have been possible without the support of the Department of Electrical Engineering and Information Technology, Institute of Digital Communication, Ruhr University, Bochum, Germany, and the University of Lagos, Nigeria. I acknowledge the sponsorship from the Nigerian Petroleum Technology Development Fund (PTDF) and the German Academic Exchange Service (DAAD) through the Nigerian-German Postgraduate Program. Special thanks to my beloved wife, Kelly, and our sons, Lucius, Luke, and Lucas. Also, I am indebted to the Deeper Life Bible Church, Essen Region, North Rhine-Westphalia, Germany, for their unwavering support. Last, I sincerely thank the Institution of Engineering and Technology (IET) for its editorial support.

Gelsenkirchen, North Rhine-Westphalia, Germany
Agbotiname Lucky Imoize

Chapter 1

An overview of artificial intelligence and blockchain technology in telehealth systems

Kingsley Theophilus Igulu[1] *and Nne Rena Saturday*[2]

Globally, healthcare services are being offered virtually with the combination of internet technologies called a telehealth system. Telehealth system focuses on delivering healthcare services to patients without physical interaction. This chapter gives the background and basic features of a telehealth system that facilitates communication between medical experts and recipients of healthcare services; exposing telecommunication protocols involved in the transmission of data in the system. It enumerates the benefits of telehealth system as well as the challenges of a telehealth system. Also, the chapter explores the integration of artificial intelligence (AI) in telehealth system, the fundamental AI models adopted in telehealth systems, the blocks that make up the blockchain, the efficacy of blockchain technology, and its pitfalls. Finally, the chapter highlights the geographical statistics of countries that are effectively adopting AI and blockchain technology in telehealth systems.

1.1 Introduction

According to recent reports [1,2], telehealth systems refer to the use of technology and telecommunications to provide remote healthcare services. These systems enable healthcare professionals to diagnose, treat, monitor, and educate patients remotely, eliminating the need for in-person visits. Telehealth systems encompass a wide range of technologies, including video conferencing, remote monitoring devices, mobile applications, and electronic health records (EHRs). They have gained significant popularity and have become an essential component of healthcare delivery, especially in situations where physical access to healthcare services may be limited or impractical [1].

Telehealth systems have revolutionized the way patients access healthcare services, providing vital connections through videoconferencing, remote monitoring, electronic consults, and wireless communications. This technology allows

[1]Department of Computer Science, Kenule Beeson Saro-Wiwa Polytechnic, Nigeria
[2]Department of Computer, Rivers State University, Nigeria

patients to receive care remotely, eliminating the need for in-person visits and improving access to healthcare services. Despite its numerous benefits, there are several barriers to the wider adoption of telehealth systems [2,3]. One of the primary challenges is the limited coverage and payment from Medicare, which hinders healthcare providers from offering telehealth services to a broader population.

Additionally, inadequate broadband access in rural areas poses a significant obstacle to the implementation of telehealth systems. To overcome these challenges, organizations like the American Hospital Association advocate for expanding Medicare coverage, resolving legal and regulatory issues, conducting more research on the cost–benefits of telehealth, and improving broadband access in rural areas. They also emphasize the importance of eliminating geographic and setting location requirements, expanding the types of technology used in telehealth systems, and covering all safe services. Legal and regulatory challenges further complicate the adoption of telehealth systems, particularly in areas such as coverage and payment, licensure, prescribing, privacy and security, as well as fraud and abuse prevention. More research is needed to evaluate the cost–benefits of telehealth for different medical conditions and to address these legal and regulatory challenges effectively [4–6].

Telehealth encompasses a broad range of digital information and communication technologies that enable patients to access healthcare services remotely and manage their health effectively. This includes virtual visits where patients can consult with healthcare providers or counselors via video or phone chats. As stated in [7], telehealth extends to web or phone-based services that provide medical care or advice, as well as remote monitoring using devices or apps to track health data. The primary goal of telehealth is to make healthcare more accessible, particularly for individuals living in remote areas who may face challenges in accessing traditional healthcare facilities [2]. Telehealth also aims to improve communication and coordination of care between patients and healthcare providers, enhancing the overall quality of care delivery. The COVID-19 pandemic has further highlighted the importance of telehealth systems, as they have become increasingly popular in ensuring continuity of care and minimizing the risk of virus transmission [8,9].

Telemedicine, a subset of telehealth, is important in providing immediate access to medical professionals, consultants, and additional education and statistics for hospitals and treatment centers. This technology enables healthcare facilities to connect with experts remotely, facilitating timely consultations and enhancing the delivery of patient care. By utilizing telemedicine, hospitals can overcome geographical barriers and leverage the expertise of medical professionals regardless of their physical location. This capability is particularly valuable in areas where specialized medical services may be limited. Telemedicine also offers opportunities for continuous education and training for healthcare professionals, ensuring they stay updated with the latest developments in their respective fields. By harnessing the capabilities of telemedicine, healthcare organizations can optimize their resources, improve patient outcomes, and enhance overall healthcare delivery.

1.1.1 Key contributions

The key contributions of the chapter are as follows:

1. The chapter provides an insightful overview of the integration of artificial intelligence (AI) and blockchain technology in telehealth systems.
2. The chapter provides a comprehensive discussion on various prospects and challenges of the integration of AI and blockchain technology in telehealth systems.
3. The chapter also discusses various solutions to the challenges of the integration of AI and blockchain technology in telehealth systems.
4. The chapter highlights several ethical and legal implications of the integration of AI and blockchain technology in telehealth systems.

1.1.2 Chapter structure

Section 1.2 presents related works of the integration AI and blockchain in telehealth. It highlights the key components and the benefits of telehealth systems. The section also discusses telehealth and general health management, evolution of telehealth systems, AI in telehealth, blockchain in telehealth as well as the synergies between AI and blockchain in telehealth. Section 1.3 presents the challenges and future directions of the integration of AI and blockchain in telehealth. Section 1.4 concludes the chapter.

1.2 Related work

1.2.1 Key components of telehealth systems

1. **Video conferencing:** Video conferencing platforms enable real-time communication between healthcare providers and patients. These platforms allow for face-to-face consultations, enabling healthcare professionals to assess patients' conditions, provide medical advice, and discuss treatment plans. Video conferencing also facilitates collaboration between multiple healthcare providers, allowing for multidisciplinary consultations and improving patient outcomes [10–13].
2. **Remote monitoring devices:** Telehealth systems often incorporate remote monitoring devices to collect and transmit patient health data from a distance. These devices can measure vital signs such as blood pressure, heart rate, glucose levels, and oxygen saturation. The data is securely transmitted to healthcare providers who can monitor the patients' health status remotely and make timely interventions when necessary. Remote monitoring is particularly beneficial for patients with chronic conditions who require continuous monitoring and management [14,15].
3. **Mobile applications:** Mobile applications are increasingly being used in telehealth systems to facilitate patient engagement and remote healthcare delivery. These apps allow patients to schedule appointments, access their medical records, receive educational materials, and communicate with healthcare

providers through secure messaging. Mobile apps also support the integration of wearable devices, enabling patients to track their health data and share it with their healthcare team [15,16].

4. **EHRs:** EHRs play a vital role in telehealth systems by providing secure and accessible storage for patient information. EHRs contain comprehensive medical records, including past diagnoses, medication history, allergies, and test results. When integrated with telehealth systems, EHRs allow healthcare providers to access and update patient records remotely, ensuring continuity of care and facilitating informed decision-making [5,10,15–17].

1.2.2 Benefits of telehealth systems

The benefits of telehealth systems are enormous. For the purpose of this work, the benefits are discussed in the following categories as also given in [3,11–13,17–19]:

Improved access to healthcare: Telehealth systems break down geographical barriers, enabling individuals in remote or underserved areas to access quality healthcare services. Patients can receive consultations, diagnosis, and treatment without the need for long-distance travel, reducing costs and improving healthcare equity.

Convenience and time savings: Telehealth eliminates the need for patients to travel to healthcare facilities, saving them time and reducing the burden of transportation. Patients can have virtual appointments from the comfort of their homes or workplaces, making healthcare more accessible and convenient.

Enhanced efficiency and workflow: Telehealth systems streamline healthcare processes by reducing waiting times, minimizing paperwork, and improving communication between healthcare providers. This leads to increased efficiency, allowing providers to see more patients and allocate their time more effectively.

Continuity of care: Telehealth enables seamless care coordination between multiple healthcare providers involved in a patient's treatment. It ensures that all relevant medical information is readily available, allowing for informed decision-making and reducing the risk of medical errors.

Cost savings: Telehealth can result in cost savings for both patients and healthcare systems. Patients save money on travel expenses, parking fees, and time away from work. Healthcare systems can reduce hospital readmissions, emergency department visits, and overall healthcare costs by proactively monitoring and managing patients remotely.

1.2.3 Telehealth and general health management

1. Telehealth modalities: The scope of telehealth systems extends beyond simply video conferencing. Store-and-forward telemedicine is one such method, and it involves the safe transmission of patient data like medical images or test results to doctors for later review. In addition, the use of wearable devices or sensors to collect and transmit real-time patient data paves the way for remote patient

monitoring, which enables healthcare professionals to remotely monitor and manage patients' conditions. Medical professionals now have access to a wider range of tools to provide care that is tailored to each patient [15,16,20].

2. Emergency telehealth services: Telehealth systems play a crucial role in emergency situations, enabling remote triage and consultation. Emergency telehealth services allow healthcare providers to assess patients' conditions quickly and determine the appropriate level of care needed. Through live video consultations, emergency telehealth systems can facilitate communication between emergency medical personnel and off-site specialists, enabling prompt decision-making and potentially lifesaving interventions [21].
3. Specialized telehealth applications: Telehealth systems have expanded beyond primary care and are increasingly being used in specialized fields. For example, teledermatology enables dermatologists to remotely diagnose and treat skin conditions through the examination of high-resolution images and patient histories. Telepsychiatry provides mental health services via video conferencing, making therapy and counseling accessible to individuals in remote areas or those with limited mobility. These specialized telehealth applications improve access to specialized care and help address healthcare provider shortages in specific disciplines [5,22].
4. Telehealth in home healthcare: The adoption of telehealth systems could have far-reaching effects on healthcare delivery in the home. Telehealth platforms allow patients who need continuous care or monitoring to receive assistance and direction remotely. Telehealth systems allow healthcare providers to remotely assess patients' conditions, manage medications, and provide advice on self-care techniques to patients in their homes. As a result, patients' quality of life improves, and healthcare costs drop due to fewer hospital readmissions and other avoidable medical visits [17,20,23–25].
5. Telehealth for health education and prevention: Health promotion and disease prevention can both benefit greatly from the use of telehealth systems. Health professionals can better advise patients on how to live a healthy lifestyle, prevent illness, and deal with chronic conditions by conducting virtual consultations. Patients can be encouraged to take an active role in their healthcare and make educated decisions with the help of telehealth platforms that provide them with educational materials, videos, and interactive tools [20,24–26].
6. Telehealth in public health and disaster response: When it comes to public health campaigns and emergency response, telehealth systems are indispensable. In the event of a pandemic or natural disaster, telehealth can be used to remotely triage patients, monitor conditions, and coordinate the distribution of medical supplies. It facilitates rapid response by public health officials to affected populations, accurate dissemination of relevant information, and effective utilization of available medical resources [27–30].
7. Advancements in telehealth technology: The potential for telehealth systems to benefit from recent technological developments is substantial, especially those involving AI, machine learning (ML), and virtual reality (VR). The use of AI algorithms in the medical field has already proven useful in areas such

as diagnosis, image analysis, and prognosis. When used for medical education and remote rehabilitation, VR can create fully immersive experiences. The capabilities and efficacy of telehealth systems have been greatly enhanced by these technological developments [10,31–34].

8. Telehealth and chronic disease management: When it comes to chronic disease management, telehealth systems have proven to be especially helpful. Patients with chronic diseases such as diabetes, high blood pressure, or cardiovascular disease typically need close observation and ongoing care. Medical professionals can monitor their patients' vital signs and medication compliance remotely with the help of telehealth platforms, and they can also offer ongoing support and education. Improved health, fewer hospitalizations, and higher levels of patient satisfaction are all possible results of taking a preventative approach to managing chronic illness [1,8,35–38].
9. Telehealth in rural and underserved areas: Providing people in rural and underserved areas with greater access to medical care is a major benefit of telehealth systems. Problems with accessibility, distance, and resources are common for these communities. Telehealth eliminates these limitations by allowing patients to receive care in the comfort of their own homes. It paves the way for people living in far-flung areas to get the medical attention they need without having to travel long distances or spend a lot of time away from home [39–42].
10. Telehealth and mental health services: As the need for mental healthcare increases, telehealth has become an important resource. There are many people who don't get help for their mental health because of things like social stigma, a lack of convenient access to mental health professionals, or their location. Patients can get private, easily accessible mental healthcare without leaving the comfort of their own homes thanks to telepsychiatry and online counseling services. Timely interventions are made possible, wait times are decreased, and more people have access to mental healthcare [36,43–47].
11. Telehealth and emergency preparedness: When it comes to being ready for and responding to disasters, telehealth systems are invaluable. Telehealth allows for the timely remote delivery of healthcare services during public health emergencies, natural disasters, or pandemics when conventional healthcare resources may be overwhelmed. It allows doctors to remotely check in on people with mild symptoms or those quarantined, triage them, and give them advice. Telehealth has the potential to enhance response times in times of crisis by improving hospital staff communication and resource management [48–50].
12. Telehealth and healthcare equity: The use of telehealth systems has the potential to reduce inequities in healthcare access and eliminate healthcare disparities. Telehealth guarantees that people with limited resources or living in underserved areas can still receive quality healthcare services by removing barriers related to geography, transportation, and socioeconomic status. It's a more equitable method of providing medical care that benefits patients of all socioeconomic backgrounds and geographic locations [17].

13. Telehealth and patient empowerment: Patients can take a more proactive approach to their healthcare with the help of telehealth systems. Patients are better able to ask questions, voice concerns, and be involved in treatment decisions thanks to the convenience of remote consultations. In order to help patients make educated decisions and participate in preventative care, many telehealth platforms now offer educational materials, individualized health information, and self-management tools [17,51].
14. Telehealth and research opportunities: Improvements in healthcare delivery and scientific understanding are possible thanks to the wealth of data made available by telehealth systems. Population health studies, outcomes research, and the creation of evidence-based practices are all made easier by the analysis of massive datasets made possible by telehealth platforms' real-time collection of patient data. Opportunities for study like these help advance the field of telehealth and pave the way for its widespread use in clinical practice [17].

1.2.4 Evolution of telehealth systems

Ancient civilizations laid the groundwork for the development of modern telehealth and telemedicine by using a variety of communication methods to access medical care. Greek and Roman physicians communicated via fires and light signals to warn of the spread of plagues in 500 BCE, as reported on www.umtrc.org. According to www.umtrc.org, however, the modern concept of telemedicine emerged in the late 1940s and early 1950s. Closed-circuit telephonic consultation between healthcare providers was one of the earliest and most well-known uses of hospital-based telemedicine at this time. This made it possible for medical professionals in different locations to evaluate and diagnose patients remotely [52].

Cardiology was the first medical specialty to make use of telemedicine in a clinical setting. As early as the 1940s, cardiologists were making use of telemedicine to consult on ECGs over the phone. This innovative application of technology-facilitated subsequent developments in telemedicine. Soon after, radiographic image transmission became feasible, enabling remote interpreting of X-rays and other diagnostic images by medical professionals [52,53].

The United States saw a proliferation of telemedicine initiatives beginning in the 1950s and continuing through the 1970s. These initiatives sought to bridge the gap in healthcare accessibility by connecting rural healthcare providers with specialists in urban areas. This first wave of telemedicine programs, however, fizzled out after nearly two decades for a variety of reasons, including technological limitations and a lack of funding.

Large-scale telemedicine initiatives did not pick backup until the late 1990s. Better and cheaper telehealth options became possible with the development of communication technologies, especially the Internet. Consultations and the transmission of diagnostic images are just the beginning of what telemedicine can do now. Robotic surgeries, remote patient monitoring, and real-time video conferencing all became part of it [54].

There have been both consistent and novel developments in the history of telehealth and telemedicine. While the primary intent of telemedicine remains the same, the means by which it is accomplished have changed considerably. These days, primary care, mental health consultations, and the management of chronic diseases are just some of the many healthcare services that can be provided via telemedicine.

Telehealth and telemedicine have seen rapid growth in popularity since the COVID-19 pandemic. With barriers to in-person contact in place, doctors and patients have increasingly turned to video conferences for healthcare. This growing reliance on telemedicine has shown the great promise of this method for expanding access to healthcare and decreasing barriers to delivery [55].

The COVID-19 pandemic prompted widespread implementation of telehealth services. Due to restrictions on in-person visits during the pandemic to prevent the spread of the virus, telehealth became the primary mode of healthcare delivery. During the pandemic, governments, healthcare organizations, and insurance companies moved quickly to increase reimbursement for telehealth services. This funding was critical to the long-term success of telehealth initiatives [48,55].

The pandemic highlighted the significance of telehealth in relieving the strain on healthcare facilities, ensuring the continuity of care, and managing chronic conditions and mental health. While the pandemic undoubtedly contributed to the initial uptick in telehealth use, the positive experiences and outcomes have led to a change in perspective. It has become an integral part of today's healthcare delivery and is expected to grow even after the pandemic ends.

Since its inception in the late 1940s, telehealth and telemedicine have undergone significant historical and evolutionary changes. Healthcare delivery has been revolutionized by telemedicine, which allows for everything from real-time video conferencing to remote patient monitoring. It has made it possible for people living in rural or otherwise underserved areas to have better access to medical care [52].

1.2.5 Telehealth statistics and projections

From 2023 to 2030, the worldwide telehealth market is expected to grow from its 2022 valuation of USD 83.5 billion at a CAGR (compound annual growth rate) of 24.0% as given in Figure 1.1 [57]. The convenience of delivering and receiving telehealth services is expanding as Internet use and smartphone technology advance. In addition, the COVID-19 pandemic and the restrictions put in place to curb the infection caused a significant increase in the demand for telehealth services over the past year. As a result of COVID-19, most hospitals and clinics had to switch from in-person to online patient care. In addition, the rising interest in virtual health management of chronic diseases is fueling the expansion of the industry.

1.2.6 Artificial intelligence in telehealth

1.2.6.1 AI and its applications in healthcare

The use of AI in healthcare is on the rise, and it has the potential to significantly improve many facets of healthcare. AI enables doctors to make more accurate diagnoses and treatment plans by equipping them with advanced decision support

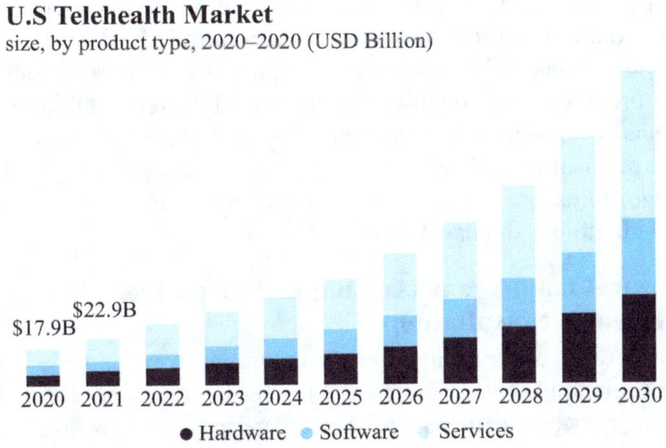

Figure 1.1 Telehealth statistics and projection [57]

systems [36]. This can eventually result in improved patient outcomes and experiences. In addition, AI can reduce healthcare expenditures by streamlining administrative processes and optimizing resource allocation. By automating time-intensive and repetitive tasks, AI can improve the work–life balance of healthcare providers, allowing them to devote more time to patient care [25,58].

For AI to be effective in healthcare, however, it must be reliable. AI systems that are legal, ethical, and robust are referred to as trustworthy. To ensure credibility, a number of factors must be considered. One of these factors is transparency, which entails making the inner workings of AI algorithms and models accessible to healthcare professionals and patients. Explainability is another essential characteristic, as it enables physicians and patients to comprehend how an AI arrived at a particular decision or recommendation. Important as well is end-user knowledge, meaning that healthcare professionals and patients should be aware of the capabilities and limitations of AI systems. Co-design entails involving end users in the development of AI systems, taking into account their needs and perspectives [25,36].

Risks associated with the application of AI in healthcare must be addressed. One such risk is the potential for AI technologies to be abused. This can include algorithms that are biased and perpetuate existing inequalities, as well as the unethical use of patient data. Inaccurate or unreliable predictions can lead to incorrect diagnoses or treatment plans, making poorly reported prediction models a further concern. In order to ensure the ethical and responsible use of AI in healthcare, it is essential to have robust guidelines and frameworks in place.

In healthcare, researchers and organizations are actively developing AI that can be trusted. The emphasis is on algorithmic fairness, ensuring that AI systems do not discriminate or introduce bias into healthcare decisions. In addition, methods for evaluating the dependability and performance of AI systems in healthcare environments are being developed. The concept of cultural mistrust in AI is also being investigated, emphasizing the need to examine various social groups and dimensions to comprehend individual differences in trust [14].

Z-Inspection is one technique used to evaluate AI systems in healthcare. This methodology provides a thorough evaluation of AI systems, taking their ethical, legal, and social dimensions into account. The auditing of algorithms is another crucial aspect of ensuring AI's credibility. This involves reviewing and monitoring healthcare algorithms on a regular basis to ensure their accuracy, fairness, and compliance with ethical standards [59].

1.2.6.2 Natural language processing and virtual assistants in telehealth consultations

In recent years, telehealth consultations have grown in popularity, and their significance has been emphasized during the COVID-19 pandemic. Ensuring effective communication between patients and healthcare providers is one of the major challenges of telemedicine [60,61]. Natural language processing (NLP) and virtual assistants can play a crucial role in this regard. NLP refers to the capacity of computers to comprehend and interpret human language, allowing for more natural and intuitive user interactions. Virtual assistants, on the other hand, are AI-powered tools that can offer users individualized assistance and direction. By incorporating NLP and virtual assistants into telehealth consultations, healthcare providers can enhance the quality of care and the patient experience as a whole [62,63].

NLP is a key component of AI, which has already made significant strides in the field of telehealth. NLP can be used to analyze and interpret spoken or written language, enabling computers to comprehend and respond to user queries as if they were human. This can be especially useful in telehealth consultations, in which patients may have questions or concerns they wish to discuss with their healthcare providers. By utilizing NLP-powered virtual assistants, patients can have more interactive and individualized conversations with their healthcare providers, resulting in improved outcomes and patient satisfaction [36].

Tele-assessment is one area where NLP and virtual assistants can be especially useful in telehealth consultations. Tele-assessment involves gathering information via remote communication about a patient's symptoms, medical history, and current condition. By extracting pertinent information from the patient's responses and generating a summary for the healthcare provider, NLP can help automate this process. This can save both the patient and the healthcare provider time and effort, allowing them to concentrate on discussing treatment options and developing a care plan.

Tele-diagnosis is another area where NLP and virtual assistants can be advantageous. NLP can assist healthcare providers in accurately diagnosing patients by analyzing their symptoms and medical history. NLP-powered virtual assistants can provide healthcare professionals with evidence-based recommendations and alerts for potential diagnoses by analyzing vast amounts of medical literature and patient data. This can help healthcare providers make more informed decisions and improve the accuracy of their diagnoses, particularly in situations where specialized knowledge or resources may be lacking [19,64].

In addition, NLP and virtual assistants can improve telehealth interactions between patients and medical professionals. These technologies can facilitate real-time communication, allowing patients to ask questions, seek clarification, and receive direction from healthcare providers. By utilizing natural language comprehension and generation capabilities, virtual assistants can provide individualized responses and explanations to patients, ensuring that they have a thorough understanding of their condition, treatment options, and required lifestyle changes [19].

Finally, NLP and virtual assistants can be beneficial for telemonitoring. Telemonitoring involves tracking and analyzing patient data remotely, including vital signs, medication adherence, and lifestyle factors. NLP can help analyze this data in real time and provide healthcare providers with timely alerts or recommendations. Based on the analyzed data, virtual assistants can also remind patients to take their medications, adhere to their treatment plans, or make necessary lifestyle changes. This can enhance patient adherence and allow for early intervention in the event of deviations from the desired health outcomes.

There is great potential for NLP and virtual assistants to improve telehealth consultations. By incorporating these technologies into telehealth platforms, healthcare providers can enhance patient communication, streamline assessment and diagnosis procedures, facilitate real-time interactions, and improve remote monitoring capabilities. However, as with any AI-enabled technology, social and ethical considerations must be taken into account to ensure patient privacy and confidentiality. NLP and virtual assistants can play a significant role in revolutionizing telehealth and addressing system-level challenges in healthcare delivery if AI algorithms are further developed and validated [64].

The following are general descriptions of how NLP and virtual assistants are utilized in telehealth as given in [49,52,55,60,62,63]:

1. **Conversational interfaces:** With the help of NLP, telehealth virtual assistants can have natural conversations with patients. With the patient's permission, virtual assistants can conduct an interview by asking questions, collecting data, and offering advice based on the patient's responses. Virtual assistants can understand and extract key information from a patient's natural language descriptions of their symptoms, concerns, and medical history.
2. **Symptom assessment and triage:** During telehealth consultations, virtual assistants powered by NLP can perform initial triage and symptom assessment. Virtual assistants can provide preliminary recommendations regarding the urgency of care, appropriate next steps, and potential treatment options by asking targeted questions and analyzing patient responses.
3. **Patient education and information:** During telehealth consultations, virtual assistants can offer patients access to educational materials, medication instructions, and healthy living suggestions. Using NLP algorithms, virtual assistants can understand patients' questions and provide them with the right answers to help them make educated decisions about their health.
4. **Documentation and EHR integration:** NLP aids in the codification of telehealth consultations' verbal and written patient information. The

conversation can be transcribed and summarized by virtual assistants, with key information like symptoms, diagnoses, and treatments extracted. By incorporating this structured data into EHRs, the administrative burden on healthcare providers can be lessened and documentation streamlined.

5. **Language translation and interpretation:** Language barriers during telehealth consultations can be reduced with the help of NLP-powered virtual assistants. With the help of these virtual assistants, healthcare providers and patients of all linguistic backgrounds and preferences can communicate effectively.
6. **Appointment scheduling and reminders:** A virtual assistant can send automated reminders and notifications to patients about their telehealth appointments. With the help of NLP algorithms, virtual assistants can now efficiently schedule appointments, check availability, and understand patient requests.
7. **Clinical decision support:** Clinical decision support for telehealth consultations can be provided by NLP algorithms that extract pertinent information from medical literature, treatment guidelines, and patient data. Using this data, virtual assistants can make recommendations supported by evidence, flag potential drug interactions and contraindications, and aid in the development of a treatment strategy.
8. **Follow-up and care coordination:** Virtual assistants can help with care coordination by providing patients with instructions after a doctor's visit, medication reminders, and other suggestions. Using NLP algorithms, virtual assistants can review patient data and plans to ensure treatment continuity and increase patient engagement in healthcare.
9. **Contextual understanding:** Using NLP algorithms, virtual assistants can grasp the gist of a telehealth consultation's conversation. They are able to decipher the intended meaning of a patient's words, make sense of unfamiliar medical terminology, and probe for clarification when necessary. Because of this awareness of context, virtual assistants can better assist doctors and patients.
10. **Risk assessment and predictive analytics:** Patient risk factors can be evaluated by virtual assistants using NLP and predictive analytics (PAs). Virtual assistants can analyze these variables to determine which users are at high risk for developing a disease or experiencing an accident. Preventative measures, alterations to one's way of life, or additional diagnostic testing can all be suggested.
11. **Emotional support and mental health:** In the context of telehealth consultations, virtual assistants with NLP capabilities can be a source of emotional support and mental health resources. They are able to have compassionate conversations, provide useful coping techniques, and point people in the direction of useful mental health resources. The emotional state of a patient can be evaluated by using NLP algorithms to analyze speech patterns and language use.
12. **Personalized treatment plans:** Using NLP, virtual assistants can examine patient information, medical history, and treatment protocols to develop

individualized care plans. During telehealth consultations, doctors can take patient preferences, demographics, and medical history into account to provide individualized treatment plans and medication suggestions.

13. **Privacy and security:** During telehealth consultations, patient privacy and data security are paramount, which is why NLP algorithms are implemented in virtual assistants. Compliance with privacy regulations and preservation of patient trust are ensured by the safe and confidential handling of individual patients' health data.
14. **Continuous learning and improvement:** With NLP, virtual assistants can learn from their patients' interactions and feedback in real time. They can enhance their performance during telehealth consultations by analyzing patterns and trends in conversations with patients in order to refine their responses, adjust to new medical information, and generally do a better job.
15. **Integration with other healthcare systems:** Virtual assistants powered by NLP can be linked to EHRs, telehealth platforms, and clinical decision support software. With this connection, virtual assistants can easily access patient information, medical records, and other pertinent details to better assist with telehealth consultations.
16. **Usability and accessibility:** Improved usability and accessibility of telehealth consultations are provided by virtual assistants powered by NLP. Patients with varying communication needs or physical limitations can benefit from using virtual assistants because they can interact with them via voice commands or text-based interfaces.
17. **Personalized treatment plans:** Using NLP, virtual assistants can examine patient information, medical history, and treatment protocols to develop individualized care plans. During telehealth consultations, doctors can take patient preferences, demographics, and medical history into account to provide individualized treatment plans and medication suggestions.
18. **Privacy and security:** During telehealth consultations, patient privacy and data security are paramount, which is why NLP algorithms are implemented in virtual assistants. Compliance with privacy regulations and preservation of patient trust are ensured by the safe and confidential handling of individual patients' health data.
19. **Continuous learning and improvement:** With NLP, virtual assistants can learn from their patients' interactions and feedback in real time. They can enhance their performance during telehealth consultations by analyzing patterns and trends in conversations with patients in order to refine their responses, adjust to new medical information, and generally do a better job.
20. **Integration with other healthcare systems:** Virtual assistants powered by NLP can be linked to EHRs, telehealth platforms, and clinical decision support software. With this connection, virtual assistants can easily access patient

information, medical records, and other pertinent details to better assist with telehealth consultations.

21. **Usability and accessibility:** Improved usability and accessibility of telehealth consultations are provided by virtual assistants powered by NLP. Patients with varying communication needs or physical limitations can benefit from using virtual assistants because they can interact with them via voice commands or text-based interfaces.

1.2.6.3 AI-powered remote monitoring and predictive analytics in telehealth

The popularity of telehealth services has led to an increase in the application of AI in the medical field. Data-driven, in-the-moment decisions made possible by AI in telemedicine have the potential to vastly improve both the patient experience and clinical outcomes [62]. Medical centers that implemented AI reported better illness management and less staff burnout, according to research out of MIT. Welltok's system is an example of AI in telehealth; it analyzes patient data in real time and makes treatment recommendations to doctors. Automated health record analysis, virtual nursing assistants, PAs for population health management, remote patient monitoring and engagement, and hospital appointment scheduling and reminders are just some of the many uses of AI in telehealth. All of these tools are designed to make healthcare better for patients, save money, and reduce waste.

AI and ML could completely alter remote patient monitoring (RPM) in the medical field. PAs can be used to anticipate the onset of specific diseases or health complications thanks to developments in AI and ML. In addition, AI algorithms can recommend treatments and care plans that are specifically designed for each patient [63]. The quality of telehealth and remote monitoring can be improved with the help of chatbots powered by AI and video conferencing. However, when implementing AI in RPM, it is important to address ethical considerations like data privacy and the impact on the doctor–patient relationship. There is not only great potential in combining AI and ML in healthcare delivery, but there are also potential obstacles that must be addressed [65].

One way that AI can be used in telehealth is to facilitate next-generation PA patient monitoring. In addition to reducing healthcare expenditures, this technology improves clinical outcomes and the quality of life for patients. Healthcare providers can prevent problems from becoming more severe by monitoring patients continuously and analyzing their data in real time. Better health outcomes can be achieved through early intervention and individualized treatment thanks to this preventative strategy. PAs can also aid in the identification of high-risk patients, allowing for more efficient resource allocation. The delivery of healthcare can be revolutionized and the quality of services improved by incorporating AI-powered remote monitoring and PAs into telehealth [60].

The use of AI in conjunction with remote monitoring and PAs could significantly improve telehealth. Care for patients, lower healthcare costs, and provide a better experience for patients in general can all result from telemedicine that makes use of AI and ML. Automated health record analysis, virtual nursing assistants, PAs for population health management, remote patient monitoring and engagement, and hospital appointment scheduling and reminders are just some of the many uses of AI in telehealth. However, when implementing AI in RPM, it is important to address ethical considerations like data privacy and the impact on the doctor–patient relationship. Using AI in telehealth, healthcare providers can revolutionize patient care by making it more individualized, efficient, and affordable [33,34,66].

1.2.7 Blockchain technology in telehealth

1.2.7.1 Blockchain technology and its relevance in healthcare

The widespread interest in blockchain technology recently can be attributed to its promising future uses in fields like healthcare. Blockchain provides a safe and transparent environment for storing sensitive medical information, alleviating concerns about privacy and security. In the healthcare industry, data security, data ownership, and data integrity are of the utmost importance, and this technology addresses these concerns. Blockchain technology allows healthcare providers to store patient data safely and restrict access to it to only those who need it [67].

Blockchain is a distributed ledger technology (DLT) that records and stores digital transactions across multiple computers in a secure and transparent manner. A series of blocks, each representing a transaction, are linked together to form the blockchain. The immutability, openness, and safety of this technology are its defining features. When discussing healthcare, the term "blockchain" is used to describe a distributed, immutable digital ledger that can be relied upon to accurately record and store relevant transactions and data [68,69].

The ability of blockchain technology to enhance the reliability and precision of EHR systems is one of its primary benefits in the healthcare sector. Paper-based systems are notorious for their inaccuracy and the length of time it can take to both update and retrieve data. Blockchain technology, however, allows healthcare providers to streamline their operations and automate processes, thereby improving efficiency, accuracy, and accessibility of data. This boosts the quality of care provided to patients generally and increases patient safety specifically [69].

By regulating access to and use of medical records, telemedicine laws put patients in charge of their own care. There is a lack of trust in third-party servers that implement consent management services for patients, and it is difficult or impossible to conduct fair audit trials using traditional consent management systems. Blockchain technology facilitates honesty by doing away with needless third parties. Consent management among multiple peers from participating organizations is encrypted by the blockchain. Consent management audit trials can benefit from the immutability, traceability, and transparency of blockchain technology. Telemedicine service providers who use blockchain and local storage systems are depicted in Figure 1.2 as given in [56].

While blockchain technology has tremendous potential in the healthcare sector, more study is required to fully understand its applicability and address any implementation challenges. Careful planning and consideration are required to

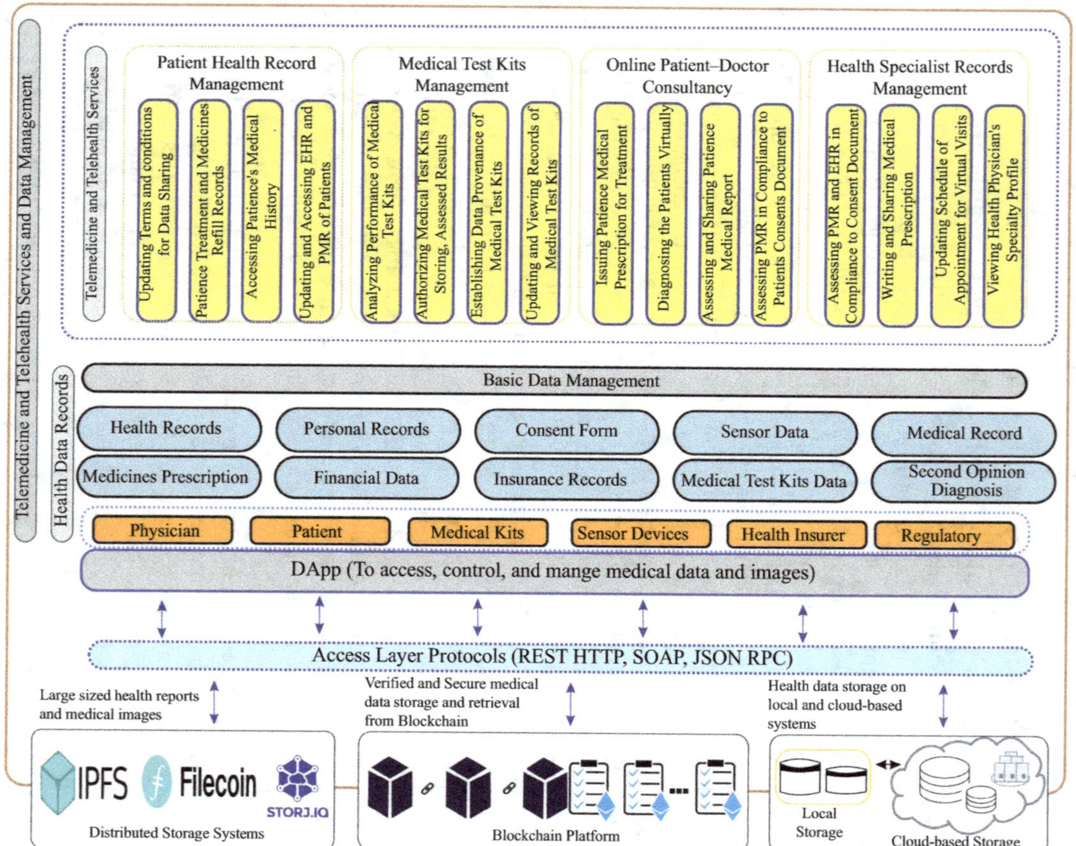

Figure 1.2 Telehealth services and data management [56]

ensure smooth interoperability and data exchange when integrating blockchain into existing healthcare systems. There may also be legal and regulatory ramifications to consider when working to meet privacy and security benchmarks [69].

1.2.7.2 Blockchain for secure and interoperable health data exchange in telehealth

To boost telehealth's interoperability and security, many healthcare organizations are looking into blockchain. Healthcare providers can use blockchain to make patient data securely shared and easily accessible across various systems and platforms [70–72]. This improves not only the effectiveness of telehealth services but also the efficiency with which health information is shared.

Among the many benefits of blockchain technology for telehealth is its potential to solve the problem of incompatible systems. One of the biggest problems in the healthcare system is the inability of different EHR systems to communicate with one another. Since it is distributed and decentralized, blockchain technology facilitates easy data transfer between various infrastructures [56,73]. Patient information can be accessed and exchanged safely across different telehealth platforms without the need for intermediaries thanks to this system's direct peer-to-peer transactions. As a result, healthcare providers will be able to provide patients with better coordinated and comprehensive care [74].

Blockchain not only solves the problem of interoperability, but it also makes telehealth data exchange more secure. The security and privacy of patients' data when stored and transmitted using conventional methods remains problematic. Blockchain technology allows healthcare providers to store patient data in a distributed ledger that is encrypted and immutable. By doing so, private medical records are protected from unauthorized access and disclosure. Because everything is recorded on the blockchain and can be easily audited, blockchain also improves accountability and trust in telehealth transactions [68].

While blockchain shows promise for facilitating secure and interoperable health data exchange in telehealth, it is not a silver bullet. Scalability, privacy, and compliance with regulations are just a few of the remaining obstacles [74]. Further study and development are required to fully realize the potential of blockchain technology in the healthcare industry, which is still in its infancy. Blockchain's potential to revolutionize the sharing, storage, and access of health data and bring about better patient outcomes and healthcare delivery is only now beginning to be explored and applied in telehealth [75].

1.2.7.3 Smart contracts and decentralized applications (DApp) in telehealth systems

In healthcare, security, privacy, transparency, and traceability are particularly important, but these features are often lacking in today's centralized systems. Blockchain technology, however, provides a distributed and unalterable system that can overcome these drawbacks. Smart contracts, which are lines of code that run automatically in response to certain conditions, can be used by telehealth systems to automate and improve many facets of healthcare deliver [71,76].

Smart contracts' ability to increase security and privacy in telehealth systems is a major benefit. When compared to older, more centralized systems, the security provided by smart contracts executed on blockchain platforms is much higher. Blockchain's distributed ledger structure eliminates the possibility of hackers gaining access to or breaching a database containing sensitive patient information. Because of blockchain's immutability and transparency, all telehealth system transactions and interactions can be retraced and audited, boosting transparency, accountability, and trust.

Smart contracts can also be extremely useful in the fight against insurance claim and medical license fraud. Smart contracts can automatically check insurance claims for authenticity and validity based on predefined conditions, cutting down on the possibility of fraud. Similarly, smart contracts can simplify the process of verifying a doctor's credentials, ensuring that only properly trained medical professionals provide treatment to their patients [71].

The immutability of medical records is another significant use of smart contracts in telehealth systems. Data integrity and accessibility problems plague conventional health record systems. Blockchain technology allows for the decentralized storage of health records, making them secure from unauthorized changes. Data integrity is improved, and health records can now be shared more easily between facilities thanks to this immutability [76].

The following are additional considerations and examples of how telehealth can benefit from the use of smart contracts and decentralized applications [71,76,77]:

Appointment scheduling and reminders: Smart contracts can automate appointment scheduling and reminders in telehealth systems. Patients can interact with the DApp to book appointments, and the smart contract can manage the availability of healthcare providers, send reminders, and handle rescheduling if needed.

Consent management: Smart contracts can facilitate consent management in telehealth consultations. Patients can provide consent for specific procedures or treatments through the DApp, and the smart contract can ensure that the consent is recorded and shared securely with relevant healthcare providers.

Secure health data exchange: Smart contracts can enable secure and transparent health data exchange in telehealth systems. When patients grant access to their health data, the smart contract can securely share the data with authorized healthcare providers, ensuring data privacy and integrity.

Prescription management: Smart contracts can streamline prescription management in telehealth. When a healthcare provider issues a prescription through the DApp, the smart contract can automatically record and track the prescription details, including medication, dosage, and refill information.

Billing and payment automation: Smart contracts can automate billing and payment processes in telehealth systems. By recording the details of telehealth services and associated fees, smart contracts can automatically generate invoices and trigger payment transactions, reducing administrative burdens and ensuring accuracy.

Provider credentialing and verification: DApps can facilitate the verification and credentialing of healthcare providers in telehealth systems. The decentralized nature of DApps enables efficient and reliable verification of qualifications, licenses, and certifications, enhancing trust and ensuring the competence of healthcare providers.

Feedback and ratings: DApps can include features for patients to provide feedback and ratings for telehealth consultations. Smart contracts can collect and aggregate feedback data, providing valuable insights for quality improvement and helping patients make informed decisions about healthcare providers.

Tokenized incentives and rewards: DApps can incorporate tokenized incentive systems to encourage patient engagement and adherence to treatment plans. Smart contracts can track patient activities, such as completing telehealth consultations or following prescribed treatments, and automatically distribute tokens or rewards as incentives.

Decentralized storage and security: DApps can leverage decentralized storage solutions, such as IPFS (InterPlanetary File System), for secure and distributed storage of sensitive health data. This reduces the reliance on centralized servers, enhancing data security and mitigating the risk of single points of failure.

Peer-to-peer consultations: DApps can facilitate peer-to-peer telehealth consultations by connecting patients directly with healthcare providers, eliminating intermediaries. Smart contracts can handle the scheduling, consent, and payment aspects of these consultations, ensuring a seamless and secure experience.

Despite the promising potential of smart contracts in telehealth systems, there are still various challenges and research problems that need to be addressed for widespread adoption. These include scalability issues, regulatory frameworks, interoperability between different blockchain platforms, and user-friendly interfaces. Furthermore, the integration of smart contracts into existing telehealth systems requires careful planning and consideration to ensure a smooth transition and minimal disruption to healthcare operations.

1.2.7.4 Privacy and security concerns in blockchain-based telehealth solutions

Privacy and security issues are crucial when implementing blockchain-based telehealth solutions. While blockchain offers inherent security features, it's important to address specific issues to protect patient data and ensure compliance with privacy regulations [2,3,7,17,25,62,78,79].

Data privacy: Blockchain-based telehealth solutions should comply with relevant data privacy regulations, such as the General Data Protection Regulation (GDPR) or the Health Insurance Portability and Accountability Act (HIPAA). Implement mechanisms that allow patients to control their data and grant specific permissions for access and use.

Identity protection: Ensure that patient identities are protected within the blockchain network. Instead of directly linking patient identities to blockchain addresses, use encryption techniques or pseudonyms to preserve patient privacy.
Data encryption: Implement strong encryption mechanisms to safeguard patient data stored on the blockchain. Encryption should be used for both data at rest and data in transit, ensuring that only authorized parties can access and decrypt the information.
Access control: Implement robust access control mechanisms to limit access to sensitive patient data. Only authorized healthcare providers or entities should have access to specific patient information, and the blockchain should enforce access restrictions based on permissions defined by patients.
Anonymization and de-identification: Consider anonymizing or de-identifying patient data before storing it on the blockchain. By removing personally identifiable information, you can further protect patient privacy while still enabling secure data sharing and analysis.
Consensus mechanism: Choose an appropriate consensus mechanism that aligns with privacy requirements. Some blockchain networks, like private or permissioned blockchains, may offer enhanced privacy features compared to public blockchains, allowing for more control over access and validation of transactions.
Secure smart contracts: Develop and audit smart contracts with security in mind. Smart contracts should undergo rigorous testing to identify and mitigate vulnerabilities or potential attack vectors. Proper code review and auditing can help ensure the integrity and security of smart contracts.
Key management: Implement secure key management practices to protect private keys used for accessing and signing transactions on the blockchain. Secure key storage, encryption, and multifactor authentication should be considered to prevent unauthorized access.
Regular security audits: Conduct regular security audits and vulnerability assessments to identify any weaknesses or potential security breaches in the blockchain-based telehealth solution. This helps maintain the integrity and confidentiality of patient data and addresses any emerging security risks [14].
Compliance with regulations: Ensure compliance with applicable regulations related to data privacy, security, and telehealth. Stay updated with evolving regulatory requirements to adapt the blockchain-based telehealth solution accordingly.
Secure integration points: Pay close attention to the integration points between the blockchain-based telehealth solution and external systems or applications. These integration points can become potential vulnerabilities if not properly secured. Implement strong authentication and encryption mechanisms to protect data exchange and communication between systems [14].
Auditability and transparency: Leverage the transparency and auditability features of blockchain to enhance accountability and transparency in telehealth transactions. The ability to trace and verify every transaction on the blockchain can help identify any unauthorized changes or access attempts, promoting trust among stakeholders.

Regular monitoring and intrusion detection: Implement robust monitoring and intrusion detection systems to identify and respond to any suspicious activities or security breaches. This includes monitoring access logs, network traffic, and system activities to promptly detect and mitigate any potential security threats [80,81].

Disaster recovery and backup: Develop a comprehensive disaster recovery plan and backup strategy to ensure business continuity and data recovery in the event of system failures or data breaches. Regularly backup blockchain data and ensure that backup copies are securely stored off-site.

Consensus protocol selection: Evaluate different consensus protocols available in blockchain technology and choose the one that best aligns with the privacy and security requirements of the telehealth solution. Consider factors such as scalability, performance, and resistance to potential attacks when selecting a consensus protocol.

Periodic security assessments: Conduct periodic security assessments and penetration testing to identify vulnerabilities in the blockchain-based telehealth solution. Engaging external security experts can provide an independent evaluation of the system's security posture and help uncover potential weaknesses that may have been overlooked [80].

Regulatory compliance monitoring: Stay updated with evolving regulations and guidelines related to telehealth and data privacy. Regularly assess the blockchain-based telehealth solution's compliance with these regulations and make necessary adjustments to ensure ongoing adherence.

User education and training: Provide training and education to all users of the telehealth system, including healthcare providers and patients. Ensure that they are aware of the security practices, privacy controls, and potential risks associated with using the blockchain-based telehealth solution.

Secure network infrastructure: Implement robust network security measures to protect the communication channels and infrastructure supporting the blockchain-based telehealth solution. This includes the use of firewalls, intrusion detection systems, and secure network protocols to safeguard against unauthorized access or data interception.

Continuous improvement and collaboration: Establish a culture of continuous improvement and collaboration among stakeholders involved in the telehealth solution. Regularly evaluate the effectiveness of privacy and security measures, gather feedback from users, and collaborate with industry experts to address emerging threats and enhance the overall security posture of the solution.

1.2.7.5 AI and blockchain in telehealth systems

Integrating AI and blockchain into telehealth systems has the potential to completely transform healthcare delivery. The combination of these two technologies can increase the efficacy, safety, and accessibility of telehealth services [68]. According to study, the most important AI–Internet of things (IoT) technologies for the healthcare sector include fog computing in IoT, deep learning, and blockchain. Fog computing facilitates the processing and analysis of data at the network's edge, hence lowering latency and guaranteeing real-time decision-making in healthcare systems. Deep learning algorithms can scan vast amounts of medical data, such as EHRs, to deliver precise diagnoses and individualized treatment recommendations [82]. Blockchain, on the other hand, provides a decentralized and immutable ledger that assures the security and confidentiality of patient information. Integrating AI and blockchain into telehealth systems enables healthcare professionals to provide more efficient and secure virtual care to patients [33,83].

Traditional healthcare systems are predominately dependent on self-managed infrastructures, which might inhibit interoperability and prevent the seamless flow of patient data. These obstacles can be solved, though, with the integration of AI and blockchain. Blockchain technology, also known as DLT, enables the construction of a shared and trustworthy network for healthcare professionals, patients, and other stakeholders [84–86]. By utilizing blockchain-based EHRs, patients can easily access their medical information while maintaining the data's integrity and confidentiality. This can promote improved coordination of treatment across various healthcare providers and enhance patient outcomes [87].

More also, AI systems can exploit the large quantity of data stored on the blockchain to give important insights and PAs. By evaluating patterns and trends in patient data, telehealth systems driven by AI are able to identify potential health hazards, predict illness development, and suggest preventative measures [82,87–89]. This proactive approach to healthcare can aid in early detection and intervention, resulting to improved patient outcomes and decreased healthcare expenses.

The creation of smart contracts for the hiring of e-healthcare specialists is an illustration of the integration of AI and blockchain in telehealth. Using blockchain technology, a framework for the construction of recruiting mechanisms was proposed. The technology produced a detailed and immutable log of the recruiting procedure, providing transparency and fostering confidence between healthcare providers and specialists. By automating the hiring process with smart contracts, healthcare firms may expedite operations and ensure that experts are fairly compensated [1,33,34,66,90–92].

This section will examine the synergies between AI and blockchain in telehealth and AI-powered data analytics and insights from blockchain-enabled telehealth data.

1.2.8 Synergies between AI and blockchain in telehealth

In telehealth, the synergies between AI and blockchain can produce strong and disruptive solutions. In the telehealth arena, AI and blockchain can complement one other in the following ways [78,93–99]:

Data privacy and security: Blockchain provides a secure and decentralized platform for storing and sharing sensitive health data. AI algorithms can be applied to analyze and process this data while preserving patient privacy. The combination of blockchain's tamper-proof and auditable nature with AI's ability to extract meaningful insights enables secure and privacy-preserving data analytics in telehealth.

Data quality and integrity: AI algorithms rely on large volumes of high-quality data to deliver accurate predictions and insights. Blockchain can ensure the integrity and reliability of data by recording every transaction and creating an immutable audit trail. This ensures that the data used by AI models in telehealth is trustworthy and has not been tampered with, enhancing the accuracy and reliability of AI-driven analyses and recommendations.

Federated learning: Federated learning is a technique where AI models are trained locally on distributed data sources while keeping the data itself private and secure. Blockchain can act as a trusted intermediary in federated learning scenarios, facilitating the aggregation of model updates from various telehealth providers while preserving the privacy of patient data. This enables collaborative AI model training without compromising data privacy.

AI-enabled decision support: AI algorithms can analyze patient data, medical literature, and treatment guidelines to provide decision support to healthcare providers during telehealth consultations. Blockchain can ensure the transparency and traceability of the AI decision-making process by recording the input data, the AI model used, and the resulting recommendations. This promotes accountability, trust, and auditability in AI-driven decision support systems.

Incentivizing data sharing: Blockchain-based tokenization mechanisms can incentivize patients to share their health data for AI research and development purposes. Patients can receive tokens or rewards in exchange for contributing their data, while maintaining control over their privacy and consent. This can help overcome data silos and encourage patient participation in AI-driven telehealth initiatives.

Clinical trials and research: Blockchain can enhance the transparency and efficiency of clinical trials and medical research in telehealth. By securely recording and sharing trial data on the blockchain, AI algorithms can analyze this data to identify patterns, discover new treatments, and improve patient outcomes. Blockchain ensures data integrity, facilitates data sharing between different organizations, and enables traceability of research findings.

Real-time monitoring and PAs: AI algorithms can leverage real-time data streams from remote monitoring devices in telehealth. Blockchain can provide a secure and transparent infrastructure for storing and analyzing this data, enabling PAs to detect health trends, predict disease progression, and facilitate proactive interventions. This combination empowers healthcare providers with timely insights for personalized patient care.

Immutable health records: Blockchain can be used to create immutable and tamperproof health records. AI algorithms can then analyze these records to extract valuable insights for telehealth. This combination ensures that the historical health data used by AI models is trustworthy, reliable, and has not been altered, enabling more accurate diagnostics, treatment planning, and personalized care.

Data sharing and interoperability: Interoperability remains a challenge in healthcare, hindering the seamless exchange of patient data across different systems. Blockchain can serve as a decentralized and standardized platform for data sharing and interoperability. AI algorithms can leverage this shared data to gain a comprehensive view of patients' health and support more informed telehealth decisions.

Enhanced trust and transparency: The combination of AI and blockchain can enhance trust and transparency in telehealth systems. Blockchain's transparent and auditable nature ensures that patients, healthcare providers, and regulatory bodies can verify the integrity of data and algorithms used in AI-driven telehealth applications. This transparency fosters trust and accountability, which are essential in healthcare.

Fraud detection and prevention: AI algorithms can analyze transactional data recorded on the blockchain to detect and prevent fraudulent activities in telehealth, such as billing fraud or identity theft. By applying ML techniques to blockchain data, AI can identify patterns and anomalies that indicate potential fraudulent behavior, protecting patients and reducing financial losses.

Personalized medicine and treatment plans: AI algorithms can analyze large volumes of patient data, including medical records, genetics, and lifestyle information, to develop personalized treatment plans in telehealth. Blockchain provides a secure and transparent platform for storing and sharing this sensitive patient data, allowing AI to deliver tailored recommendations and interventions based on individual needs and characteristics.

Smart contracts for automated processes: Smart contracts, powered by blockchain, can automate various processes in telehealth, such as appointment scheduling, billing, and consent management. AI algorithms can be integrated into these smart contracts to provide decision support and automate routine tasks, improving efficiency and reducing administrative burdens for healthcare providers.

Patient-driven data governance: Blockchain can empower patients with greater control over their health data. Patients can securely store their data on the blockchain and grant access to healthcare providers or researchers based on their preferences. AI can then analyze this patient-controlled data to generate insights that directly benefit the individual's health and well-being.

Continuous learning and improvement: AI algorithms can continuously learn and improve from the data stored on the blockchain. The feedback loop between AI and blockchain enables the refinement of algorithms over time, leading to more accurate predictions, diagnoses, and treatment recommendations in telehealth.

Ethical and bias mitigation: AI algorithms in telehealth need to be developed and deployed ethically, ensuring fairness and mitigating biases. Blockchain's transparency and traceability can help identify potential biases in the data used to train AI models. This enables proactive measures to address biases and ensures equitable and unbiased delivery of telehealth services.

1.2.8.1 AI-powered data analytics and insights from blockchain-enabled telehealth data

The combination of AI-powered data analytics with blockchain technology in telehealth data presents various prospects to improve patient care, research, fraud detection, policymaking, and overall healthcare results. The integration of these technologies has the potential to revolutionize the management, analysis, and utilization of healthcare data for the benefit of patients, providers, and society as a whole. The extraction of meaningful insights from blockchain-enabled telemedicine data can rely heavily on AI-powered data analytics. Telehealth can profit from the integration of AI, data analytics, and blockchain technology in the following ways [33,60,68,89,100–108]:

Data management and security: Blockchain technology ensures secure and tamperproof storage of telehealth data. It allows for decentralized storage and cryptographic techniques, which enhance data privacy and integrity. AI algorithms can be employed to monitor and audit the blockchain network for any potential security breaches or anomalies, ensuring data protection.

Real-time analytics: AI algorithms can analyze telehealth data in real time, providing immediate insights and actionable recommendations. For instance, AI can detect patterns in patient data, identify health risks, and provide alerts to healthcare providers. Real-time analytics can help improve patient monitoring, diagnosis, and treatment decisions.

PAs: By leveraging historical telehealth data stored on the blockchain, AI algorithms can identify patterns, trends, and correlations that may not be apparent to human analysts. This enables PAs, where AI models can forecast disease outbreaks, predict patient outcomes, and personalize treatment plans based on individual patient data.

Treatment optimization: AI-powered data analytics can assist healthcare providers in optimizing treatment plans by analyzing a large volume of telehealth data. By considering various patient characteristics, treatment outcomes, and evidence-based guidelines, AI algorithms can recommend personalized treatment options, dosage adjustments, or alternative therapies.

Population health management: Aggregating and analyzing blockchain-enabled telehealth data at a population level can provide valuable insights for public health initiatives. AI algorithms can identify high-risk populations, track disease prevalence, and support proactive interventions, such as targeted vaccination campaigns or resource allocation in specific regions.

Research and development: Blockchain-enabled telehealth data can facilitate medical research by providing access to a diverse range of patient data while maintaining privacy and data ownership. AI can assist researchers in analyzing this data to discover new disease patterns, validate treatment efficacy, or identify potential drug interactions. Such insights can expedite the development of new therapies and improve healthcare outcomes.

Regulatory compliance: Blockchain technology provides transparency and auditability to telehealth data, ensuring compliance with privacy regulations such as HIPAA. AI algorithms can assist in automating compliance processes, flagging potential breaches, and ensuring adherence to data protection standards.

Fraud detection: Blockchain technology's transparency and immutability can be leveraged by AI algorithms to detect fraudulent activities in telehealth data. By analyzing patterns, anomalies, and discrepancies within the blockchain network, AI can identify potentially fraudulent claims, unauthorized access, or misuse of patient data, contributing to a more secure and trustworthy telehealth ecosystem.

Continuous monitoring and remote care: AI-powered data analytics can enable continuous monitoring and remote care in telehealth. By analyzing real-time patient data streamed from wearables, sensors, or remote monitoring devices, AI algorithms can alert healthcare providers to any concerning changes in a patient's health status, facilitating timely interventions and personalized care management.

Clinical decision support: AI algorithms can assist healthcare providers in making informed clinical decisions by analyzing blockchain-enabled telehealth data. By integrating patient-specific data, evidence-based guidelines, and medical literature, AI can provide decision support tools that offer treatment recommendations, drug interactions, or risk assessments, thereby improving the accuracy and efficiency of clinical decision-making.

Patient engagement and empowerment: AI-powered data analytics can empower patients by providing personalized health insights derived from their telehealth data. AI algorithms can analyze patient-generated data, such as symptoms, lifestyle behaviors, or medication adherence, and deliver personalized health recommendations, educational resources, or behavior change interventions, fostering patient engagement and proactive self-management.

Data sharing and interoperability: Blockchain technology can facilitate secure and standardized data sharing among different healthcare entities involved in telehealth. AI can play a role in analyzing and integrating disparate data sources, such as EHRs, wearables, or genomic data, allowing for a holistic view of patient health. This interoperability enables comprehensive data analytics and insights generation, leading to more informed decision-making and improved patient outcomes.

Privacy-preserving analytics: AI algorithms can be designed to perform data analytics directly on the blockchain without accessing the actual raw data. This technique, known as federated learning or differential privacy, allows for privacy-preserving analytics, where sensitive patient information remains encrypted or anonymized. By ensuring privacy protection, patients can have confidence in sharing their data while still benefiting from advanced analytics.

Continuous quality improvement: AI-powered data analytics can contribute to continuous quality improvement in telehealth services. By analyzing aggregated telehealth data, AI algorithms can identify areas for improvement, such as reducing wait times, optimizing resource allocation, or enhancing service delivery. These insights can drive evidence-based decision-making and help healthcare organizations refine their telehealth practices.

Health policy and planning: Blockchain-enabled telehealth data, when combined with AI-powered analytics, can inform health policy and planning at a macro level. By analyzing population-level data, policymakers can gain insights into disease prevalence, healthcare utilization patterns, and resource allocation needs. These insights can guide the development of targeted policies, interventions, and infrastructure investments to address public health challenges effectively.

It is important to note that while the combination of AI, data analytics, and blockchain technology offers significant potential benefits, there are also challenges to address, such as data quality, interoperability, and ethical considerations surrounding data usage and privacy. Nonetheless, these technologies can empower healthcare providers and researchers with valuable insights derived from blockchain-enabled telehealth data, leading to improved patient care, population health, and medical research.

1.2.8.2 Trust and transparency through blockchain-enabled AI algorithms in telehealth

Trust and transparency are critical factors in the successful implementation of telehealth services. Blockchain-enabled AI algorithms have the potential to enhance trust and transparency in telehealth by providing secure and auditable data management, improving data accuracy, facilitating patient consent, ensuring data privacy, enabling traceability, enhancing accountability, and promoting open collaboration [56]. Various aspects of trust and transparency through blockchain-enabled AI algorithms in telehealth are discussed in this section [93,109,110].

Secure and auditable data management: By leveraging blockchain, AI algorithms can access and analyze data while maintaining data integrity. Every transaction and access to the data can be recorded on the blockchain, providing an auditable trail of data management activities. This transparency enhances trust among stakeholders, as they can verify the integrity of the data and have confidence in the analytics derived from it.

Improved data accuracy: AI algorithms can leverage blockchain's consensus mechanism to validate and verify the accuracy of telehealth data. By cross-referencing data from multiple sources on the blockchain, AI can identify inconsistencies or discrepancies, ensuring the accuracy and reliability of the data being analyzed. This verification process helps in mitigating errors or fraudulent activities, further enhancing trust in the telehealth ecosystem.

Facilitated patient consent: Blockchain-enabled smart contracts can provide patients with greater control and transparency over their data. AI algorithms can leverage these smart contracts to seek patient consent, define data usage permissions, and enable patients to manage access to their telehealth data.

Patients can have a clear understanding of how their data is being utilized, empowering them to make informed decisions and fostering trust in telehealth services.

Data privacy: Blockchain technology can enable privacy-preserving analytics by allowing data analysis without exposing sensitive patient information. AI algorithms can perform computations on encrypted or anonymized data stored on the blockchain, preserving privacy while still deriving valuable insights. This privacy-enhancing feature helps address concerns regarding data security and privacy, building trust among patients who are hesitant about sharing their personal health information.

Traceability and auditability: Blockchain's decentralized and transparent nature enables the traceability of telehealth data. Every transaction and update to the data can be recorded and traced back to its origin on the blockchain. AI algorithms can leverage this traceability to provide an auditable record of data access, sharing, and analytics performed. This auditability ensures accountability and transparency in telehealth practices, fostering trust among patients, healthcare providers, and regulators.

Accountability and quality assurance: By leveraging blockchain and AI, telehealth platforms can implement accountability mechanisms that promote high-quality care delivery. AI algorithms can monitor and analyze telehealth interactions, treatment outcomes, and adherence to protocols, ensuring accountability among healthcare providers. Blockchain technology can record and verify these interactions, providing an immutable record that supports quality assurance initiatives and builds trust in the telehealth ecosystem.

Open collaboration and research: Blockchain-enabled AI algorithms can facilitate open collaboration and data sharing in telehealth research. Blockchain provides a secure and standardized platform for sharing anonymized patient data, enabling researchers and institutions to collaborate and access a diverse range of data for studies and innovation. This open collaboration fosters transparency, accelerates research, and promotes trust among the research community and patients who contribute their data.

Fraud prevention and detection: Blockchain-enabled AI algorithms can contribute to fraud prevention and detection in telehealth. By analyzing data patterns, AI algorithms can identify potential fraud indicators, such as duplicate claims, inappropriate billing, or unauthorized access to patient data. The transparency and immutability of blockchain technology provide a reliable audit trail, enabling the detection of fraudulent activities and enhancing trust by ensuring the integrity of the telehealth ecosystem.

Patient data ownership and control: Blockchain technology combined with AI algorithms can empower patients by giving them ownership and control over their telehealth data. Through blockchain-based consent management systems, patients can determine who has access to their data, for what purposes, and for how long. This increased control over personal health information fosters trust and transparency in telehealth, as patients are actively involved in the decision-making process regarding their data.

Provider credentialing and verification: Blockchain-enabled AI algorithms can streamline and enhance provider credentialing and verification processes in telehealth. By leveraging blockchain's decentralized and transparent nature, AI algorithms can verify and validate provider credentials, licenses, and qualifications. This ensures that only authorized and qualified healthcare professionals participate in telehealth services, promoting trust and transparency in the quality and legitimacy of care being delivered.

Supply chain integrity: AI-powered data analytics in conjunction with blockchain can ensure supply chain integrity in telehealth. By leveraging blockchain's transparency, AI algorithms can track and verify the provenance of medical devices, pharmaceuticals, or supplies used in telehealth. This allows for better traceability, reducing the risk of counterfeit or substandard products entering the telehealth supply chain. Patients can have confidence in the authenticity and quality of the products and services they receive, enhancing trust in telehealth.

Dispute resolution and mediation: Blockchain-enabled AI algorithms can facilitate efficient and transparent dispute resolution and mediation in telehealth. By recording interactions, treatment decisions, and patient outcomes on the blockchain, AI algorithms can assist in resolving disputes by providing an immutable and auditable record of events. This transparency and accountability can help address any conflicts or misunderstandings that may arise, ensuring fair and equitable resolution and maintaining trust among all stakeholders involved in telehealth.

1.3 Challenges and future directions

1.3.1 Technical challenges and limitations of AI and blockchain in telehealth systems

There are a number of technological obstacles and limits that need to be taken into consideration, despite the fact that the incorporation of AI and blockchain into telehealth delivers a number of benefits. This section will go over some of the more significant challenges and constraints [29,41,48,50,59,61,79,93,94,96,109–112].

1.3.1.1 Scalability

Both AI and blockchain technologies can generate and process large volumes of data. Ensuring scalability to handle the increasing volume of telehealth data is a challenge. AI algorithms require significant computational resources, while blockchain networks may face scalability issues due to the consensus mechanisms and storage requirements. Efforts are needed to optimize resource allocation and design scalable architectures to accommodate the growing demands of telehealth systems.

1.3.1.2 Data quality and standardization

AI algorithms heavily rely on high-quality and standardized data for accurate analysis and decision-making. However, telehealth data may come from diverse sources, including different medical devices, EHRs, and wearables, leading to data heterogeneity and inconsistencies. Ensuring data quality, interoperability, and adherence to standardized formats is crucial to enable effective AI analytics and meaningful insights.

1.3.1.3 Data privacy and security

While blockchain technology provides enhanced security and privacy features, challenges remain in ensuring the protection of sensitive patient data in telehealth systems. Ensuring proper encryption, secure data access, and robust identity management solutions are essential to safeguard patient privacy. Additionally, AI algorithms may be susceptible to adversarial attacks or unauthorized access, necessitating the implementation of robust security measures.

1.3.1.4 Integration and interoperability

Integrating AI algorithms and blockchain technology into existing telehealth systems can be complex due to interoperability challenges. Legacy systems, different data formats, and varying communication protocols make seamless integration a significant technical hurdle. Developing standardized interfaces and protocols that enable interoperability among AI, blockchain, and existing telehealth systems is essential for their successful implementation.

1.3.1.5 Ethical and regulatory considerations

The use of AI algorithms and blockchain technology in telehealth raises ethical and regulatory considerations. Transparent and explainable AI models are necessary to ensure accountability and trust. Additionally, complying with data protection regulations, such as HIPAA, and addressing ethical concerns regarding data ownership, informed consent, and algorithmic biases require careful attention.

1.3.1.6 Cost and infrastructure requirements

Implementing AI and blockchain in telehealth systems can require substantial investments in infrastructure, computational resources, and skilled personnel. Upgrading existing systems, deploying blockchain networks, and training AI models can be costly and resource-intensive, especially for smaller healthcare providers or organizations with limited budgets.

1.3.1.7 User adoption and acceptance

The successful implementation of AI and blockchain in telehealth relies on user adoption and acceptance. Healthcare professionals, patients, and other stakeholders need to understand and trust the technologies to fully embrace them. Providing proper training, education, and user-friendly interfaces that align with existing workflows can facilitate user adoption and ensure a smooth transition to AI and blockchain-enabled telehealth systems.

1.3.1.8 Computational complexity

AI algorithms, especially deep learning models, can be computationally intensive and require significant processing power. Running these algorithms in real time for telehealth applications can pose challenges, particularly in resource-constrained environments or for mobile telehealth solutions. Optimizing AI models for efficient computation and developing hardware or cloud-based solutions that can handle the computational demands are areas of focus to overcome this challenge.

1.3.1.9 Algorithmic bias and fairness

AI algorithms can be susceptible to bias, which can have implications for equitable healthcare delivery. If training data used to develop AI models are biased or not representative of diverse patient populations, the algorithms may perpetuate disparities or produce inaccurate results for certain demographic groups. Ensuring fairness, inclusivity, and addressing algorithmic bias in AI models is crucial for equitable telehealth services.

1.3.1.10 Regulation and legal considerations

The regulatory landscape for AI and blockchain in telehealth is still evolving. Compliance with existing regulations, such as data privacy laws (e.g., GDPR, HIPAA), cybersecurity requirements, and licensure considerations for telehealth providers, presents challenges. Developing appropriate regulatory frameworks and standards specific to AI and blockchain in telehealth is necessary to ensure legal compliance and protect patient rights.

1.3.1.11 Energy consumption

Blockchain networks, especially those based on proof-of-work consensus mechanisms (e.g., Bitcoin), require significant computational power and energy consumption. This can be a concern for sustainable and environmentally conscious telehealth systems. Exploring alternative consensus mechanisms with lower energy requirements, such as proof-of-stake or proof-of-authority, can help mitigate the energy consumption associated with blockchain-based telehealth solutions.

1.3.1.12 Governance and decision-making

Blockchain networks in telehealth require effective governance models for decision-making and consensus. Determining the governance structure, roles, and responsibilities of participants and mechanisms for resolving conflicts or making protocol changes can be complex. Developing governance frameworks that involve key stakeholders and ensure transparency, inclusivity, and accountability is essential for the successful implementation of blockchain-enabled telehealth systems.

1.3.1.13 Education and skills gap

The integration of AI and blockchain in telehealth requires a skilled workforce with expertise in both technologies. However, there is currently a shortage of professionals who possess the necessary knowledge and skills. Bridging the education and skills gap through training programs, certifications, and academic initiatives can help address this limitation and ensure a competent workforce capable of implementing and managing AI and blockchain in telehealth effectively.

1.3.1.14 Interdisciplinary collaboration

The successful integration of AI and blockchain in telehealth systems necessitates collaboration among healthcare professionals, data scientists, computer engineers, and legal experts. Fostering interdisciplinary collaboration and creating platforms for knowledge sharing and communication among these different domains are vital to overcoming technical challenges and achieving the full potential of AI and blockchain in telehealth.

1.3.1.15 Long-term sustainability

Ensuring the long-term sustainability of AI and blockchain in telehealth systems requires continuous support, maintenance, and upgrades. Technological advancements, evolving standards, and changing user needs necessitate ongoing investments in research and development. Creating sustainable business models and strategies for the maintenance and evolution of AI and blockchain-based telehealth systems is essential to ensure their long-term viability.

1.3.2 Opportunities for research and innovation in AI and blockchain-based telehealth systems

The future of telehealth is promising, with ongoing advancements and innovations [12,13,48,49,60,97,99,111,113]:

1. AI and ML will play a significant role in improving telehealth capabilities. AI algorithms can assist in diagnostics, triage, and personalized treatment recommendations.
2. VR and augmented reality (AR) technologies have the potential to enhance telehealth experiences, allowing for immersive simulations, virtual training, and improved visualization of medical information.
3. The integration of telehealth with other emerging technologies, such as 5G networks, IoT devices, and blockchain, will further enhance its capabilities and facilitate secure data exchange.
4. Telehealth will likely continue to expand into various specialties, including remote surgery, teleoncology, telepediatrics, and telecritical care, enabling access to specialized care regardless of geographic location.

1.4 Concluding remarks

1.4.1 Implications for the future of AI and blockchain in telehealth systems

The future of AI and blockchain in telehealth systems holds significant implications for healthcare delivery and patient outcomes. Here are some key implications to consider:

Enhanced diagnostic accuracy: AI algorithms can analyze vast amounts of patient data, including medical records, imaging results, and genetic information, to assist healthcare professionals in making more accurate diagnoses. By leveraging AI's pattern recognition capabilities, telehealth systems can provide healthcare providers with valuable insights and support in diagnosing complex conditions, leading to earlier detection and improved treatment outcomes.

Personalized treatment plans: AI algorithms can analyze patient data and generate personalized treatment plans based on individual characteristics, medical history, and response to therapies. This personalized approach enables tailored interventions, optimized medication regimens, and targeted healthcare interventions, improving patient adherence and outcomes. Blockchain can facilitate secure storage and sharing of patient treatment plans, ensuring continuity of care across different healthcare providers and settings.

Remote patient monitoring: The integration of AI and blockchain in telehealth enables remote patient monitoring on a continuous basis. IoT devices, wearables, and sensors collect real-time patient data, which can be securely transmitted, stored on the blockchain, and analyzed by AI algorithms. This continuous monitoring allows healthcare providers to identify early warning signs, intervene promptly, and provide remote care, reducing hospital readmissions and improving patient management.

Decentralized and secure health records: Blockchain technology can revolutionize the management of health records by providing a decentralized and tamperproof system for storing and sharing patient information. Patient health records stored on the blockchain can be accessed securely by authorized healthcare providers, ensuring data integrity, privacy, and interoperability. AI algorithms can leverage this secure data to derive insights, facilitate research, and improve care coordination.

Real-time decision support: AI algorithms can provide real-time decision support to healthcare professionals during telehealth consultations. By analyzing patient data, clinical guidelines, and medical literature, AI systems can offer evidence-based recommendations, assist in treatment planning, and alert healthcare providers to potential risks or contraindications. This real-time support enhances clinical decision-making and helps optimize patient care in telehealth settings.

Improved population health management: AI and blockchain in telehealth enable population health management at a broader level. By analyzing aggregated and anonymized patient data stored on the blockchain, AI algorithms can identify trends, risk factors, and population health patterns. This information can guide public health initiatives, disease prevention strategies, and resource allocation, ultimately improving the health of communities.

Research and clinical trials: AI and blockchain integration in telehealth can streamline and enhance research and clinical trial processes. Blockchain-based smart contracts can automate consent management, ensure data integrity, and facilitate transparent and auditable research protocols. AI algorithms can support the analysis of large-scale clinical trial data, identify patient eligibility criteria, and optimize trial design, accelerating the discovery of new treatments and interventions.

Collaborative healthcare ecosystems: The integration of AI and blockchain in telehealth fosters collaboration among healthcare stakeholders. Blockchain networks can facilitate secure data sharing and incentivization models, allowing patients, healthcare providers, researchers, and pharmaceutical companies to collaborate and contribute to improved healthcare outcomes. AI algorithms can analyze shared data and generate insights that benefit the entire ecosystem, promoting a collective approach to healthcare innovation.

1.4.2 Conclusions and future scope

The chapter provides an insightful overview of the integration of AI and blockchain technology in telehealth systems. It highlights the potential benefits, challenges, and future implications of these technologies in healthcare delivery.

The chapter begins by introducing the concept of telehealth and the increasing role of technology in transforming healthcare. It then delves into the applications of AI in telehealth, emphasizing its ability to enhance diagnostic accuracy, personalize treatment plans, enable remote patient monitoring, and provide real-time decision support. The integration of blockchain technology is also explored, showcasing its potential for secure and decentralized health record management, consent management, and data sharing.

However, the chapter also acknowledges the technical challenges and limitations associated with AI and blockchain in telehealth systems. Computational complexity, algorithmic bias, regulatory compliance, and infrastructure requirements are among the considerations that organizations must address for successful implementation.

The chapter concludes by highlighting emerging trends and advancements in the field, including federated learning, explainable AI, and tokenization models. It emphasizes the importance of interoperability, user acceptance, and ethical considerations in the adoption of AI and blockchain telehealth solutions. Collaboration among stakeholders and the development of sustainable business models are seen as crucial factors for the future growth and effectiveness of these technologies in telehealth.

In summary, the article provides a comprehensive overview of AI and blockchain technology in telehealth systems. It showcases the transformative potential of these technologies in improving healthcare delivery, enhancing patient outcomes, and fostering collaborative healthcare ecosystems. By addressing challenges and embracing emerging trends, the future of AI and blockchain in telehealth holds great promise for revolutionizing the healthcare landscape and shaping a patient-centric approach to care.

References

[1] American Telemedicine Association (ATA), *Telehealth: Defining 21st Century Care*, American Telemedicine Association, 2022.

[2] A. Jasper, "Telehealth Basics," *Optometric Management*, vol. 55, no. 6, 2020.

[3] L. Berkowitz, S. Vyas, I.O. Korolev, *et al.*, "Predictions for Telehealth in 2021: We Can't Wait for It!," *Telehealth and Medicine Today*, vol. 6, no. 1, 2021, doi: 10.30953/tmt.v6.248.

[4] D. Al-Thani, S. Monteiro, and L. S. Tamil, "Design for eHealth and Telehealth," in *Design for Health: Applications of Human Factors*, Cambridge: Academic Press, 2020. doi: 10.1016/B978-0-12-816427-3.00004-X.

[5] E. Andrikopoulou, "The Rise of AI in Telehealth," in *Emerging Practices in Telehealth: Best Practices in a Rapidly Changing Field*, Cambridge: Academic Press, 2023. doi: 10.1016/B978-0-443-15980-0.00011-9.

[6] G. Bansal, K. Rajgopal, V. Chamola, Z. Xiong, and D. Niyato, "Healthcare in Metaverse: A Survey on Current Metaverse Applications in Healthcare," *IEEE Access*, vol. 10, 2022, doi: 10.1109/ACCESS.2022.3219845.

[7] M. Seneviratne and D. Peiris, "Digital Health in Low- and Middle-Income Countries," in *Revolutionizing Tropical Medicine: Point-of-Care Tests, New Imaging Technologies and Digital Health*, New York: Wiley, 2019. doi: 10.1002/9781119282686.ch32.

[8] M. Liyanage, A. Braeken, P. Kumar, and M. Ylianttila, *IoT Security: Advances in Authentication*, New York: Wiley, 2019.

[9] V. Li, I. Roos, M. Monif, *et al.*, "Impact of Telehealth on Health Care in a Multiple Sclerosis Outpatient Clinic During the COVID-19 Pandemic," *Multiple Sclerosis and Related Disorders,* vol. 63, 2022, doi: 10.1016/j.msard.2022.103913.

[10] D. V. Gunasekeran, R. M. W. W. Tseng, Y. C. Tham, and T. Y. Wong, "Applications of Digital Health for Public Health Responses to COVID-19: A Systematic Scoping Review of Artificial Intelligence, Telehealth and Related Technologies," *NPJ Digital Medicine*, vol. 4, no. 1. 2021. doi: 10.1038/s41746-021-00412-9.

[11] E. G. S. Nascimento, A. N. Furtado, R. Badaró, and L. Knop, "The New Technologies in the Pandemic Era," *Journal of Bioengineering and Technology Applied to Health*, vol. 3, no. 2, 2020, doi: 10.34178/jbth.v3i2.122.

[12] M. Magnus, N. Sikka, T. Cherian, and S. Q. Lew, "Satisfaction and Improvements in Peritoneal Dialysis Outcomes Associated with Telehealth," *Applied Clinical Informatics*, vol. 8, no. 1, 2017, doi: 10.4338/ACI-2016-09-RA-0154.

[13] A. While and G. Dewsbury, "Nursing and Information and Communication Technology (ICT): A Discussion of Trends and Future Directions," *International Journal of Nursing Studies*, vol. 48, no. 10, 2011, doi: 10.1016/j.ijnurstu.2011.02.020.

[14] S. T. Wynn, "Achieving Patient Satisfaction: Utilizing Telehealth Via an Academic–Practice Partnership," *Journal of the American Psychiatric Nurses Association*, vol. 27, no. 2, 2021, doi: 10.1177/1078390320902828.

[15] H. Zerga, A. Amraoui, and B. Benmammar, "Distributed, Dynamic and Trustworthy Access Control for Telehealth Systems," *Concurrency and Computation,* vol. 34, no. 28, 2022, doi: 10.1002/cpe.7352.

[16] X. Ren, Y. Zhai, X. Song, Z. Wang, D. Dou, and Y. Li, "The Application of Mobile Telehealth System to Facilitate Patient Information Presentation and Case Discussion," *Telemedicine and e-Health*, vol. 26, no. 6, 2020, doi: 10.1089/tmj.2020.0084.

[17] L. Gurbeta, A. Badnjevic, M. Maksimovic, E. Omanovic-Miklicanin, and E. Sejdic, "A Telehealth System for Automated Diagnosis of Asthma and Chronical Obstructive Pulmonary Disease," *Journal of the American Medical Informatics Association*, vol. 25, no. 9, 2018, doi: 10.1093/jamia/ocy055.

[18] M. Faisal, H. ElGibreen, N. Alafif, and C. Joumaa, "Reducing Children's Obesity in the Age of Telehealth and AI/IoT Technologies in Gulf Countries," *Systems*, vol. 10, no. 6, 2022, doi: 10.3390/systems10060241.

[19] S. D. Das and P. K. Bala, "Artificial Intelligence in Telemedicine: A Brief Survey," in *Studies in Computational Intelligence*, Singapore: Springer, 2022. doi: 10.1007/978-981-19-1076-0_23.

[20] G. Marquez, H. Astudillo, and C. Taramasco, "Exploring security issues in telehealth systems," in *Proceedings – 2019 IEEE/ACM 1st International Workshop on Software Engineering for Healthcare, SEH 2019*, 2019. doi: 10.1109/SEH.2019.00019.

[21] C. Botrugno, "Towards an Ethics for Telehealth," *Nursing Ethics*, vol. 26, no. 2, 2019, doi: 10.1177/0969733017705004.

[22] P. S. Whitten and M. S. Mackert, "Addressing Telehealth's Foremost Barrier: Provider as Initial Gatekeeper," *International Journal of Technology Assessment in Health Care*, vol. 21, no. 4. 2005. doi: 10.1017/S0266462305050725.

[23] C. W. Delaney, C. A. Weaver, J. Sensmeier, L. Pruinelli, and P. Weber, *Nursing and Informatics for the 21st Century – Embracing a Digital World, 3rd Edition, Book 3: Innovation, Technology, and Applied Informatics for Nurses*. Milton Park: Taylor & Francis Group, 2022. doi:10.4324/9781003281016.

[24] C. Tedeschi, "Ethical, Legal, and Social Challenges in the Development and Implementation of Disaster Telemedicine," *Disaster Med Public Health Prep*, vol. 15, no. 5, 2021, doi: 10.1017/dmp.2020.118.

[25] Y. C. Huang and Y. L. Hsu, "Social Networking-based Personal Home Telehealth System: A Pilot Study," *Journal of Clinical Gerontology and Geriatrics*, vol. 5, no. 4, 2014, doi: 10.1016/j.jcgg.2014.05.004.

[26] A. R. Dewar, T. P. Bull, D. M. Malvey, and J. L. Szalma, "Developing a Measure of Engagement With Telehealth Systems: The mHealth Technology Engagement Index," *Journal of Telemedicine and Telecare*, vol. 23, no. 2, 2016, doi: 10.1177/1357633X16640958.

[27] A. Garavand, N. Aslani, H. Nadri, S. Abedini, and S. Dehghan, "Acceptance of Telemedicine Technology Among Physicians: A Systematic Review," *Informatics in Medicine Unlocked*, vol. 30. 2022. doi: 10.1016/j.imu.2022.100943.

[28] T. P. Bull, A. R. Dewar, D. M. Malvey, and J. L. Szalma, "Considerations for the Telehealth Systems of Tomorrow: An Analysis of Student Perceptions of Telehealth Technologies," *JMIR Medical Education*, vol. 2, no. 2, 2016, doi: 10.2196/mededu.5392.

[29] A. Haleem, M. Javaid, R. P. Singh, and R. Suman, "Telemedicine for Healthcare: Capabilities, Features, Barriers, and applications," *Sensors International*, vol. 2. 2021. doi: 10.1016/j.sintl.2021.100117.

[30] B. Calton, N. Abedini, and M. Fratkin, "Telemedicine in the Time of Coronavirus," *Journal of Pain and Symptom Management*, vol. 60, no. 1, 2020, doi: 10.1016/j.jpainsymman.2020.03.019.

[31] H. Hah and D. Goldin, "Moving Toward AI-Assisted Decision-Making: Observation on Clinicians' Management of Multimedia Patient Information in Synchronous and Asynchronous Telehealth Contexts," *Health Informatics Journal*, vol. 28, no. 1, 2022, doi: 10.1177/14604582221077049.

[32] J. F. Echelard, F. Méthot, H. A. Nguyen, and M. P. Pomey, "Medical Student Training in eHealth: Scoping Review," *JMIR Medical Education*, vol. 6, no. 2, 2020, doi: 10.2196/20027.

[33] H. Ghunaim, T. R. Weekes, and T. C. Eskridge, "Designing an AI Assistant for Student Telehealth: A Case Study Using Human-Centered Design," in *Proceedings of the 2022 IEEE International Conference on Human-Machine Systems, ICHMS 2022*, 2022. doi: 10.1109/ICHMS56717.2022.9980800.

[34] L. Hong-tan, K. Cui-hua, B. A. Muthu, and C. B. Sivaparthipan, "Big Data and Ambient Intelligence in IoT-Based Wireless Student Health Monitoring System," *Aggression and Violent Behavior*, 2021. doi: 10.1016/j.avb.2021.101601.

[35] A. Papa, M. Mital, P. Pisano, M. Del Giudice, (2020). "E-health and well-being monitoring using smart healthcare devices: An empirical investigation," *Technological Forecasting and Social Change*, vol. 153, p. 119226.

[36] A. Asadzadeh, Z. Mohammadzadeh, Z. Fathifar, S. Jahangiri-Mirshekarlou, and P. Rezaei-Hachesu, "A Framework for Information Technology-Based Management Against COVID-19 in Iran," *BMC Public Health*, vol. 22, no. 1, 2022, doi: 10.1186/s12889-022-12781-1.

[37] K. Furlepa, A. Tenderenda, R. Kozłowski, M. Marczak, W. Wierzba, and A. Śliwczyński, "Recommendations for the Development of Telemedicine in Poland Based on the Analysis of Barriers and Selected Telemedicine Solutions," *International Journal of Environmental Research and Public Health*, vol. 19, no. 3, 2022, doi: 10.3390/ijerph19031221.

[38] P. Jain and P. Chawla, "A Novel Smart Healthcare System Design for Internet of Health Things," in *Proceedings of the 2021 IEEE International Conference on Innovative Computing, Intelligent Communication and Smart Electrical Systems, ICSES 2021*, 2021, doi: 10.1109/ICSES52305.2021.9633869.

[39] H. Mahmud and T. Rahman, "An Application of Blockchain to Securely Acquire, Diagnose and Share Clinical Data Through Smartphone," *Peer-to-Peer Networking and Applications*, vol. 14, no. 6, 2021, doi: 10.1007/s12083-021-01210-6.

[40] R. Kumar, Arjunaditya, D. Singh, K. Srinivasan, and Y. C. Hu, "AI-Powered Blockchain Technology for Public Health: A Contemporary Review, Open Challenges, and Future Research Directions," *Healthcare (Switzerland)*, vol. 11, no. 1, 2023, doi: 10.3390/healthcare11010081.

[41] P. Deka, G. Singh, and G. Kaur, "Artificial Intelligence Powered Healthcare Internet of Things Devices and Their Role," in *Artificial Intelligence to Solve Pervasive Internet of Things Issues*. Cambridge: Academic Press, 2020, doi: 10.1016/B978-0-12-818576-6.00012-5.

[42] A. A. Malik, H. Hussain, R. Maniar, *et al.*, "Integrated Tuberculosis and COVID-19 Activities in Karachi and Tuberculosis Case Notifications," *Tropical Medicine and Infectious Disease*, vol. 7, no. 1, p. 12, 2022, doi: 10.3390/tropicalmed7010012.

[43] B. Zohuri and P. McDaniel, "Artificial Intelligence–Driven Mental Health and Depression Treatment," in *Transcranial Magnetic and Electrical Brain Stimulation for Neurological Disorders*. Amsterdam: Elsevier, 2022, doi: 10.1016/b978-0-323-95416-7.00003-1.

[44] G. Nittari, R. Khuman, S. Baldoni, *et al.*, "Telemedicine Practice: Review of the Current Ethical and Legal Challenges," *Telemedicine and e-Health*, vol. 26, no. 12, pp. 1427–1437, 2020, doi: 10.1089/tmj.2019.0158.

[45] M. Intan Sabrina and I. R. Defi, "Telemedicine Guidelines in South East Asia—A Scoping Review," *Frontiers in Neurology*, vol. 11. 2021, doi: 10.3389/fneur.2020.581649.

[46] I. Hunter, C. Lockhart, V. Rao, B. Tootell, and S. Wong, "Enabling Rural Telehealth for Older Adults in Underserved Rural Communities: Focus Group Study," *JMIR Formative Research*, vol. 6, no. 11, 2022, doi: 10.2196/35864.

[47] P. Boydston, R. Redner, and K. Wold, "Examination of a Telehealth-Based Parent Training Program in Rural or Underserved Areas for Families Impacted by Autism," *Behavior Analysis in Practice*, 2022, doi: 10.1007/s40617-022-00763-z.

[48] K. F. Johnson and L. B. Mahan, "Interprofessional Collaboration and Telehealth: Useful Strategies for Family Counselors in Rural and Underserved Areas," *Family Journal*, vol. 28, no. 3, 2020, doi: 10.1177/1066480720934378.

[49] K. Allen Watts, E. Malone, J. N. Dionne-Odom, *et al.*, "Can You Hear Me Now?: Improving Palliative Care Access Through Telehealth," *Research in Nursing & Health*, vol. 44, no. 1, pp. 226–237, 2021, doi: 10.1002/nur.22105.

[50] R. L. Wilson, O. Higgins, J. Atem, *et al.*, "Artificial Intelligence: An Eye Cast Towards the Mental Health Nursing Horizon," *International Journal of Mental Health Nursing*, vol. 32, no. 3, pp. 938–944, 2023, doi: 10.1111/inm.13121.

[51] A. Alevizopoulos, J. Kritikos, and G. Alevizopoulos, "Intelligent Machines and Mental Health in the Era of COVID-19,"*Psychiatrike = Psychiatriki*, vol. 32, no. 2. 2021, doi: 10.22365/jpsych.2021.015.

[52] M. A. Sizer, D. Bhatta, B. Acharya, and K. P. Paudel, "Determinants of Telehealth Service Use among Mental Health Patients: A Case of Rural Louisiana," *International Journal of Environmental Research and Public Health*, vol. 19, no. 11, 2022, doi: 10.3390/ijerph19116930.

[53] R. E. Reay, J. C. L. Looi, and P. Keightley, "Telehealth Mental Health Services During COVID-19: Summary of Evidence and Clinical Practice," *Australasian Psychiatry*, vol. 28, no. 5, 2020, doi: 10.1177/1039856220943032.

[54] F. A. Wilson, S. Rampa, K. E. Trout, and J. P. Stimpson, "Telehealth Delivery of Mental Health Services: An Analysis of Private Insurance Claims Data in the United States," *Psychiatric Services*, vol. 68, no. 12, 2017, doi: 10.1176/appi.ps.201700017.

[55] D. Mahtta, M. Daher, M. T. Lee, S. Sayani, M. Shishehbor, and S. S. Virani, "Promise and Perils of Telehealth in the Current Era," *Current Cardiology Reports*, vol. 23, no. 9. 2021, doi: 10.1007/s11886-021-01544-w.

[56] A. Hadadi, C. Guillet, J. R. Chardonnet, M. Langovoy, Y. Wang, and J. Ovtcharova, "Prediction of Cybersickness in Virtual Environments Using Topological Data Analysis and Machine Learning," *Frontiers in Virtual Reality*, vol. 3, 2022, doi: 10.3389/frvir.2022.973236.

[57] L. Uscher-Pines, J. Sousa, A. Mehrotra, L. H. Schwamm, and K. S. Zachrison, "Rising to the Challenges of the Pandemic: Telehealth Innovations in U.S. Emergency Departments," *Journal of the American Medical Informatics Association*, vol. 28, no. 9, 2021, doi: 10.1093/jamia/ocab092.

[58] R. M. Zimbroff, K. A. Ornstein, and O. C. Sheehan, "Home-Based Primary Care: A Systematic Review of the Literature, 2010–2020," *Journal of the American Geriatrics Society*, vol. 69, no. 10, 2021, doi: 10.1111/jgs.17365.

[59] W. Jiang, S. Majumder, S. Kumar, *et al.*, "A Wearable Tele-Health System Towards Monitoring COVID-19 and Chronic Diseases," *IEEE Reviews in Biomedical Engineering*, vol. 15, pp. 61–84, 2022, doi: 10.1109/RBME.2021.3069815.

[60] J. P. Lyons, K. Watson, and A. Massacci, "The Evolution of Elderly Telehealth and Health Informatics," in *Recent Advances in Digital System Diagnosis and Management of Healthcare*. London: IntechOpen Limited, 2021, doi: 10.5772/intechopen.88416.

[61] N. D. Shah, E. A. Krupinski, J. Bernard, and M. F. Moyer, "The Evolution and Utilization of Telehealth in Ambulatory Nutrition Practice," *Nutrition in Clinical Practice*, vol. 36, no. 4. 2021, doi: 10.1002/ncp.10641.

[62] C. Der-Martirosian, T. Wyte-Lake, M. Bault, *et al.*, "Implementation of Telehealth Services at the US Department of Veterans Affairs During the COVID-19 Pandemic: Mixed Methods Study," *JMIR Formative Research*, vol. 5, no. 9, e29429, 2021, doi: 10.2196/29429.

[63] D. R. Campbell and H. Goldstein, "Evolution of Telehealth Technology, Evaluations, and Therapy: Effects of the COVID-19 Pandemic on Pediatric Speech-Language Pathology Services," *American Journal of Speech-Language Pathology*, vol. 31, no. 1, 2022, doi: 10.1044/2021_AJSLP-21-00069.

[64] R. V. Zicari, J. Brodersen, J. Brusseau, *et al.*, "Z-Inspection ®: A Process to Assess Trustworthy AI," *IEEE Transactions on Technology and Society*, vol. 2, no. 2, 2021, pp. 83–97, doi: 10.1109/tts.2021.3066209.

[65] S. M. Meystre, P.M. Heider, Y. Kim, *et al.*, "Natural Language Processing Enabling COVID-19 Predictive Analytics to Support Data-Driven Patient Advising and Pooled Testing," *Journal of the American Medical Informatics Association*, vol. 29, no. 1, pp. 12–21, 2022, doi: 10.1093/jamia/ocab186.

[66] E. Sezgin, Y. Huang, D. Lin, U. Ramtekkar, L. Pauline, and S. Lin, "Documented Reasons of Cancellation and Rescheduling of Telehealth Appointments during the Pandemic," *Telemedicine and e-Health*, vol. 27, no. 10, 2021, doi: 10.1089/tmj.2020.0454.

[67] E. Massaad and P. Cherfan, "Social Media Data Analytics on Telehealth During the COVID-19 Pandemic," *Cureus*, 2020, doi: 10.7759/cureus.7838.

[68] T. Champagne-Langabeer, M. W. Swank, S. Manas, Y. Si, and K. Roberts, "Dramatic Increases in Telehealth-Related Tweets During the Early Covid-19 Pandemic: A Sentiment Analysis," *Healthcare (Switzerland)*, vol. 9, no. 6, 2021, doi: 10.3390/healthcare9060634.

[69] T. Kamei, "Telenursing and Artificial Intelligence for Oncology Nursing," *Asia-Pacific Journal of Oncology Nursing*, vol. 9, no. 12, 2022, doi: 10.1016/j.apjon.2022.100119.

[70] K. Joy, *5 Healthcare Technology Trends to Watch in 2020*. Patient-Centered Care, 2019.

[71] P. Bhattacharya, M. S. Obaidat, D. Savaliya, S. Sanghavi, S. Tanwar, and B. Sadaun, "Metaverse Assisted Telesurgery in Healthcare 5.0: An Interplay of Blockchain and Explainable AI," in *Proceedings of the 2022 International Conference on Computer, Information and Telecommunication Systems, CITS 2022*, 2022, doi: 10.1109/CITS55221.2022.9832978.

[72] N. R. S. Narikimilli, A. Kumar, A. D. Antu, and B. Xie, "Blockchain Applications in Healthcare – A Review and Future Perspective," in *Lecture Notes in Computer Science (including subseries Lecture Notes in Artificial Intelligence and Lecture Notes in Bioinformatics)*. Cham: Springer, 2020, doi: 10.1007/978-3-030-59638-5_14.

[73] N. Naik, B.M. Hameed, N. Sooriyaperakasam, *et al.*, "Transforming Healthcare Through a Digital Revolution: A Review of Digital Healthcare Technologies and Solutions," *Frontiers in Digital Health*, vol. 4, p. 919985, 2022, doi: 10.3389/fdgth.2022.919985.

[74] M. Reddy, "Digital Transformation in Healthcare in 2021: 7 Key Trends," Digital Authority Partners, 4, 2021.

[75] H. R. Hasan, K. Salah, R. Jayaraman, I. Yaqoob, M. Omar, and S. Ellahham, "Blockchain-Enabled Telehealth Services Using Smart Contracts," *IEEE Access*, vol. 9, 2021, doi: 10.1109/ACCESS.2021.3126025.

[76] S. Shi, M. Luo, Y. Wen, L. Wang, and D. He, "A Blockchain-Based User Authentication Scheme with Access Control for Telehealth Systems," *Security and Communication Networks*, vol. 2022, 2022, doi: 10.1155/2022/6735003.

[77] C. Krittanawong, M. Aydar, H.U.H. Virk, *et al.*, "Artificial Intelligence-Powered Blockchains for Cardiovascular Medicine," *Canadian Journal of Cardiology*, vol. 38, no. 2, pp. 185–195, 2022, doi: 10.1016/j.cjca.2021.11.011.

[78] R. W. Ahmad, K. Salah, R. Jayaraman, I. Yaqoob, S. Ellahham, and M. Omar, "The Role of Blockchain Technology in Telehealth and Telemedicine," *International Journal of Medical Informatics*, vol. 148, 2021, doi: 10.1016/j.ijmedinf.2021.104399.

[79] M. T. Oyshi, M. Z. Bonny, S. Saha, and Z. N. Tumpa, "IoT Security Issues and Possible Solution Using Blockchain Technology," in *Lecture Notes in Networks and Systems*. Singapore: Springer, 2021, doi: 10.1007/978-981-15-4218-3_12.

[80] A. B. Mahammad and R. Kumar, "Progression of Digital Healthcare with Deep Learning and Blockchain Methods for Smart Cities," In *Advances in Deep Learning Applications for Smart Cities*, IGI Global, pp. 248–266, 2022, doi: 10.4018/978-1-7998-9710-1.ch012.

[81] K. N. Griggs, O. Ossipova, C. P. Kohlios, A. N. Baccarini, E. A. Howson, and T. Hayajneh, "Healthcare Blockchain System Using Smart Contracts for Secure Automated Remote Patient Monitoring," *Journal of Medical Systems*, vol. 42, no. 7, 2018, doi: 10.1007/s10916-018-0982-x.

[82] I. T. Javed, F. Alharbi, B. Bellaj, T. Margaria, N. Crespi, and K. N. Qureshi, "Health-id: A blockchain-based decentralized identity management for remote healthcare," *Healthcare (Switzerland)*, vol. 9, no. 6, 2021, doi: 10.3390/healthcare9060712.

[83] T. Alam and M. Benaida, "Internet of Things and Blockchain-Based Framework for Coronavirus (COVID-19) Disease," *International Journal of Online and Biomedical Engineering*, vol. 18, no. 6, 2022, doi: 10.3991/ijoe.v18i06.29919.

[84] B. Zaabar, O. Cheikhrouhou, M. Ammi, A. I. Awad, and M. Abid, "Secure and Privacy-aware Blockchain-based Remote Patient Monitoring System for Internet of Healthcare Things," in *International Conference on Wireless and Mobile Computing, Networking and Communications*, 2021, doi: 10.1109/WiMob52687.2021.9606362.

[85] M. Abomhara, M. Gerdes, and G. M. Køien, "A STRIDE-Based Threat Model for Telehealth Systems," in *Norwegian Information Security Conference (NISK)*, vol. 8, January 2016, 2015.

[86] M. Aazam, E. N. Huh, S. Zeadally, K. A. Harras, E. AbuKhousa and N. Mohamed, "Fog Computing – Glimps of Upcoming Research Area (#4)," *Future Generation Computer Systems*, vol. 5, no. 2, 2017.

[87] E. Molina, C. E. S. Torres, R. Salazar-Cabrera, D. M. López, and R. Vargas-Cañas, "Intelligent Telehealth System to Support Epilepsy Diagnosis," *Journal of Multidisciplinary Healthcare*, vol. 13, 2020, doi: 10.2147/JMDH.S247878.

[88] E. Long, J. Chen, X. Wu, *et al.*, "Artificial Intelligence Manages Congenital Cataract with Individualized Prediction and Telehealth Computing," *NPJ Digital Medicine*, vol. 3, no. 1, p. 112, 2020, doi: 10.1038/s41746-020-00319-x.

[89] T. Darwish, S. Korouri, M. Pasini, M. V. Cortez, and W. W. Ishak, "Integration of Advanced Health Technology Within the Healthcare System

to Fight the Global Pandemic: Current Challenges and Future Opportunities," *Innovations in Clinical Neuroscience*, vol. 18, no. 1–3, 2021.

[90] H. M. P. Morales, M. Guedes, J. S. Silva, and A. Massuda, "COVID-19 in Brazil—Preliminary Analysis of Response Supported by Artificial Intelligence in Municipalities," *Frontiers in Digital Health*, vol. 3, 2021, doi: 10.3389/fdgth.2021.648585.

[91] A. Thurzo, V. Kurilová, and I. Varga, "Artificial Intelligence in Orthodontic Smart Application for Treatment Coaching and Its Impact on Clinical Performance of Patients Monitored with AI-Telehealth System," *Healthcare (Switzerland)*, vol. 9, no. 12, 2021, doi: 10.3390/healthcare9121695.

[92] A. Rana and S. Malik, "A Review of Computational Intelligence Technologies for Tackling Covid-19 Pandemic," in *Internet of Things*. Cham: Springer, 2021. doi: 10.1007/978-3-030-75220-0_11.

[93] Geetanjali, R. Malviya, R. Awasthi, *et al.*, "Applications of Artificial Intelligence, Blockchain, and Internet-of-Things in Management of Chronic Disease," in *Cognitive Intelligence and Big Data in Healthcare*. New York: Wiley, 349–365, 2022, doi: 10.1002/9781119771982.ch13.

[94] P. Bhattacharya, D. Saraswat, D. Savaliya, *et al.*, "Towards Future Internet: The Metaverse Perspective for Diverse Industrial Applications," *Mathematics*, vol. 11, no. 4, p. 941, 2023, doi: 10.3390/math11040941.

[95] A. Pal, K. Gudimetla, Riyazuddin Md Y, and Akkalakshmi M, "Digital Technology in Management of Covid-19: A New Ray to Healthcare," *International Journal of Research in Pharmaceutical Sciences*, vol. 11, no. SPL1, pp. 1426–1436, 2020, doi: 10.26452/ijrps.v11ispl1.3684.

[96] S. L. Burton, "Artificial Intelligence (AI) and Augmented Reality (AR): Disambiguated in the Telemedicine/Telehealth Sphere," *Scientific Bulletin*, vol. 26, no. 1, 2021, doi: 10.2478/bsaft-2021-0001.

[97] C. Pistorius, "Developments in Emerging Digital Health Technologies," *DeltaHedron Innovation Insight,* no. 1, 2017.

[98] C. Pistorius, *Developments in Emerging Digital Health Technologies*. Innovation Insight, 2017.

[99] M. Tiik, "The Road to eHealth in Estonia: Lessons Learned and Future Opportunities and Challenges...14th European Public Health Conference (Virtual), Public Health Futures in a Changing World, November 10–12, 2021," *European Journal of Public Health*, vol. 31, 2021.

[100] R. S. V. Sharma, "Success of Indian National Health Protection Scheme Needs Creative Destruction of Mines of Healthcare Corruption," *International Journal of Business & Management Science*, vol. 4, no. 4, 2018.

[101] C. Dilibal and Y. Tur, "Implementation of Developed Esantem Smart Healthcare System in Metaverse," in *ISMSIT 2022 – 6th International Symposium on Multidisciplinary Studies and Innovative Technologies, Proceedings*, 2022, doi: 10.1109/ISMSIT56059.2022.9932849.

[102] H. Dar and K. Kashyap, "Smart Healthcare System (SHS): Medical Tourism Delivering, Consumption, and Elevating Tool in the Ages of Smart Technologies," *Tourism Planning and Development*, vol. 20, no. 3, 2023, doi: 10.1080/21568316.2022.2109206.

[103] M. J. Chehade, L. Yadav, D. Kopansky-Giles, *et al.*, "Innovations to Improve Access to Musculoskeletal Care," *Best Practice and Research: Clinical Rheumatology*, vol. 34, no. 5, 101559, 2020, doi: 10.1016/j.berh.2020. 101559.

[104] C. El Morr, H. Ali-Hassan, C. El Morr, and H. Ali-Hassan, "Healthcare, Data Analytics, and Business Intelligence," *Analytics in healthcare: a practical introduction*, pp. 1–13. 2019, doi: 10.1007/978-3-030-04506-7_1.

[105] K. Batko and A. Ślęzak, "The Use of Big Data Analytics in Healthcare," *Journal of Big Data*, vol. 9, no. 1, 2022, doi: 10.1186/s40537-021-00553-4.

[106] S. J. Alsunaidi, A. M. Almuhaideb, N. M. Ibrahim, *et al.*, "Applications of Big Data Analytics to Control Covid-19 Pandemic," *Sensors*, vol. 21, no. 7, p. 2282, 2021, doi: 10.3390/s21072282.

[107] M. Srivathsan and A. K. Yogesh, "Health Monitoring System by Prognotive Computing Using Big Data Analytics," *Procedia Computer Science*, 2015, doi: 10.1016/j.procs.2015.04.092.

[108] W. Wang, Z. Zhang, N. Gao, and Y. Zhao, "Progress of Big Data Analytics Methods Based on Artificial Intelligence Technology," *Jisuanji Jicheng Zhizao Xitong/Computer Integrated Manufacturing Systems, CIMS*, vol. 25, no. 3, 2019, doi: 10.13196/j.cims.2019.03.001.

[109] M. S. Hunt, S. J. Weiss, and A. Y. Lee, "The Role of Data Analytics and Artificial Intelligence (AI) in Ocular Telehealth," in *Ocular Telehealth*. Amsterdam: Elsevier, 2023, doi: 10.1016/b978-0-323-83204-5.00018-4.

[110] R. S. H. Istepanian and T. Al-Anzi, "m-Health 2.0: New Perspectives on Mobile Health, Machine Learning and Big Data Analytics," *Methods*, vol. 151, 2018, doi: 10.1016/j.ymeth.2018.05.015.

[111] A. Jain and A. K. Tripathi, "Blockchain Enable Smart Contract Based Telehealth and Medicines System," in *Communications in Computer and Information Science*. Cham: Springer, 2022, doi: 10.1007/978-3-031-07012-9_60.

[112] K. A. Colón, "Creating a Patient-Centered, Global, Decentralized Health System: Combining New Payment and Care Delivery Models with Telemedicine, AI, and Blockchain Technology," *Blockchain in Healthcare Today,* vol. 1, 2018, doi: 10.30953/bhty.v1.30.

[113] M. Y. Jabarulla and H.-N. Lee, "A Blockchain and Artificial Intelligence-Based, Patient-Centric Healthcare System for Combating the COVID-19 Pandemic: Opportunities and Applications," *Healthcare*, vol. 9, no. 8, 2021, doi: 10.3390/healthcare9081019.

Chapter 2

Taxonomy of artificial intelligence and blockchain technology in telehealth systems

Abdulwaheed Musa[1,2,3], *Abdulhakeem Abdulfatai*[1], *Daniel Oluyemi*[1], *Segun Jacob*[1] *and Agbotiname Lucky Imoize*[4]

Telehealth systems have rapidly emerged as a critical component of modern healthcare, enabling remote patient care, real-time monitoring, and improved access to medical services. With the advent of artificial intelligence (AI) and blockchain technology, telehealth systems have witnessed significant advancements in terms of efficiency, security, and interoperability. AI and blockchain technologies have emerged as powerful tools with immense potential in healthcare. However, there exists the problem of effectively categorizing and classifying the various applications and implementations of AI and blockchain technology in the context of telehealth systems. There is a need for a comprehensive taxonomy to organize and understand the diverse applications of AI and blockchain technology in telehealth due to the rapid growth in these fields. Therefore, this chapter presents a taxonomy that explores the integration of AI and blockchain in telehealth systems. The taxonomy aims to categorize, classify, and analyze the various applications, benefits, challenges, and future directions of this integration, providing a comprehensive understanding of the synergistic relationship among AI, blockchain, and telehealth. The chapter, thus, contributes to the advancement and adoption of these technologies in healthcare settings.

2.1 Introduction

Telehealth systems encompass a wide range of applications, including teleconsultations, remote monitoring, telesurgery, and telepsychiatry [1]. They

[1]Department of Electrical and Computer Engineering, Kwara State University, Nigeria
[2]Centre for Artificial Intelligence and Machine Learning Systems, Kwara State University, Nigeria
[3]Institute for Intelligent Systems, University of Johannesburg, South Africa
[4]Department of Electrical and Electronics Engineering, Faculty of Engineering, University of Lagos, Nigeria

leverage advancements in artificial intelligence (AI), machine learning (ML), and Internet of Things (IoT) technologies to enhance diagnosis accuracy, personalize treatment plans, and streamline healthcare workflows [2]. AI has the potential to enhance telehealth systems by improving diagnosis accuracy, enabling remote monitoring, personalizing care, and enhancing the overall patient experience. One of the primary applications of AI in telehealth systems is in improving diagnosis accuracy [3]. AI algorithms can analyze vast amounts of patient data, including medical records, lab results, and imaging studies, to identify patterns and detect abnormalities that may be missed by human clinicians. This can lead to more accurate and timely diagnoses, enabling earlier interventions and improved patient outcomes. AI-powered diagnostic systems have shown promising results in various medical specialties, including radiology, pathology, and dermatology [4].

Furthermore, [5–8] proposed blockchain-based frameworks that enable patients to maintain control over their medical data, granting permission to healthcare providers for access and ensuring transparency in data handling. By eliminating the need for intermediaries, blockchain can streamline the sharing of patient records across different healthcare institutions, ultimately leading to improved care coordination and reduced medical errors. The combination of AI and blockchain in telehealth systems has shown promising results.

However, there exists the problem of effectively categorizing and classifying the various applications and implementations of AI and blockchain technology in the context of telehealth systems. Because of the rapid growth in these fields, there is a need for a comprehensive taxonomy to organize and understand the diverse applications of AI and blockchain technology in telehealth. By establishing taxonomy for this rapidly evolving field, we can attain a deeper understanding of the interconnected elements, enabling us to explore their synergistic potential and foster future developments at the intersection of AI, blockchain, and telehealth. This chapter presents a taxonomy that explores the integration of AI and blockchain in telehealth systems. The taxonomy aims to categorize and analyze the various applications, benefits, challenges, and future directions of this integration, providing a comprehensive understanding of the synergistic relationship among AI, blockchain, and telehealth.

2.1.1 Key contributions of the chapter

The following are the significant contributions of this chapter:

1. Review of recent and related works on AI and blockchain technology used for telehealth systems was conducted.
2. The chapter examines the history and evolution of telehealth systems.
3. The chapter explains AI and blockchain technology in telehealth systems.
4. The security and privacy issues in telehealth systems have been discussed.
5. The chapter presents a taxonomy for AI and blockchain technology in telehealth systems. The taxonomy can be used to better understand and classify the different ways that these technologies are being used in telehealth systems.
6. The chapter also provides recommendations on how to improve the taxonomy of AI and blockchain technology in telehealth systems.

2.1.2 Chapter organization

The remaining sections of this chapter are structured as follows: Section 2.2 reviews relevant related works on blockchain and AI in telehealth systems. Section 2.3 provides the evolution of telehealth systems, including their transformation and potential during COVID-19. Section 2.4 discusses AI for telehealth systems and Section 2.5 highlights blockchain technology for telehealth systems. In Section 2.6, security and privacy issues in telehealth systems are presented. Section 2.7 presents the taxonomy of AI and blockchain technology in telehealth systems. Section 2.8 highlights and discusses the lessons learned. Finally, Section 2.9 concludes the chapter with some recommendations.

2.2 Related work

Telehealth systems have gained prominence in recent years, especially during the COVID-19 pandemic, as they enable remote delivery of healthcare services. Several studies have demonstrated the use of AI in telehealth systems to improve diagnostic accuracy, patient monitoring, and personalized treatment. For instance, [9–12] in their studies mentioned the developed AI algorithms that analyze medical images, such as X-rays or MRIs, to assist healthcare professionals in diagnosing various conditions. These algorithms leverage deep learning techniques to identify patterns and anomalies in the images, providing valuable insights and aiding in faster and more accurate diagnoses. Additionally, AI-powered chatbots and virtual assistants have been employed to offer personalized health advice, answer patient queries, and monitor symptoms, leading to improved patient engagement and self-management [13–16].

The authors [5–8] also proposed blockchain-based frameworks that enable patients to maintain control over their medical data, granting permission to healthcare providers for access and ensuring transparency in data handling. By eliminating the need for intermediaries, blockchain can streamline the sharing of patient records across different healthcare institutions, ultimately leading to improved care coordination and reduced medical errors. Furthermore, the combination of AI and blockchain in telehealth systems has shown promising results. The authors [17–20] explored the potential synergies between these technologies to enhance the efficiency and effectiveness of healthcare services. These reviewed works highlight the significant potential of integrating AI and blockchain technology in telehealth systems.

Meanwhile, there are also specific related works on the taxonomy of AI and blockchain technology in telehealth systems that are worth mentioning. One of them was the work by [21] that proposed a taxonomy for the use of AI in medicine. He identified several categories, such as AI-assisted diagnostics, AI-assisted therapeutics, and AI-assisted monitoring, and provided examples of how these categories could be applied to telehealth systems. Another related work is by [22], who proposed a taxonomy for the use of AI in telemedicine. They identified several use cases, such as automated diagnosis, personalized treatment, and remote monitoring, and categorized them based on the type of AI used. Hasan *et al.* [23] proposed a taxonomy for the use of AI in remote patient monitoring. They identified several categories, such as physiological monitoring, behavioral monitoring, and environmental monitoring, and provided examples of how these categories could be applied to telehealth systems.

Similarly, [24] proposed a taxonomy for the use of AI in telemedicine during the COVID-19 pandemic. They identified several categories, such as AI-assisted diagnosis, AI-assisted treatment planning, and AI-assisted remote monitoring, and provided examples of how AI could be used to address the challenges of the pandemic. Hussien *et al.* [25] proposed a taxonomy for the use of blockchain technology in telemedicine. They identified use cases, such as secure data sharing, authentication, and patient consent management, and categorized them into different groups based on the role of blockchain.

The work [26] proposed a taxonomy for the use of blockchain technology in healthcare systems, including telehealth systems. Their taxonomy categorized blockchain use cases into six different areas, including data management, identity management, and payment systems. The work by [27] proposed a taxonomy for the use of blockchain technology in healthcare supply chains, which could be relevant in the context of telehealth systems. They identified some categories, such as interoperability, data security, and supply chain management, and provided examples of how blockchain could be used to address the challenges in these areas. Table 2.1 is a comprehensive table that presents a summary of some literature on AI and blockchain technology in telehealth systems, stating their coverage, scope of work, limitations, and how the current work has addressed the identified gaps.

Table 2.1 Related literature on artificial intelligence and blockchain technology in telehealth systems

Literature	Coverage	Scope of work	Limitations	Addressing identified gaps
[22]	Examines various AI technologies in telehealth	Proposes taxonomy for AI and blockchain technology	Small sample size limits and limited generalizability	Expands on previous taxonomies to include blockchain technology in telehealth
[25]	Investigates the impact of AI and blockchain on telehealth	Analyzes the impact of AI and blockchain on telehealth systems	Lack of real-world implementation challenges	Provides insights on practical implications and challenges of implementing AI and blockchain in telehealth
[26]	Explores the use of blockchain technology in telehealth	Evaluates the use of blockchain in telehealth systems	Limited focus on technical feasibility	Identifies gaps in the existing literature and proposes a framework for integrating AI and blockchain in telehealth
[21]	Reviews existing literature on AI and blockchain	Reviews the existing literature on AI and blockchain in healthcare	Lack of standardization and interoperability challenges	Highlights the potential benefits and challenges of AI and blockchain in telehealth systems and suggests future directions for research

These key literature sources provide valuable insights into the coverage, scope of work, limitations, and how the current work addresses the identified gaps in the research article. By synthesizing and building upon these existing studies, the article aims to contribute to the development of a comprehensive taxonomy for understanding the application of AI and blockchain technology in telehealth systems. This has been leveraged and developed in this current work.

2.3 Evolution of telehealth systems

Telehealth systems have evolved significantly over the years, opening up new avenues for efficient, effective, and affordable healthcare services. Telehealth systems, also known as telemedicine or remote healthcare, have emerged as a transformative solution in the field of healthcare delivery. These systems utilize advanced communication technologies to enable healthcare professionals to remotely diagnose, treat, and monitor patients, bridging the gap between patients and healthcare providers. The evolution of telehealth systems has been driven by advancements in technology, changes in healthcare policies, and the need for improved accessibility and efficiency in healthcare services.

The roots of telehealth can be traced back to the early twentieth century when telegraph and telephone technologies were first employed for medical consultations and guidance. One of the pioneering instances of telehealth occurred in 1925 when a radio connection was used to transmit radiographic images for diagnostic purposes.

In the 1960s and 1970s, significant progress was made in the field of telemedicine, with the National Aeronautics and Space Administration (NASA) playing a crucial role. The space agency implemented telemedicine technology to monitor astronauts' health during space missions, providing real-time vital signs monitoring and video consultations [28]. These early experiments demonstrated the potential of telehealth systems in extending healthcare services beyond traditional settings and across vast distances.

The 1990s marked a turning point for telehealth systems with the rapid expansion of the Internet and the development of videoconferencing technologies [29]. This enabled real-time audiovisual communication between healthcare providers and patients, facilitating remote consultations and diagnosis. Additionally, advancements in medical imaging technology allowed for the transmission of high-quality images, facilitating remote radiology and pathology consultations.

In the early 2000s, telehealth systems gained further momentum with the proliferation of broadband Internet and the widespread availability of affordable digital devices. This led to the development of remote patient monitoring systems, which allowed healthcare providers to remotely track patients' vital signs, chronic conditions, and medication adherence [30]. Moreover, telehealth systems started to integrate electronic health records (EHRs), facilitating seamless information exchange and continuity of care [31].

The COVID-19 pandemic, which emerged in 2019, acted as a catalyst for the widespread adoption of telehealth systems. To minimize in-person contact and curb

Table 2.2 Evolution of telehealth

Period	Key developments
Early twentieth century	Use of telegraphy to transmit radiographic images for diagnostic purposes
1960s–1970s	Development of telephonic transmission of medical data, such as electrocardiograms
1980s–1990s	Introduction of teleconferencing and video communication technologies in telehealth
2000s	Integration of electronic health records (EHRs) into telehealth systems for seamless information sharing
Mid-2000s	Adoption of telehealth for remote patient monitoring, including vital signs and chronic condition management
The late 2000s	The emergence of mobile health (mHealth) applications, leveraging smartphones and wearables for health tracking and remote consultations
2010s	Integration of artificial intelligence (AI) and machine learning (ML) algorithms for data analysis, diagnosis support, and personalized treatment plans
Present day	Advancements in telecommunication infrastructure, high-speed Internet, and improved video conferencing software. Expansion of telehealth services globally

the spread of the virus, healthcare providers rapidly scaled up their telehealth capabilities. Virtual visits became the norm, allowing patients to receive medical advice, prescriptions, and follow-up care from the safety and convenience of their homes. This shift highlighted the potential of telehealth systems in improving healthcare accessibility, especially for underserved populations and remote areas.

Today, telehealth systems encompass a wide range of applications, including teleconsultations, remote monitoring, telesurgery, and telepsychiatry [1]. They leverage advancements in AI, ML, and IoT technologies to enhance diagnosis accuracy, personalize treatment plans, and streamline healthcare workflows [2]. Telehealth systems have become an integral part of the modern healthcare ecosystem, delivering cost-effective, efficient, and patient-centered care.

Table 2.2 provides an overview of the evolution of telehealth systems. The history of telehealth systems is a testament to the transformative power of technology in healthcare. From the early telephonic experiments to the current era of advanced digital platforms, telehealth has evolved to overcome geographical barriers, improve access to care, and enhance patient outcomes. As technology continues to advance, telehealth systems will play an increasingly pivotal role in shaping the future of healthcare, ensuring that high-quality medical services are accessible to all, regardless of location or circumstance.

2.4 Artificial intelligence for telehealth systems

One area where AI impact has been particularly significant is telehealth systems. AI has the potential to enhance telehealth systems by improving diagnosis accuracy, enabling remote monitoring, personalizing care, and enhancing the overall patient experience. One of the primary applications of AI in telehealth systems is in improving diagnosis accuracy [3]. AI algorithms can analyze vast amounts of patient data, including medical records, lab results, and imaging studies, to identify patterns and detect abnormalities that may be missed by human clinicians. This can lead to more accurate and timely diagnoses, enabling earlier interventions and improved patient outcomes. AI-powered diagnostic systems have shown promising results in various medical specialties, including radiology, pathology, and dermatology [4].

Another key area where AI can be utilized in telehealth is remote patient monitoring. With the help of wearable devices and sensors, AI algorithms can continuously monitor patients' vital signs, such as heart rate, blood pressure, and glucose levels [32]. These algorithms can detect deviations from normal values and alert healthcare providers in real time, enabling timely interventions and proactive care. Remote monitoring systems powered by AI can be particularly beneficial for patients with chronic conditions who require regular monitoring and for those who are geographically distant from healthcare facilities [33].

Personalizing care is another advantage of AI in telehealth systems. AI algorithms can analyze patient data, including medical history, genetic information, lifestyle factors, and treatment responses, to develop personalized treatment plans [34]. This can help healthcare providers make more informed decisions about the most appropriate interventions for individual patients. By considering a patient's unique characteristics, AI-powered telehealth systems can optimize treatment outcomes and minimize the risk of adverse effects. Furthermore, AI can support shared decision-making by providing patients with evidence-based information and recommendations tailored to their specific circumstances [35].

AI also plays a crucial role in improving the overall patient experience in telehealth. Natural language processing (NLP) algorithms enable AI chatbots and virtual assistants to engage in interactive conversations with patients, addressing their queries and concerns [36]. These AI-powered systems can provide basic healthcare information, schedule appointments, remind patients about medication schedules, and offer emotional support. They can also assist in triaging patients, directing them to the most appropriate level of care based on their symptoms and urgency. By automating routine tasks and providing round-the-clock support, AI enhances accessibility and convenience for patients, leading to increased patient satisfaction.

Table 2.3 and Figure 2.1 show various AI algorithms used in healthcare, along with their methodologies and common applications. In Table 2.3 and Figure 2.1, some key AI algorithms, namely: Convolutional Neural Networks (CNN), Support Vector Machines (SVM), Random Forests, and Naive Bayes, that are used in the healthcare system are highlighted and further elaborated. The CNN is designed to learn complex patterns and features within images, enabling them to detect abnormalities, identify specific conditions, and aid in diagnostic decision-making. SVM is a powerful algorithm that finds an optimal hyperplane to separate different classes of data based on features extracted from patient data. Random forests are

Table 2.3 Artificial intelligence algorithms for healthcare

Reference	Algorithm	Methodology	Uses
[37]	Decision trees	A tree-based model that makes decisions based on conditions	Diagnosing diseases, predicting outcomes, and risk assessment
[38]	Random forests	Ensemble of decision trees that improves predictive accuracy	Disease classification, identifying important features
[39]	Support Vector Machines (SVM)	Constructs hyperplanes to separate data into classes	Image recognition, cancer diagnosis, patient monitoring
[40]	Artificial Neural Networks (ANN)	Interconnected layers of artificial neurons	Disease prediction, medical imaging analysis, genomics
[41]	Convolutional Neural Networks (CNN)	Designed for image processing and pattern recognition	Medical image analysis, tumor detection, radiology
[42]	Recurrent Neural Networks (RNN)	Designed to analyze sequential data with memory	Time series analysis, patient monitoring, clinical notes
[43]	Long Short-Term Memory (LSTM)	Type of RNN with memory units to retain information	Predicting patient outcomes, anomaly detection
[44]	Generative Adversarial Networks (GAN)	Comprises generator and discriminator models	Synthetic data generation, medical image synthesis
[45]	Reinforcement Learning (RL)	Learning from trial and error through rewards and penalties	Optimizing treatment plans, personalized medicine
[46]	Naive Bayes	A probabilistic classifier based on Bayes' theorem	Disease prediction, diagnosis, risk assessment
[47]	k-Nearest Neighbors (k-NN)	Classifies data points based on similarity to neighbors	Disease diagnosis, patient stratification, data clustering
[48]	Hidden Markov models (HMM)	A probabilistic model with hidden states and observed outputs	Speech recognition, gesture analysis, disease modeling
[49]	Gaussian Mixture Models (GMM)	Represents probability distributions as a combination of Gaussian components	Clustering patient populations, anomaly detection

ensemble learning algorithms used in disease diagnosis to analyze patient data and classify individuals into different disease categories. While the Naive Bayes calculates the probability of a patient having a particular disease based on the presence or absence of various symptoms or features.

Despite the numerous benefits of AI in telehealth systems, there are also challenges that need to be addressed. Data privacy and security are paramount

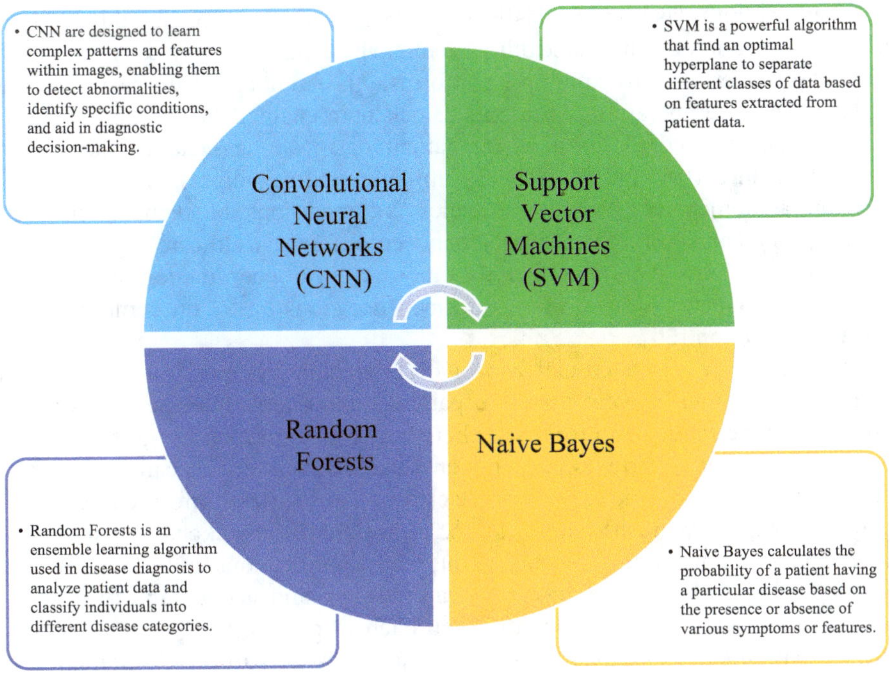

Figure 2.1 Some AI algorithms in healthcare

concerns, as telehealth systems involve the transmission and storage of sensitive patient information. Robust security measures, including encryption and authentication protocols, need to be implemented to protect patient data from unauthorized access. Additionally, ensuring the ethical use of AI algorithms and addressing issues of bias and fairness in healthcare decision-making are critical considerations.

2.5 Blockchain technology for telehealth systems

Traditional healthcare systems often suffer from data breaches and unauthorized access due to centralized storage and vulnerabilities in existing infrastructure. Blockchain, on the other hand, employs a distributed ledger that records transactions across multiple nodes, ensuring that data are replicated and secured in a decentralized manner [50]. This decentralized architecture makes it extremely difficult for malicious actors to tamper with or compromise patient data. Each transaction recorded on the blockchain is cryptographically secured and linked to previous transactions, creating an immutable audit trail that can be audited and verified by authorized participants [51]. This transparency and immutability contribute to a higher level of trust in the telehealth system.

Interoperability is another challenge in healthcare that can be addressed by blockchain technology. In telehealth systems, where patients may seek care from different providers or across multiple platforms, it is essential to have seamless data exchange and interoperability standards. Blockchain enables the creation of a unified and standardized platform where patient data can be securely shared and accessed by authorized parties [52]. By utilizing smart contracts, which are self-executing agreements with predefined rules and conditions, blockchain can facilitate automated and secure data sharing between different healthcare organizations. This interoperability can significantly improve care coordination and enable healthcare providers to make more informed decisions based on comprehensive patient information [20].

Patient privacy is a crucial aspect of telehealth systems, and blockchain technology can help protect sensitive patient data. Blockchain networks allow patients to have greater control over their health information by granting them ownership and consent rights [23]. Patients can determine who can access their data and under what conditions, empowering them to make informed decisions about sharing their health information. Additionally, blockchain can enable secure and auditable consent management, where patient consent transactions are recorded on the blockchain, ensuring transparency and accountability in data-sharing practices. This patient-centric approach to data privacy can foster trust between patients and healthcare providers and encourage greater participation in telehealth services.

Blockchain technology can also facilitate the secure integration of IoT devices into telehealth systems [23]. IoT devices, such as wearables and remote monitoring sensors, generate vast amounts of patient data [53]. By connecting these devices to a blockchain network, the data can be securely transmitted, stored, and analyzed [20]. This integration ensures data integrity and authenticity, as each data transaction is recorded on the blockchain, making it highly resistant to tampering or manipulation [52]. Furthermore, blockchain can enable the creation of smart contracts that automate data processing and incentivize data contributors, fostering a decentralized ecosystem of health data sharing and analysis [54].

Figure 2.2 depicts a taxonomy that outlines key dimensions of blockchain technology in telehealth systems. The key dimensions include blockchain-based data management; smart contracts and automation; privacy, security, and consent; and a decentralized telehealth ecosystem. The blockchain-based data management, for instance, highlights immutable data storage, patient identity, and consent management, as well as interoperability and data exchange. While the decentralized telehealth ecosystem includes teleconsultation and remote monitoring, telemedicine payments and incentives, as well as patient-driven data marketplaces.

The blockchain use cases in the healthcare industry are shown in Table 2.4. They include health data exchange, clinical trials, drug traceability, medical billing and claims processing, telemedicine, and remote monitoring, as well as research and intellectual property.

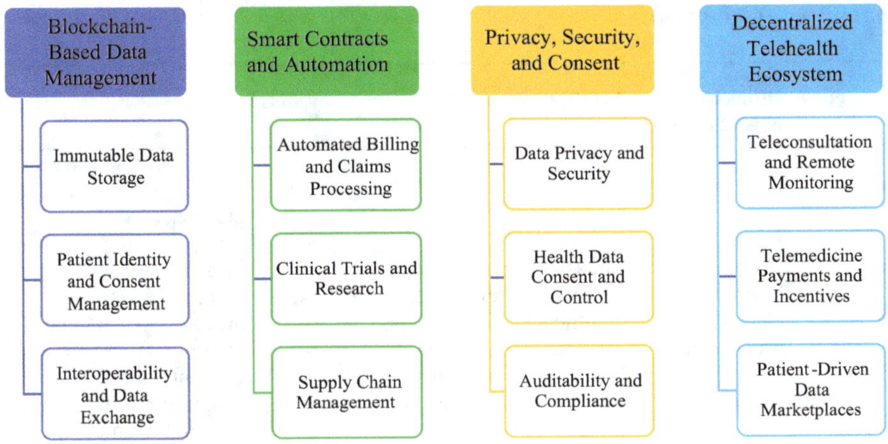

Figure 2.2 Key dimensions of blockchain technology in telehealth systems

Table 2.4 Blockchain use cases in healthcare industry

Reference	Blockchain use case	Methodology	Uses
[55]	Health data exchange	Permissioned blockchain networks where multiple healthcare providers, researchers, and patients participate. Data are encrypted and stored in blocks linked to each other, forming a chain	1. Secure and interoperable exchange of patient data between healthcare providers 2. Streamlined access to medical records for researchers and clinicians 3. Improved patient care coordination and continuity
[56]	Clinical trials	Smart contracts are used to automate trial protocols, consent management, and data collection. Trial data are stored on a blockchain, ensuring immutability and transparency.	1. Enhanced transparency and accountability in clinical trials 2. Streamlined patient recruitment and consent management 3. Efficient tracking of trial data, ensuring integrity and auditability
[57]	Drug traceability	Blockchain-based supply chain solutions track the movement of drugs from manufacturing to distribution, ensuring transparency and authenticity. Unique identifiers are used to record drug transactions.	1. Preventing counterfeit drugs by ensuring authenticity and traceability 2. Efficient recalls and targeted investigations in case of safety issues

(Continues)

Table 2.4 (Continued)

Reference	Blockchain use case	Methodology	Uses
			3. Enhanced transparency and accountability in the pharmaceutical supply chain
[58]	Medical billing and claims processing	Smart contracts automate the verification and execution of healthcare claims. Billing information is stored on a blockchain, ensuring transparency and accuracy	1. Streamlined and automated claims processing, reducing administrative costs 2. Prevention of fraudulent claims through immutable and auditable records 3. Faster reimbursement for healthcare providers
[59]	Telemedicine and remote monitoring	Blockchain-based platforms securely store and share patient-generated health data. Smart contracts facilitate automated payments and consent management	1. Secure and private sharing of patient data during telemedicine consultations 2. Efficient remote monitoring of patients, enabling proactive healthcare interventions 3. Transparent and automated payment processes for telemedicine services
[60]	Research and intellectual property	Blockchain platforms enable secure and traceable sharing of research data. Smart contracts enforce data usage agreements and facilitate intellectual property protection	1. Collaborative research with secure and auditable data sharing 2. Transparent attribution and ownership of research findings 3. Efficient intellectual property management and licensing

2.6 Security and privacy issues in telehealth systems

The widespread adoption of telehealth systems has also brought to light significant security and privacy concerns that must be addressed. The sensitive nature of patient health data makes it a prime target for cybercriminals, and any breach of this data can have severe consequences for both patients and healthcare providers. To mitigate this risk, telehealth systems must be designed with robust security measures in place. By classifying the security and privacy issues in telehealth systems into access control, data protection, third-party security, human factors, compliance, and network security, healthcare providers can better understand the risks and develop appropriate measures to mitigate them [61]. This approach can help to improve patient trust and confidence in telehealth systems and ultimately enhance patient health outcomes.

2.6.1 Access control

One major security issue in telehealth is access control. Access control refers to the measures taken to ensure that only authorized individuals can access sensitive information or systems. In the context of telehealth, access control is crucial for protecting patient health information (PHI) from unauthorized access, disclosure, or modification [62].

1. Weak passwords: One common access control issue in telehealth is weak passwords [63]. Many telehealth platforms require users to create passwords to access their accounts, but if these passwords are weak or easily guessable, they can be easily compromised by hackers. To address this issue, telehealth providers should implement strong password policies that require users to create complex passwords and change them regularly.
2. Shared devices: Another access control issue in telehealth is the use of shared devices [64]. Many patients may access telehealth services from shared devices, such as computers in public libraries or community centers. This can make it difficult to ensure that only authorized individuals are accessing PHI. To address this issue, telehealth providers should implement multifactor authentication, which requires users to provide additional authentication factors beyond a password, such as a fingerprint or a one-time code sent to their mobile device.
3. Role-based access control (RBAC): Telehealth providers should also implement RBAC to ensure that users can only access the information and systems that are necessary for their job function. RBAC assigns access permissions based on a user's role in the organization, ensuring that users only have access to the information and systems that are relevant to their job function. This can help prevent unauthorized access and reduce the risk of data breaches [65].

2.6.2 Data protection

PHI includes personal details such as patient names, addresses, and medical records, and it is highly sensitive and valuable to cybercriminals. To protect PHI, telehealth providers must use secure data encryption techniques to protect patient information while it is being transmitted between devices or stored on servers [66]. Encryption technology ensures that data are transmitted securely and prevents unauthorized access to the data during transmission. Telehealth systems must also ensure the accuracy and completeness of patient data, and that data are not tampered with or altered in any way. This requires mechanisms to prevent data tampering and to detect any attempts at data tampering. Data breaches and cyberattacks can also occur when telehealth providers use third-party vendors for services such as cloud storage or telehealth software [67]. These vendors may not have the same level of security measures in place, which can put patients' PHI at risk. To mitigate this risk, telehealth providers must conduct thorough security assessments of third-party vendors before engaging their services and ensure that these vendors meet the same security and data protection standards as their organization.

2.6.3 Network security

Telehealth systems rely on network infrastructure to transmit patient data, which makes them vulnerable to network-based attacks [68]. To address the issue of data breaches which can occur when cybercriminals gain unauthorized access to the telehealth platform or network and steal patients' personal and medical information, telehealth providers must implement robust network security measures, such as firewalls, intrusion detection and prevention systems, and network segmentation. Distributed denial of service (DDoS) attacks can overwhelm the telehealth platform or network with a flood of traffic, making it inaccessible to users and disrupting medical care delivery. To address this issue, telehealth providers must implement DDoS mitigation measures, such as traffic filtering and rate limiting, to prevent and mitigate the impact of DDoS attacks [69]. Telehealth providers must also ensure that their networks are properly configured and patched to address known vulnerabilities and security issues. Unpatched or improperly configured networks can be vulnerable to cyberattacks, which can compromise the security of patient's health information.

2.6.4 Compliance

Compliance with regulatory requirements is another critical security and privacy issue in telehealth systems. Telehealth providers must comply with laws and regulations governing the collection, storage, and transmission of patients' personal and medical information, such as the Health Insurance Portability and Accountability Act (HIPAA) in the United States [70]. HIPAA sets specific standards for protecting patients' health information, and telehealth providers must ensure that their platforms and practices are compliant with these regulations. They must also obtain patients' consent to collect, store, and use their personal and medical information. Telehealth providers must ensure that their services are accessible and inclusive to all patients, including those with disabilities. They must comply with the Americans with Disabilities Act and other laws and regulations governing accessibility and inclusivity in healthcare. Telehealth providers must ensure that their platforms and services are accessible to patients with disabilities, and they must provide reasonable accommodations to ensure that all patients can access their services. They must also comply with ethical and professional standards governing their practice. They must adhere to ethical principles such as confidentiality, informed consent, and respect for patient autonomy, and they must maintain a high standard of professionalism in their interactions with patients.

2.6.5 Human factors

One major human factor issue in telehealth is the potential for miscommunication or misunderstandings between patients and providers. Telehealth communication can be impacted by various factors, such as poor Internet connectivity, technology glitches, cultural and linguistic differences, and limitations of virtual consultations [71]. These factors can lead to misinterpretations, inaccuracies, or incomplete information, which can compromise patient safety and the quality of care provided. Telehealth providers must be aware of these potential communication barriers and take steps to mitigate their impact, such as using clear and simple language, confirming understanding, and using visual aids or interpreter services when necessary. Another human factor issue in telehealth is the potential for technical difficulties or user errors. Telehealth technology can be complex [72], and providers and patients may experience difficulty in operating and troubleshooting the platforms and devices used for remote consultations. User errors, such as inputting incorrect data, misunderstanding instructions, or using incorrect settings, can lead to inaccurate diagnoses, incorrect treatments, or other adverse outcomes. Telehealth providers must ensure that they and their patients are trained to use the technology effectively, and they must have contingency plans in place to address technical difficulties or user errors. Telehealth also poses a risk of patients experiencing social isolation and a lack of connection to their healthcare providers. The lack of physical interaction and nonverbal communication may lead to a decrease in empathy and trust between patients and providers, reducing the perceived quality of care. Providers must be conscious of this potential issue and take steps to establish a meaningful connection with their patients by utilizing methods such as active listening, emotional validation, and utilizing different communication channels.

2.6.6 Third-party security

Third-party security is a significant concern in telehealth, as it involves the sharing of sensitive medical information with outside organizations and individuals. Telehealth providers often rely on third-party vendors, such as cloud service providers and software developers, to host and maintain their platforms and services [67]. These third-party vendors may have access to sensitive patient data, and any security breaches or data breaches that occur on their systems can have severe consequences for patients and the telehealth provider. One of the main third-party security issues in telehealth is the potential for data breaches or cyberattacks. Cybercriminals may target third-party vendors to gain access to sensitive patient data, or they may exploit vulnerabilities in third-party systems to launch attacks on the telehealth provider's platform. The consequences of a data breach can be severe, ranging from financial losses to reputational damage and legal liability. Telehealth providers must ensure that their third-party vendors have adequate security measures in place to protect patient data, such as strong access controls, encryption, and regular security audits. Another third-party security issue in telehealth is the potential for third-party vendors to violate data protection and privacy laws. Third-party vendors may not be subject to the same legal and regulatory requirements as the telehealth provider, and they may not have the same level of commitment to patient privacy. Telehealth providers must ensure that their third-party vendors comply with applicable data protection and privacy laws and that they have appropriate contractual arrangements in place to protect patient data. Telehealth providers must also ensure that their third-party vendors are compliant with industry-specific standards and regulations. For example, in the United States, telehealth providers must comply with the HIPAA when handling patient data. Third-party vendors that handle patient data on behalf of telehealth providers must also comply with HIPAA and other industry-specific standards. Telehealth providers must ensure that their third-party vendors have appropriate policies and procedures in place to comply with these standards.

2.7 Taxonomy of AI and blockchain technology in telehealth systems

Taxonomy refers to the classification of different elements into categories based on their characteristics or attributes. Telehealth, or the use of technology to provide remote medical care, has become increasingly popular in recent years as a way to increase access to care and reduce costs. AI has the potential to revolutionize healthcare by enabling quicker, more accurate diagnoses, and providing more personalized treatment recommendations. Similarly, blockchain technology has also gained traction in the healthcare industry as a secure and transparent method for managing health data. When AI and blockchain technology are combined in telehealth, the result is a powerful tool and system that can improve patient outcomes and streamline workflows.

In this section, we will discuss the taxonomy of AI and blockchain technology used in telehealth systems, as it plays a crucial role in comprehending and structuring the convergence of AI and blockchain technology in the realm of telehealth systems. Taxonomy offers a framework to categorize and classify the various applications, methodologies, and components of AI and blockchain technology that contribute to the advancement of telehealth systems as depicted in Figure 2.3.

2.7.1 Taxonomy for AI

The AI-powered telehealth systems use AI to improve patient outcomes and workflows. AI-powered telehealth systems can be classified into several different categories based on their applications, functionality, and the type of AI that is used. The application categories presented here encompass various AI use cases in telehealth, highlighting the diverse ways in which AI technology is employed in this field. These categories may include diagnostic and decision support systems, remote monitoring and wearable devices, virtual assistants and chatbots, predictive analytics and population health management, NLP and speech recognition, fraud detection and security, personalized medicine and precision healthcare, and mental health support [73]. Figure 2.4 shows a taxonomy for AI in telehealth systems.

1. Diagnostic tools: AI-powered diagnostic tools use ML algorithms to analyze medical images, such as X-rays or CT scans, and provide automated diagnoses.

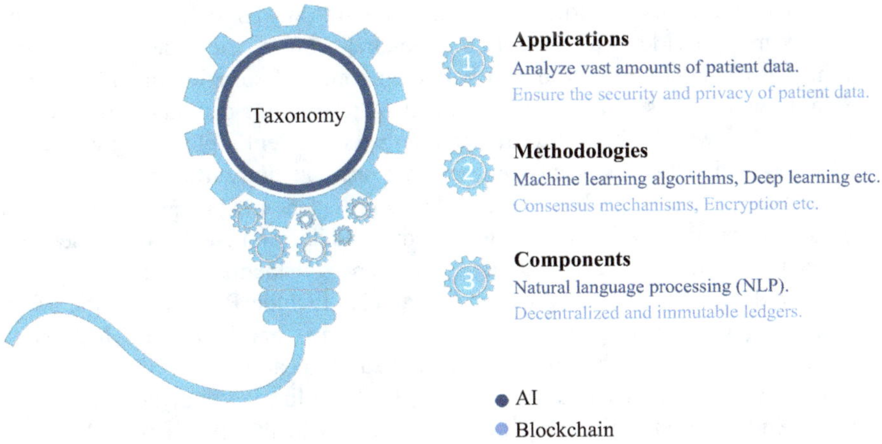

Figure 2.3 Applications, methodologies, and components of AI and blockchain technology for taxonomy

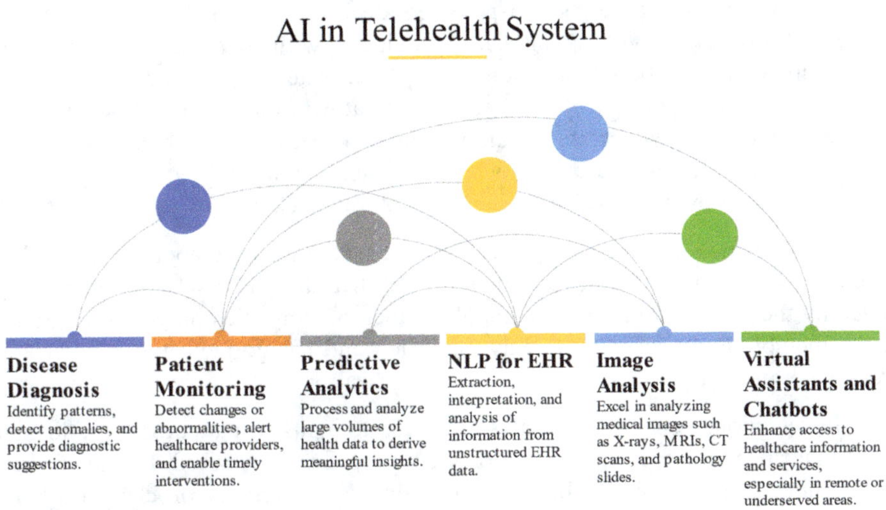

Figure 2.4 Taxonomy for AI in a telehealth system

These tools can help to reduce the workload of radiologists and other specialists and improve the accuracy of diagnoses. Examples include Enlitic, which uses deep learning to analyze medical images, and Zebra Medical Vision, which uses computer vision to detect abnormalities in medical imaging.

2. Remote monitoring systems: AI-powered remote monitoring systems use sensors and ML algorithms to monitor patients' vital signs and detect changes

that may indicate deterioration in their condition. These systems can alert healthcare providers to potential problems before they become critical, enabling earlier intervention and better outcomes. Examples include Current Health, which uses wearable sensors and AI to monitor patients remotely, and Biofourmis, which uses AI to detect changes in patient's physiological data.

3. Chatbots and virtual assistants: AI-powered chatbots and virtual assistants facilitate remote interactions between healthcare providers and patients, and they can be used to provide patients with basic medical advice and answer their questions. These tools can improve patient engagement and satisfaction, while also reducing the workload of healthcare providers. Examples include Babylon Health, which uses AI-powered chatbots to provide medical advice, and Florence, which uses a virtual assistant to remind patients to take their medication.
4. EHRs: AI-powered EHR systems use ML algorithms to analyze patient data and identify patterns that may indicate potential health problems [74]. These systems can help healthcare providers to make more informed and personalized treatment recommendations, improving patient outcomes. Examples include Careskore, which uses AI to analyze patient data and predict readmissions, and KenSci, which uses ML to identify patients at risk of developing sepsis.
5. Decision support systems: AI-powered decision support systems use ML algorithms to provide healthcare providers with personalized treatment recommendations based on patient data. These systems can help to improve the accuracy and efficiency of diagnoses and treatment plans, while also reducing the risk of medical errors. Examples include MaxQ AI, which uses AI to analyze medical images and provide automated diagnoses, and Sensely, which uses AI to provide virtual triage and symptom checking.

On the other hand, AI methodology refers to the techniques and approaches used to develop AI systems. The advancement of telehealth systems has been greatly fueled by the diverse array of AI technology methodologies employed in the field. These methodologies can be broadly classified and categorized into several key areas, each playing a crucial role in enhancing healthcare delivery.

1. ML techniques enable the analysis of vast amounts of patient data, aiding in diagnostics and decision support. ML may be Supervised Learning, i.e., training models using labeled data to make predictions or classifications, Unsupervised Learning, i.e., extracting patterns and insights from unlabeled data without predefined outcomes, or Reinforcement Learning, i.e., training models to make decisions and take actions based on feedback from the environment [75].
2. Deep learning algorithms excel in processing complex medical images and sequential patient data. Deep learning involves CNN, i.e., analyzing and processing visual data such as medical images, Recurrent Neural Networks (RNN), i.e., handling sequential data like time-series patient monitoring data, and Generative Adversarial Networks (GAN), i.e., generating synthetic medical data for training or research purposes [76].

3. NLP capabilities facilitate effective communication and understanding of patient text data. These may include Text Classification, i.e., categorizing and analyzing text data, such as medical records or research papers, Named Entity Recognition, i.e., identifying and extracting specific entities from text, such as medical conditions or drug names, and Sentiment Analysis, i.e., analyzing the sentiment or emotion expressed in text, such as patient feedback or social media posts.
4. Computer vision techniques empower the interpretation of medical images and the identification of anomalies. Computer vision involves Image Classification, i.e., categorizing and analyzing medical images, such as X-rays or MRIs, Object Detection, i.e., identifying and localizing specific objects within images or video streams, such as tumors or anatomical structures, and Image Segmentation, i.e., partitioning images into meaningful regions for detailed analysis or surgical planning.

The categorization areas also include data analytics and big data methodologies, which extract valuable insights from healthcare datasets; knowledge representation and reasoning techniques, which involve capturing and utilizing medical knowledge; Bayesian networks and probabilistic modeling for probabilistic predictions and analysis, and finally, robotics and automation technologies which bring about innovations in surgical procedures and remote patient care [77].

The integration of these AI methodologies propels telehealth systems to new heights, revolutionizing healthcare delivery and paving the way for improved patient outcomes. The methodology encompasses a range of AI systems in telehealth, including the following examples.

2.7.2 Taxonomy for blockchain technology

The blockchain-based telehealth systems use blockchain technology to secure and manage health data. Blockchain can help ensure the privacy and security of patient data [78], while also improving interoperability between different healthcare providers. Unlike traditional centralized systems, blockchain offers transparency, immutability, and enhanced security. In telehealth, blockchain can address challenges such as data security, interoperability, and privacy by providing a tamper-proof and auditable system for storing and sharing health-related information [20]. The blockchain-based telehealth systems can be classified into different categories based on their functionality and the type of blockchain that is used. These categories include:

1. Health data management systems: Blockchain-based health data management systems enable secure and efficient sharing of patient health data across different healthcare providers. These systems can improve interoperability and enable better collaboration between healthcare providers, ultimately leading to better patient outcomes. Examples include Medicalchain, which uses blockchain technology to store and share patient health data, and Hashed Health, which uses blockchain technology to create a secure and transparent healthcare ecosystem. Blockchain's efficient coordination features, such as smart

contracts and interoperability standards, streamline administrative processes, automate tasks, and enhance collaboration among various stakeholders within the telehealth ecosystem.

2. Patient identity management systems: Blockchain-based patient identity management systems enable secure and efficient management of patient identities, reducing the risk of fraud and identity theft. These systems can also enable patients to control their health data and share it with healthcare providers as needed. Examples include Civic, which uses blockchain technology to create secure digital identities, and Patientory, which uses blockchain technology to create a secure and decentralized electronic medical record system.
3. Supply chain management systems: Blockchain-based supply chain management systems enable tracking and verification of medical supplies and pharmaceuticals, reducing the risk of counterfeit or adulterated products [79]. These systems can also enable more efficient distribution of medical supplies and pharmaceuticals, ultimately leading to better patient outcomes. Examples include Chronicled, which uses blockchain technology to create a secure and transparent supply chain for pharmaceuticals, and Blockpharma, which uses blockchain technology to track the authenticity of drugs.
4. Payments and billing systems: Blockchain-based payments and billing systems enable secure and efficient payment processing for healthcare services, reducing the risk of fraud and reducing administrative costs. These systems can also enable quicker payment processing and reduce the administrative burden on healthcare providers. Examples include SimplyVital Health, which uses blockchain technology to create a secure and efficient payment system for healthcare providers, and Gem Health, which uses blockchain technology to create a secure and transparent billing system for healthcare services.
5. The blockchain-based telehealth systems also include decentralization and traceability and auditability. Blockchain technology enables decentralized telehealth systems by eliminating the need for central authorities or intermediaries. It allows for direct and secure peer-to-peer communication between patients and healthcare providers, fostering trust and reducing reliance on centralized platforms. Finally, blockchain's transparent nature allows for the traceability and auditability of healthcare transactions in telehealth systems. Every transaction recorded on the blockchain can be verified and audited, ensuring accountability and compliance with regulations such as HIPAA.

The methodology categories of blockchain technology encompass distributed ledger technology (DLT), consensus mechanisms, cryptography, and tokenization. DLT forms the foundation of blockchain systems, enabling decentralized and immutable record-keeping of patient data and healthcare transactions. Consensus mechanisms ensure the security and trustworthiness of the blockchain network by achieving agreement among participants. Cryptography secures patient data, authenticates participants, and ensures confidentiality and integrity. Last, tokenization and cryptocurrencies incentivize and reward desired behaviors, fostering active participation and value exchange within the telehealth ecosystem. The methodology categories of blockchain technology contribute significantly to the advancement of telehealth systems. They empower telehealth systems with transparency, security, privacy, automation, interoperability, and patient-centricity [80].

In Table 2.5, the application categories represent the different areas of telehealth where AI and blockchain technologies make significant contributions. The methodologies column highlights the specific techniques and approaches used within each category. The AI components column outlines the key AI technologies and tools utilized. Finally, the blockchain components column specifies the relevant components of blockchain technology that enhance telehealth systems. The specific methodologies and components used may vary depending on the implementation and requirements of telehealth systems.

As AI and blockchain technology continue to evolve, we can expect to see even more innovative telehealth systems that leverage the power of both

Table 2.5 Overview of application categories, methodologies, and components in telehealth systems

Application categories	Methodologies	AI components	Blockchain components
Diagnostic and decision support systems	Machine learning, deep learning, NLP	Medical image analysis, symptom checkers, virtual assistants	Patient data privacy, data integrity
Remote monitoring	Machine learning, data analytics	Vital sign monitoring, continuous glucose monitoring, remote patient monitoring	Secure data transmission, immutable records
Virtual assistants and chatbots	NLP, machine learning	Virtual consultations, medication reminders, patient education	Secure messaging, patient consent
Predictive analytics and population health management	Machine learning, data analytics, Bayesian networks	Disease outbreak forecasting, readmission risk assessment, population health management	Data privacy, consent management
Natural language processing (NLP) and speech recognition	NLP, speech recognition	Transcription services, language translation, sentiment analysis	Speech-to-text data privacy, language translation integrity
Fraud detection and security	Machine learning, data analytics	Fraud detection, cybersecurity	Secure transactions, access control
Personalized medicine and precision healthcare	Genomic analysis, machine learning	Genomic analysis, precision medicine, drug discovery	Patient consent management, genomic data privacy
Mental health support	NLP, machine learning	Mental health screening, emotional well-being monitoring, virtual therapy	Confidentiality, consent management

technologies to improve healthcare. By classifying the AI and blockchain-based telehealth systems into different categories, we can better understand their functionality, capabilities, methodology, and potential applications.

2.7.3 Taxonomy on security issues in telehealth systems

Telehealth systems offer immense potential for transforming healthcare delivery, but they also introduce security challenges that must be addressed to ensure patient data privacy and system integrity. By understanding the taxonomy of security issues in telehealth systems and implementing appropriate security measures, healthcare organizations and technology providers can enhance the security posture of telehealth systems, fostering trust and confidence among patients, and healthcare professionals alike. Figure 2.5 presents a taxonomy of security issues in telehealth systems, highlighting the key areas where vulnerabilities may arise.

1. Data privacy: Data privacy is a crucial concern in telehealth systems. Healthcare providers collect and store sensitive patient information, such as medical records, test results, and personal details. The following security issues may arise in this context:
   i. Unauthorized access: Unauthorized individuals gaining access to patient data can lead to privacy breaches and identity theft. Weak authentication mechanisms, inadequate access controls, or compromised user accounts can all contribute to this issue.
   ii. Data leakage: Data leakage refers to the unintentional disclosure of sensitive information. It can occur through various means, such as insecure communication channels, insecure storage systems, or accidental sharing of information with unauthorized parties.
   iii. Inadequate encryption: Encryption is crucial for protecting the confidentiality of data transmitted over telehealth systems. Weak encryption algorithms, improper implementation, or missing encryption of sensitive data can expose it to unauthorized interception and decryption.

2. Network security: Telehealth systems rely on networks, both wired and wireless, to transmit data between healthcare providers and patients. Network security

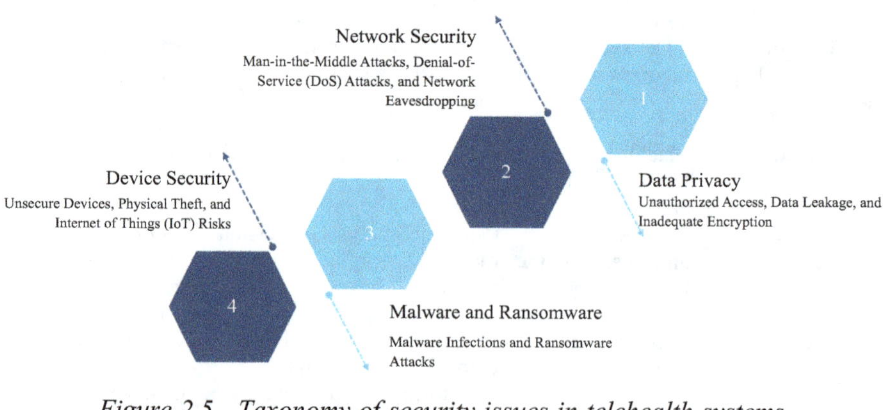

Figure 2.5 Taxonomy of security issues in telehealth systems

issues can pose significant risks to the confidentiality, integrity, and availability of patient information. The following security challenges may arise in this domain:

  i. Man-in-the-middle attacks: A man-in-the-middle attack occurs when an attacker intercepts the communication between two parties, potentially gaining unauthorized access to sensitive data. In telehealth systems, such attacks can compromise the privacy and integrity of patient information.
  ii. Denial-of-service (DoS) attacks: DoS attacks aim to disrupt the availability of telehealth services by overwhelming the system's resources or network infrastructure. This can lead to service interruptions, rendering patients unable to access healthcare services when needed.
  iii. Network eavesdropping: Network eavesdropping involves capturing and monitoring network traffic to obtain sensitive information. If telehealth systems do not employ adequate encryption or secure communication protocols, attackers can intercept and collect patient data.

3. Malware and ransomware: Telehealth systems can be vulnerable to malware and ransomware attacks, which can have severe consequences for both patients and healthcare providers. The following security issues are associated with malicious software:
  i. Malware infections: Malicious software, such as viruses, worms, and trojans, can infect telehealth systems, compromising their integrity and potentially leading to unauthorized access, data loss, or system disruption.
  ii. Ransomware attacks: Ransomware is a type of malware that encrypts the victim's data and demands a ransom for its release. If telehealth systems fall victim to ransomware attacks, they can disrupt healthcare operations and compromise patient records.
4. Device security: Telehealth systems rely on various devices, including computers, smartphones, tablets, and medical devices [78], to facilitate remote consultations and monitoring. Device security issues can introduce vulnerabilities that compromise the overall security of telehealth systems:
  i. Unsecure devices: Insecure devices can serve as entry points for attackers. Outdated operating systems, lack of security patches, or weak security configurations can all contribute to device vulnerabilities.
  ii. Physical theft: The loss or theft of devices used in telehealth systems can lead to unauthorized access to sensitive patient data. Without proper security measures like device encryption or remote data wipe capabilities, stolen devices pose a significant risk.
  iii. Internet of things (IoT) risks: Telehealth systems increasingly integrate IoT devices [81] for remote monitoring and patient care. However, IoT devices often have weaker security controls compared to traditional computing devices, making them potential targets for exploitation.

2.8 Lessons learned

The chapter provides valuable insights into the taxonomy for AI and blockchain technology in telehealth systems, capable of enabling researchers and practitioners to make informed decisions and drive advancements in this field. By understanding these lessons, the full potential of these technologies for improving patient care can be realized. Some of the lessons learned are highlighted in this section.

1. The history and evolution of telehealth systems.
2. The taxonomy for AI and blockchain technology in telehealth systems: The taxonomy can be used to better understand and classify the different ways that these technologies are being used in telehealth systems.
3. Importance of standardization: One key lesson is the importance of standardizing terminologies, and frameworks in the context of AI and blockchain technology for telehealth systems. Without clear and consistent standards, it becomes challenging to compare, integrate, and collaborate on different implementations. The chapter underscores standardization and its impact on the interoperability and scalability between different AI and blockchain systems in telehealth systems.
4. Technical feasibility: Another lesson is the technical feasibility of integrating AI and blockchain technology into telehealth systems. The chapter highlights the challenges faced in terms of computational resources, data privacy, security, and scalability. It also outlines approaches and solutions to overcome these challenges, such as optimized algorithms, and secure data storage.
5. Real-world implementation challenges: Lessons can also be derived from the real-world implementation challenges of AI and blockchain technology in telehealth systems. These include regulatory compliance, ethical considerations, user acceptance, and integration with existing healthcare infrastructures. The regulatory environment for telehealth is still evolving, and it is important to understand the regulatory requirements before deploying AI and blockchain technology for telehealth.
6. Privacy and security issues: Patient data are sensitive, and it is important to take steps to protect it from unauthorized access. Blockchain technology can help to improve privacy and security, but it is important to implement them correctly.
7. Benefits: The chapter discusses some of the benefits of using AI and blockchain technology in telehealth systems. This includes improved patient outcomes, enhanced data security, streamlined workflows, and reduced costs. However, it is important to address the limitations, such as potential biases in AI algorithms, scalability issues, and the complexity of blockchain implementation.

2.9 Conclusions and future scope

The integration of AI and blockchain technology in telehealth systems presents significant opportunities for transforming the healthcare industry. These advanced technologies offer numerous benefits, including enhanced data security, improved interoperability, streamlined processes, and personalized patient care. However, to fully leverage their potential and ensure responsible deployment, the development of a comprehensive taxonomy is crucial. The taxonomy provides a structured framework for categorizing and organizing AI and blockchain technologies, enabling stakeholders to gain a deeper understanding of their capabilities, limitations, and potential applications in telehealth.

It is recommended to establish a collaborative effort involving healthcare professionals, technology experts, policymakers, and other relevant stakeholders to develop an inclusive taxonomy that reflects diverse perspectives and addresses the specific needs of the healthcare industry. Standardization, granularity, and the incorporation of ethical considerations should be key considerations in taxonomy development. Regular updates, education, and awareness initiatives, along with pilot projects and evaluations, will further refine and enhance the taxonomy over time. By following these recommendations, a more robust and comprehensive taxonomy can be created, facilitating responsible implementation and maximizing the benefits of AI and blockchain technology in telehealth systems, ultimately improving healthcare delivery and patient outcomes.

References

[1] E. Dorsey and E. Topol, "State of Telehealth," *New England Journal of Medicine*, vol. 375, no. 2, pp. 154–611, 2016.

[2] L. Omrčen, H. Leventić, K. Romić and I. Galić, "Integration of Blockchain and AI in EHR Sharing: A Survey," *International Symposium ELMAR*, vol. 2021, pp. 155–160, 2021.

[3] S. Jayakumar, V. Sounderajah, P. Normahani, L. Harling, S. Markar, H. Ashrafian and A. Darzi, "Quality Assessment Standards in Artificial Intelligence Diagnostic Accuracy Systematic Reviews: A Meta-Research Study," *NPJ Digital Medicine*, vol. 5, 2022.

[4] C. W. Rundle, P. Hollingsworth and R. P. Dellavalle, "Artificial Intelligence in Dermatology." *Clinics in Dermatology*, vol. 37, no. 4, pp. 657–666, 2021.

[5] R. Gupta, S. Tanwar, S. Tyagi, N. Kumar, M. S. Obaidat, and B. Sadoun, "HaBiTs: Blockchain-based Telesurgery Framework for Healthcare 4.0," in *2019 International Conference on Computer, Information and Telecommunication Systems (CITS)*, 2019.

[6] H. Kordestani, K. Barkaoui and W. Zahran, "HapiChain: A Blockchain-based Framework for Patient-Centric Telemedicine," in *2020 IEEE 8th International Conference on Serious Games and Applications for Health (SeGAH)*, 2020.

[7] N. Bawany, T. Qamar, H. Tariq and S. Adnan, "Integrating Healthcare Services Using Blockchain-Based Telehealth Framework," *IEEE*, vol. 10, pp. 36505–36517, 2022.

[8] Y. Ji, J. Zhang, J. Ma, C. Yang and X. Yao, "BMPLS: Blockchain-Based Multi-level Privacy-Preserving Location Sharing Scheme for Telecare Medical Information Systems," *Journal of Medical Systems*, vol. 42, pp. 1–13, 2018.

[9] S. Suganyadevi, V. Seethalakshmi and K. Balasamy, "A Review on Deep Learning in Medical Image Analysis," *International Journal of Multimedia Information Retrieval*, vol. 11, pp. 19–38, 2022.

[10] A. Fourcade and R. Khonsari, "Deep Learning in Medical Image Analysis: A Third Eye for Doctors," *Journal of Stomatology, Oral and Maxillofacial Surgery*, vol. 120, pp. 279–288, 2019.

[11] J. N. Averitt, S. Rahman, S. Rahman, H. Wimmer, L. Chen and C. Aasheim, "Applying Artificial Intelligence to Medical Data," *Georgia Southern University*, 2020. [Online]. Available: https://digitalcommons.georgiasouthern.edu/etd/2111/. [Accessed: Nov. 2, 2023]

[12] J. Olveres, G. González, F. Torres, *et al.*, "What Is New in Computer Vision and Artificial Intelligence in Medical Image Analysis Applications," *Quantitative Imaging in Medicine and Surgery*, vol. 11, no. 8, pp. 3830–3853, 2021.

[13] M. Vasileiou and I. Maglogiannis, "The Health ChatBots in Telemedicine: Intelligent Dialog System for Remote Support," *Journal of Healthcare Engineering*, vol. 2022, pp. 1–12, 2022.

[14] U. Bharti, D. Bajaj, H. Batra, S. Lalit, S. Lalit and A. Gangwani, "Medbot: Conversational Artificial Intelligence Powered Chatbot for Delivering Tele-Health after COVID-19," in *2020 5th International Conference on Communication and Electronics Systems (ICCES)*, 2020.

[15] T. Jadczyk, W. Wojakowski, M. Tendera, T. Henry, G. Egnaczyk and S. Shreenivas, "Artificial Intelligence Can Improve Patient Management at the Time of a Pandemic: The Role of Voice Technology," *Journal of Medical Internet Research*, vol. 23, 2020.

[16] E. M. Boucher, N. Harake, H. E. Ward, *et al.*, "Artificially Intelligent Chatbots in Digital Mental Health Interventions: A Review," *Expert Review of Medical Devices*, vol. 18, pp. 37–49, 2021.

[17] P. Tagde, S. Tagde, T. Bhattacharya, *et al.*, "Blockchain and Artificial Intelligence Technology in e-Health," *Environmental Science and Pollution Research*, vol. 28, pp. 52810–52831, 2021.

[18] C. P. S. K, "Enabling the Efficiency of Blockchain Technology in Tele-Healthcare with Enhanced EMR," *2020 International Conference on Computer Science, Engineering and Applications (ICCSEA)*, pp. 1–6, 2020.

[19] S. Shi, M. Luo, Y. Wen, L. Wang and D. He, "A Blockchain-Based User Authentication Scheme with Access Control for Telehealth Systems," *Security and Communication Networks*, vol. 2, pp. 1–18, 2022.

[20] R. Ahmad, K. Salah, R. Jayaraman, I. Yaqoob, S. Ellahham and M. A. Omar, "The Role of Blockchain Technology in Telehealth and Telemedicine," *International Journal of Medical Informatics*, vol. 148, pp. 104399–104399, 2021.

[21] E. J. Topol, "High-Performance Medicine: The Convergence of Human and Artificial Intelligence," *Nature Medicine*, vol. 25, no. 1, pp. 44–56, 2019.

[22] A. Garg, A. Aggarwal, S. Khera and R. Singh, "Artificial Intelligence in Telemedicine: Opportunities for Future Research," *Telemedicine and e-Health*, vol. 25, no. 1, pp. 3–13, 2019.

[23] H. R. Hasan, K. Salah, R. Jayaraman, I. Yaqoob, M. A. Omar and S. Ellahham, "Blockchain-Enabled Telehealth Services Using Smart Contracts," *IEEE Access*, vol. 9, pp. 151944–151959, 2021.

[24] S. Muzammil, "Telehealth: Is It Only for the Rural Areas? A Review of Its Wider Use," *Telehealth and Medicine Today*, vol. 5, 2021.

[25] H. M. Hussien, S. M. Yasin, S. N. I. Udzir, A. A. Zaidan and B. B. Zaidan, "A Systematic Review for Enabling of Develop a Blockchain Technology in Healthcare Application: Taxonomy, Substantially Analysis, Motivations, Challenges, Recommendations and Future Direction," *Journal of Medical Systems*, vol. 43, no. 10, pp. 320–320, 2019.

[26] W. Bialy, A. Abulaish and M. Ashouri, "Blockchain Technology for Healthcare Systems," *Healthcare Informatics Research*, vol. 26, no. 2, pp. 136–154, 2020.

[27] L. Chen, X. Zhang, Q. Li, J. Sun and H. Wang, "Blockchain Technology for Healthcare Supply Chains," *International Journal of Production Research*, vol. 58, no. 12, pp. 3886–3913, 2020.

[28] W. Horner and S. Sabia, *Development of Real-Time Software Environments for NASA's Modern Telemetry Systems,* in Proceedings of the 1989 NASA Goddard Conference on Spacecraft Control, pp. 53–62, 1989.

[29] J. Winters, "Videoconferencing and Telehealth Technologies Can Provide a Reliable Approach to Remote Assessment and Teaching Without Compromising Quality," *Journal of Cardiovascular Nursing*, vol. 22, no. 1, pp. 51–57, 2007.

[30] S. Mohammed and A. J. Alzubaidi, "Remote Patient Monitoring (RPM)," *Encyclopedia of the UN Sustainable Development Goals*, vol. 15, pp. 115–124, 2019.

[31] M. Cowie, J. Blomster, L. Curtis, *et al.*, "Electronic Health Records to Facilitate Clinical Research," *Clinical Research in Cardiology*, vol. 106, pp. 1–9, 2016.

[32] M. Ha, S. Lim and H. Ko, "Wearable and Flexible Sensors for User-Interactive Health-Monitoring Devices," *Journal of Materials Chemistry. B*, vol. 6, no. 24, pp. 4043–4064, 2018.

[33] A. Spournias, P. Bountas, E. Faliagka, *et al.*, "Smart Health Monitoring using AI Techniques in AAL Environments," in *Mediterranean Conference on Embedded Computing*, 2021.

[34] H. S. Adnan, S. Matthews, M. Hackl, *et al.*, "Human Centered AI Design for Clinical Monitoring and Data Management," *European Journal of Public Health*, vol. 30, pp. 165–225, 2020.

[35] M. Joshi, A. Pal and M. Sankarasubbu, "Federated Learning for Healthcare Domain - Pipeline, Applications and Challenges," *ACM Transactions on Computing for Healthcare*, vol. 3, pp. 1–36, 2022.

[36] B. Kavitha and C. R. Murthy, "Chatbot for Healthcare System using Artificial Intelligence," *International Research Journal of Modernization in Engineering Technology and Science*, vol. 5, pp. 1304–1307, 2019.

[37] N. Pawar, "Decision Tree-based Health Prediction System," *International Journal for Research in Applied Science and Engineering Technology*, vol. 8, pp. 552–557, 2020.

[38] P. Prihandoko, B. Bertalya and L. Setyowati, "City Health Prediction Model Using Random Forest Classification Method," in *2020 Fifth International Conference on Informatics and Computing (ICIC)*, 2020.

[39] S. Modak, S. Mehta, D. Sehgal and J. Valadi, "Application of Support Vector Machines in Viral Biology," *Global Virology III: Virology in the 21st Century*, Springer Nature, pp. 361–403, 2019.

[40] A. Pandit and A. Garg, "Artificial Neural Networks in Healthcare: A Systematic Review," *Confluence*, vol. 1, pp. 1–6, 2021.

[41] A. A. Dutta, T. Batabyal, M. Basu and S. Acton, "An Efficient Convolutional Neural Network for Coronary Heart Disease Prediction," *ArXiv*, vol. abs/1909.00489, 2019.

[42] M. Usama, B. Ahmad, W. Xiao, M. S. Hossain and M. Ghulam, "Self-Attention based Recurrent Convolutional Neural Network for Disease Prediction using Healthcare Data," *Computer Methods and Programs in Biomedicine*, vol. 190, pp. 105–191, 2019.

[43] G.-H. Shin, Y.-S. Kweon and M. Lee, "Predicting the Transition from Short-term to Long-term Memory based on Deep Neural Network," in *Balkan Conference in Informatics*, 2020.

[44] X. Yi, E. Walia and P. Babyn, "Generative Adversarial Network in Medical Imaging: A Review," *Medical Image Analysis*, vol. 58, p. 101552, 2018.

[45] A. Coronato, M. Naeem, G. Pietro and G. Paragliola, "Reinforcement Learning for Intelligent Healthcare Applications: A Survey," *Artificial Intelligence in Medicine*, vol. 109, p. 101964, 2020.

[46] A. Desiani, R. Primartha, M. Arhami and O. Orsalan, "Naive Bayes Classifier for Infant Weight Prediction of Hypertension Mother," *Journal of Physics: Conference Series*, vol. 1282, pp. 1–12, 2019.

[47] Y. F. Safri, R. Arifudin and M. A. Muslim, *K-Nearest Neighbor and Naive Bayes Classifier Algorithm in Determining the Classification of Healthy Card Indonesia Giving to The Poor,* Sci. J. Informatics, vol. 5, pp. 18, 2018.

[48] Y. Liao, Y. Xiang and M. Wang, "Health Assessment and Prognostics based on Higher-Order Hidden Semi-Markov Models," *Naval Research Logistics*, vol. 68, pp. 259–276, 2020.

[49] A. Nada and Z. I. K. Alqahtani, "Gaussian Mixture Models Based on Principal Components and Applications," *Mathematical Problems in Engineering*, vol. 1, pp. 1–13, 2020.

[50] R. Mishra and K. V. Pallavi, "Decentralized Blockchain Based ISP Networks," *Advances in Intelligent Systems and Technologies*, vol. 1, pp. 345–354, 2022.

[51] A. Gaikwad, "Overview of Blockchain," *International Journal for Research in Applied Science and Engineering*, 2020.

[52] W. J. Gordon and C. Catalini, "Blockchain Technology for Healthcare: Facilitating the Transition to Patient-Driven Interoperability," *Computational and Structural Biotechnology Journal*, vol. 16, pp. 224–230, 2018.

[53] S.-J. Wu, R.-D. Chiang, S.-H. Chang and W.-T. Chang, "An Interactive Telecare System Enhanced with IoT Technology," *IEEE Pervasive Computing*, vol. 16, pp. 62–69, 2017.

[54] K. P. Satamraju and B. Malarkodi, "Proof of Concept of Scalable Integration of Internet of Things and Blockchain in Healthcare," in *Italian National Conference on Sensors*, 2020.

[55] M. Koscina, M. D, C. N. Ribalta and O. Perez, "Enabling Trust in Healthcare Data Exchange with a Federated Blockchain-based Architecture," in *IEEE/WIC/ACM International Conference on Web Intelligence-Companion Volume*, 2019.

[56] Y. Zhuang, L. Sheets, X. Gao, Y. Shen, Z. Shae, J. Tsai and C. Shyu, "Development of A Blockchain Framework for Virtual Clinical Trials," in *AMIA ... Annual Symposium Proceedings. AMIA Symposium*, 2020.

[57] M. Uddin, K. Salah, R. Jayaraman, S. Pesic and S. Ellahham, "Blockchain for Drug Traceability: Architectures and Open Challenges," *Health Informatics Journal*, vol. 27, 2021.

[58] A. Alnuaimi, A. Alshehhi, K. Salah, R. Jayaraman, I. A. Omar and A. Battah, "Blockchain-Based Processing of Health Insurance Claims for Prescription Drugs," *IEEE Access*, vol. 10, pp. 118093–118107, 2022.

[59] J. J. Hathaliya, P. Sharma, S. Tanwar and R. Gupta, "Blockchain-Based Remote Patient Monitoring in Healthcare 4.0," *IEEE International Advance Computing Conference*, 2019.

[60] J. Hugendubel, "Blockchain Technology and Intellectual Property – A Basic Introduction," *Social Science Research Network*, vol. 2021, pp. 1–36, 2021.

[61] G. Márquez, H. Astudillo and C. Taramasco, "Security in Telehealth Systems From a Software Engineering Viewpoint: A Systematic Mapping Study," *IEEE Access*, vol. 8, pp. 10933–10950, 2020.

[62] R. Valecha, S. Upadhyaya and H. Rao, "An Activity Theory Approach to Leak Detection and Mitigation in Patient Health Information (PHI)," *Journal of the AIS*, vol. 22, pp. 1–6, 2021.

[63] J.-W. Lo, C.-Y. Wu and S. Chiou, "A Lightweight Authentication and Key Agreement Scheme for Telecare Medicine Information System," *Journal of Internet Technology*, vol. 21, pp. 263–272, 2020.

[64] K. M. Tsiouris, D. A. Gatsios, V. D. Tsakanikas, *et al.*, "Designing Interoperable Telehealth Platforms: Bridging IoT Devices with Cloud Infrastructures," *Enterprise Information Systems*, vol. 14, pp. 1194–1218, 2020.

[65] M. Vega-Barbas, F. Seoane and I. Pau, "Characterization of User-Centered Security in Telehealth Services," *International Journal of Environmental Research and Public Health*, vol. 16, 2019.

[66] H. Li, Y. Yang, Y.-S. Dai, S. Yu and Y. Xiang, "Achieving Secure and Efficient Dynamic Searchable Symmetric Encryption over Medical Cloud Data," *IEEE Transactions on Cloud Computing*, vol. 8, pp. 484–494, 2020.

[67] H. Shah, J. Shah and U. Desai, "Third Party Public Auditing Scheme for Security in Cloud Storage," *International Journal of Trend in Scientific Research and Development*, vol. 2, pp. 179–184, 2019.

[68] A. M. Kandan, G. J. Kathrine and A. R. Melvin, “Network Attacks and Prevention techniques – A Study,” in *IEEE International Conference on Electrical, Computer and Communication Technologies (ICECCT)*, 2019.

[69] S. Kumar, D. N. P. Singh and D. N. Kumar, “Literature Review of Distributed Denial of Service (DDoS) Attacks, its Detection Techniques and Prevention Mechanisms,” *International Journal for Research in Applied Science and Engineering Technology*, vol. 10, pp. 1681–1685, 2022.

[70] T. Floyd-Carney, “Health Insurance Portability and Accountability Act of 1996 (HIPAA) administrative simplification,” in American Academy of Pediatrics eBooks. American Academy of Pediatrics, pp. 143–144, 2022. [Online].

[71] S. N. Gajarawala and J. N. Pelkowski, “Telehealth Benefits and Barriers,” *The Journal for Nurse Practitioners*, vol. 17, pp. 218 – 221, 2020.

[72] O. John, “Maintaining and Sustaining a Telehealth-based Ecosystem,” in Fundamentals of Telemedicine and Telehealth, Elsevier, pp. 127–143, 2020.

[73] J. Batsis, P. DiMilia, L. Seo, *et al.*, “Effectiveness of Ambulatory Telemedicine Care in Older Adults: A Systematic Review,” *Journal of the American Geriatrics Society*, vol. 67, no. 8, pp. 1737–1749, 2019.

[74] G. Fagherazzi, C. Goetzinger, M. Rashid, G. Aguayo and L. Huiart, “Digital Health Strategies to fight COVID-19 Worldwide: Challenges, Recommendations, and a Call for Papers,” *Journal of Medical Internet Research*, vol. 16, 22(6), e19284, 2020.

[75] A. Rajkomar, J. Dean and I. Kohane, “Machine Learning in Medicine,” *New England Journal of Medicine*, vol. 4, 380(14), pp. 1347–1358, 2019.

[76] A. Beam and I. Kohane, “Big Data and Machine Learning in Health Care,” *JAMA*, vol. 319, no. 13, pp. 1317–1318, 2018.

[77] K. Yeow, A. Gani, R. Ahmad, J. Rodrigues and K. Ko, “Decentralized Consensus for Edge-Centric Internet of Things: A Review, Taxonomy, and Research Issues,” *IEEE Access*, Vol. 6, 1513–1524, 2017.

[78] A. L. Imoize, P. A. Gbadega, H. I. Obakhena, D. O. Irabor, K. V. N. Kavitha and C. Chakraborty, “Artificial Intelligence-Enabled Internet of Medical Things for COVID-19 Pandemic Data Management,” *Explainable Artificial Intelligence in Medical Decision Support Systems*, The Institution of Engineering and Technology (IET), pp. 357–380, 2022.

[79] L. K. Ramasamy, F. K. KP, A. L. Imoize, J. O. Ogbebor, S. Kadry and S. Rho, “Blockchain-Based Wireless Sensor Networks for Malicious Node Detection: A Survey,” *IEEE Access*, vol. 9, pp. 128765–128785, 2021.

[80] M. Sookhak, M. Jabbarpour, N. Safa and F. Yu, “Blockchain and Smart Contract for Access Control in Healthcare: A Survey, Issues and Challenges, and Open Issues,” *Journal of Network and Computer Applications*, vol. 178, 102950, 2021.

[81] R. L. Kumar, Y. Wang, T. Poongodi and A. L. Imoize, “Internet of Things, Artificial Intelligence and Blockchain Technology,” *Cham*: *Springer*, 2021.

Chapter 3

A review of AI-based wireless communication channels, models and protocols for telehealth systems

Samuel Ibukun Olotu[1] *and Agbotiname Lucky Imoize*[2]

Healthcare service provided with the application of communication technologies is known as telehealth. The delivery in telehealth ranges from a phone consultation between a medical professional and a patient to a more complex remotely controlled surgical operation using robotic technology. Existing telehealth systems usually rely on Internet of Things and sensors to monitor the health status of patients and transmit the collected data to the healthcare provider using wireless technology. Different standard channels, models and protocols have been developed to support the functions of existing wireless communication technologies. This chapter reviews wireless communication channels, models and protocols used in telehealth systems. The study aims to enable researchers and healthcare providers to decide on the telehealth system that best suits their needs and requirements.

3.1 Introduction

Telehealth enables access to healthcare remotely through the use of digital information and communication technology [1]. A few examples of telehealth include a virtual meeting between healthcare providers and patients via video calls and chats, medical surgery carried out by robots controlled from a remote location and the use of sensors to monitor patients' health conditions [2]. The advancements in healthcare information technology and the demand for unlimited access to healthcare services have facilitated the growth of telehealth and united providers and patients in many ways. Among the services provided by telehealth are remote monitoring of patients, medical imaging, videoconferencing, patient consultation, wireless health applications, report transmission and medical education [3].

[1]Department of Information Technology, School of Computing, Federal University of Technology Akure, Nigeria
[2]Department of Electrical and Electronics Engineering, Faculty of Engineering, University of Lagos, Nigeria

Artificial intelligence innovations have been used to support telehealth in analytic precision, upgrading patient results, expanding the effectiveness of medical care conveyance and so on [4]. An advantage of artificial intelligence in telehealth is the ability to handle vast amounts of information rapidly and precisely. The patterns in the health conditions of patients can be detected from medical records and series of laboratory results and medical scans using artificial intelligence [5]. Another significant use of artificial intelligence is the improvements of chatbots and virtual assistants which can assist patients with preliminary medical diagnosis and give essential clinical counsel. Additionally, these tools are not only of benefit to patients but also assist healthcare providers in appointment scheduling and medication prescription workflows [6]. In telehealth, the remote observation and early identification of medical conditions can be achieved with the use of sensors and wearable devices that capture the medical data of the patients and transmit it to artificial intelligence algorithms for analysis. These applications enable the system to detect changes in the medical patterns of a patient and provide some fundamental medical diagnosis and possible early medication. Computer-based intelligence can assist in reducing certain surgical costs via the use of robots for routine assignments and even medical surgeries [7].

The transmission of data without a physical cable connection is referred to as wireless communication. Wireless communication assists medical service experts in providing telehealth services such as remote diagnosis and monitor patients using audio, video and messaging wireless technologies. Wireless communication channels are used for signal transmission in open space. It is unpredictable, highly variable, random and susceptible to interference, distortion, noise, scattering etc. Wireless channels are usually characterized by path loss which is determined by transmission distance, shadowing and multipath fading. This work aims to review research works on wireless communication channels, models and protocols in telehealth systems. The study aims to enable researchers and healthcare providers to decide on the telehealth system that best suits their needs and requirements.

3.1.1 Key contributions of the chapter

This chapter presents the following contributions:

1. Examine existing and emerging wireless communication technologies applied in telehealth systems in use to date.
2. Establish that most telehealth systems rely on one or more wireless communication technologies.

3.1.2 Chapter organization

The overview of wireless communication in telehealth systems is presented in Section 3.2. Section 3.3 discusses existing and emerging wireless technologies and protocols. Sections 3.4 and 3.5 present classifications of wireless communication technologies based on transmission ranges. Section 3.6 discusses the communication standards and protocols used in telehealth systems. Section 3.7 presents a review of related surveys on wireless communication technologies in telehealth.

Section 3.8 presents some performance measures of wireless technologies in telehealth systems, and finally, Section 3.9 presents the concluding discussions for the chapter.

3.2 Wireless communication in telehealth systems

Wireless communication is the exchange of data with the use of radio signals over space instead of physical conductors. Some common applications of wireless communication in telehealth have been implemented in wireless body area networks (WBANs), wireless sensor networks (WSNs) and Health Internet of Things (HIoTs). A survey on related works on wireless communication technologies in telehealth is presented in Section 3.7, and the summary is shown in Table 3.1.

3.2.1 Wireless sensor network

A WSN comprises sensor-based nodes that sense one or more physical variables such as pressure, body temperature, bone growth and blood pressure, to mention a few, as shown in Figure 3.1. WSNs are low-cost, low-power, quick to deploy, self-organizing and cooperative in their data processing with applications in intelligent agriculture, home automation, habitat monitoring and telehealth. The nodes usually have low processing, broadcasting or storage capabilities. The information acquired by the sensor nodes is sent to the user through the wireless link and gateway to a sink node.

3.2.2 Wireless body area network

A WBAN is a network of sensor nodes that monitor signals in the human body. WBAN consists of sensors and actuators that acquire data from the body, transmit it from a central unit (smartphone) to a remote data centre via the Internet and forward it to a medical centre as shown in Figure 3.2. The devices in WBAN are sensors, actuators and personal devices. The actuator acts on the data received from the sensors or instruction from the user. Personal devices, such as smartphones, are used to collect and process information from sensors and actuators. The WBAN uses wireless communication technologies to link the sensors in the body and the data centre to remotely monitor the health conditions of patients.

3.2.3 Health Internet of Things

The HIoTs comprises medical IoT devices which are equipped with intelligent sensors that sense the environment [18] as shown in Figure 3.3.

The IoT devices acquire data from patients that are processed by a smart gateway device or cloud service, while the collected health information is transferred to relevant stakeholders where the appropriate decision about the condition of the patient is made [20].

Some of the applications of HIoT are the monitoring of temperature, blood pressure, oxygen level, respiratory conditions, mood, medication and walking patterns [21].

Table 3.1 Review of wireless technologies in telehealth

Author (s)	Wireless technology	Communication paradigm	Years of publication	Major challenges	Aim
Chakraborty and Rodriques [8]	Bluetooth, ZigBee, Wi-Fi	D2D communication	2020	Interference, power consumption and security	Review of D2D service and application for healthcare
Karthick and Pankajavalli [9]	Wi-Fi, Bluetooth, LoRa, ZigBee, WiMAX, UWB	Internet of Things (IoT)	2020	Security and privacy	Review of wireless communication technologies in IoT-based healthcare
Selvaraj and Sundaravaradhan [10]	IoT healthcare, IoT-cloud integration	IoT-cloud integration	2020	Power consumption, resources availability and security issues	Review of IoT-based healthcare monitoring system
Alshehri and Muhammad [11]	Wi-Fi, BLE, ZigBee	IoT	2021	Sensor interoperability, device communication, security and privacy etc.	Review of IoMT-based healthcare system with edge and cloud computing
Tun *et al.* [12]	Not specified	IoT and wearable technologies	2021	Not stated	Review of IoT/wearable technologies
Taleb *et al.* [13]	LPWAN, 5G, B5G and 6G	Wireless body area network (WBAN)	2021	Power consumption, interference, security and privacy	Review of WBAN systems and technologies
Verma *et al.* [14]	ZigBee, LoRaWAN and RFID	IoT-based communication	2022	Compatibility of IoT devices, sensor accuracy and cost, volume of data, interoperability	Review of real-time monitoring and prediction of diseases common in elderly people
Alenoghena *et al.* [15]	Bluetooth, ZigBee, Wi-Fi, UWB, RFID, satellite, Internet, mobile network	Wireless body area network (WBAN)	2023	Review of standards and protocols in telemedicine	Data security and privacy, energy consumption, scheduling, medical video streaming

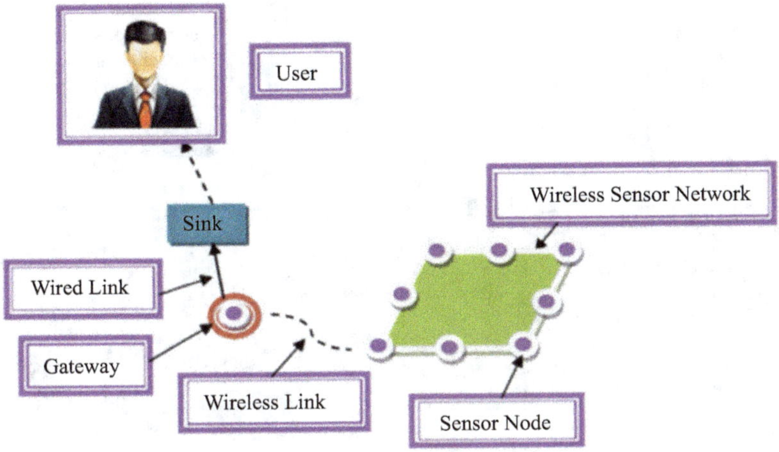

Figure 3.1 Wireless sensor network [16]

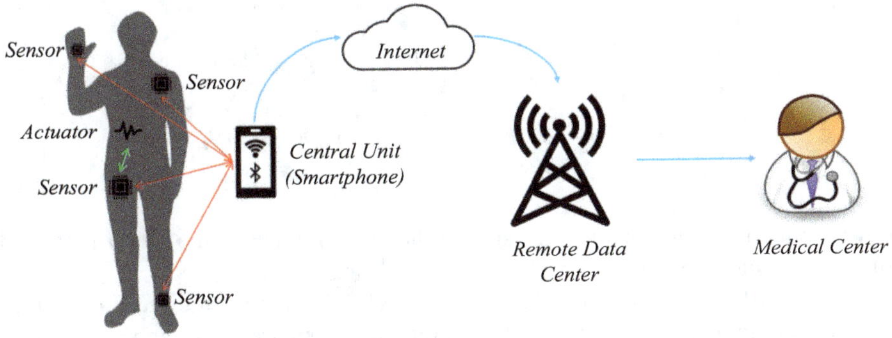

Figure 3.2 Wireless body area network [17]

In the first application, the system keeps track of the change in temperature over time to assist doctors in making inferences about the health condition of the patient. The conventional way of using a thermometer in the mouth, armpit or rectum can result in discomfort to the patient and a high chance of contracting an infection. A recent innovation has resulted in wearable sensors that can track body temperature on desktop or mobile phones using different wireless technologies. The second application involves diagnostic procedure is the measurement of blood pressure. The application of IoT and sensing technology has improved the method of measuring blood pressure. With the use of wearable sensors, systolic and diastolic pressure information can be measured and stored in the cloud. In the third application, IoT-based technology is used to measure oxygen saturation necessary for analysis in healthcare. Pulse and tissue oximeters are used to measure the heart rate, oxygen level and pulse parameters in real time and eliminate the challenges of

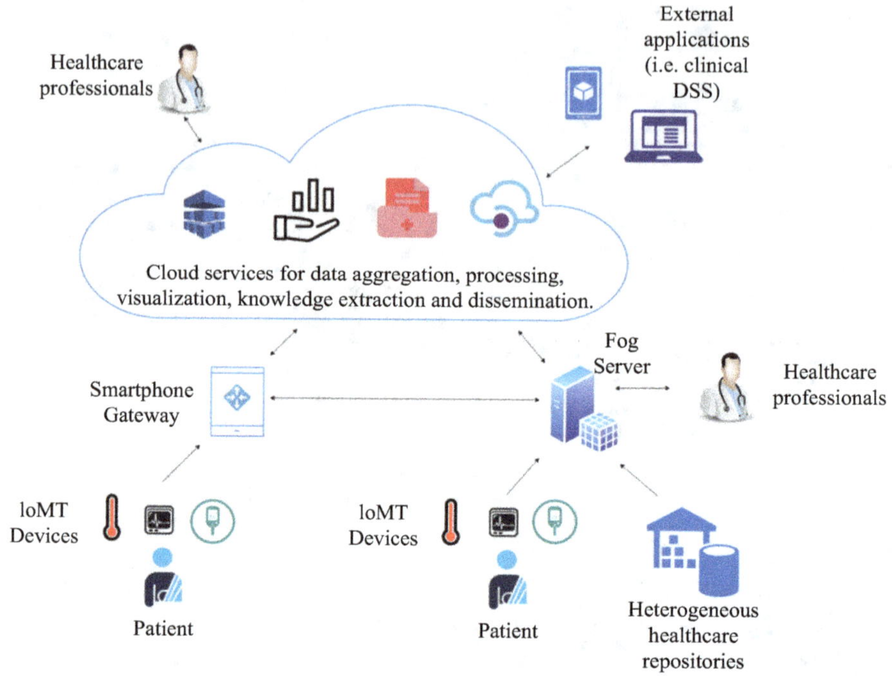

Figure 3.3 IoT-based telehealth system [19]

conventional methods. The transmission of the recorded data to the server is carried out using wireless technologies.

The fourth application involves the use of IoT-based solutions to monitor asthma patients by recording respiratory rates using a smart sensor and storing it in a cloud server. An example is the respiratory monitoring alarm system that monitors the respiratory rate using a sensor and transmits the data to a health centre. Another system is proposed to monitor, warn and suggest a medication to be administered to patients with asthma conditions.

In the fifth application, wearable devices used to capture real-time mood measurements have been proposed to detect stress conditions and negative emotions or moods which are analysed and used to prevent accidents.

The sixth application uses an IoT-based smart medication system to monitor and track patients' medication. The system is developed for patients on a strict medical schedule such as the elderly and women on in vitro fertilization treatment. A smart wheelchair is developed to assist patients with restricted mobility and their caregivers. The steering system uses sensor-based hand gloves to control the wheelchair and transmits the sensor data to the server and the cloud.

The seventh application uses a smart walker to monitor the walking patterns of patients by integrating a wearable armband and robotic hand to help the patient during the stroke recovery period. A low-power wearable system is used to monitor galvanic skin response (GSR) to detect psychophysiological conditions by assessing stress and emotions in humans.

3.3 Wireless communication technologies and protocols

Wireless communication technologies function according to sets of protocols and standards. However, making the right choice for wireless technology is an essential component of telehealth systems, as using the wrong technology can waste time and effort. Wireless communication technologies can be grouped based on communication ranges such as short-range and long-range [15,22]. Table 3.2 shows a summary of existing short-range and long-range technologies.

3.4 Short-range communication technologies

Short-range technologies are network protocols that enable nodes to connect over very short distances. The distance of communication, in short-range communication, ranges from a few centimetres to hundreds of metres. The technology is associated with reduced low power and low cost. Examples of short-range technologies are radio frequency identification (RFID), Bluetooth Low Energy, ZigBee, ultra-wideband (UWB), near-field communication and wireless fidelity (Wi-Fi) [22,23].

3.4.1 Radio frequency identification

RFID is used for short-range communications such as 10 cm–200 m. It is utilized to remarkably recognize an article/gadget (medical services gear) in the IoT climate. It is made up of tag and reader components. An antenna and a microchip are used to create the tag. Radio waves are used by the reader to communicate with a tag and exchange information with the object. The information utilized in the tag is referred to as an electronic item code. RFID technology assists healthcare providers in quickly locating and tracking medical equipment. A primary advantage of RFID technology is that it does not require an external power source. However, it may exhibit compatibility issues when connecting to a smartphone and is a highly insecure protocol.

3.4.2 Bluetooth

Bluetooth technology is an open standard intended for fixed and cell phones to shape remote individual region organizations (WPANs) with high security. It is a packet-based, connection-oriented, master–slave (client-server) protocol. Utilizing ultra-high frequency radio waves, Bluetooth is a technology for wireless communication over short distances. In the 2.4 GHz frequency range, this technology makes it possible to connect two or more medical devices wirelessly. The Bluetooth convention presents a correspondence scope of up to 100 m. Bluetooth gives information security as validation and encryption. The primary determinations had restricted applications as a result of moderately high-power utilization,

Table 3.2 Overview of wireless technologies

Technology	Standard	Deployment	Frequency band	Max. data rate	Range	Power consumption	Encryption
RFID/NFC	ISO/IEC 14443	1959	13.56 MHz	106 kbps, 212 kbps, 424 kbps	10 cm	Very low	Public key generated by AES algorithm
Bluetooth (BLE)	IEEE 802.15.1	1999	2.4 GHz	3 Mbps	0.1 km	Low	EO stream cypher
Wi-Fi	IEEE 802.11	1997	2.4 and 2.5 GHz	1 Gbps	50 m	Low high	RC4 stream cypher (WEP), AES block cypher
ZigBee	IEEE 802.15.4	2004	2.4 GHz	500 kbps	10–100 m	Very low	Stream cypher, AES block cypher
WiMAX	IEEE 802.16	2010	10–66 GHz	11–100 Mbps	50 km	Medium	3DES, AES block cypher
LoRa/ LoRaWAN	IEEE 802.15g	2010	868/915 MHz	50 kbps	25 km	High	AES block cypher
Sigfox	IEEE 802.15	2018	868/915 MHz	300 kbps	50 km	Low	AES
DASH7	ISO/IEC 180000-7	2017	433.92 MHz	200 kbps	1–2 km	Low	AES symmetric key cryptography
GSM	ETSI	1991	850–900 MHz	9.6 kbps	25 km	Moderate	A5/1 stream cypher
3G	Cellular	2001	2,100 MHz	14 Mbps	10 km	Low	A5/1
4G	Cellular	2010	1,700–2,100 MHz, 2,500–2,700 MHz	100 Mbps	3–6.5 km	Moderate	SNOW 1.0/2.0/3G
LTE	LTE	2008	1,625.5–1,637.5 MHz	0.1–1 Gbps	3–6.5 km	High	SNOW 1.0/2.0/3G
5G	Cellular/NR	2020 and later	1–6GHz	20 Gbps	1.6–5 km	High	NEA and NIA
6G	Long	2025	7–15 GHz	9.6 Gbps	1 km	High	AESs
NB-IoT	3GPP	2016	900 MHz	250 kbps	20 km	Moderate	AES
UWB	Long	2002	3.1–10.66 Gsbps		4–20 m	Low	AES block cypher

high transmission idleness (around 100 ms) and long correspondence set-up time (primarily because of the sluggish revelation method, in the request for seconds). To overcome these limitations and specifically target wearable devices for health, sport and fitness applications, Bluetooth low energy (BLE) was introduced. The benefit of Bluetooth lies in its minimal expense and energy proficiency, in any case, when the medical care application requests long-range correspondence, this innovation neglects to meet the prerequisite.

3.4.3 ZigBee

ZigBee is a wireless technology for short distances. It is inexpensive, moves at a slow speed and uses little power. ZigBee is used in smart homes, smart tags, remote control, network sensors and medical monitoring. The ZigBee stack has two stack profiles. The first, stack profile 1, is used in wireless networks in homes and small businesses, while stack profile 2, referred to as ZigBee Pro, makes use of a symmetric key exchange protocol to make multicast, many-to-one routing and enhanced security possible.

3.4.4 Ultra-wideband

UWB is a low-power remote transmission technique that operates over short distances. It is capable of sending information at very high speeds. It achieves this by transmitting over a much wider bandwidth than is typically provided by conventional narrowband radio transmission systems. For personal area networks (PANs), UWB technology offers numerous advantages. Among the benefits of this technology are fast data rates (up to 480 Mbps) and low-power consumption (1 mW/Mbps). UWB is a good choice for WBAN applications that require a lot of transmission capacity but not a lot of force. The Industrial Scientific Medicine (ISM) (industrial scientific and medical) band is referred to as the UWB technology used in PANs in IEEE 802.15.3. It is intended for use in baseband processors and RF short-distance communication.

3.4.5 Near-field communication

Near-field communication (NFC) wireless technology enables smartphones, wearable devices, payment devices and other devices to communicate smartly. It is a peer-to-peer technology that has a data transfer rate of 424 kbit/s and operates within a range of 4–10 cm.

NFC operates in active and passive modes. NFC consumes no energy in the passive mode, while it attracts the same energy as BLE in the active mode. To process cardless payments, smart devices with NFC can be worn on the body like smart suits and jackets. They can also be utilized to lock and unlock doors and convey medical information. Some other applications of NFC are smart jewellery, e-skin, wrist-worn wearables and e-tattoos.

3.4.6 Wireless fidelity

Wi-Fi is based on the IEEE 802.11 wireless standard. The protocol is used for local area networks (LANs) and operates over the 2.4 GHz ISM band and the 5 GHz

Unlicensed National Information Infrastructure band. Its basic transmission rate of 2 Mbps makes it possible to use wireless LANs over a short distance. A network based on Wi-Fi technology can transmit data at up to 6.75 Gbps to a maximum range of 383 km. Wi-Fi can operate using four configurations: infrastructure, ad hoc, bridge and repeater. The method of direct or indirect communication between Wi-Fi devices is defined by the first two modes, while the method of extending the range of Wi-Fi network is defined by the last two. An access point coordinates some wireless stations or clients which are associated and authenticated for connecting to the network. The basic service set (BSS), composed of the wireless stations and the access point, is tagged with a BSSidentifier. An extended service set structure is formed when the BSSs are connected. The ad hoc mode involves the wireless connection of devices in a network such as a mobile or mesh network. In this configuration, the devices can serve as both a wireless station and an access point. The independent BSS structure is formed from the set of all connection stations and is identified by SSID. The carrier sense multiple access with collision avoidance is adopted in Wi-Fi to access the wireless channel. The protocol enables wireless devices to transmit data without collisions by using the exponential back-off algorithm. The process compels the devices to sense the radio channel for busyness, start transmitting if idle, or wait for some random time when the channel is in a busy state.

3.5 Long-range communication technologies

The long-range technology enables connectivity for voice and data services over a long distance of up to 40 mi. Some long-range communication technologies used in telehealth include satellite, Global System for Mobile Communication (GSM) and cellular and lower power WAN (LPWAN).

3.5.1 Satellite

This communication system transmits information between two places by using a communication satellite moving in orbit around the Earth. The communication satellite transmits signals to a transponder by creating channels between the transmitter and receiver far apart from each other on the Earth. It achieves this by bouncing signals (e.g. radio, television and Internet data) from one location to another in three stages: uplink, transponder and downlink. In the uplink, the signal from the ground station on the Earth is beamed up to the satellite. The transponder is used to boost the signals using radio receivers, amplifiers and transmitters. In the downlink, data is sent to the receiving end of the Earth.

3.5.2 Cellular communication

Cellular technology enables mobile phones to be used for wireless communication. One of the second-generation (2G) telecommunications standards is the GSM. The technology uses Time Division Multiple Access (TDMA) and Frequency Division Multiple Access techniques for mobile data and voice services between devices. The 2G technology improves voice quality by utilizing 20–200 kHz and digital modulation as an improvement over the 1G. After 2G came the General Packet Radio Service and then the Enhanced Data Rate for GSM evolution termed 2.5G and 2.75G, respectively.

The Universal Mobile Telecommunication Service was introduced by the third-generation technology (3G). It provides quality audio, multimedia service, video and data using Code Division Multiple Access.

The 4G brought about improvements in the Internet and high data rates with a throughput of over 100 Mbps. The technology utilized orthogonal frequency division multiple access to improve the efficiency of the spectrum for more data rates, narrowband interference and mitigation of frequency-selective fading. Further improvements came with the introduction of long-term evolution technology and WiMAX protocols based on the IEEE 802.16 standard.

The fifth generation (5G) technology offers low latency, high throughput, unbounded connectivity and high-definition video. The technology uses mm-Wave spectrum spanning from 3 to 300 GHz. The OFDM is improved in the physical layer to meet the 5G requirements on capacity and bandwidth.

Device-to-device (D2D) is a communication technique provided in 5G [24]. It operates in two ways: where communications between nodes are via a base station and the other where there is direct communication without the base station. Some benefits of the direct communication approach include increased cell traffic capacity and improved SNR, low energy consumption and link latency [25,26].

A terahertz signal transmission is introduced in 6G with improvements in data rate and bandwidth. The technology also promises to fulfil the requirements of low latency, high mobility support, high reliability and high bandwidth.

3.5.3 Low-power wide area network

The LPWAN enables low, wide-area coverage and low data rate. The technology can establish a lot of connections at a lower cost than other conventional cellular systems and is suitable for IoT applications such as intelligent cities [27]. LPWAN is a classification of remote correspondence that goes about as a network empowering influence to help different IoT applications by supplementing short and cell remote correspondence. Cell-based arrangements have long networks yet consume more energy [28]. LPWAN technology supports the connection of a lot of end devices to the gateway (infrastructure) and offers a connection range of up to multiple kilometres [28]. The types of LPWAN technologies are LoRaWAN, DASH7, Sigfox and NB-IoT [27].

LoRa (long range) uses the ISM bands and uses six spreading factors to balance the trade-off of the range and data rate. Lora utilizes the ISM band and chirp spread spectrum technology. LoRa adjusts the information rate and reaches a trade-off by utilizing six spreading factors. By using the spreading factor, an increase in the range decreases the data rate and vice versa.

The base station can receive messages simultaneously with the spreading factors in LoRa. LoRaWAN enables all messages sent by any end device to be received by all the base stations. LoRaWAN boosts the proportion of messages successfully received by taking advantage of this redundant reception. LoRaWAN also takes advantage of multiple base stations receiving the same message to localize end devices. The localization method for the time difference of arrival is utilized, and it is backed up by extremely precise time synchronization between multiple base stations. In addition, the LoRaWAN network avoids handover when multiple base stations receive the same message. Different types of end devices are provided in LoWaWAN to meet the latency requirements for IoT applications.

DASH7 Union Convention (D7A) characterizes an ISM band-worked correspondence convention that depends on the ISO/IEC 18000-7 norm for RFID labels and sensor hubs. DASH7 is worked around the idea of Impact Innovation. Bursty, Light, Asynchronous, Stealthy and Transitive are spelt BLAST. Light is used to describe the small size of a packet with a typical limit of 256 bytes per transaction. Nonconcurrent is one of the significant ideas based on the D7A standard; any time, the gateways and end devices can send and receive commands and responses. Stealth reflects the fact that the end devices are connected to the gateway and do not require periodic beacons to indicate their presence. The D7A upholds three classes of gadgets: the entryway, sub-regulator and end point. Out of the three, the passage and the end points are the broadly carried out gadget classes. The end point only uses a small amount of the protocol and uses the least amount of energy. End-gadget utilizes discontinuous channel examining to check for any approaching parcel and invests the greater part of its energy in rest. Although it is essentially an end point, the sub-controller is a fully functional DASH7 device. The D7A stack should be implemented by the gateway, which links the low-power network to another network.

Sigfox offers a start-to-finish IoT availability arrangement in light of its protected advancements. The IP-based network is utilized in Sigfox to connect its base stations to the back-end servers, which are outfitted with cognitive software-defined radios. The unlicensed ISM band is utilized in Sigfox. Sigfox utilizes the recurrence transmission capacity proficiently and encounters a decrease in noise levels, resulting in low-power utilization, high recipient responsiveness and low-cost radio antenna design to the detriment of the greatest throughput of just 100 bps.

An uplink communication is first carried out by Sigfox and now developed bidirectional innovation with a huge connection lopsidedness. Following an uplink communication, a downlink of data from the base station to the end devices is done.

The length of the payload for each message in the uplink can reach a maximum of about 12 bytes. There is no support for the acknowledgement of uplink messages since only four messages can be sent over the downlink per day. The maximum payload length of each downloaded message is 8 bytes. Each message is sent multiple times to the end device over various frequency channels [29].

3.6 Wireless communication standards and protocols in telehealth

The standards and protocols refer to the set of rules that ensures the successful transmission of data from the source to the destination with communication devices. Some of the techniques involved in protocols and standards are error detection and correction authentication, demodulation, signalling and modulation. Common examples of protocols are ZigBee stack, Bluetooth stack, wireless application protocols, Hypertext Transfer Protocol, TCP, File Transfer Protocol and User Datagram Protocol (UDP). The ZigBee protocol links data computing devices, such as PCs and PDAs, directly connected to medical devices. With the simplicity, low power and ability to integrate a lot of devices, of the protocol, the protocol is expected to take the lead in home automation applications. Bluetooth is intended to replace the cable connection within a short range. The technology operates at 2.4 GHz of the ISM frequency band. WiMAX is a protocol developed to replace the need for a cable to provide long-distance connectivity for mobile stations of 30 mi. Wi-Fi is a wireless protocol that comprises access points to connect clients to a backbone network. The UDP functions as a transport protocol for streaming videos with no acknowledgement received. TCP/IP is another transport protocol that ensures transmission from source to destination is achieved using the mechanism of acknowledgement to confirm delivery.

3.7 Review of related works

Chakraborty and Rodriques [8] present a review of D2D for healthcare. The study classified the reviewed works based on power control, resource allocation algorithms and security mechanisms. The work also identifies some challenges in D2D communications as neighbour discovery, synchronization, cellular mode selection between transceiver pairs, spectrum access, spectrum use, interference management, channel modelling, state acquisition, resource allocation, power control, energy efficiency, security, joint resource allocation, optimal resource allocation and user satisfaction ratio.

Karthick and Pankajavalli [9] explore the Human Healthcare IoT (H^2IoT). The work discusses the techniques which enable the transmission of data used in H^2IoT systems. The application of IoT in the healthcare domain is highlighted, and how the technologies enhance the intelligence of H^2IoT is examined. The work further discusses the H^2IoT frameworks in three different areas: network topology, architecture and platform. The authors identify and compare the available wireless communication technologies for H^2IoT such as Wi-Fi, Bluetooth, WiMAX, LoRa, ZigBee and UWB. The work further studies the H^2IoT sensing devices and technologies such as wearable sensors, and inertial sensors like accelerometers, gyroscopes and magnetic field sensors. The work also highlights the threat issues and security challenges in H^2IoT. The work discusses the applications of H^2IoT in body temperature monitoring, blood pressure monitoring, blood glucose monitoring, GSR monitoring, ECG monitoring, oxygen saturation monitoring, rehabilitation system, activity monitoring, medication control system and smart wheelchair system.

Alshehri and Muhammad [11] present a review of IoT-based smart healthcare systems. The review is discussed based on (i) IoMT or medical signals fusion,

(ii) IoMT and medical signals, (iii) security concerns in the application of IoT in healthcare and (iv) edge- and cloud-based smart healthcare. The study also identifies significant difficulties of IoT and simulated intelligence-based brilliant medical services such as sensors' interoperability, gadget correspondence, security and protection, gadgets for the executives, data for the board hindrance and effective utilization of computer-based intelligence.

Selvaraj and Sundaravaradhan [10] discuss existing research on improving the performance of IoT-based healthcare to monitor elder patients. Some areas covered by the survey are (i) IoT-based architecture that can detect heart diseases in patients with arthritis at an early stage, (ii) systems that utilize and plot the sensor devices to replace cameras to monitor the household of patients with chronic disease and (iii) collection of real-time data from IoT-based systems using advanced sensors and detection of health problems by analysing physical and behavioural patterns in homes to assist the aged people suffering from age-related illnesses and having medication needs.

Tun *et al.* [12] present a study on emerging IoT-based healthcare systems for the elderly. The research classifies monitoring data types, IoT/wearable device types and IoT technologies in elderly healthcare. The study highlights the applications, data types and devices for IoT-based healthcare for the elderly.

Verma *et al.* [14] present monitoring systems for healthcare based on blood pressure, diabetes, heart disease, cancer and sleep apnoea in the elderly. The work highlights the communication methods required for real-time health monitoring system as ZigBee, RFID and LoRaWAN.

Taleb *et al.* [13] present a survey of wireless technologies applied to WBAN systems. The work discusses the applications of WBAN in telemedicine based on methodologies, wireless technologies and the sensors used. The suitability of LPWAN, 5G, B5G and 6G technologies are investigated.

Alenoghena *et al.* [15] present a survey of reviews of communication technologies in telemedicine and highlight the challenges and potential future directions. The work reviewed various standards and protocols in telemedicine and identified some challenges present in the application.

3.8 Performance measures of wireless technologies in telehealth systems

A taxonomy of the performance of wireless communication in telehealth is discussed in this subsection.

3.8.1 Latency

The delay in the time it takes for the transmission of data between the sensor node to a gateway in a network is known as latency. By and large, idleness concludes the speed of the H^2IoT organization, when the inertness of an organization diminishes then the organization's speed will increment. Increasing the data rate, which is made possible by some coding and higher bandwidths, reduces latency.

Considering that forwarding and routing may introduce more delays, multi-hop topologies increase latency. Additionally, computing a new route whenever a link fails may introduce some delay, rendering multi-hop topologies time-consuming when time-sensitive applications require low latency.

In IoT technologies, where devices aim to sleep as long as possible to save energy, the design of medium access control (MAC) may have a significant on latency, delaying transmissions and receptions. MAC protocols can be categorized as (i) Fixed Assignment Protocols, in which resources are distributed among the nodes for a predetermined amount of time; (ii) Demand Assignment Protocols, in which resources are made available to a node at any time; (iii) Random Access Protocols, in which resources are distributed at random; and (iv) Hybrid Protocols, in which resources are distributed at random and fixed or demand assignment are combined. Under very high loads, Fixed Assignment Protocols, like TDMA, introduce determinism and achieve lower latency than Random Access Protocols. However, under low load, they use up channel time inefficiently and achieve lower latency. Because explicitly asking for resources each time takes up bandwidth and increases latency, demand-based protocols are not suitable for low-latency, time-sensitive communications. For heterogeneous industry applications, mixture approaches are the most encouraging given that they expect to join the advantages of both fixed task and irregular access conventions while outperforming their cutoff points simultaneously and adjusting to the organization conditions. Retransmissions must also be kept to a minimum because they also add latency.

3.8.2 Communication range

The transmission power, which is typically restricted by regulations, the radio and propagation properties, as well as the complexity of coding and modulation, determine the majority of the transmission range. If a radio sends at consistent power, bringing down this intricacy rate allows the right unravelling of a more fragile or more misshaped signal by a collector, subsequently expanding the transmission range. Also, higher frequency bands with more bandwidth allow for higher data rates and faster data transmission. However, higher frequency bands also have lower penetration capabilities, which reduces the range in an industrial site with many obstacles. Topology is also a major factor in determining the range. Multi-jump geographies broaden the reach to the detriment of inertness, plan intricacy and energy utilization due to the requirement for synchronization of hubs, directing etc. In conclusion, multi-hop topologies and low data rates at low frequencies are both extending the range but increasing latency.

3.8.3 Reliability

Unwavering not entirely settled by geography, Macintosh plan and Tweak and Coding plan. Inter- and intra-technology interference in the air, which can result in collisions and increase packet loss, is one of the major reliability shortcomings of wireless technologies in comparison to wired counterparts. Advancements that work in authorized groups hold a piece of the range for themselves, relieving the issue. However, spectrum is a pricey resource with limited availability. Confidential organizations are impractical in the held range, crippling the chance of neighbourhood command over an organization. Shared range, then again, can be shared by quite a few innovations that can attempt to relieve impedance by channel jumping or utilizing some Macintosh layer systems, for example Tune in Before Talk (LBT). Besides, in a solitary jump organization, the achievement likelihood is completely reliant upon a solitary connection, rather than different connections in multi-bounce organizations. The reliability in the MAC layer can be improved via retransmission and repetition

Retransmissions and repetitions can be used to improve reliability at the MAC layer, which also increases latency. To lessen the number of retransmissions, mistake control procedures like forward blunder revision (FEC) can be utilized. Coding plans and balance generally characterize unwavering quality. Modulation's reliability is enhanced by the addition of error-checking bits produced by coding rates. Although they are slower, modulation schemes are more reliable because they have fewer points on the constellation diagram. Given that it can only accommodate two points (one bit per burst), binary phase shift keying is the modulation that is both the slowest and the most reliable when compared to quadrature amplitude modulation (QAM) and quadrature phase shift keying (QPSK). QAM can have any number of points, whereas QPSK uses four constellations. The space between the points on the constellation diagram narrows as the number of points increases, reducing error margins. As a result, QAM is the most efficient modulation method, but it is less reliable over longer distances.

3.8.4 Energy consumption

The utilization of energy utilization depends upon information rate, geography and the Macintosh plan, as well as the equipment plan. Transmission times at low data rates are long and can cause an increase in the power consumption at the node and a decrease in battery life. Nodes in multi-hop networks use more energy than in single-hop networks because they have to forward packets from other nodes in addition to sending and receiving packets.

The routing protocols determine the energy consumption and the energy efficiency along the forwarding paths of the data. Complex coding and interpreting tasks additionally add to energy utilization. Due to the energy consumption of the decoding operation, commercial 802.15.4-based networks have omitted FEC. By the by, utilizing FEC could decrease generally energy utilization as less energy would be spent on retransmissions and rescheduling. Additionally, the scheduling and radion control is determined by this process the energy consumption is significantly impacted by the MAC design [30].

3.8.5 Scalability

Versatility is not entirely settled by Macintosh's plan. To maximize network capacity, scheduling, contention resolution and other MAC mechanisms collaborate. When the upper capacity of a single-hop network reaches its limit, it can only be increased by adding more base stations. Nonetheless, by and by, the thickness of such base stations is restricted. This issue is addressed by multi-hop networks, which permit wireless data forwarding at the expense of overall throughput. In TDMA-based conventions, network thickness is restricted by the requirement for synchronization and time division in a blend with QoS prerequisites.

3.8.6 *Spectrum regulations*

The choice between licensed bands and unlicensed ISM bands is another design choice. Worldwide permitted unlicensed operation, on the one hand, reduces run-time costs but lacks regulatory protection from interference from other wireless networks operating in the same frequency band. However, licensed bands typically rely on an external operator, even though they prevent interference. Therefore, the external operator must resolve network issues because they cannot be resolved on-site immediately. This presents authoritative postpones which are excessively expensive in time-basic modern applications. Locally managed and maintained communication technologies use the unlicensed spectrum. However, multiple co-located or overlapping wireless networks in the same frequency band will interfere with one another, resulting in packet loss and a decrease in QoS.

The regulatory bodies have issued standards to alleviate coexistence issues in unlicensed spectrum and a clear channel assessment check before any transmission by all devices.

This means that a device must determine whether the channel is free using energy detection or other types of detect and avoid (DAA) mechanisms. Even though the DAA mechanisms make it easier for competing wireless nodes and networks to coexist, collisions can still happen. Aside from crashes, medium detecting adds to the idleness and acquaints non-determinism due to the medium clog. The previously mentioned realities altogether limit the utilization of remote arrangements in shut circle control applications in the mechanization business. Additionally, the unlicensed sub-GHz spectrum is subject to a limiting regulation. If they support LBT and adaptive frequency agility, devices with operating ranges of 863–868 MHz in Europe, 916.5–927.5 MHz in Japan and 902–928 MHz in the United States must adhere to the maximum duty cycle limit of 2.8% and 10%, respectively, for the access point [30].

3.9 Conclusion

The use of wireless technologies to provide healthcare services and information is known as telehealth. The delivery of telehealth may be a simple process of healthcare providers deliberating on a medical case over the phone or a more complex process using robotic technology to carry out surgery from a remote location. WBAN, HIoTs and WSNs are typical IoT-based networks that are used in current telehealth systems. The health status of the patient is tracked by these systems, which typically use wireless technology to send data to a healthcare provider. The communication range, power consumption and speed of current wireless communication technologies are necessary trade-offs while dealing with telehealth transmission. This work presents a review of wireless communication channels, models and protocols in telehealth systems. The review discusses telehealth systems based on wireless technology and communication paradigm. It is observed that most of the existing works on telehealth systems utilized the IoT-based system and WBAN and transmitted the acquired medical data to the healthcare provider using one or more wireless communication technologies. The identified challenges are power consumption, data security and privacy and interference. This study has provided a brief overview of the various telehealth framework, empowering specialists and medical services suppliers to settle on the telehealth framework that best suits their necessities and prerequisites.

References

[1] E. R. Dorsey and E. J. Topol, "State of telehealth," *N. Engl. J. Med.*, vol. 375, no. 2, pp. 154–161, 2016, doi: 10.1056/nejmra1601705.

[2] A. L. Imoize, J. Hemanth, D. T. Do, and S. N. Sur, (Eds.). (2022). *Explainable artificial intelligence in medical decision support systems*, IET.

[3] S. N. Gajarawala and J. N. Pelkowski, "Telehealth benefits and barriers," *J. Nurse Pract.*, vol. 17, no. 2, pp. 218–221, 2021, doi: 10.1016/j.nurpra.2020.09.013.

[4] J. Hendy, T. Chrysanthaki, J. Barlow, *et al.*, "An organisational analysis of the implementation of telecare and telehealth: the whole systems demonstrator," *BMC health services research*, vol. 12, pp. 1–10, 2020.

[5] A. Barak, B. Klein, and J. G. Proudfoot, "Defining internet-supported therapeutic interventions," *Ann. Behav. Med.*, vol. 38, no. 1, pp. 4–17, 2009, doi: 10.1007/s12160-009-9130-7.

[6] J. Weizenbaum, "ELIZA-A computer program for the study of natural language communication between man and machine," *Commun. ACM*, vol. 9, no. 1, pp. 36–45, 1966, doi: 10.1145/365153.365168.

[7] L. C. Klopfenstein, S. Delpriori, S. Malatini, and A. Bogliolo, "The rise of bots: a survey of conversational interfaces, patterns, and paradigms," *DIS 2017—Proc. 2017 ACM Conf. Des. Interact. Syst.*, pp. 555–565, 2017, doi: 10.1145/3064663.3064672.

[8] C. Chakraborty and J. J. C. P. Rodrigues, "A comprehensive review on device-to-device communication paradigm: trends, challenges and applications," *Wireless Pers. Commun.*, vol. 114, no. 1, pp. 185–207, 2020, doi: 10.1007/s11277-020-07358-3.

[9] G. S. Karthick and P. B. Pankajavalli, "A review on human healthcare Internet of Things: a technical perspective," *SN Comput. Sci.*, vol. 1, no. 4, pp. 1–19, 2020, doi: 10.1007/s42979-020-00205-z.

[10] S. Selvaraj and S. Sundaravaradhan, "Challenges and opportunities in IoT healthcare systems: a systematic review," *SN Appl. Sci.*, vol. 2, no. 1, pp. 1–8, 2020, doi: 10.1007/s42452-019-1925-y.

[11] F. Alshehri and G. Muhammad, "A comprehensive survey of the Internet of Things (IoT) and AI-based smart healthcare," *IEEE Access*, vol. 9, pp. 3660–3678, 2021, doi:10.1109/ACCESS.2020.3047960.

[12] S. Y. Y. Tun, S. Madanian, and F. Mirza, "Internet of Things (IoT) applications for elderly care: a reflective review," *Aging Clin. Exp. Res.*, vol. 33, no. 4, pp. 855–867, 2021, doi: 10.1007/s40520-020-01545-9.

[13] H. Taleb, A. Nasser, G. Andrieux, N. Charara, and E. Motta Cruz, "Wireless technologies, medical applications and future challenges in WBAN: a survey," *Wireless Networks*, vol. 27, no. 8, pp. 5271–5295, 2021, doi: 10.1007/s11276-021-02780-2.

[14] N. Verma, S. Singh, and D. Prasad, "A review on existing IoT architecture and communication protocols used in healthcare monitoring system," *J. Inst. Eng. Ser. B*, vol. 103, no. 1, pp. 245–257, 2022, doi: 10.1007/s40031-021-00632-3.

[15] C. O. Alenoghena, H. O. Ohize, A. O. Adejo, *et al.*, "Telemedicine: a survey of telecommunication technologies, developments, and challenges," *J. Sens. Actuator Networks*, vol. 12, no. 2, p. 20, 2023, doi: 10.3390/jsan12020020.

[16] L. K. Ramasamy, F. Khan K. P., A. L. Imoize, J. O. Ogbebor, S. Kadry, and S. Rho, "Blockchain-based wireless sensor networks for malicious node detection: a survey," *IEEE Access*, vol. 9, pp. 128765–128785, 2021, doi: 10.1109/ACCESS.2021.3111923.

[17] A. Alhayajneh, A. N. Baccarini, G. M. Weiss, T. Hayajneh, and A. Farajidavar, "Biometric authentication and verification for medical cyber physical systems," *Electronics*, vol. 7, no. 12, pp. 3–19, 2018, doi: 10.3390/electronics7120436.

[18] J. B. Awotunde, A. L. Imoize, O. B. Ayoade, *et al.*, "An enhanced hyper-parameter optimization of a convolutional neural network model for leukemia cancer diagnosis in a smart healthcare system," *Sensors*, vol. 22, no. 24, p. 9689, 2022, doi: 10.3390/s22249689.

[19] M. Elhoseny, N. N. Thilakarathne, M. I. Alghamdi, *et al.*, "Security and privacy issues in medical Internet of Things: overview, countermeasures, challenges and future directions," *Sustainability*, vol. 13, no. 21, p. 11645, 2021, doi: 10.3390/su132111645.

[20] A. L. Imoize, P. A. Gbadega, H. I. Obakhena, D. O. Irabor, K. V. N. Kavitha, and C. Chakraborty, "Artificial intelligence-enabled internet of medical things for covid-19 pandemic data management," in *Explainable Artificial Intelligence in Medical Decision Support Systems*. London: IET, 2022, pp. 357–380.

[21] O. C. Abikoye, E. T. Oladipupo, A. L. Imoize, J. B. Awotunde, C. C. Lee, and C. T. Li, "Securing critical user information over the internet of medical things platforms using a hybrid cryptography scheme," *Future Internet*, vol. 15, no. 3, pp. 1–33, 2023, doi: 10.3390/fi15030099.

[22] K. R. Laskhmana, W. Yichuan, T. Poongodi, and L. I. Agbotiname, *Internet of Things, artificial intelligence and blockchain technology*. Cham: Springer, September 2021.

[23] B. Pradhan, S. Bhattacharyya, and K. Pal, "IoT-based applications in healthcare devices," *J. Healthc. Eng.*, vol. 2021, p. 6632599, 2021, doi: 10.1155/2021/6632599.

[24] S. Li, L. Da Xu, and S. Zhao, "5G Internet of Things: a survey," *J. Ind. Inf. Integr.*, vol. 10, pp. 1–9, 2018, doi: 10.1016/j.jii.2018.01.005.

[25] A. Muthanna, P. Masek, J. Hosek, *et al.*, "Analytical evaluation of D2D connectivity potential in 5G wireless systems," in *Internet of Things, Smart Spaces, and Next Generation Networks and Systems*. 16th International Conference, NEW2AN 2016, and 9th Conference, ruSMART 2016, St. Petersburg, Russia. Springer International Publishing, 2016, pp. 395–403.

[26] A. Ahad, M. Tahir, M. Aman Sheikh, K. I. Ahmed, A. Mughees, and A. Numani, "Technologies trend towards 5G network for smart health-care using IoT: a review," *Sensors*, vol. 20, no. 14, p. 4047, 2020, doi: 10.3390/s20144047.

[27] K. Mekki, E. Bajic, F. Chaxel, and F. Meyer, "A comparative study of LPWAN technologies for large-scale IoT deployment," *ICT Express*, vol. 5, no. 1, pp. 1–7, 2019, doi:https://doi.org/10.1016/j.icte.2017.12.005.

[28] R. K. Singh, P. P. Puluckul, R. Berkvens, and M. Weyn, "Energy consumption analysis of LPWAN technologies and lifetime estimation for IoT application," *Sensors*, vol. 20, no. 17, p. 4794, 2020, doi: 10.3390/s20174794.

[29] Y.-P. E. Wang, X. Lin, A. Adhikary, *et al.*, "A primer on 3GPP narrowband Internet of Things," *IEEE Commun. Mag.*, vol. 55, no. 3, pp. 117–123, 2017, doi: 10.1109/MCOM.2017.1600510CM.

[30] A. Seferagić, J. Famaey, E. De Poorter, and J. Hoebeke, "Survey on wireless technology trade-offs for the industrial Internet of Things," *Sensors*, vol. 20, no. 2,p.448, 2020, doi: 10.3390/s20020488.

Chapter 4

Artificial intelligence and blockchain technology for efficient electronic medical record management

Akoramurthy Balasubramaniam[1] *and Surendiran Balasubramaniam*[1]

Over the past decade, blockchain technology has expanded at a staggering rate. The clandestineness and anonymity that "B" provides led to its primer as the underpinning of cryptocurrencies like Bitcoin, but it quickly found efficacy in other contexts as well. Secure data logging, transactions, and maintenance via smart contracts (SCs) are just a few examples of how blockchain technology has been put to use in the healthcare sector. Artificial intelligence (AI) has been extensively incorporated into blockchain to make it smart, bringing together the best of the two technologies. Many people have many physicians and receive multiple prescriptions and reports over the course of their therapy. Physicians and medical personnel can use the medical information of a patient to better care for them in the event of a life-threatening situation. However, time constraints prevent them from reviewing the person's medical record and a variety of past findings and prescriptions. In this chapter, we put forward a blockchain-based framework that incorporates AI to streamline the process of compiling a patient's medical history from disparate sources such as prescriptions (printed or handwritten) and imprinted documents into a single record. The report is kept safely via a decentralized blockchain network and displays just the most important facts in a succinct style for ease of access and reading.

4.1 Introduction

Since health informatics [1] is so centered around data, it stands to benefit greatly from the rapid development of technological and scientific advances. Medical professionals throughout the planet still use pen and paper to keep track of patient information, filing their records away in massive piles whenever they are not being used. It is expected that B5G/6G networks [2] would address the problems

[1]Department of CSE, National Institute of Technology Puducherry, India

experienced by current 5G networks, allowing them to better satisfy the needs of smart and intelligent environments. Complex interactions, the possibility of calculations on devices, etc. [3] are all examples. For secure applications, a blockchain is an attractive option due to its proven ability to maintain immutable and auditable data records [4–6]. It is widely believed that the electronic medical record, or EMR, which is used to store private patient information, may play a pivotal role in modernizing medical knowledge and enhancing the standard of the end-user experience. It has been estimated that electronic medical records may save over a billion dollars annually [7], and applying cutting-edge technologies, like 6G networking, artificial intelligence (AI), and blockchain, will further boost those estimates [8,9]. Critical conditioned individuals with disorders are sometimes predisposed to several additional ailments, as is widely seen by researchers [10]. In such cases, the patient may be seen repeatedly by several specialists. Due to a possible link between the disorders, treatment might be lengthy and protracted overall [11]. A number of studies [12,13] argue that most of the information needed to make a diagnosis may be gleaned from a thorough medical history. Over 50% of the doctors polled in one research agreed that patient history was the most important factor in making an assessment [14]. Patients with chronic conditions sometimes see several specialists throughout the duration of their treatment. Every kind of test result, prescription form, and other supplementary information is included. Oftentimes, the collection and storage of such information are chaotic, leading to the loss of certain paper documents and the storage of others without regard to the chronology of events in the patient's medical history. It is becoming increasingly difficult to provide high-quality medical care and treatment when patients, especially those with complicated conditions, lack familiarity with the relevant science of medicine [15]. As a result, doctors are not always able to get a clear picture of a patient's medical background, leading to things like unnecessary medication administration and overlooked details. This carelessness might cause untimely deaths over time. It can be very difficult and time-consuming for a newly minted physician to offer adequate care in the event of an emergency, especially in remote location hospitals. In most situations, clinicians who are presented with patients who lack complete health records decline to treat them and instead send the individuals to other facilities [16]. There is a need for a secure system that allows for the decentralized exchange of data among doctors, nurses, patients, and other interested parties in the healthcare industry. Electronic medical records (EMRs) include personal information that might cause serious harm if disclosed. Modern medical facilities are built on an integrated framework that necessitates confidence between all parties involved across a secure and quick channel for interaction [17]. An effective EMR alliance and cooperation between the existing systems remains a challenging task. Furthermore, patients have very little control over their personal information [18]. Optical character recognition (OCR) and other AI-assisted approaches are able to make the process entirely computerized and user-friendly. The previously mentioned flaws highlight the necessity for a client-centric management framework that also reliably protects patients and data security. It is clear that the blockchain system will be used in medical, diagnostic, and therapeutic procedures, which will produce tenfold more value [19]. Based on Bitcoin's [20] key privacy in public key encryption, the concept of blockchain protects the privacy of its final user, in this case, the person receiving treatment. In this work, we propose a unified platform that incorporates 5G connectivity, blockchain technology, AI, and machine learning (ML) methods to improve the lives of patients as well as doctors by digitally depicting the full history of the patient in one convenient digital format. To do this, a decentralized network is developed using the Ethereum platform.

4.1.1 Key contributions of the chapter

The following are the significant contributions of this chapter:

1. An efficient patient-driven distributed framework for preserving medical records, which is concerned with confidentiality, safety, credibility, seamless integration, and sustainability at the same time.
2. In this work, we suggested a simplified system that can be used by patients and healthcare professionals to assist them by digitally illuminating the full medical record comprehensively. The system will integrate blockchain with AI, with the network support of 5G and ML techniques.
3. Using the Hyperledger Fabric (HF) platform, a network of nodes is built to accomplish the purpose.

4.1.2 Chapter organization

Section 4.2 presents the related works on the applications of blockchain, AI, and ML for medical image processing and storing. Section 4.3 discusses the procedures and challenges in the applicability of medical images in the Ethereum blockchain. Section 4.4 presents the proposed BAI-SCs-based medical information chain network architecture and discusses its development, deployment, and assessment. Section 4.5 discusses the health chain network created using HF, Section 4.6 presents the results and the implications of the proposed system, and finally, Section 4.7 concludes the chapter with future direction.

4.2 Related work

The work of [21] discusses the SG and applications of AI, IoT, and BC. This work throws light on some of the major challenges in providing affordable, efficient, secure, and reliable healthcare from the viewpoint of computer and medical sciences. Tuli *et al.* [22] explain a conceptual model that can provide a complete solution for these increasing demands. In order to help secure the smart farm ecosystem, Chukkapalli *et al.* [23] develop a smart farming ontology. Abdul Robby *et al.* [24] investigate the opportunities for such system development under the use of proven agile process models. Cao *et al.* [25] presents a highly dense research overview of smart financial businesses and their challenges, the smart FinTech ecosystem, the DSAI techniques to enable smart FinTech, and some research directions of smart FinTech futures to the DSAI communities. Iftekhar *et al.* [26] aim to present a holistic reference architecture as well as fundamentals, recent advancements, promises, and challenges in order to foster investigations on cutting-edge research and allow one to contribute to advancing the convergence of blockchain and IoT [27]. The introduction of the Internet of Things (IoT) to the blockchain will offer tremendous advantages as well as the study of IoT combined with blockchain and 5G infrastructure for its application and development: a review. Blockchain integration offers a detailed exploration of how to combine the IoT technology with the IoT scheme. The subject of [15] was to develop a conceptual framework for responding to the COVID-19 pandemic via IT management, based on an extensive literature review and expert knowledge. Liu *et al.* [28] presents a comprehensive survey on the application and implementation of blockchain-enabled federated learning frameworks for IoVs. Other influential work includes [29]. An insightful privacy-aware energy-efficient architecture using AIoMT for COVID-19 pandemic data handling is presented in this chapter. The goal is to secure sensitive medical records of patients and other stakeholders in the healthcare domain. Additionally, this chapter presents an elaborate discussion on improving energy efficiency and minimizing communication costs to improve healthcare information security [30].

4.3 Procedures

The procedures followed by the suggested system model are shown in Figure 4.1. When a user signs up for the service, they must provide digital images of their medical records, including prescriptions and test results. All of the material is kept safely on the blockchain, which is hosted on the Ethereum platform, and the information is fed into the deep learning model on demand. Several recent

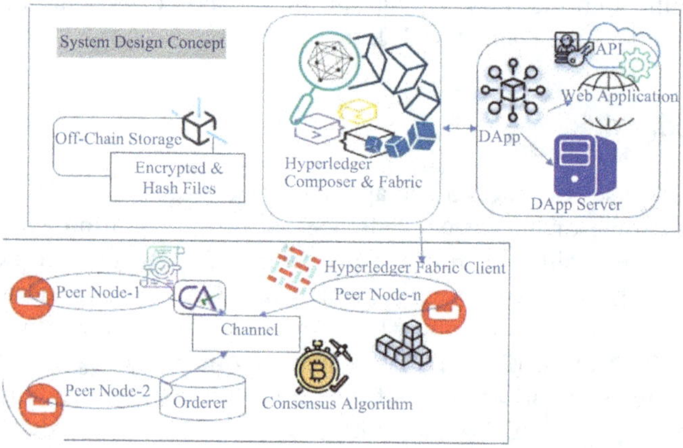

Figure 4.1 System design concept

publications [31,32] apply various ML [33] and deep learning ideas to medical applications such as human ear biometrics [34], with the goal of making these tools more useful to clinicians and also securing patient data using cryptographic techniques [35]. Many researchers have directed healthcare toward XAI [36,37] which can find trends that doctors would miss, helping in the early detection of diseases by analyzing large amounts of patient data. A single report is created for each patient once the data given by all patients have been compiled, improved, and analyzed by the system of smart procedures. The report may be read and modified by medical professionals, staff members, and patients, and it gives a concise and graphic account of each patient's biobank. The following procedures are required to put the previously mentioned structure into action:

1. On the Ethereum blockchain, a decentralized network has been formed. Everyone involved in the health informatics system, from physicians and nurses to patients and to any interested party, is welcome to apply for membership in the community.
2. A protected entry system with credentials is used by all users to enter the ecosystem. When adding a fresh patient to the system through 5G, they just need to submit digital images of their medical records and medications. For a current patient, this means entering any new medications they may have been given into the system.
3. Every file is transferred to the BitTorrent File System (BTFS) using Ethereum SCs, and the transactional ledger is updated with the eternal and irreversible BTFS connections. It occurs due to the fact that takes a lot of fuel to store things like pictures. Nevertheless, the privacy of the app is maintained through BTFS hashing.
4. Depending on the file's format, the hash numbers are recorded on the Ethereum network's blockchain. The fresh BTFS hash linkages are obtained by scanning the database in Py for use in the consolidated reports. These point to the decentralized applications (DApp)-stored media files.
5. The summary reports are examined by the model in stages, as shown in Figure 4.1; initially, pictures of handwritten prescriptions (HPs) are cleaned up to enhance performance, making them as suitable as possible for the method that is used. Keywords in the texts are then extracted using a variety of AI-based deep learning methods, followed by OCR and the storage of Unicode data.
6. Microsoft Azure Cognitive Service for Vision analyzes the printed medications and other printed materials to extract the necessary data, which is then saved in an encoded NoSQL database.
7. Health conditions, histories of care, current medication(s), indications, diagnoses, lab and test results, results, transcripts, etc. are collected. The information collected from many sources is compiled into a single report. No matter where the data are or how long they have been there, you can be assured that it is safe.
8. The concise history of the patient is easily accessible to physicians as well as patients. If the patient goes to a different doctor or gets a new prescription, the

summary record will reflect that. For the convenience of medical experts, an intuitive front-end framework is made available, which provides a visual summary of the complete case. The physician may then swiftly and readily review the patient's whole medical history. This could additionally relieve the patients and their caretakers of the burden of keeping track of, safeguarding, and producing all the necessary documentation when called upon. Using simply an identification card, the patient may see the medical professional, and the physician will have access to the patient's whole medical history right there in the portal. All interactions and data transfers take place through a lightning-fast 5G network.

In the subsequent part, we will talk about the chapter's model of networks with respect to the suggested services and the detailed procedure for implementation.

The soft estimate received by user k can be remodeled as (4.1). The samples are defined in (4.2).

4.4 System design

In its broadest sense, the network design consists of four parts: a web fore part that acquires and acts the information, a rear that stores files in BTFS, a rear that stores files in a blockchain, and a rear that processes an in-depth deep learning model to produce outcomes. Figure 4.1 provides a concise overview of the network model's suggested design. We then go on to detail how various parts of the network model are really put into action.

4.4.1 Fore part

4.4.1.1 Blockchain-based on Hyperledger Fabric

HF is a permissioned blockchain network, meaning that users must register to participate. HF's modeling and user management tools manage who has the authorization to do what on the network's infrastructure. HF is a shared ledger system with an extensible architecture that provides high levels of privacy, security, robustness, adaptability, and durability. As health data are often politically and legally delicate, an isolated blockchain like HF is useful for protecting patient confidentiality. Since HF supports several levels of permission, the information's possessor may decide which data elements are accessible to others. This makes it an ideal choice to control the accessibility of medical information. The SC contains regulations for the drafting of said contract.

We are using HF, a permissioned blockchain that relies on predetermined events, to provide secure and private communication between healthcare providers and patients. The Byzantium fault tolerance consensus technique may be used to reach a consensus on HF without resorting to mining or a dedicated currency. For its state database, HF employs a tree-like Merkle directed acyclic graph topology that can be duplicated with BTFS objects. As a result, BTFS can serve as a prototype for both off-chain and on-chain blockchain implementations for medical records. Combining an HF blockchain and the proposed system, we were able to develop a system for access control that was both open and granular enough to prevent hackers without the agreement of individual patients.

With an attractive user interface, the fresh user may sign up for the network safely as a surgeon or a patient. The credentials may be verified by either a centralized or decentralized security mechanism, giving users a permanent ID, so the patients are allowed to access ubiquitous. The patient or user can upload pictures or scanned PDFs that will be processed by this top-tier service. Also, the patients are encouraged to avoid uploading rotated images and instead post them in the correct orientation. Participants are also advised to utilize a portable copier to achieve the best possible outcomes. Because the material must be fed into a blockchain trio according to the picture kind, the user-patient must tag every picture as it is uploaded. Printed prescription, HP, and printed medical report are the three main categories of tags. Patients have access to an overview of their created health records, and physicians with the proper permissions can examine the full records of their patients by querying for them by ID.

4.4.1.2 Blockchain and BTFS

BTFS is designed to work on top of the Interplanetary File System and integrates the peer-to-peer file-sharing capabilities of the BitTorrent protocol. Here is a high-level overview of how BTFS works:

- File chunking: When a file is added to BTFS, it is divided into smaller chunks. Each chunk is typically 256 kilobytes in size, although this can vary. The chunking process ensures that files can be efficiently distributed across the network.
- Content addressing: BTFS uses content addressing to uniquely identify each chunk of data. Each chunk is assigned a cryptographic hash called a content identifier (CID) based on its content. This CID serves as a unique reference to the chunk, allowing nodes in the network to locate and retrieve it.
- Distributed storage: BTFS leverages a distributed network of nodes to store and share files. When a file is added to BTFS, it is divided into chunks and distributed across multiple nodes in the network. This distribution increases redundancy and availability, as multiple nodes hold copies of the file.
- Peer-to-peer file sharing: BTFS utilizes the BitTorrent protocol to facilitate file sharing among peers. Nodes in the network can request chunks from other nodes that have copies of the file. This peer-to-peer sharing mechanism helps improve download speeds and ensures that files can be accessed even if some nodes go offline.
- File retrieval: When a user requests a file from BTFS, the system retrieves the necessary chunks from the network. It locates nodes that have copies of the chunks and downloads them in parallel. Once all the required chunks are obtained, the file is reassembled and made available to the user.
- Decentralization and redundancy: BTFS's decentralized nature and redundancy make it more resistant to censorship and failures. Since files are distributed across

multiple nodes, even if some nodes are inaccessible or compromised, the data can still be accessed and reconstructed from other available nodes.

- A label is associated with each submitted file, and the system's algorithm uses those tags to determine which blockchain that every file should be connected to in BTFS.

The React Truffle Box (RTB) is installed in a new directory that is utilized for the build process. Truffle is a background in developing DApps on Ethereum, which speeds up the development process. In this case, RTB will by default deploy an SC named store.sol, which will be labeled according to our specifications and modified as needed. This SC records the BTFS reference (hash) on the blockchain. The SC for health records was created and blockchain integration is achieved by changing the network's config file to utilize the identical address that Ganache used for operating the blockchain. Tatum and Ganache are employed for development. Using Ganache, you can easily set up and operate your own personal blockchain right on your computer. Whenever we need to save a BTFS hash on the blockchain, it helps the blockchain link up, making it possible to use SCs. Tatum, a decentralized platform that supports both Ethereum and BTFS nodes, is the BTFS node instance with which a link is established. It connects external Ethereum and BTFS machines automatically through the RPC protocol, so the individual using it does not have to. The file is then transformed into an encrypted stream of information that may be used to carry out the exchange of information. To do this, we make use of a buffer to upload the picture to BTFS. A BTFS hash is returned after effective registration and upload. The Internet protocol layer has been updated so that it will now record the BTFS hash that was obtained alongside the picture submission.

ZenGo will ask for payment from the user whenever a blockchain transaction is requested. The cost of gas is calculated with the help of the following formula to determine the cost of a transaction on Ethereum, denoted by Tc:

$$\mathrm{Tc} = \mathrm{Gp} \times \mathrm{Gl} \tag{4.1}$$

where Gp is the price of the gas and Gl is the limit of the gas.

Wherein miners set and adjust the settings for the limit and price of the gas with each new block. When juxtaposed with preserving the actual photos, the cost of maintaining the BTFS hash on the digital ledger is far lower. The space needed to keep track of the value of the hash (Hs) is represented by the formula that follows:

$$\mathrm{Hs} = \frac{\mathrm{Hsize} + H \times N}{\sum_{1}^{N} T + H} \tag{4.2}$$

where Hsize is the BTFS hash size, N is the aggregate number of hashes or events on the blockchain, and T is the number of original transactions involved. The BTFS-returned hash is also added to a patient ID table.

In accordance with what the system has described, the patient, $\mathrm{P_n}$, authorizes access to their electronic medical record ($\mathrm{EMR_n}$) to the physician, Phyn, as illustrated in

Algorithm 4.1. As a result, the system generates a patient-centric view of the electronic medical record (EMR_n). As opposed to sending entire patient medical information, the function retrieves attribute-specific data depending on the physician's (Phy_n's) request. A patient-focused perspective on a single medical record enables individuals to view and alter just the information they require. The patient-focused view, in a nutshell, is a portion of the medical data. Furthermore, the software creates a session key S_k that is utilized by both the physician and the patient for a particular appointment.

Algorithm 4.1: Model_Function ()

Input: When a physician Phy logs into their electronic medical record (EMR_n) using their PHK_{pri} and PHK_{pub} and a session key S_k, P_n is a patient, PK_{pri} and PK_{pub} are their private and public keys, and S_k is the session key to their electronic medical record (EMR_n).

Output: Boolean (Hit or Miss)

Procedure:
Methodology for Maintaining Current Medical Records
For every access (A) who has the authorization to see the Medical Chart
Check the Proposed Model
If (Access==" Approved" && role==" Physician") then
Create patient-centric Accessing PCA of EMRn in BTFS
PCA → D(E(EMRn))
Create () Sk
send Encrypted (PKpub (Sk), PHKpub(Sk), PCA(Sk)) to Pn, Dn and PCA
create_Update ()
EMRn [(Decryption PKpub (Encrypted PHKpub (EMRn)) + Encryption (APCA)]
PCA Pledge (BTFS (EMRn))
BTFS EMRn(hash)
EMRn(hash) HF Blocks
Return True
Else
Authorization=Refute
Return False End if
End For ()
End procedure

4.4.1.3 Assistance offered to subscribers

In [38], we have a description of a cryptographic technique that does all of the above: validates the client's identities, creates and confirms signing and credentials, and creates and validates credentials. As can be seen in Figure 4.2, the HF relies on the Fabric-Certificate Authority (CA) of [26] as its interface for delivering resources to the network's authorized subscribers.

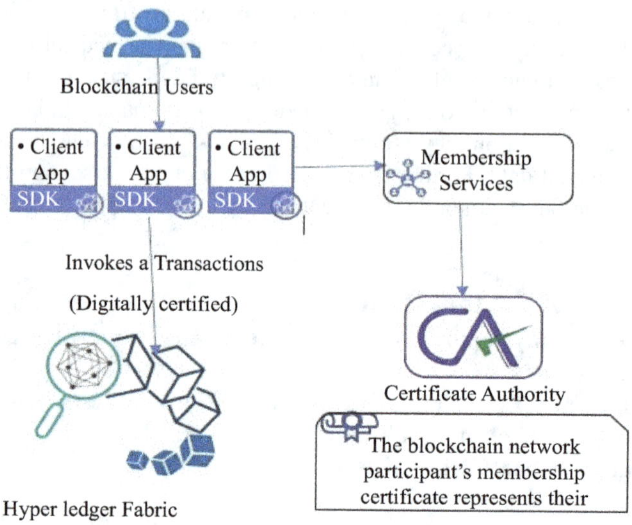

Figure 4.2 Validation service for HF certificates

4.5 Health chain

Figure 4.3 depicts the proposed framework for the health chain. The DApp's composer API sends requests from users to the fabric network, and the DApp's administrator can manage these requests in real time. The current state is returned by the API and is used by the Angular framework when making GET calls to the composer in order to retrieve data from the on-chain database. Composing SCs allows for the development of blockchain-based, distributed applications. Stakeholders in the HF [39] network can use blockchain codes, which are SCs, to verify the validity of entered medical data. This innovation was made for use in decentralized ledger applications. Hyperledger was developed for preserving medical records, while Bitcoin [20] was designed for online financial transactions.

In Figure 4.3, we can see how the suggested system architecture makes use of a blockchain with restricted access built on the HF framework and utilized by Hyperledger Composer users in order to create web apps for a single enterprise by means of three peer nodes. The organization uses three peer nodes; one acts as a validating node, whereas the other acts as an ordering node for registering interested parties. Several peers in this framework can reach the relevant database, BTFS for decentralized data storage, a Solitary Ordering Node, CA, a Membership Service Provider, and SCs for blockchain interoperability. For the purpose of ensuring the system can scale, additional peers can be placed in multiple places and on multiple machines. Through this infrastructure, intelligent contractors have control over ledgers and can access ledgers. When the app is linked to peer nodes, the ledger is updated in real time via SCs. There are n peer nodes in the network: peernode1 (P1), peernode2 (P2), and peernoden (Pn). Each individual peer node has a copy of the ledger and the SCs.

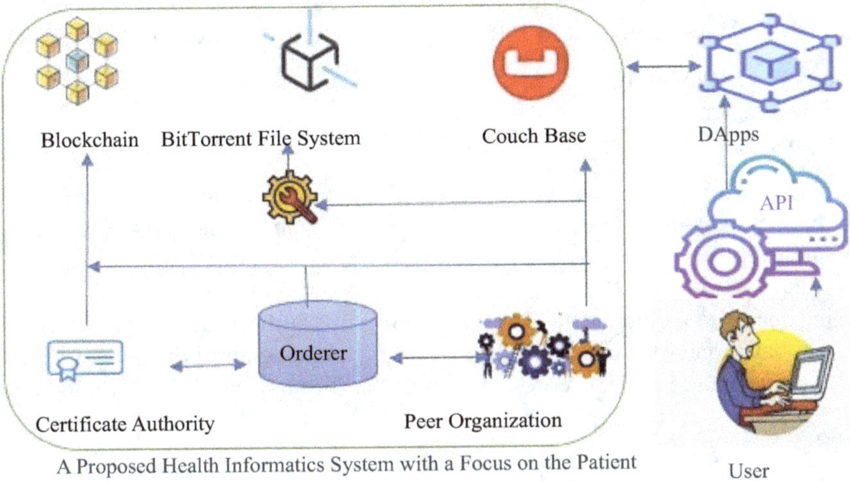

Figure 4.3 Health informatics chain

4.5.1 Metadata server

The metadata server details the BTFS file namespace, including file and directory-related data like size and modification time. The metadata server must have every file added, and all data removed, once their existence is no longer required. If the specified directory has not been previously in use by a different file in the same namespace, then the registration will succeed. The metadata server's responsibilities involve enforcing file permissions and providing customers with torrent data related to the desired items. In BTFS, every file is linked to a certain torrent. Filename, size, hashing data, fragments, seeder and monitor URLs, and so on are all included in the torrent information, just like they are in any other Torrent that will be utilized for sharing files among peers thanks to the BitTorrent protocol [40]. In the present setup, metadata for all namespaces is stored in just one server.

4.5.2 Working with data files

The hash values of medications, whether written by hand or imprinted, or reports, are entered into the relevant blockchains. We use the Python module web3.py that allows users to work with Ethereum. It is widely used in DApps to facilitate transaction transmission, SC interaction, block information learning, and other similar tasks. An SC is invoked to set up a link to Ethereum. The secret key of the ledger account, the location of the SC once it has been deployed, and the application binary interface (a JSON array describing the SC's format) are all necessities. These parameters help retrieve BTFS hash data from the blockchain and allow the SC to be reconstructed in a Python scenario. For gathering data, a Python script is frequently called to process freshly supplied hash values on each blockchain.

Before sending the retrieved BTFS hash values to their relevant sub-utility, these values are checked against those already recorded in the database with tags.

In accordance with the tags allocated to them, the hash values of the three distinct categories of files submitted to BTFS are each kept on a different blockchain:

Category 1: Handwritten
Category 2: Imprinted
Category 3: Medical report

The BTFS hash and the document tag type are used as inputs to the appropriate data extraction parts. Here, we break down how each of the parts contributes to the whole.

Figure 4.4 depicts the way medical professionals and patients connect when gaining access to medical data. The physician wants authorization for reviewing the medical data contained in the BTFS. Instead of releasing all of the patient's data, it generates a focused patient representation of the files in accordance with the query.

4.5.3 Set up

The BTFS python library is set up, and a Tatum link is made to BTFS Peer. Following that, the BTFS hash is used to get the content from BTFS. The photograph is cleaned up in the manners that follow to provide the best possible outcome.

Tesseract [24] uses the Leptonica library to perform a number of image processing tasks while beginning the OCR process. In most situations, it performs admirably, however in others, it may fall short, leading to a noticeable drop in efficiency.

An acceptable baseline size for text has been determined. As important as point size is, a resolution is essential. Precision decreases significantly under eight points×300 dpi, and it stops altogether below ten points×300 dpi. You may quickly examine the x_height of your characters by counting their pixels. Elevation of the lowercase x is referred to as "x_height." Depending on the typeface, the x_height at 10 pt and 300 dpi might be as little as a few pixels or as high as a few dozen. There is a high probability of getting inaccurate results if the x_height is less than ten

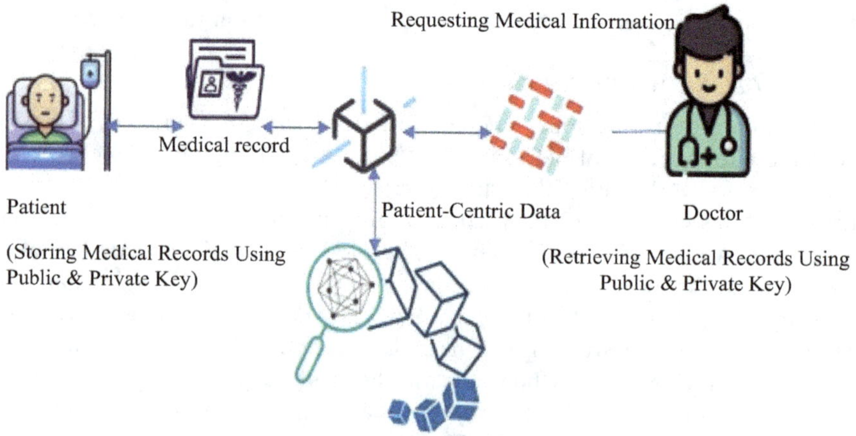

Figure 4.4 Interaction between patient and physician

pixels, and below roughly eight pixels, the majority of the content will be "noise cleaned."

- **Resizing:** Imagery with a dpi of 300 or higher is recommended for use with Tesseract, thus scaling them down may be useful.

```
# Use leptonic to read a picture.
img = lep.imread(/content/drive)
print(img.shape)
```

- **Lightening up:**
  The sporadic changes in luminance or color that constitute noise might obscure the image's text. Tesseract's inability to eliminate all sources of noise during the binarization process can lead to decreased accuracy.
- **Eliminating extraneous noise:**
  The methods used to improve contrast and remove noise can vary from one particular kind of image to another. Certain areas that are relevant may be made clearer after noise removal, especially if the original image had a poor resolution. Therefore, noise removal should only be used when the picture quality is great.

```
# noise removal
def rem_noise(Medical_image):
return cv2.medianBlur(Medical_image,7)
```

- **Digitization:**
  To a machine, an image is simply a collection of numbers called "pixels." Our tesseract pal will be able to discern and see details more clearly if they only exist in two colors, black and white. So that it will not muddle things up. When the brightness of an image is poor or there is a dark backdrop, it is easier for Tesseract to detect text.

Figure 4.5 exhibits the preprocessing of the medical prescription using Tesseract to store it in a blockchain system, and the text will be extracted from the HP with the help of AI concepts.

4.6 Results and discussions

The expense of keeping a large amount of information on the blockchain is high, hence BTFS hashes are used instead. Cost differentials are expected to appear as the volume of blockchain operations grows, as seen in Figure 4.3. Since putting data into the blockchain is more costly than reading it, that is what it focuses on most in terms of cost projections. As can be seen in Figure 4.3, storage costs are drastically reduced when the BTFS hash is saved rather than the whole picture.

The DApp uses BTFS to keep media with the help of peers. As illustrated in Figure 4.6, the time required for execution or time necessary to purchase the media grows in proportion to the number of neighbors viewing the transaction or the number of rivals contributing to the archiving of an image. It is additionally apparent that the time required to obtain a picture or report grows proportionally with its size. Enabling the intent of OCR in Category 2 documents, different

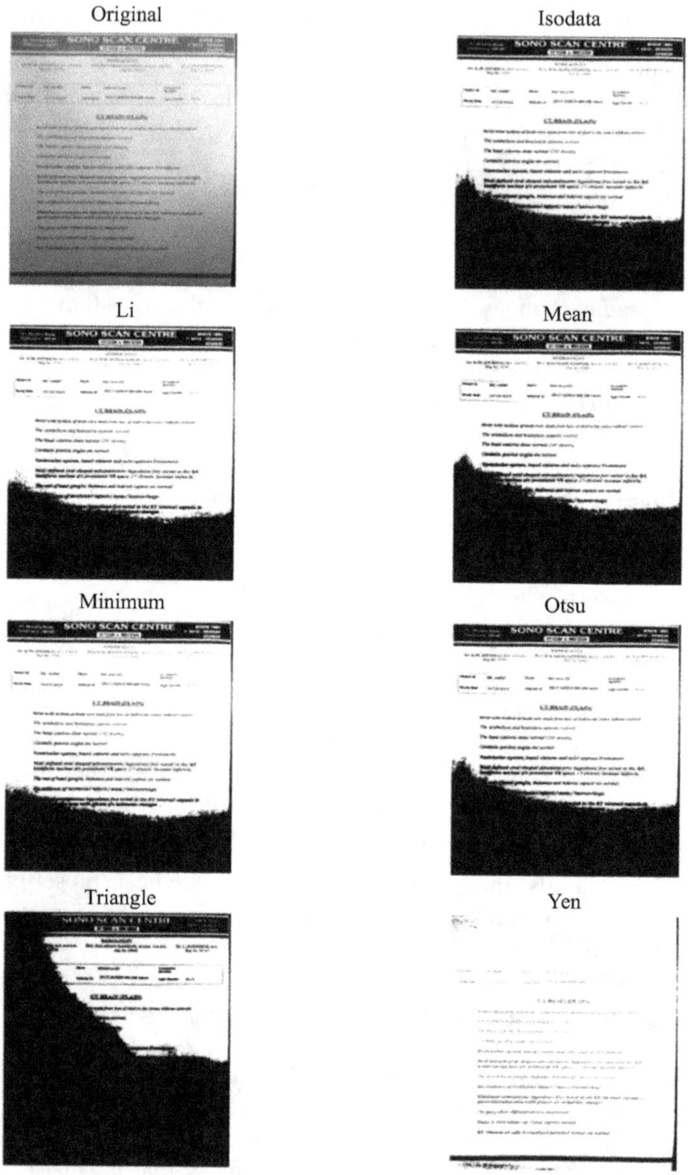

Figure 4.5 Handwritten prescription preprocessing

AI-based cloud services have been investigated in addition to the use of 5G integration for comprehensive swift as well as effective connectivity throughout the system and creation of replies. All of the systems are accessible through APIs, and while they all provide state-of-the-art performance, we need to make sure that the one we pick to run our design is reliable enough to produce a Category 1 document. It is also worth noting that there is constantly room for enhancement in the design.

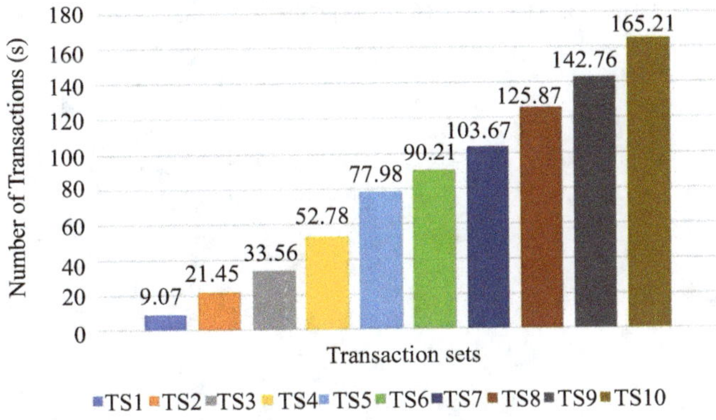

Figure 4.6 Time delay for the transaction sets

Categories 1 and 3 documents go through a series of preprocessing filters prior to being sent to the AI OCR system Tesseract for analysis. The effectiveness of character recognition prior to and subsequent to preprocessing is shown in Figure 4.6.

The overall efficiency of the model is enhanced by 5.976% once picture preprocessing is applied. The amount of online content accessed by medical practitioners is also noteworthy. Physicians need data regarding their patients; nevertheless, they only have so much duration, so it must be clear and simple. Figure 4.7 displays a decrease in the amount of patient data as medical professionals perceive only the summaries produced by the framework rather than all the records; huge quantities of evidence are averted as the number of patients goes up, but only essential data are maintained for medical professionals to peruse, thereby decreasing the period taken for evaluation.

John Hopkins Medicine's Medical Information Mart for Intensive Care III (MIMIC-III) patient records were mined for a dataset. The collection included both small and large images and texts. It was put to the test by verifying the accuracy of the current medical files. An application built on the blockchain was tested using MixBytes Tank [41]. Throughput, latency, and success rate (average, minimum, maximum, and percentile) are just a few of the measures that MixBytes Tank uses to test Hyperledger's performance. It also shows how the system's resources, including CPU memory, will be divided up. The indicators that follow are used in the analysis and generation of the result from MBT reports benchmarks:

1. Hit and loss rate
2. Transaction throughput and latency
3. The use of available resources

It is crucial that the suggested application may be easily expanded. Thus, the suggested architecture was evaluated via service orders against a range of peer counts. This network's efficiency was first measured using a single enterprise and three peer nodes. The effectiveness of the framework was calculated, assisted by peer-to-peer comparisons made possible by the standard report.

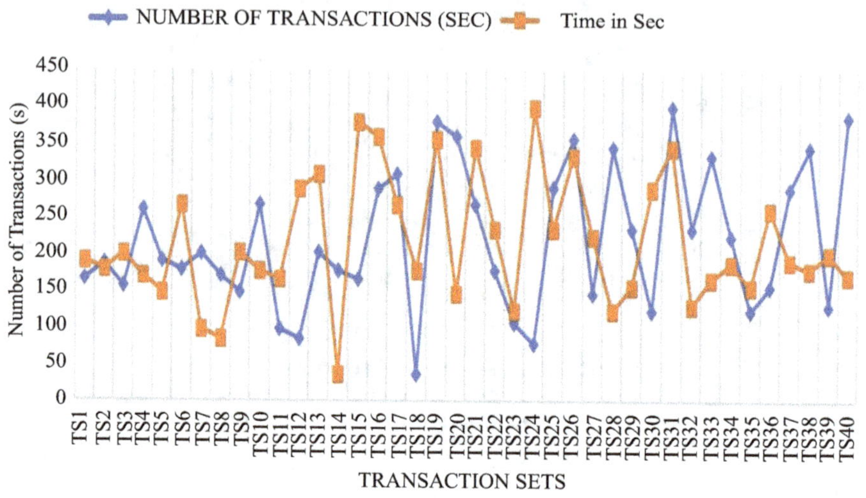

Figure 4.7 Time delay with total number of transactions (400)

In the initial test, transaction latency was calculated using the HF blockchain platform, which is represented as TL. This TL indicates the period it requires to make a final decision [42]. The value of this attribute is shared by all of the connected devices. The Tl is defined as the differences in the times it takes to submit a transaction (TL_s) and have it confirmed (TL_c) in a health chain composed of size n nodes.

$$TL = TL_s - TL_c \tag{4.3}$$

As can be seen in Figures 4.6 and 4.7, the network ledger was modified by means of ten sets of activities in peer node 1 of organization 1 with numbers ranging from 10 to 100. In this setup, the primary 10 network-wide transactions were recorded in 100+ s, but the last 90 needed an average time of 165 s to complete. To achieve this pilot result, we included the time required to complete 100–400 transactions. As shown in Figure 4.8, the average time required to commit 400 transactions over 3 organizational peer nodes was 430 s. This resulted in a transaction delay that was mostly unaffected by a spike in transaction volume. Examining the difference in commit transaction latency between nodes in the first, second, and third stages of a quad-node comparison, such as Organization 1, Organization 2, and so on. As can be seen in Figure 4.6, there is a negligible rise in latency as the amount of peer nodes grows. Following this series of studies, efficiency was measured. The number of legitimate, executed transactions divided by the number of total transactions done is transaction yield.

$$TLP = TL_{vc}/TL_c \tag{4.4}$$

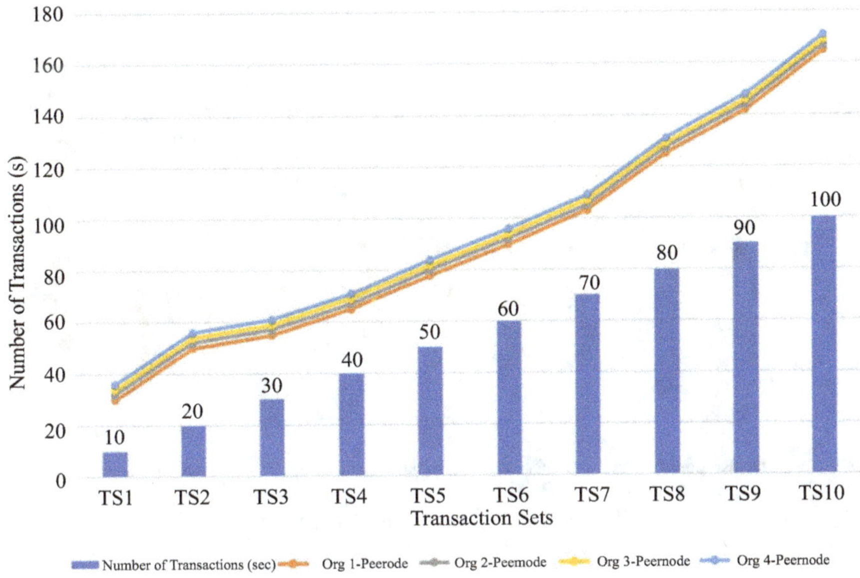

Figure 4.8 Evaluation of network delay between four peer groups of an organization

Experimental results from eight different sets of transactions are presented in Figure 4.6 to demonstrate the suggested system's transaction performance. It took 81 s to commit the initial ten transactions to the blockchain. This means that there are a total of four legitimate transactions in the test network. Similarly, with 29 valid transactions per minute, the last transaction in the system takes around 105 s to commit in the network. One group with one peer node, one group with two peer nodes, and one group with three peer nodes all undergo the identical set of tests. Figure 4.8 shows that the performance of the first organization's peer node is a bit greater than that of the other three peers. Measurement of asset delay occurs after assets have been satisfactorily imported and committed to a database. An n-node blockchain network's asset latency is denoted by ALAT. For both the response time TR and the asset submit time TALATs, milliseconds are used as the unit of measurement.

$$\text{ALAT} = \text{TR} - \text{TALATs} \quad (4.5)$$

Figure 4.9 depicts a representative sample of the transactions in the blockchain's asset time-to-commit format. That is why it is possible to process a massive dataset quickly with this technique. Extending the experiment to encompass 20–120 users and 200–20,570,000 bytes of data allowed for a more thorough analysis of the range of ALAT. Figure 4.9 shows that the median time it took for the ledger's resources to be updated was 2.9 s.

Even with an increase from 100 to 120 users, the system's efficiency would be improved and its asset size would grow, but the process of updating assets throughout the network would take a little longer time due to the configuration of

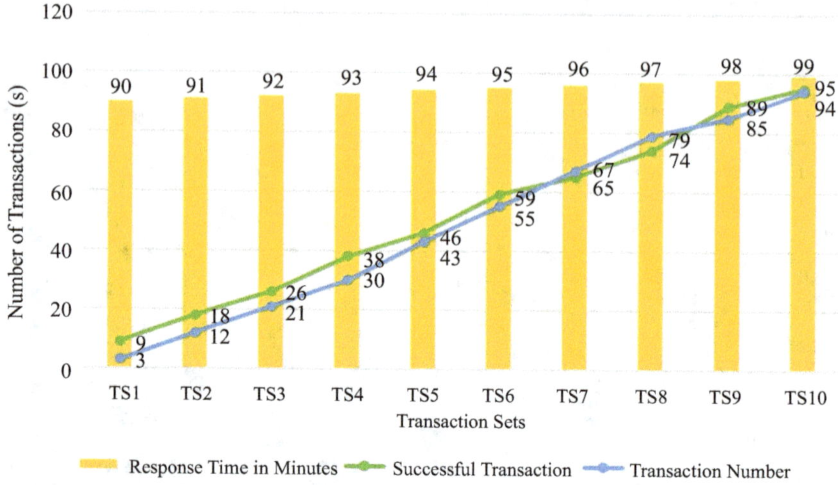

Figure 4.9 First two peer nodes in an organization

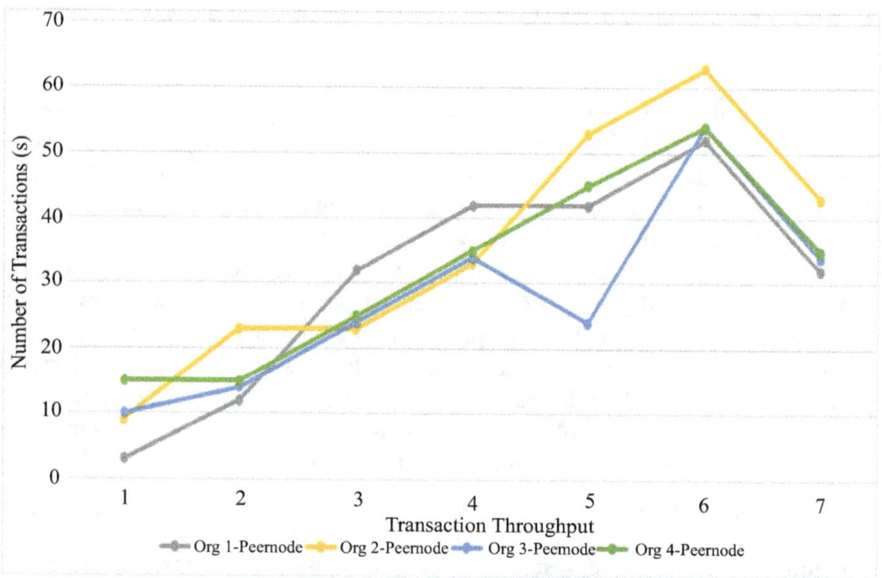

Figure 4.10 Comparison of all nodes' throughput

the system. In an outcome, this approach can handle massive datasets with negligible delays. Additional investigation, such as BTFS data upload and download operations totaling of 0.14 GB and 1 min, respectively, is warranted. According to Figure 4.10, the median time to upload 100,000 kB of healthcare image data to BTFS is 0.49167 min, while the median time for downloading 100,000 kB of medical image data is 0.7166 min. According to Figure 4.11, the typical transfer times for a 100,000 kB sample of a health record document are 40 and 52 s. As can be seen in Figures 4.10 and 4.11, the median uploading and downloading latency remains stable across all transaction sets. This demonstrates that the system's scalability has increased thanks to the proposed approach. The MBT report is displayed in Figure 4.12 related to the use of materials. Resource consumption was consistent across all experiments. Therefore, the tested system will not be affected.

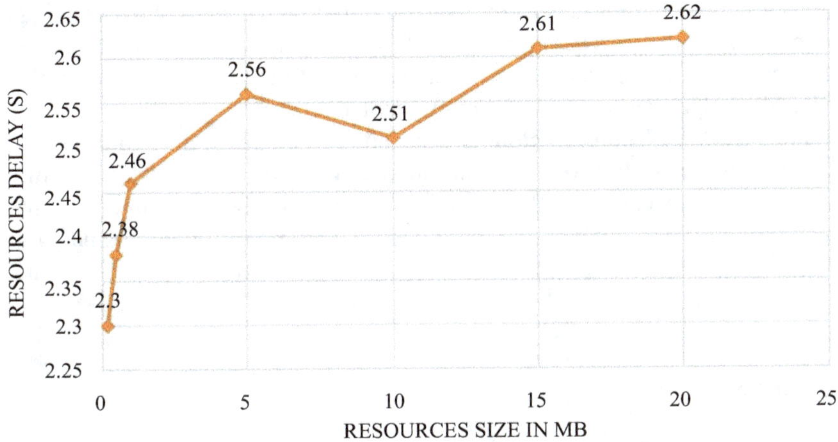

Figure 4.11 The typical delay between submitting an asset and receiving feedback

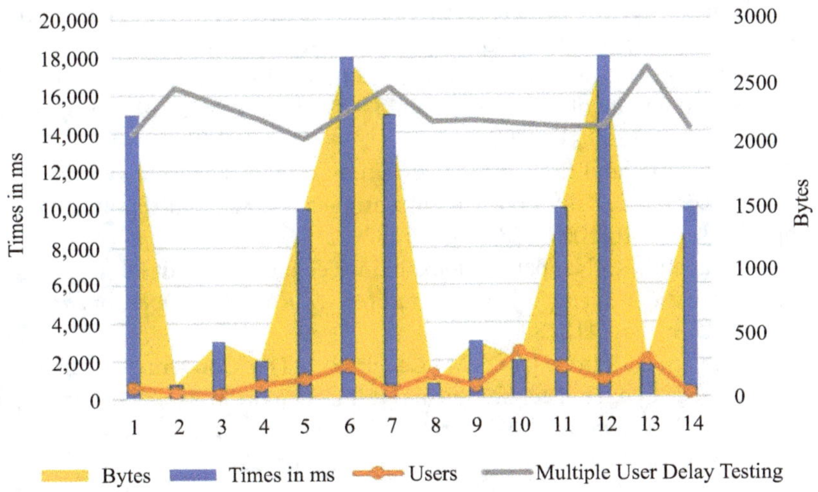

Figure 4.12 Multiple user delay testing of resources simulation

4.7 Conclusions and future scope

We present the framework, a BAI-SCs-based medical information chain network architecture and discuss its development, deployment, and assessment. This architecture protects sensitive medical information by using a combination of BTFS, SCs, and medical prescription chain systems. It also has a novel authentication method that is in line with privacy regulations and the comfort levels of individual patients. According to the findings of the investigation, the current system is effective and meets several security standards. It is possible to attain great levels of anonymity, safety, secrecy, and sustainability. This study has certain caveats that ought to be worked out in subsequent studies. The implementation of multiple blockchain systems is extremely labor-intensive.

Future work will be on including non-fungible tokens (NFT) into the framework in the future so that we can send video and audio recordings as information from NFT to the backers. With NFTs, users are going to determine who has to access their data, decide whether or not to sell it, and monitor how it is being used. Reliable NFT administration services can help with data transfers and tracking for patients.

References

[1] S. Dakshit, S. Dakshit, N. Khargonkar, and B. Prabhakaran, "Bias Analysis in Healthcare Time Series (BAHT) Decision Support Systems from Meta Data," *Journal of Healthcare Informatics Research*, vol. 7, no. 2, pp. 225–253, 2023, doi: 10.1007/s41666-023-00133-6.

[2] C. Suraci, S. Pizzi, A. Molinaro, and G. Araniti, "Business-Oriented Security Analysis of 6G for eHealth: An Impact Assessment Approach," *Sensors*, vol. 23, no. 9, p. 4226, 2023, doi: 10.3390/s23094226.

[3] H. Yoon and C. Shin, "Cross-Device Computation Coordination for Mobile Collocated Interactions with Wearables," *Sensors*, vol. 19, no. 4, p. 796, 2019, doi: 10.3390/s19040796.

[4] A. Luntovskyy and D. Gütter, "Definition: Highly-Distributed Systems," in *Highly-Distributed Systems*, Cham: Springer International Publishing, 2022, pp. 3–23. doi: 10.1007/978-3-030-92829-2_1.

[5] P. Arora and R. Nagpal, "Blockchain Technology and Its Applications: A Systematic Review of the Literature," *SSRN Electronic Journal*, 2022, doi: 10.2139/ssrn.4121824.

[6] B. Farahani, F. Firouzi, and M. Luecking, "The Convergence of IoT and Distributed Ledger Technologies (DLT): Opportunities, Challenges, and Solutions," *Journal of Network and Computer Applications*, vol. 177, p. 102936, 2021, doi: 10.1016/J.JNCA.2020.102936.

[7] J. W. Beasley, R. J. Holden, and F. Sullivan, "Electronic Health Records: Research into Design and Implementation," *British Journal of General Practice*, vol. 61, no. 591, pp. 604–605, 2011, doi: 10.3399/bjgp11X601244.

[8] A. Asadzadeh, Z. Mohammadzadeh, Z. Fathifar, S. Jahangiri-Mirshekarlou, and P. Rezaei-Hachesu, "A Framework for Information Technology-based Management Against COVID-19 in Iran," *BMC Public Health*, vol. 22, no. 1, p. 402, 2022, doi: 10.1186/s12889-022-12781-1.

[9] K. B. Letaief, W. Chen, Y. Shi, J. Zhang, and Y.-J. A. Zhang, "The Roadmap to 6G: AI Empowered Wireless Networks," *IEEE Communications Magazine*, vol. 57, no. 8, pp. 84–90, 2019, doi:10.1109/MCOM.2019.1900271.

[10] P. A. Dennis, K. M. Stechuchak, C. H. Van Houtven, *et al.*, "Informing a Home Time Measure Reflective of Quality of Life: A Data Driven Investigation of Time Frames and Settings of Health Care Utilization," *Health Services Research*, 2023, doi: 10.1111/1475-6773.14196.

[11] J. R. Brown, G. S. Goda, and K. McGarry, "Long-Term Care Insurance Demand Limited by Beliefs About Needs, Concerns About Insurers, and Care Available from Family," *Health Affairs*, vol. 31, no. 6, pp. 1294–1302, 2012, doi: 10.1377/hlthaff.2011.1307.

[12] G. G. Fillenbaum and M. A. Smyer, "The Development, Validity, and Reliability of the Oars Multidimensional Functional Assessment Questionnaire," *Journal of Gerontology*, vol. 36, no. 4, pp. 428–434, 1981, doi: 10.1093/geronj/36.4.428.

[13] J. Siette, G. T. Knaggs, Y. Zurynski, J. Ratcliffe, L. Dodds, and J. Westbrook, "Systematic Review of 29 Self-Report Instruments for Assessing Quality of Life in Older Adults Receiving Aged Care Services," *BMJ Open*, vol. 11, no. 11, p. e050892, 2021, doi: 10.1136/bmjopen-2021-050892.

[14] N. M. Kumar, A. A. Chand, M. Malvoni, *et al.*, "Distributed Energy Resources and the Application of AI, IoT, and Blockchain in Smart Grids," *Energies (Basel)*, vol. 13, no. 21, p. 5739, 2020, doi: 10.3390/en13215739.

[15] M. E. Kruk, A. D. Gage, C. Arsenault, *et al.*, "High-Quality Health Systems in the Sustainable Development Goals Era: Time for a Revolution," *Lancet Global Health*, vol. 6, no. 11, pp. e1196–e1252, 2018, doi: 10.1016/S2214-109X(18)30386-3.

[16] F. Al-Jabri, T. Kvist, R. Sund, and H. Turunen, "Quality of Care and Patient Safety at Healthcare Institutions in Oman: Quantitative Study of the Perspectives of Patients and Healthcare Professionals," *BMC Health Services Research*, vol. 21, no. 1, p. 1109, 2021, doi: 10.1186/s12913-021-07152-2.

[17] I. Alrashdi, "Evaluation of Quality of Healthcare: To What Extent can We Rely on Patient Expectations and Preferences," *Oman Medical Journal*, vol. 27, no. 6, pp. 448–449, 2012, doi: 10.5001/omj.2012.107.

[18] S. N. D'Costa, I. L. Kuhn, and Z. Fritz, "A Systematic Review of Patient Access to Medical Records in the Acute Setting: Practicalities, Perspectives and Ethical Consequences," *BMC Medical Ethics*, vol. 21, no. 1, p. 18, 2020, doi: 10.1186/s12910-020-0459-6.

[19] H. Saeed, H. Malik, U. Bashir, *et al.*, "Blockchain Technology in Healthcare: A Systematic Review," *PLoS One*, vol. 17, no. 4, p. e0266462, 2022, doi: 10.1371/journal.pone.0266462.

[20] P. Kayal and P. Rohilla, "Bitcoin in the Economics and Finance Literature: A Survey," *SN Business & Economics*, vol. 1, no. 7, p. 88, 2021, doi: 10.1007/s43546-021-00090-5.
[21] A. Kumar, D. Sundar, and D. Agarwal, "Commentary: Electronic Medical Record System – Should Complement but Not Replace Traditional Health Care," *Indian Journal of Ophthalmology*, vol. 68, no. 3, p. 432, 2020, doi: 10.4103/ijo.IJO_1474_19.
[22] S. Tuli, S. Tuli, G. Wander, *et al.*, "Next Generation Technologies for Smart Healthcare: Challenges, Vision, Model, Trends and Future Directions," *Internet Technology Letters*, vol. 3, no. 2, p. e145, 2020, doi: 10.1002/itl2.145.
[23] S. S. L. Chukkapalli, A. Piplai, S. Mittal, M. Gupta, and A. Joshi, "A Smart-Farming Ontology for Attribute Based Access Control," in *2020 IEEE 6th Intl Conference on Big Data Security on Cloud (BigDataSecurity), IEEE Intl Conference on High Performance and Smart Computing, (HPSC) and IEEE Intl Conference on Intelligent Data and Security (IDS)*, IEEE, May 2020, pp. 29–34. doi: 10.1109/BigDataSecurity-HPSC-IDS49724.2020.00017.
[24] G. Abdul Robby, A. Tandra, I. Susanto, J. Harefa, and A. Chowanda, "Implementation of Optical Character Recognition using Tesseract with the Javanese Script Target in Android Application," *Procedia Computer Science*, vol. 157, pp. 499–505, 2019, doi: 10.1016/J.PROCS.2019.09.006.
[25] L. Cao, Q. Yang, and P. S. Yu, "Data Science and AI in FinTech: An Overview," *International Journal of Data Science and Analytics*, vol. 12, no. 2, pp. 81–99, 2021, doi: 10.1007/s41060-021-00278-w.
[26] A. Iftekhar, X. Cui, Q. Tao, and C. Zheng, "Hyperledger Fabric Access Control System for Internet of Things Layer in Blockchain-Based Applications," *Entropy*, vol. 23, no. 8, p. 1054, 2021, doi: 10.3390/e23081054.
[27] V. R. Balaji, and J. R. Dinesh Kumar, (2021). Electronic Health Record Maintenance (EHRM) using Blockchain Technology. In: R. Lakshmana Kumar, Y. Wang, T. Poongodi, and A. L. Imoize. (eds.), *Internet of Things, Artificial Intelligence and Blockchain Technology*. Cham: Springer International Publishing, 2021. doi: 10.1007/978-3-030-74150-1.
[28] K. Liu, Z. Yan, X. Liang, R. Kantola, and C. Hu, "A Survey on Blockchain-Enabled Federated Learning and Its Prospects with Digital Twin," *Digital Communications and Networks*, 2022, doi: 10.1016/J.DCAN.2022.08.001.
[29] K. Bhugaonkar, R. Bhugaonkar, and N. Masne, "The Trend of Metaverse and Augmented & Virtual Reality Extending to the Healthcare System," *Cureus*, 2022, doi: 10.7759/cureus.29071.
[30] A. L. Imoize, P. A. Gbadega, H. I. Obakhena, D. O. Irabor, K. V. N. Kavitha, and C. Chakraborty, *Artificial Intelligence-Enabled Internet of Medical Things for COVID-19 Pandemic Data Management*. London: Institution of Engineering and Technology, 2022. doi:10.1049/PBHE050E_ch13.
[31] G. Varoquaux and V. Cheplygina, "Machine Learning for Medical Imaging: Methodological Failures and Recommendations for the Future," *NPJ Digital Medicine*, vol. 5, no. 1, p. 48, 2022, doi: 10.1038/s41746-022-00592-y.

[32] D. Placido, B. Yuan, J. X. Hjaltelin *et al.* "A Deep Learning Algorithm to Predict Risk of Pancreatic Cancer from Disease Trajectories," *Nature Medicine*, vol. 29, no. 5, pp. 1113–1122, 2023, doi: 10.1038/s41591-023-02332-5.

[33] K. V. N. Kavitha, S. Ashok, A. L. Imoize *et al.*, "On the Use of Wavelet Domain and Machine Learning for the Analysis of Epileptic Seizure Detection from EEG Signals," *Journal of Healthcare Engineering*, vol. 2022, pp. 1–16, 2022, doi: 10.1155/2022/8928021.

[34] O. G. Oyebiyi, A. Abayomi-Alli, O. 'Tale Arogundade, A. Qazi, A. L. Imoize, and J. B. Awotunde, "A Systematic Literature Review on Human Ear Biometrics: Approaches, Algorithms, and Trend in the Last Decade," *Information*, vol. 14, no. 3, p. 192, 2023, doi: 10.3390/info14030192.

[35] O. C. Abikoye, E. T. Oladipupo, A. L. Imoize, J. B. Awotunde, C.-C. Lee, and C.-T. Li, "Securing Critical User Information over the Internet of Medical Things Platforms Using a Hybrid Cryptography Scheme," *Future Internet*, vol. 15, no. 3, p. 99, 2023, doi: 10.3390/fi15030099.

[36] O. B. Ayoade, T. Oladele, A. L. Imoize *et al.*, "Explainable Artificial Intelligence (XAI) in Medical Decision Systems (MDSSs): Healthcare Systems Perspective," in *Explainable Artificial Intelligence in Medical Decision Support Systems*, London: Institution of Engineering and Technology, 2022, pp. 1–43. doi: 10.1049/PBHE050E_ch1.

[37] A. T. Rufai, K. F. Dukor, O. M. Ageh, and A. L. Imoize, "XAI Robot-Assisted Surgeries in Future Medical Decision Support Systems," in *Explainable Artificial Intelligence in Medical Decision Support Systems*, London: Institution of Engineering and Technology, 2022, pp. 167–195. doi: 10.1049/PBHE050E_ch6.

[38] Y. Sei, A. Ohsuga, and A. L. Imoize, "Statistical Test with Differential Privacy for Medical Decision Support Systems," in *Explainable Artificial Intelligence in Medical Decision Support Systems*, London: Institution of Engineering and Technology, 2022, pp. 401–433. doi: 10.1049/PBHE050E_ch15.

[39] E. Androulaki, C. Cachin, C. Ferris *et al.*, "Hyperledger Fabric," in *Proceedings of the Thirteenth EuroSys Conference*, New York, NY, USA: ACM, Apr. 2018, pp. 1–15. doi: 10.1145/3190508.3190538.

[40] A. Bori and P. Ekler, "The Analysis of BitTorrent Protocol Reliability in Modern Mobile Environment," in *2013 3rd Eastern European Regional Conference on the Engineering of Computer Based Systems*, IEEE, Aug. 2013, pp. 120–126. doi: 10.1109/ECBS-EERC.2013.23.

[41] N. K. Tran, M. A. Babar, and A. Walters, "A Framework for Automating Deployment and Evaluation of Blockchain Networks," *Journal of Network and Computer Applications*, vol. 206, p. 103460, 2022, doi: 10.1016/j.jnca.2022.103460.

[42] A. L. Imoize, J. Hemanth, D.-T. Do, and S. N. Sur, *Explainable Artificial Intelligence in Medical Decision Support Systems*, London: Institution of Engineering and Technology, 2022. doi:10.1049/PBHE050E.

Chapter 5

Artificial intelligence and blockchain enabling data access authorization in telehealth systems

Peace Busola Falola[1], Joseph Bamidele Awotunde[2], Abidemi Emmanuel Adeniyi[3], Rasheed Gbenga Jimoh[2], Aminat Omotayo Adebayo[4], Ezekiel K. Olatunji[5] and Agbotiname Lucky Imoize[6]

Artificial intelligence (AI) and blockchain (BC) technologies have emerged as powerful tools in revolutionizing data access authorization in telehealth applications. This chapter explores the integrations of AI and BC and their implications for secure and transparent data access in telehealth. Through real-life case studies, the benefits and applications of AI-driven access authorization mechanisms and BC-enabled data storage and verification can be analyzed. The integration of AI in telehealth systems enables advanced data analysis, interpretation, and decision-making. AI algorithms can process vast amounts of patient data, providing accurate diagnoses, personalized treatment recommendations, and valuable insights. This integration enhances the efficiency and effectiveness of healthcare processes, leading to improved patient care outcomes. With its decentralized and immutable nature, BC technology ensures data integrity, privacy, and transparency. By leveraging BC, telehealth systems can establish trust and accountability in data access authorization. Managing individuals' health data grants access only to authorized individuals or organizations. BC-enabled smart contracts facilitate the secure sharing of healthcare data, enabling stakeholder collaboration while preserving data privacy. The real-life applications of AI and BC in telehealth, such as

[1]Department of Computer Sciences, Faculty of Pure and Applied Sciences, Precious Cornerstone University, Nigeria
[2]Department of Computer Science, Faculty of Communication and Information Sciences, University of Ilorin, Nigeria
[3]Department of Computer Science, College of Computing and Communication Studies, Bowen University, Nigeria
[4]Department of Computer Science, Faculty of Sciences, Al-Hikmah University, Nigeria
[5]Department of Computer Science, Faculty of Computing and Applied Sciences, Thomas Adewumi University, Nigeria
[6]Department of Electrical and Electronics Engineering, Faculty of Engineering, University of Lagos, Nigeria

Medicalchain, Nebula Genomics, and Shivom, demonstrate the successful integration of AI and BC in telehealth systems. This chapter discusses potential areas of research and development, including enhancing interoperability between AI algorithms and BC systems, incorporating privacy-preserving techniques, and exploring federated learning approaches. Combining BC and AI technologies enables secure, transparent, and patient-centric data access authorization in telehealth systems. By leveraging AI advanced data analysis capabilities and BC secure and immutable ledger, telehealth systems can enhance healthcare delivery, empower patients, foster research collaboration, and improve patient outcomes.

5.1 Introduction

The rapid advancements in technology have revolutionized the healthcare industry, particularly in telehealth. Telehealth systems offer convenient access to medical services remotely, bridging the gap between patients and healthcare professionals. However, with this convenience comes the critical challenge of ensuring the confidentiality and safety of sensitive patient information. Information and communication technology development has simplified and streamlined data collecting for health and the environment [1]. For instance, the growing storage capacity of clusters of computers now allows portable sensors to gather data continually. Nonetheless, the obtained data is often not used to its full ability. Nonetheless, low-cost data storage and the growing processing capability of technologies encourage the generation of enormous databases containing untapped health and environmental data [2].

The growing explosion in medical information has prompted the establishment of firms offering cloud and quantum computing data storage amenities. The preservation of safety and confidentiality while promoting connectivity is a fundamental concern for these services, especially for sensitive information related to genetics, habits, and other factors in digital medical records. The distributed blockchain (BC) idea, which underpins the trade of digital currencies, has found adoption in the healthcare industry and is promising to enhance clinical and cloud-based medical studies.

Data access authorization is crucial to telehealth systems, as it governs who can access and modify patient information [3]. Traditional authorization methods, such as centralized databases and role-based access control, have limitations when it comes to scalability, security, and transparency. To address these challenges, BC technology and artificial intelligence (AI) are emerging as promising solutions.

AI can improve the accuracy and productivity of data access authorization in telehealth systems. AI algorithms can learn from patterns and historical data to identify potential security breaches or unauthorized access attempts, thus bolstering the system's overall security. Additionally, AI can carry out challenging computational tasks and swiftly analyze huge amounts of patient data. Despite AI's remarkable abilities, some physicians are still wary about utilizing it in medical care, especially in roles that might affect a patient's wellness. After all, AI has proven that it can perform various flexible and mental tasks quicker than a person can. The capacity of the auto industry to use AI to create autonomous vehicles has already been shown. However, some businesses have discovered methods to use machine learning to spot fraud or detect financial dangers. Only a few examples show the sophistication of AI [4].

BC technology, on the other hand, provides a decentralized and immutable ledger that records all transactions and interactions within a telehealth system [5]. It ensures transparency and trust by eliminating the need for intermediaries, such as centralized authorities or third-party auditors. By leveraging BC, telehealth systems can maintain a tamperproof record of data access requests, granting access only to authorized individuals or entities. BC technology can confirm authentication and rights by enabling distributed copies of documents or bioinformatic programming codes and enabling users to control selective intellectual property transmission. While maintaining the confidentiality of patient data archives (unique descriptors taken from electronic health records (EHRs), wearable technology, genomic or exomic profiles, etc.), BC computing (i.e., distributed Hyperledger technology) can be used in medical care to achieve the advantages of sophisticated analytics and electronic currency trading [6–9].

The integration of AI and BC in telehealth systems for data access authorization offers several advantages. First, it enhances security by detecting and preventing unauthorized real-time access attempts. Additionally, it gives patients greater influence on their data by enabling them to approve or remove access as necessary. Moreover, it enables healthcare providers to streamline their operations by automating the authorization process and reducing administrative overhead.

Employing BC, AI, and other readily available technology is the key to achievement [10,11]. In order to advance clinical innovation and achieve patient-centricity, the sector would leverage technology user- and customer-focused platforms and info-driven options for innovative data-handling approaches and enhanced outcomes [12]. Medical trial data was tracked utilizing quantitative drug development techniques and AI for reinventing commercial drugs, investigating the efficacy of pharmaceutical formulations, and dosage monitoring [13–15]. Governments must choose the best strategies for leveraging resources and advancing change in this quickly changing environment while guaranteeing data's essential uniformity, conformity, or privacy [16].

This chapter explores the potential of combining AI and BC technologies to enable robust data access authorization in telehealth systems. We delve into the technical aspects of integrating these technologies and discuss the advantages and difficulties of implementing them. Additionally, we examine real-world use cases and present examples of AI and BC-enabled data access authorization systems in the telehealth domain.

5.1.1 Key contributions of the chapter

The points that follow are the chapter's main contributions:

1. The chapter highlights how the integration of AI and BC can enhance the safety and confidentiality of patient data in telehealth systems. Utilizing BC technology ensures the inviolability and transparency of data access records,

providing patients with greater control over their health information. By leveraging AI algorithms, the system can proactively detect and prevent efforts at unwanted entry, lowering the likelihood of data thefts.

2. Combining AI and BC eliminates the need for intermediaries, enabling faster and more efficient authorization workflows.
3. The chapter explores real-world use cases and examples of AI and BC-enabled data access authorization systems in telehealth.
4. The contribution of this chapter lies in its exploration of how the combination of AI and BC technologies enables robust data access authorization in telehealth systems. It provides a thorough awareness of the prospective advantages, difficulties, and real-world applications, paving the way for further advancement in the field. This chapter significantly contributes to the knowledge and development of secure and efficient healthcare systems (HSs).

5.1.2 Chapter organization

Section 5.2 presents the related works on integrating AI and BC technologies for data authorization in telehealth systems. Section 5.3 discusses the AI applications in telehealth systems and its role in data access authorization. Section 5.4 presents BC technology in telehealth systems and its overview in telehealth systems. Section 5.5 discusses the integration of AI and BC for data access authorization in telehealth systems. Section 5.6 presents real-life case studies of AI and BC integration for data access authorization in telehealth systems. Section 5.7 concludes the chapter and presents future research directions.

5.2 Related work

This section gives a brief presentation of related work. In the existing literature, Elvas *et al.* [17] noted how confidentiality and safety concerns make exchanging medical information a significant challenge. Companies and crooks value medical data highly. Because medical information may be used for both past and future studies at a low cost, the European Commission has designated it as a special asset. This research suggested using a BC platform to facilitate safe, open clinical data sharing across healthcare organizations. The authors used design science research methodology (DSRM) to create a lab-based prototype. According to the authors' patient-centric approach, individuals are the proprietors of their data and may provide clinics and medical personnel entry.

According to [18], technology developments and growing use in medical care operations, including data collecting, archiving, diagnoses, and medical care, are the main reasons healthcare has substantially evolved in the past few years. The growth of linked medical facilities has advanced electronic healthcare thanks to the emergence of the Industrial Internet of Things (IIoT), which may greatly increase data connection, exposure, and interoperability, resulting in a better standard of care provided to patients.

However, the widespread use of future e-healthcare infrastructure is being hampered by increasing worries about the protection and secrecy of medical data, particularly when it is gathered, distributed, and handled via innovative linked sensor gadgets. Due to the restricted abilities of the IoT devices used, there is a safety concern about the confidentiality, honesty, authorization, and access management of the data throughout the front-end and back-end data transmission in medical records chat. The authors looked at how distributed ledger technology (DLT) may be used to tackle these safety concerns for new HSs. To establish safe data exchange inside a HS and demonstrate the viability of the suggested method for protecting healthcare data in a linked IIoT context, they employed masked authenticated messaging (MAM) via the Tangle. Additionally, they evaluated and analyzed data transfer concerning operation time productivity and encryption criteria.

Electronic-Healthcare is one of the emerging concepts in the healthcare sector, according to [19]. Doctors want a single-patient database that contains a wealth of helpful information to analyze patient records. Changing the healthcare data of healthcare and its unique entities will create a severe risk of sensitive e-Health data leakage. A major barrier for the healthcare sector will be safeguarding patients' private information. The social services field is quite progressive, and a lot of data collected from different sensors and saved in the cloud is also used extensively in this field. Processing patient data daily and allocating its memory is necessary to deal with the enormous amount of data generated in the electronic-healthcare sector. Instead of keeping this medical information on one server, the cloud is the greatest solution for dispersed storage. Therefore, whatever data was collected from it was encrypted with BC technology, and before the data were sent to the cloud storage, a private electronic ring signature was employed to confirm the identity of the intended user and protect patient privacy in distributed EHRs. This study improved the e-healthcare cloud's private data privacy by utilizing BC technology and anonymous ring signatures, making it appropriate for actual time applications.

According to [20], e-HSs are extensively used in hospitals thanks to the numerous applications of the IoT and the popularity of wearable technology. The electronic medical record (EMR), a major bearer of medical data, is easy to save and recover, considerably simplifying the process of medical care and reducing the unnecessary labor of paramedics. EMRs typically contain a lot of private data, including patient ID numbers or home addresses, which is easily accessible to unapproved physicians and cloud servers. Based on this worry, attribute-based encryption (ABE) may be used by e-HSs to safeguard private data while establishing fine-grained access control of encrypted EMRs. However, most ABE schemes do not enable keyword search and policy concealing. Inner product encryption (IPE) can hide access policies and specify access rights so that only individuals with matching characteristics can access the intended files.

Additionally, the suggested approach coupled federated BC (FB) with searchable encryption (SE) to perform an effective and reliable multi-keyword search. MK-IPSE demonstrated superior compute and storage performance in comparison to the previous systems. Security studies also revealed that the plan could withstand IND-CKA and collusion assaults.

Digitalization and automation have always had a significant influence on healthcare, according to [21]. It encompasses all cutting-edge and novel technologies. Recently, the metaverse, a novel digital technology, has been developed globally. The metaverse has a wealth of expertise and has great potential to provide patients and healthcare practitioners with an extensive selection of health services. In order to deliver better, quicker healthcare facilities in cyberspace that are safer with an authentic user experience, this study suggested combining BC technology with AI in the metaverse. BC technology helps physicians and patients interact in a metaverse environment while protecting the secrecy, confidentiality, and protection of patient data. The primary component of their suggested design is the metaverse platform. The nurses, physicians, and patients all access this setting by signing up on the BC, and they are all portrayed in the metaverse environment by avatars. The doctor and patient's session will be documented, and all the data—including pictures, audio, text, videos, and clinical information—will be collected, sent to, and kept on the BC. Explainable AI (XAI) models employ these data to forecast and diagnose diseases. GradCAM and LIME approaches from XAI employ logical thinking to build confidence, explainability, understanding, and openness in diagnosing and prognosis disorders. BC technology protects patient data while making it visible, traceable, and unchangeable. These BC features ensure that patients can trust the information they provide.

As a consequence, the recommended design ensures transparency and dependability in terms of both disease diagnostics and patient data security. The writers also looked at the metaverse's foundational technologies. They also looked at the benefits and difficulties of a healthcare metaverse.

According to [22], virtual health monitoring can aid in illness prevention at an early phase. Recently developed IoT ideas allow for constant surveillance. Due to the dire circumstances, these systems require high-quality attributes, such as availability and accuracy. Deep learning algorithms have potential in such health applications when there is a lot of data available. These approaches are perfect for an IoT system built on a distributed BC. The frequency of these system answers depends heavily on the Internet connection quality. Smart gateway devices cannot use deep learning algorithms due to their restricted computing power. The deep learning model categorized the brain conditions as benign or malignant. The study included AD, moderate cognitive impairment, and typical mental level as three separate classifications to categorize the brain illness as benign or malignant. The study includes several processing steps, most of which were used to train these classifiers, and an ensemble model followed by a metaclassifier to group the final resulting class. The model was then trained and evaluated using the UDS dataset from ADNI. The findings demonstrated that the suggested approach answered the query with a high level of accuracy (98%) and quick retrieval of results that were categorized, with an improved training accuracy of 0.539 and testing accuracy of 0.559.

According to [23], telehealth systems have developed into more commonplace solutions that can provide care to patients at home and in faraway locations via smart devices and 5G networks. In these online systems, preserving users' safety and confidentiality is essential. Despite the numerous protocols that offer safety through reliable authentication mechanisms, advanced IoT assaults are rising. According to the authors, solving authentication issues for human and IoT devices requires machine learning to deal with biometric data or physical layer properties. The study included the uses of machine learning to suggest reliable verification mechanisms. These dynamic verification models may be more trustworthy than conventional techniques since machine learning techniques are developed using hidden ideas in biometric and physical layer data. The fundamental benefit of these techniques is how difficult it is to imitate human and technological behavior. Machine learning also makes it possible to authenticate continuously while considering the context.

A critical component of a patient's follow-up is the use of a medical record, according to [24]. It includes the opinions, recommendations, evaluations, and patient data of healthcare specialists. The client, physician, and pharmacist are among those involved in exchanging and handling this information. The EMR is accessible by anybody with authorization from any location, and the information is shared with a variety of healthcare service providers. Sharing the EMR is subject to a variety of criteria, including privacy and safety. According to the authors, present medical systems make it difficult to offer trustworthy services and may be vulnerable to malware infiltration and system failure. This fusion makes decentralized, granular, and dynamic access control management possible for EMR administration. Such a solution is made possible by BC technology, which functions as a safely distributed ledger and access control system to offer participants in the system transparency, reliability, immutability, and trustworthiness.

To provide patients with safe, decentralized control over their medical data, Ghosh *et al.* [25] set out to create a PHR management solution using smart contracts on the Ethereum BC. Personal health records (PHRs) are useful tools because they allow people to handle and combine their medical data. Patients can monitor their health data using a PHR, an electronic tool. The chance to rebalance the doctor–patient relationship is attractive when patients are given access to their medical records. However, according to the authors, present PHR operating systems fall short of giving patients reliable, traceable, and secure power over their health information, posing serious dangers to their validity and sensitive nature.

Furthermore, the majority of PHR management methods and platforms now in use are centralized, increasing the risk of exchanging medical data and the possibility of a sole opinion of disaster. In this study, patients have authority over their data using decentralized, unchanging, open identifiable, trustworthy, and secure smart contracts developed on the Ethereum BC. The project aims to create a PHR management system built on Ethereum BC smart contracts that give patients safe, decentralized control of their medical data. The authors concluded that the recommended system might be a Web3 application that securely collects, stores, and exchanges patient medical data using decentralized IPFS storage and the Ganache, Truffle, and MetaMask tools.

In their paper, Zaman *et al.* [26] addressed how the healthcare industry's information processing paradigm is changing as a consequence of the improvement of computing and communication technology. Since medical data is kept electronically, saving and accessing patient data remotely is simple. However, transforming HSs into intelligent healthcare settings presents difficulties and added demands. The IoT creates a network by connecting objects, including computing devices, via wired or wireless connections. Due to the absence of intrinsic security features, there are several security flaws and threats in the current IoT-based systems. For instance, gathering and maintaining EHRs is thought impossible without considering patient medical data, confidentiality of information, data exchange, and ease. However, because of varying security standards and data access patterns, typical IoT-based EHR systems cannot handle these paradigms. BC technology is a distributed ledger that is useful for preserving patient data and overcoming problems with data integrity and privacy. As a result, it is a workable solution to the problems with IoT data safety and confidentiality that are now present. By boosting data security, confidentiality, and transparency, BC opens a significant way for revolutionizing established IoT systems. The scientific community has demonstrated a range of AI-based healthcare applications that enhance health diagnosis and monitoring procedures.

Additionally, entrepreneurs and technology businesses are transforming the healthcare industry using AI and associated technologies. This study demonstrated the value of integrating BC, IoT, and AI technologies to address expanding healthcare concerns. This study analyzed the developments of these novel paradigms in the medical care industry and looked at how BC technology and IoT were integrated. Additionally, their research study provided a thorough analysis of the technologies that are needed to create the smart, safe, and future Internet of health things (IoHT). The uniqueness of the IoHT environment, as well as the advancement, efficiency, and security of the supporting technologies, is all thoroughly studied in this paper. First, BC technologies' security and performance advantages are mapped to identify the research needs. Second, practical concerns about integrating BC and IoT devices are highlighted. Third, IoT, BC, and ML in healthcare contexts are examined for healthcare applications. Lastly, study deficiencies, potential directions, and enabling technology limits are highlighted.

Deebak *et al.* [27] talked about how sustainable urbanization projects employ ICT-based innovation to boost smart city service efficiency and uncover new business prospects. Smart sustainable cities prefer IoT connectivity and data integration to satisfy the requirements of new computing paradigms with supporting technologies. Digital applications (DApps) entail the continual creation of IoT data across a dedicated gateway to provide broad connectivity and enhanced access control. Conversely, it remains difficult to guarantee device safety due to a critical privacy-preserving IoT concern. Significantly, the current procedures don't make any safety claims about user anonymity and the exchange of authentication keys with formal evidence. Therefore, this research presents the seamless authentication framework with a privacy-preserving (SAF-PP) protocol to address smart e-Health intelligence's security and privacy concerns.

Dubey and Verma [28] discussed that telemedicine is effective for treating unreachable sufferers in hospitals or private clinics. These four pillars are important: instant communication, accumulate and forwards, telemonitoring or distant patient care, and mobile health (mHealth). The wearables are very important in providing essential signs, which are respiratory rate, oxygen saturation, the temperature of the body, and breathing patterns to diagnose any disease. These wearables have sensors, and all vital signs are captured in these. With the progression of information technology, cloud computing has come into existence, and all these sensors are connected to a network so that medical practices will respond properly to patients on time through Tele-calling. This study began with the prologue of AI, IoT, and BC, concerning telemedicine. Digital health transmission through these cutting-edge technologies was also discussed. The AI-based bot "aapka sawasthaya salahkar" was developed for primary disease diagnosis for patients (malaria was addressed here). It's easy to use virtual assistants or message-based methods. In this way, patients can book an appointment with a doctor or utilize a questionnaire to understand their disease for treatment. This will also allow video calls if needed. An AI-based BC model called innovative AI-based secure telemedicine model (IAISTM) is developed. This model is a promising tool to protect all kinds of data of patients and is available on demand, capable of working on time. AI in healthcare is rapidly making its path to provide the whole chain of clinical practice and patient-focused care. With the assessment of BC technology, security to all kinds of communications and data recordings of healthcare was enhanced. IAISTM can store all the EHRs that are shared between patients and healthcare providers. This could work from patient disease identification, monitoring, and treatment to proper care with personal assistance, including follow-ups and providing medicines at doorsteps. Hence, easy to use, trustable, and significant use of AI-based telemedicine can reach any remote place where patients hesitate to reach medical professionals due to social stigma. This study also explored the different applications of the model with existing techniques. And prospects were also highlighted.

Geetanjali *et al.* [29] addressed how a variety of cutting-edge technology might lower the cost of treating chronic diseases. There are several options for monitoring health, including wearable technologies and mobile applications (apps). Researchers, patients, and physicians all utilize these technologies to assess a subject's health. AI has several useful uses in the administration of healthcare. AI systems simplify detecting diseases, including cardiac abnormalities, lung and heart issues, strokes, and neurological disorders. The AI system gathers data, sends it to analysts, and assists in lowering healthcare risks. Devices for discipline and self-monitoring are helpful for the elderly and those who are unable to see doctors often. It helps patients and healthcare professionals establish a safe, confidential, and reliable relationship. BC technology supports the analysis, protection, and transparency of massive data in the healthcare industry. The quick development of analytics techniques can govern healthcare data and enhance living.

Tolba and Al-Makhadmeh [30] discussed how current HSs depend on system-aided exploration and communication technologies to give end users trustworthy medical services. Healthcare and grid data will be handled only when necessary to increase safety measures to prevent unwelcome access to private information. In order to stop unauthorized access to medical data, this study introduced the predictive data analysis (PDA) method to HSs. The various medical and grid data are studied in this PDA study to communicate knowledge via the transfer learning function. To categorize the loss and forecast correct analytical data, the data matching procedure was repeatedly carried out. The suggested method's extensive learning and training procedure distinguishes between legitimate and unauthorized access to healthcare data. The effectiveness of the suggested technique is assessed using the metrics accuracy, data loss, and processing time by changing the number of users and the quantity of the data accordingly.

According to [31], upon request access to medical data and the requirement for high-quality patient care are the primary drivers of digital health trends (DHTs). With the development of AI, the advancement of electronic healthcare has accelerated and is anticipated to accelerate further as the sector moves toward BC technology. BC is a DLT that may be encrypted and decentralized. There have been a growing number of uses outside of finance for this technology, most of which are important for medical imaging. It was first developed for cryptocurrencies and is most frequently used.

Along with potential implementation challenges, including public–private key access, distributed book size constraints, speed and complexity issues, and safety flaws. Common pictures, image ownership of a patient, device tracking for medical devices, research, teleradiology, and AI are examples of potential BC applications that are especially pertinent for medical imaging. BC technology opens wonderful possibilities for safe and immutable data, trust-free cooperation, and the elimination of complexity. The writers of this report included a thorough analysis of the BC in healthcare, including its benefits and drawbacks, applications, and guiding principles. Based on diverse technologies, they also briefly reviewed the problems and their solutions, guiding researchers in new directions.

The most prominent international catchphrase for the year 2020, according to [32], is "Stay Home; Stay Safe." In the COVID-19 epidemic, the IoT has filled the distance between the physical and digital worlds. With its scientific, social, and economic potential, it offers a viable answer to contemporary health problems. The quick rise in instances confirmed by laboratory testing makes it possible for individuals to safeguard themselves against diseases thanks to this technical innovation. Even if a person contracts COVID-19 virus, IoT-based medical equipment aids in virtual surveillance during quarantine to stop the spread of illnesses to the general population. The security of patient data is in danger because of the countless bogus news stories concerning COVID-19 that are exposed daily. BC and AI technologies are being investigated to further solve these issues. A comprehensive evaluation of the state of telemedicine, the Internet of medical things, and the IoHT industries is also given. The study suggested a brand-new classification called "Internet of Covid Things," along with several difficulties. The framework for the evaluation also covered industry factors related to the production of medical gadgets and mobile applications that will help practically everyone assist with remote surveillance during quarantine to stop the spread of infection to the general population.

According to [33], information technology advancements are transforming the healthcare industry to provide better medical services, diagnostics, constant surveillance through wearable technologies, etc. at a lower cost. This digitalization makes it easier to compute, store, and access medical records, which helps patients to receive better care. However, there is a chance for cyberattacks and safety and confidentiality issues concerning this digital data. Therefore, to address the safety and confidentiality issues presently lacking in current e-Health systems, the authors of their study gave a BC-based approach to healthcare data.

Patient authentication is considered a crucial safety need in an online health monitoring system, according to [34]. Credential-based verification methods that rely on sensors—such as orientation, a user's finger, or a camera—from a usability standpoint are not very practical for medical applications. Additionally, patients could give their credentials to a third party, going against the privacy rules. Therefore, further research is needed to emphasize the problems and discuss how complete the remedies are. This work explored the unresolved problems with multilayer systematic review-based mHealth authentication methods. The study also explored the architecture and assessed patient usability using a novel sensor-based smartphone verification method. For real-time mHealth monitoring systems, a new verification mechanism that utilizes 3D touch and microphone sensors was put forth. Three separate and succeeding phases of the suggested strategy were given, and the methodological components of the strategy were explored.

Health information exchange (HIE) has been shown by [35] to provide outstanding advantages for patient care, including enhancing healthcare value and accelerating coordinated treatment. Patient-centric HIE is now faced with several challenges, such as concerns over security and privacy, conflicting data, and sluggish entry to the necessary information across many healthcare institutions. After examining the present HIE workflow, this study offered a workable solution to these problems by leveraging BC. This method accomplishes patient-centric HIE by customizing data segmentation and creating an "allowed list" for doctors to acquire their data. Using a large-scale simulation of this patient-centric HIE process, the authors statistically assessed the model's viability, steadiness, safety, and resilience.

BC technology is one of the most modern and disruptive innovations in the world, according to [36]. The authors of this paper used BC technology to perform a current investigation of applications and advances in the healthcare sector. Along with some present difficulties and potential remedies, they also talked about several strong applications and numerous businesses now employing BC technology to secure their data.

5.2.1 Summary of related work

Table 5.1 gives a summary of the related work of this chapter. It displays the methodology used by each study, the result obtained, and the gap identified or the future research direction of each study reviewed.

Safety precautions in e-Health using BC and AI are mentioned in Figure 5.1. With safe and automated data analysis, ledgers, or content blocks, may be created

Table 5.1 Summary of related work

Author	Methodology	Result	Gap/future direction
Elvas *et al.* [17]	A blockchain framework to enable the transparent sharing of medical information among health entities in a secure environment	A patient-centric approach holds that patients are the owners of their information and may grant permission to their information to clinics and other healthcare providers	AI can be incorporated into the system for more robust features
Abdullah *et al.* [18]	They used masked authenticated messaging (MAM) over the Tangle for the healthcare industry to ensure safe data exchange	The Tangle offered tamperproof solutions and helped in attaining security	AI can be incorporated into the system for more robust features
Grover and Kushwaha [19]	Blockchain technology and an anonymous digital ring signature were used to authorize the intended user and maintain, before transmitting information to remote storage, the confidentiality of individual cloud-based data dispersed in digital health record systems	The protection of personal data of the patient health data was enhanced with blockchain and anonymous ring signatures in the e-healthcare cloud	AI can be incorporated into the system for more robust features
Liu *et al.* [20]	An inner product searchable encryption scheme with multi-keyword search (MK-IPSE) using blockchain technology to enable complete confidentiality protection and effective ciphertext retrieval for EMRs	Security analysis demonstrated that the scheme can resist IND-CKA and collusion attacks	AI can be incorporated into the system for more robust features
Ali *et al.* [21]	Metaverse environment assisted by blockchain technology that ensures the safety, security, and privacy of data	The architecture ensured transparency and trust regarding both the diagnosis of illnesses and the patient's data safety	AI can be incorporated into the system for more robust features
Hannah *et al.* [22]	Deep neural networks based on blockchain for faster healthcare data transmission in a healthcare management platform	The results showed that the proposed method accurately (98%) responded to the request with rapid extraction of categorized answers and improved training and testing accuracy of 0.539 and 0.559	The training and testing accuracy is low. Security of the data was not discussed

Hazratifard *et al.* [23]	Using machine learning to manage biometric data or physical layer attributes to solve verification issues for people and Internet of Things devices	Gadgets and human behavior were difficult to imitate. Also, machine learning facilitated continuous and context-aware authentication	Blockchain can be incorporated into the system for more robust features
Mhamdi *et al.* [24]	SEMRAchain is a system based on access control [role-based access control (RBAC), attribute-based access control (ABAC)] and a smart contract approach	Decentralized, fine-grained, and dynamic access control management for EMR management plus a secure distributed ledger and such an approach is provided by access control, which thanks to blockchain technology gives system stakeholders not just transparency but also reliability, trustworthiness, and immutability	AI can be incorporated into the system for more robust features
Ghosh *et al.* [25]	Ethereum blockchain-based smart contracts PHR management solution to supply patients with secure, decentralized ownership over their medical data	The proposed system was successful	AI can be incorporated into the system for more robust features
Deebak *et al.* [27]	A seamless authentication framework with privacy-preserving (SAF-PP) protocol to deal concerning smart e-Health intelligence safety and confidentiality problems	SAF-PP can adhere to significant security properties while improving the system efficiency rate. The suggested SAF-PP is more effective at expanding the number of active users thanks to an enhanced packet delivery ratio and network life span, according to the effectiveness analysis	Issues with blockchain technology in the healthcare industry were identified
Dubey and Verma [28]	An AI-based blockchain model was developed called innovative AI-based secure telemedicine model (IAISTM)	IAISTM can store all the electronic health records that are shared between patients and healthcare providers	The security of patients' data needs to be emphasized
Tolba and Al-Makhadmeh [30]	A predictive data analysis (PDA) approach for HSs to prevent illegal access to medical data was developed	The intensive learning and training process of the proposed method differentiated authenticated and illegal access to healthcare data	Blockchain can be incorporated into the system for more robust features

(Continues)

Table 5.1 (Continued)

Author	Methodology	Result	Gap/future direction
Jennath *et al.* [33]	A blockchain-based solution for healthcare records to address security and privacy concerns. Also, constructing reliable AI algorithms on top of blockchain for e-Health	A transparent platform for consent-based data sharing by the users was designed	The security of patients' data needs to be emphasized
Shuwandy *et al.* [34]	A new microphone and 3D touch for verification sensors were proposed for real-time health monitoring systems	The proposed methodology was intended to be modeled and put into practice later on as an example of confidentiality protection in verification methods, leading to long-lasting and highly functional utilization in mHealth apps	AI and blockchain can be incorporated into the system for more robust features
Zhuang *et al.* [35]	A patient-centric health information exchange (HIE) using blockchain technology to establish data provenance, safeguard patient confidentiality and safety, and give patients complete authority over their medical information	The model's feasibility, stability, security, and robustness were attained	AI can be incorporated into the system for more robust features

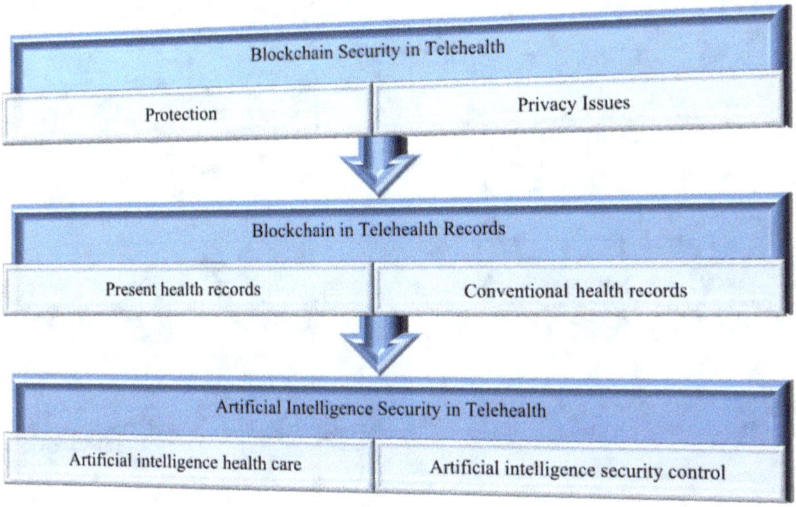

Figure 5.1 Blockchain and AI safety in telehealth

and managed thanks to BC technology. AI started to learn and think like a physician to understand health trends and patterns [37,38]. It collects unorganized information from a variety of sources, such as the patient, the radiologist, and the pictures.

5.3 Artificial intelligence applications in telehealth systems

AI is the scientific and technological method of creating intelligent computer systems that can perform tasks that would otherwise put people under stress at work. To respond to a query or make a conclusion, these computer systems use a variety of recommended algorithms, decision-making power, and vast amounts of data [13].

The effectiveness of autonomous automobiles, developments in medical research, and personal wearable devices have shown how far technology has progressed in recent years [39]. Healthcare is expected to continue to be the first industry, given the advancements achieved in many other sectors, where AI could have an impact that goes above usefulness and positively impacts human lives [40]. The use of AI in telehealth systems is expanding in several areas, including online patient surveillance and medical image analysis, among others (see Figure 5.2).

The figure describes how AI is applied in telehealth. Table 5.2 provides an overview of these applications and their relevance in improving telehealth systems.

5.3.1 Role of AI in data access authorization

The role of AI in data access authorization in telehealth is crucial for enhancing security, efficiency, and accountability within the system. AI performs various roles

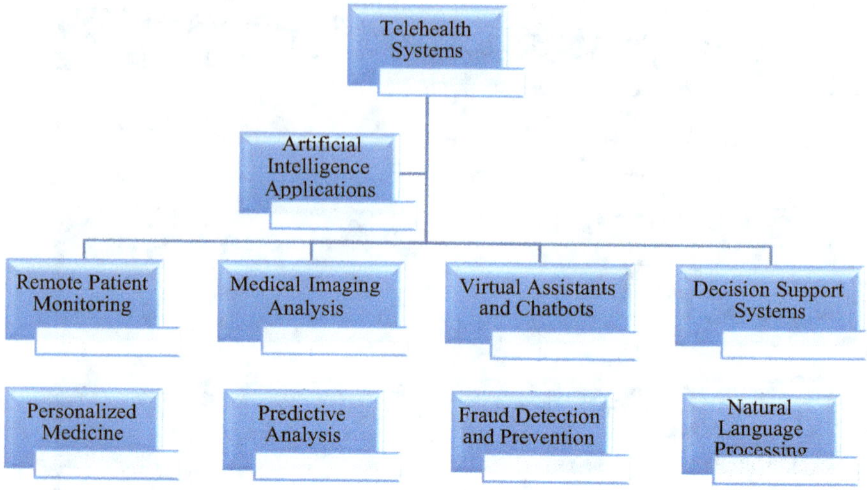

Figure 5.2 Artificial intelligence applications in telehealth

Table 5.2 Artificial intelligence applications in telehealth [41]

Application	Description
Remote patient monitoring	AI algorithms can analyze patient data collected remotely, such as vital signs, symptoms, and behavior, to detect patterns and provide insights to healthcare providers
Medical imaging analysis	AI can analyze medical images (X-rays, MRIs, among others) to aid in illness identification and diagnosis, such as cancer or abnormalities in scans, aiding radiologists in their assessments
Virtual assistants and chatbots	AI-powered virtual assistants and chatbots can provide patient support, answer queries, and offer basic medical advice, improving accessibility and convenience for patients seeking information
Predictive analytics	AI algorithms can utilize patient data to predict potential health risks, disease progression, or adverse events enabling proactive interventions and personalized treatment plans
Decision support systems	AI can assist healthcare professionals in making clinical decisions by analyzing patient data, medical records, research literature, and treatment guidelines, and providing evidence-based recommendations
Natural language processing	AI algorithms can process and understand natural language, facilitating the extraction of relevant information from medical texts, clinical notes, and patient records for analysis and decision-making
Personalized medicine	AI can analyze large datasets to identify patient-specific treatment options, considering factors like genetics, medical history, and lifestyle, leading to personalized and targeted interventions
Fraud detection and prevention	AI can analyze healthcare data to identify patterns of fraudulent activities, such as billing fraud or insurance abuse, helping in the prevention and early detection of fraudulent practices.

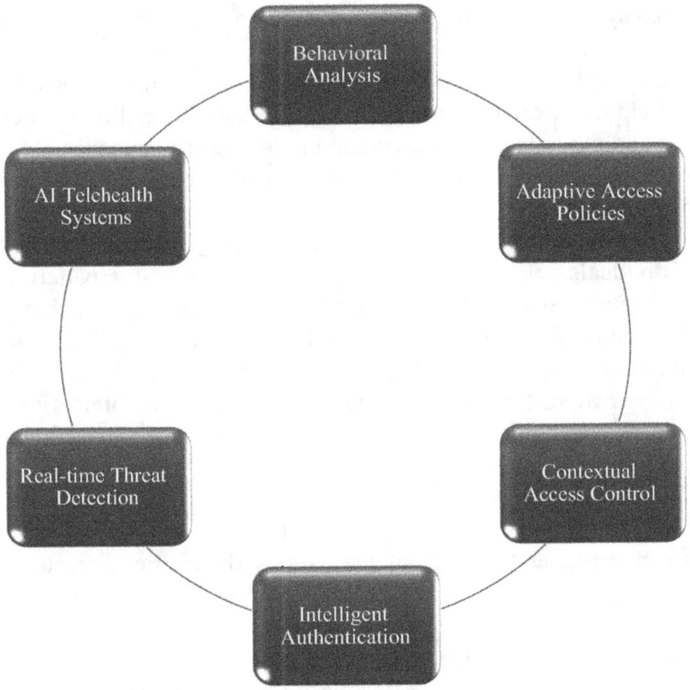

Figure 5.3 AI for data access authorization in telehealth

to ensure authorized access and protect patient data [41]. AI enables real-time threat detection by continuously monitoring access requests and analyzing patterns to identify potential security threats or unauthorized access attempts. It incorporates intelligent authentication methods, such as facial or voice recognition, to enhance the authentication process and ensure that only authorized individuals can access patient data. AI plays a crucial role in auditing and compliance by automating the auditing process. It generates detailed logs of data access activities, ensuring transparency, accountability, and compliance with data protection regulations. The AI techniques facilitate predictive authorization by analyzing historical data and user behavior patterns [42]. It predicts future access authorization needs, streamlining the authorization process and improving efficiency. This strengthens data access authorization in telehealth systems, safeguarding patient information and ensuring secure and accountable access to healthcare data. The visual representation of AI for data access authorization in a telehealth system is provided in Figure 5.3.

5.3.2 Artificial intelligence algorithms for user authentication and authorization

AI algorithms for user authentication and authorization in a telehealth system are designed to increase the system's effectiveness and safety by leveraging AI techniques [43]. These algorithms utilize machine learning, pattern recognition, and advanced biometric technologies to authenticate and authorize users to access telehealth services and sensitive patient data.

The process of telehealth verification involves confirming a user's identification of an individual before granting access to the system. Traditional methods such as usernames and passwords can be vulnerable to security breaches. AI algorithms introduce more robust and sophisticated authentication mechanisms, such as which are as follows:

Biometric authentication: AI algorithms leverage biometric characteristics unique to individuals, such as fingerprints, facial features, iris patterns, or voiceprints, to authenticate users. These algorithms compare captured biometric data with stored reference templates to verify identity, providing higher security.

Behavioral authentication: AI algorithms analyze user behavior patterns, including typing patterns, mouse movements, or touchscreen interactions, to create a unique behavioral profile. This profile authenticates users by comparing their real-time behavior with the established profile.

Multi-factor authentication (MFA): AI algorithms can incorporate multiple authentication factors, such as something the user knows (password), something the user has (smart card), and something the user is (biometric characteristic). MFA improves safety by allowing users to submit many forms of identification verification.

Telehealth authorization is granting specific access rights and permissions to authenticated users based on their roles and responsibilities. AI algorithms for user authorization in telehealth systems offer the following capabilities:

Role-based access control (RBAC): AI algorithms implement RBAC models, adding access rights based on predefined roles. Users are granted access to specific resources and functionalities based on their assigned roles, ensuring appropriate access privileges.

Contextual access control: AI algorithms analyze contextual information, such as user location, time of access, and device used, to determine the appropriate level of access authorization. This ensures that access is granted only in specific contexts and reduces the risk of unauthorized access.

Adaptive access policies: AI algorithms dynamically adjust access policies based on changing circumstances. The algorithms can modify access privileges in real time by considering factors like user behavior, network conditions, and security threats, providing a flexible and adaptive authorization framework.

The AI algorithms for user authentication and authorization in telehealth systems help mitigate security risks, protect patient data, and ensure that only people with permission can access private medical information. They contribute to building a trustworthy and safe environment for telehealth services, enhancing patient data's overall privacy and confidentiality.

5.4 Blockchain technology in telehealth systems

HSs are created to meet our needs in terms of health, and as our populace ages, so do our needs in terms of efficiency [44]. Concerning COVID-19, health-related information about a patient, such as their temperature or symptoms, is very helpful [44–46]. There is a heightened understanding of medical concerns and a requirement for improved client care as society matures and more individuals suffer chronic illnesses [47]. The safety of all Internet-enabled devices is the other significant concern in digital and ubiquitous healthcare [44].

BC integration in the healthcare industry results in decentralized computing, archiving, and enhanced safety. Due to the reliability of its data and the breadth of its uses, BC has recently gained popularity [43]. BC offers a framework for decentralization and confidence in various programs, including banking, business, IoT, reputation management, and healthcare [43]. The trust deficit in traditional HIE intermediations continues to be exposed by EHRs, conflicting passions, and several other reasons [43]. Therefore, BC technology has made healthcare an ideal choice and has lately attracted attention.

Safety, connectivity, non-repudiation, authorization of entry, authorization, medical data exchange, and mobility are just a few of the special needs the healthcare sector faces. EHRs, EMRs, and PHRs are the three types of computerized health records. It is crucial to offer authentication-appropriate access control to such data. Additionally, the query to get healthcare data must be verified with the proper access control to prevent manipulation attempts [48]. Furthermore, encryption is not a reliable method of securing medical documents. Interoperability problems arise if several encryption techniques are available to encrypt various medical documents [49,50]. Numerous privacy problems result from inadequate security of healthcare data [43]. Another important criterion for healthcare data is connectivity. Connectivity is the capacity to share and transmit data between different sources [51]. Connectivity is based on the use of centralized data storage. Healthcare data is difficult to store centrally since doing so might cause access delays, safety hazards, and confidentiality issues. Since medical information expands with time, sending all of the information to a single location is impossible via unreliable connections.

Additionally, because the information is stored centrally, getting prompt and safe access might be difficult. Numerous health investigations depend on the sharing of medical data. Thus, it's critical to ensure uniformity, accessibility, and flexibility while exchanging data [43].

As patients grow increasingly mobile and demand their data to be portable, mobility in the healthcare industry is becoming more and more necessary. With the prevalence of smart devices, sensors, and other Internet-connected devices rising, the ability to transport data is becoming increasingly important. According to [43], one mobility category is mobile health. Another category is wireless. Smartphones, wireless body area networks (WBAN), and sensors are all part of mobile health. Managing user permission, trust, access control, and safe data exchange are the problems in mobile health [43].

5.4.1 Overview of blockchain technology in healthcare

The need for expansion in the healthcare sector is growing at unprecedented rates. Tremendous-quality medical facilities supported by advanced technology are in popular demand nowadays. In this case, BC may play a significant role in transforming the medical sector. Moreover, the medical system is changing in support of a patient-centered approach that stresses two crucial components: readily accessible services and an adequate supply of medical supplies at all times [52]. Owing to the BC, hospitals and clinics may better provide correct patient care and first-rate medical facilities. Another laborious, repetitive activity that raises expenses in the health sector is HIE, which may be resolved swiftly with this technology [52]. BC technology enables public participation in health research projects. Enhanced data sharing and public health studies will lead to better treatments in many fields. The whole medical system and enterprises are managed by a single database [52]. The largest difficulties in managing community health have been related to information transmission, confidentiality, and connection. For this specific problem, BC technology is trustworthy. When utilized appropriately, this technology enhances accessibility, connectedness, honesty, real-time modifications, and information exchange.

Additionally, there are significant worries about the safety of data, especially in the fields of wearable technology and personalized medicine. To record, transport, and consult data over networks without worrying about security, patients and medical professionals require easy, secure methods [52]. The overview of the use of BC technology in medical settings is summarized with some of its key points below.

5.4.1.1 Improved data security

BC technology offers enhanced data security by leveraging cryptographic algorithms and decentralized storage [53]. It enables healthcare organizations to securely store and transmit sensitive patient data, minimizing the risk of unauthorized access, data breaches, and tampering [54]. BC's decentralized structure makes hacking the system challenging for malevolent parties.

5.4.1.2 Data integrity and trust

BC offers a permanent, open ledger where all activities and information inputs are tracked. Without the network's participants' consent, there is no way to alter or erase the data uploaded to the BC [52]. This ensures medical records' accuracy, clinical trials, and research data, fostering trust among healthcare providers, patients, and researchers.

5.4.1.3 Interoperability and data exchange

BC can address the interoperability challenges faced by HSs. It enables seamless sharing and exchange of patient health information across different platforms, EHR systems, and healthcare providers. Smart contracts and standardized data formats ensure compatibility and streamline data exchange, improving care coordination and decision-making [55].

5.4.1.4 Patient identity management

BC technology can enhance patient identity management and authentication. By assigning a unique identifier to each patient and linking it to their health records, healthcare organizations can verify patient identities accurately [56]. This helps prevent identity theft, reduce medical errors, and streamline patient registration processes.

5.4.1.5 Consent management and privacy

BC enables to give patients greater power over their health data and privacy. Smart contracts can automate consent management, allowing or disallowing patients access to their medical records for specific providers or researchers [57]. Patient consent preferences are securely recorded on the BC, ensuring privacy and data-sharing compliance.

5.4.1.6 Clinical trials and research

BC has the potential to transform clinical trials and medical research. It can facilitate the secure and transparent sharing of research data, enabling collaboration among researchers and institutions globally [58]. BC-based systems can improve the integrity of trial data, enhance participant recruitment, automate consent processes, and ensure transparency in trial outcomes [59].

5.4.1.7 Supply chain management

In the healthcare industry, BC can revolutionize supply chain management for pharmaceuticals, medical devices, and equipment. It enables end-to-end traceability of products, ensuring authenticity and reducing the risk of counterfeit drugs or equipment entering the market [60,61]. BC-based supply chain systems can improve inventory management, reduce costs, and enhance patient safety.

5.4.1.8 Billing and insurance

BC can streamline billing processes and prevent fraudulent activities in healthcare insurance claims. Smart contracts can automate claims processing, verification, and payment execution, reducing administrative costs and improving efficiency [61]. BC-based insurance systems enable the secure sharing of patient data between providers and insurers, enhancing accuracy and transparency.

5.4.1.9 Telehealth and remote monitoring

BC technology can support the growth of telehealth and remote monitoring services. It enables secure storage and transmission of patient health data during virtual consultations [62]. Smart contracts can automate payment processes for telehealth services, ensuring transparency and trust between patients and providers.

5.4.1.10 Regulatory compliance

BC can assist in meeting regulatory compliance requirements [63] that provides transparent and auditable nature that simplifies compliance audits, data governance, and consent management.

5.4.2 Use of blockchain for secure data access management

In telehealth systems, secure data access management is crucial to ascertain the honesty, reliability, and accessibility of patient health information. BC technology offers a decentralized and immutable platform that can revolutionize data access management, providing enhanced security, privacy, and control over patient data. By leveraging the BC in telehealth systems, healthcare providers can address critical challenges such as data breaches, unauthorized access, and data-sharing inefficiencies [52]. Some of the utilization of BC for secure data access administration are as follows:

- Decentralized and immutable storage: BC provides a decentralized storage solution where patient health data can be securely stored across multiple nodes or devices in the network. The data is encrypted and distributed, making it highly resistant to unauthorized access and tampering. The immutability of the BC guarantees that information is not changeable once it has been recorded retroactively, maintaining data integrity and auditability.
- Patient-controlled access: Thanks to BC, patients can manage exactly who may access their health data. Using smart contracts, patients can grant or revoke access permissions to specific healthcare providers, researchers, or third-party applications [64]. This decentralized approach ensures patients have full visibility and authority over who can access their data, enhancing patient privacy and consent management.
- Identity verification and authentication: BC technology can streamline telehealth systems' identity verification and authentication processes. Patients can have a BC-based distinct electronic identity linked to their health records. This helps ensure that only permitted people or organizations have control over patient information reducing the risk of impersonation and fraud.
- Auditability and transparency: BC's transparency allows for real-time auditability and transparency in data access management. Every access request, permission change, or data-sharing event is recorded on the BC, creating an immutable audit trail [65]. This enables healthcare providers and regulators to track and verify data access activities, enhancing accountability and compliance.
- Data encryption and security: BC can facilitate end-to-end encryption of patient health data in telehealth systems. Before being saved, the information is encoded on the BC, and decryption keys are securely shared with authorized parties. This ensures that even if the BC is compromised, the encrypted data remains protected, adding an extra layer of security to sensitive patient information.
- Interoperability and data exchange: BC can facilitate data sharing and connectivity. Various healthcare organizations and methods can securely share patient data using standardized data formats and BC protocols. This facilitates seamless integration and communication between disparate systems, improving care coordination and patient outcomes [66].
- Smart contracts for access control: Smart contracts, programmable code executed on the BC, can automate access control processes in telehealth systems. Access permissions can be defined and enforced using smart contracts, and we can do away with the necessity for intermediaries and reduce administrative

overhead. Smart contracts can also enforce data-sharing agreements and consent management rules, ensuring compliance with privacy regulations.

- Enhanced security and resilience: BC technology offers enhanced security and resilience against cyber threats and system failures. The decentralized nature of the BC makes it more resistant to single points of failure and distributed denial-of-service (DDoS) attacks [67]. Additionally, consensus algorithms ensure that data modifications require agreement among network participants, further enhancing the security of patient data.

Using BC to govern safe data access in telehealth systems can solve significant confidentiality and safety issues. By utilizing BC's distributed and unchangeable characteristics, healthcare providers can ensure secure storage, controlled access, and interoperable sharing of patient health data.

5.4.3 Blockchain-based access control mechanisms

Techniques for access control are essential for assuring the safety and privacy of patient data in telehealth systems. BC technology offers innovative solutions to enhance access control by leveraging its decentralized, immutable, and transparent nature [68]. BC-based access control mechanisms provide robust authentication, authorization, and audibility, addressing the challenges of data breaches, unauthorized access, and data-sharing inefficiencies. Some key aspects of BC-based access control mechanisms in telehealth systems are as follows:

- Decentralized identity management: BC enables decentralized identity management by allowing patients to keep a special digital ID on the BC. Each patient can have a public–private key pair as their digital signature. This eliminates the need for centralized identity management systems and reduces the risk of single points of failure or data breaches.
- Digital identity verification: BC-based access control mechanisms provide a reliable and tamperproof method for verifying the digital identity of healthcare providers, patients, and other participants in telehealth systems [69]. The BC can store and validate digital certificates or credentials issued by trusted entities, ensuring the authenticity and integrity of users' identities.
- Smart contracts for access policies: Smart contracts, programmable code executed on the BC, can be utilized to define and enforce access control policies in telehealth systems. Access policies can be encoded in smart contracts, specifying who has access to specific information and under what circumstances. These smart contracts automatically enforce access permissions, eliminating the need for centralized intermediaries and improving efficiency.
- Consent management: BC-based access control mechanisms facilitate patient-centric consent management. Smart contracts can be used to automate consent processes, ensuring that patient consent is explicitly obtained before granting access to their health data [69]. Patients have control over granting or revoking consent, and these consent decisions are securely recorded on the BC, promoting transparency and compliance with privacy regulations.

- Immutable audit trail: BC provides an immutable and transparent audit trail of access control activities. Each access request, permission change, or data-sharing event is recorded on the BC, creating a tamperproof and auditable log [69]. This enables healthcare providers, patients, and regulators to track and verify access control activities, enhancing accountability and facilitating compliance audits.
- Fine-grained access control: BC-based access control mechanisms allow for fine-grained control over data access. Access permissions can be defined at the individual data field level, ensuring that only authorized individuals can access specific parts of patient records [70]. This granularity helps protect sensitive information and ensures that only relevant data is shared with authorized parties.
- Interoperability and data sharing: BC enhances interoperability and secure data sharing among telehealth systems and healthcare providers. BC protocols and smart contracts enable seamless and standardized data exchange, ensuring access control policies are consistently enforced across disparate systems. This promotes care coordination and enables efficient sharing of patient information for improved healthcare outcomes.
- Enhanced security and privacy: BC-based access control mechanisms provide enhanced security and privacy for patient data. BC's decentralized structure lessens the possibility of single points of breakdown and illegal access [64]. The immutability of the BC ensures that access control policies and permissions cannot be tampered with, maintaining data integrity and confidentiality.
- BC-based access control mechanisms offer significant advantages in telehealth systems by providing decentralized identity management, secure authentication, fine-grained access control, consent management, and auditable data trails. These mechanisms enhance security, privacy, interoperability, and trust among healthcare providers and patients.

5.5 Integration of AI and blockchain for data access authorization in telehealth systems

A consolidated health information BC might use AI to hasten tailored treatment discovery, creation, and dissemination. Patients and organizations may allow AI to search for records if the BC is filled with defined, extracted, and distributed health data and has unchangeable privacy controls. This represents the patient's databank to look for health-related warning signs, patterns, findings, epidemics, and undiscovered treatments.

Health information represents our genetic makeup, the treatments we take, and their results. That accessible data structure on the BC can be useful for businesses and academic institutions. Given the amount of medical information and BC's openness, it might not be practical. However, as far as the documents are not explicitly kept on the BC, there is no explanation for why the more significant learning capability can't be exploited in the data created in the medical industry with the appropriate model. Instead, entry to and authorization of medical records might be provided through the BC.

AI algorithms use semi-structured datasets. Connecting thousands of dissimilar items reveals concealed trends and produces meaning. For the first time, these highly skilled, trustworthy, narrow AI agents might have access to a large range of executable datasets by legally disseminating health information via BC. The main objective would be to improve patient care worldwide, not only collect and analyze data. Figure 5.4 shows the prospect and implementation strategy of integrating AI and BC in telehealth systems.

5.5.1 Synergies between AI and blockchain in telehealth systems

The combination of AI and BC technology can transform various industries, and one area where this synergy is particularly promising is telehealth systems. Telehealth, which involves the remote delivery of healthcare services, has significantly increased in popularity in recent years. By harnessing the power of AI and BC, telehealth systems can enhance efficiency, security, and accessibility while improving patient outcomes. Table 5.3 shows the benefits of combining AI and BC in telehealth systems.

5.5.2 Examination of AI-driven access authorization mechanisms in blockchain-based telehealth systems

One critical aspect of telehealth systems is access authorization mechanisms, which control and manage secure access to patient data. Telehealth systems, which involve the remote delivery of healthcare services, have recently received great interest due

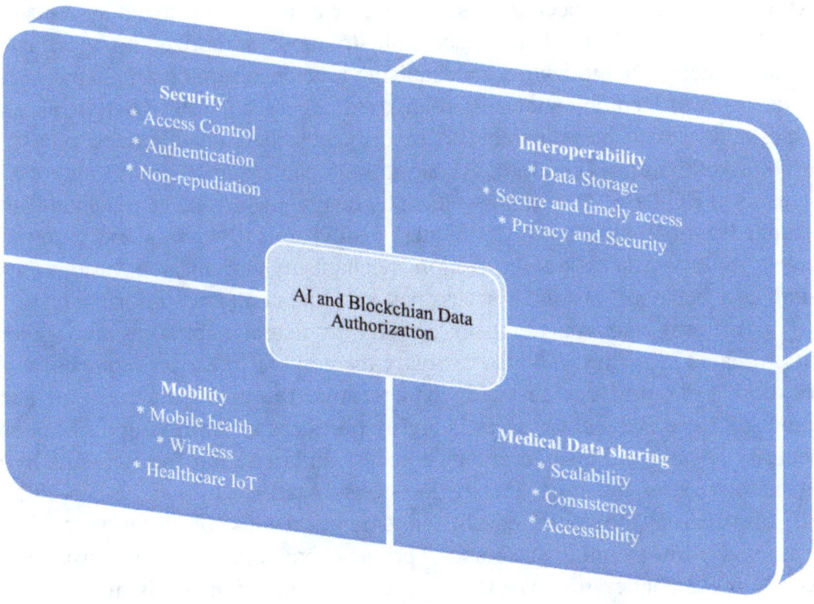

Figure 5.4 Prospect of AI and blockchain integration in telehealth

Table 5.3 Benefits of AI and blockchain integration

Benefits	Description
Enhanced data security	Blockchain ensures secure and immutable storage of patient data [71]
Improved data privacy	Patient-controlled access to health records through smart contracts [72]
Interoperability	Seamless integration and sharing of data from multiple sources [73]
AI-powered diagnosis	AI algorithms analyze medical data for accurate diagnosis and treatment [74]
Streamlined payments	Transparent and automated payment processes through blockchain and smart contracts [75]
Research and development	AI and blockchain facilitate data sharing and collaboration for medical research

to their ability to provide healthcare accessibility, efficiency, and patient outcomes. BC technology has surfaced as an optimistic remedy for open and safe data management in telehealth systems. AI algorithms also offer advanced capabilities for analyzing and interpreting medical data. By using BC technology, healthcare data may be shared and stored securely on a distributed, unchangeable ledger. It offers several advantages, including data security, privacy, interoperability, and auditability. In a BC-based telehealth system, stakeholders, such as patients, insurance firms, and healthcare providers, can safely access and update patient records.

Access authorization mechanisms play a crucial role in telehealth systems, guaranteeing that patient data is only accessible to those authorized to view it [76]. Traditionally, access authorization mechanisms rely on centralized systems, such as username–password combinations or role-based access control (RBAC). However, these mechanisms can be vulnerable to security breaches, unauthorized access, and single points of failure. Therefore, AI algorithms can enhance access authorization mechanisms in BC-based telehealth systems by leveraging advanced machine learning and natural language processing techniques. To dynamically assess and grant access privileges, AI-driven access authorization mechanisms can analyze various factors, including user behavior, historical access patterns, and contextual information.

AI algorithms can analyze user activity to detect anomalies and potential security threats [77]. They can also evaluate the context of access requests, such as the location, time, and device used, to determine the appropriateness of access. Combining AI and BC technologies is highly pertinent in improving access control and security. AI algorithms can enhance access authorization mechanisms by providing adaptive and dynamic access decisions based on user behavior and contextual information. However, careful consideration must be given to challenges such as algorithm reliability, biases, privacy concerns, and governance. By addressing these challenges, AI-driven access authorization mechanisms can contribute to secure and efficient telehealth systems that protect patient data while facilitating authorized access.

5.5.3 Analysis of trust and transparency aspect of data access authorization in telehealth systems

Trust and transparency are fundamental in data access authorization within telehealth systems. Building trust through secure and transparent data access authorization processes is crucial for patient confidence, regulatory compliance, and the establishment of positive healthcare provider–patient relationship. Technology reliability, data security and privacy, healthcare provider competence, and clear communication and empathy are the factors that contribute to establishing trust in telehealth systems. Transparency promotes accountability and allows patients to make informed decisions: access to information, consent and authorization, documentation and audibility, and communication of policies and practices. Complex authorization mechanisms, lack of patient awareness, and third-party involvement are the challenges in ensuring data access authorization transparency. These challenges come with potential solutions such as patient education, clear consent processes, enhanced communication and auditing, and accountability.

5.6 Real-life case studies of AI and blockchain integration for data access authorization in telehealth systems

The integration of AI and BC technologies has paved the way for innovative solutions in data access authorization. AI offers advanced data analysis capabilities, while BC ascertains transaction security, openness, and immutability [78]. The integration of AI and BC for data access authorizations opens up new possibilities for personalized services, research collaboration, and improved patient outcomes. As these technologies continue to advance, it is expected that further transformative applications in data access authorization will be in the future. The following are real-life case studies demonstrating the successful integration of AI and BC for data access authorization in telehealth systems.

5.6.1 Medicalchain

This BC-based telehealth platform utilizes AI and BC technology to enhance data access authorization and security. The platform enables to provide people authority over their health data through smart contracts. AI algorithms analyze and interpret medical data, providing accurate diagnoses and treatment recommendations. Access to patient data is made safe and open while preserving confidentiality and data integrity thanks to the integration of BC and AI. Figure 5.5 displays the architecture of the Medicalchain platform. The platform shows the integration of user interfaces, AI data analysis engines, and BC for data storage with the data pool.

5.6.2 Nebula genomics

This genomics data-sharing platform leverages BC and AI for data access authorization. The platform allows individuals to confidentially share their genomic data with researchers while maintaining control over their data. This integration

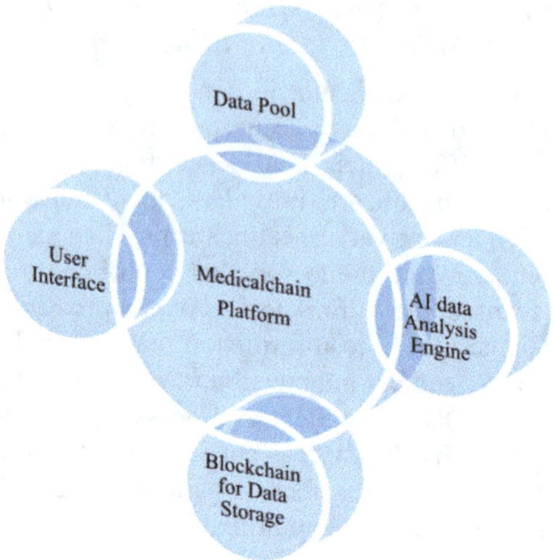

Figure 5.5 Medicalchain application of AI and blockchain

Table 5.4 Data access authorization process

Steps	Description
Step 1	Patient consent
Step 2	Blockchain-based data sharing
Step 3	AI data analysis

provides transparency and trust in data access and fosters collaborations between individuals and researchers. Table 5.4 outlines Nebula Genomics' data access authorization process, highlighting the steps of patent consent, BC-based data sharing, and AI data analysis.

5.6.3 Shivom

Shivom is another noteworthy case study demonstrating the integration of AI and BC for data access authorization. The platform allows secure sharing of genomic data among patients and researchers. Figure 5.6 shows the data access control flow in the Shivom platform with the interaction between patients, researchers, and the BC-based platform, emphasizing the utilization of smart contracts for authorization and AI algorithms for data analysis.

5.6.4 Lessons learned

This chapter looks at how sophisticated technologies may be used to improve data security and access control in telehealth systems. The relevance of data security,

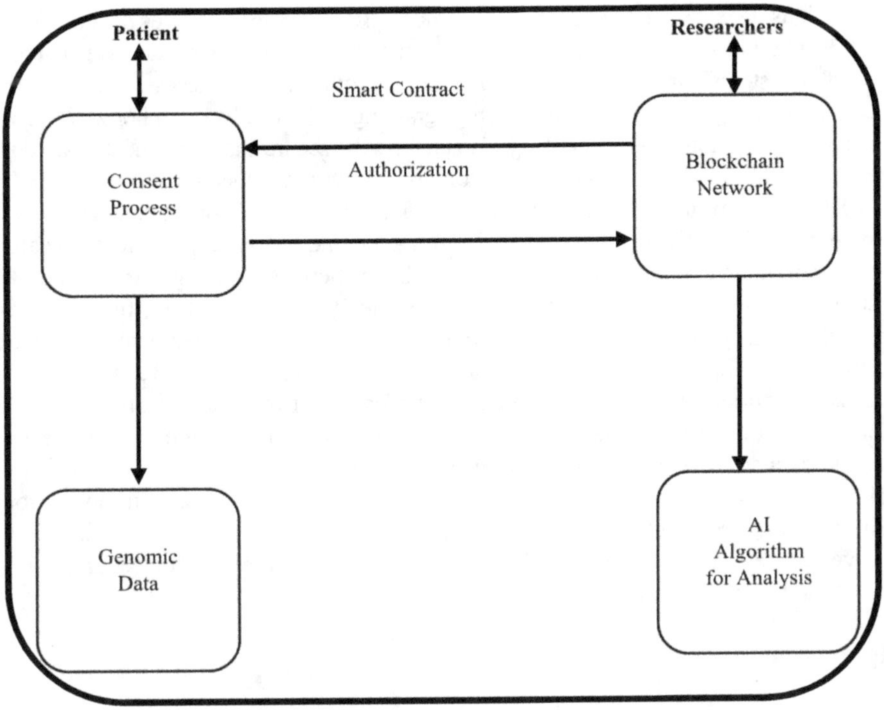

Figure 5.6 Shivom architecture for AI and blockchain integration

access control, privacy, trust, interoperability, ethics, scalability, and regulatory compliance is also emphasized in the chapter. By considering these factors, healthcare institutions can maximize the potential of new technologies to improve patient care while protecting sensitive health data.

5.7 Conclusions and future scope

The combination of AI and BC technologies has showcased its possibilities in revolutionizing data access authorization in telehealth systems. Through real-life case studies, it was discovered how AI and BC work together to enhance security, transparency, and patient control over their data. These technologies have demonstrated their ability to empower individuals, facilitate research collaboration, and improve patient outcomes in telehealth systems.

AI-driven access authorization mechanisms have proven to be effective in ensuring secure and authorized access to sensitive healthcare data. By leveraging AI algorithms, organizations can analyze and interpret vast amounts of data, providing accurate diagnoses, personalized treatment recommendations, and valuable insights. This integration allows for streamlined and efficient healthcare processes, ultimately improving patient care.

With its decentralized and immutable nature, BC technology ensures data integrity, privacy, and transparency. By utilizing BC for data storage and transaction verification, telehealth systems can establish trust and accountability in data access authorization. Patients can control their medical records, granting access only to authorized individuals or organizations. BC technology also enables the secure sharing of healthcare data among stakeholders, fostering collaboration and research advancements.

The integration of AI and BC for data access authorization in telehealth systems presents significant potential for future scope advancements. Future research can be conducted to enhance the interoperability between AI algorithms and BC systems. Privacy remains a crucial concern in healthcare. Therefore, future development can focus on incorporating privacy-preserving techniques, such as secure multi-party computation and differential privacy, into AI and BC integration. Finally, federated learning techniques can be explored to leverage distributed AI models without compromising data privacy. By training AI models on decentralized data sources while preserving privacy, telehealth systems can benefit from collective intelligence while maintaining control over data access authorization. With ongoing research and development, these technologies will continue to evolve, addressing challenges and unlocking new opportunities for secure, transparent, and patient-centric healthcare delivery.

References

[1] Awotunde, J. B., Ajamu, G. J., Abdulraheem, M., *et al.* (2023, April). Plant Disease Diagnosis and Detection Using Type-2 Fuzzy Logic System. In 2023 International Conference on Science, Engineering and Business for Sustainable Development Goals (SEB-SDG) (vol.1, pp. 1–11). IEEE.

[2] Yang, C. T., Chen, C. J., Tsan, Y. T., Liu, P. Y., Chan, Y. W., and Chan, W. C. (2019). An implementation of real-time air quality and influenza-like illness data storage and processing platform. *Computers in Human Behavior*, vol.100, pp. 266–274.

[3] Talal, A. H., Sofikitou, E. M., Jaanimägi, U., Zeremski, M., Tobin, J. N., and Markatou, M. (2020). A framework for patient-centered telemedicine: application and lessons learned from vulnerable populations. *Journal of Biomedical Informatics*, vol.112, p.103622.

[4] Akkiraju R., Sinha V., Xu A., *et al.* (2020) Characterizing machine learning processes: a maturity framework. In: Fahland D., Ghidini C., Becker J., Dumas M. (eds.) *Business Process Management.* BPM 2020. Lecture Notes in Computer Science, vol.12168. Springer, Cham.

[5] Yaqoob, I., Salah, K., Jayaraman, R., and Al-Hammadi, Y. (2021). Blockchain for healthcare data management: opportunities, challenges, and future recommendations. *Neural Computing and Applications*, vol. 34, pp. 11475–11490.

[6] Adeniyi, J. K., Adeniyi, T. T., Awotunde, J. B., Abiodun, M. K., and Atanda, O. G. (2023, April). Agrolend: a blockchain implementation approach of smart contract farming platform. In *2023 International Conference on*

Science, Engineering and Business for Sustainable Development Goals (SEB-SDG) (vol.1, pp. 1–7). IEEE.

[7] Casado-Vara, R., Prieto-Castrillo, F., and Corchado, J. M. (2018). A game theory approach for cooperative control to improve data quality and false data detection in WSN. *International Journal of Robust and Nonlinear Control*, vol.28, issue 16, pp.5087–5102.

[8] Awotunde, J. B., Ogundokun, R. O., Adeniyi, A. E., *et al.* (2022). Cloud-IoMT-based wearable body sensors network for monitoring elderly patients during the COVID-19 pandemic. In *Biomedical Engineering Applications for People with Disabilities and the Elderly in the COVID-19 Pandemic and Beyond* (pp. 33–48). Academic Press, New York.

[9] Adeniyi, A. E., Abiodun, K. M., Awotunde, J. B., Olagunju, M., Ojo, O. S., and Edet, N. P. (2023). Implementation of a block cipher algorithm for medical information security on cloud environment: using modified advanced encryption standard approach. *Multimedia Tools and Applications*, vol. 82, pp. 20537–20551.

[10] Awotunde, J. B., Misra, S., Ayo, F. E., Agrawal, A., and Ahuja, R. (2023). Hybridized support vector machine and Adaboost technique for malaria diagnosis. In *Frontiers of ICT in Healthcare: Proceedings of EAIT 2022* (pp. 25–38). Springer Nature Singapore, Singapore.

[11] Bragazzi, N. L., Dai, H., Damiani, G., Behzadifar, M., Martini, M., and Wu, J. (2020). How big data and artificial intelligence can help better manage the covid-19 pandemic. *International Journal of Environmental Research and Public Health,* vol.17, issue 9, p.3176.

[12] Sahoo, M. S. and Baruah, P. K. (2018). HBasechainDB – a scalable blockchain framework on Hadoop Ecosystem. In: Yokota R., Wu W. (eds) *Supercomputing Frontiers. SCFA 2018. Lecture Notes in Computer Science*, vol.10776. Springer, Cham.

[13] Paul, D., Sanap, G., Shenoy, S., Kalyane, D., Kalia, K., and Tekade, R. K. (2021). Artificial intelligence in drug discovery and development. *Drug Discovery Today,* vol.26, pp.80–93.

[14] Cha, Y., Erez, T., Reynolds, I. J., *et al.* (2018) Drug repurposing from the perspective of pharmaceutical companies. *British Journal of Pharmacology,* vol.175, issue 2, pp.168–180.

[15] Awotunde, J. B., Adeniyi, A. E., Ajagbe, S. A., Jimoh, R. G., and Bhoi, A. K. (2022). Swarm intelligence and evolutionary algorithms in processing healthcare data. In *Connected e-Health: Integrated IoT and Cloud Computing* (pp. 105–124). Springer International Publishing, Cham.

[16] Siyal, A. A., Junejo, A. Z., Zawish, M., Ahmed, K., Khalil, A., and Soursou, G. (2019). Applications of blockchain technology in medicine and healthcare: challenges and future perspectives. *Cryptography,* vol.3, issue 1, p.3.

[17] Elvas, L. B, SerrÃ£o, C., and Ferreira, J. C. (2023). Sharing health information using a blockchain. *Healthcare (Basel)*, vol.11, issue 2, p.170.

[18] Abdullah, S., Arshad, J., Khan, M. M., Alazab, M., and Salah, K. (2023). PRISED tangle: a privacy-aware framework for smart healthcare data

sharing using IOTA tangle. *Complex & Intelligent Systems*, vol.9, issue 3, pp.3023–3041.

[19] Grover, B., and Kushwaha, D. K. (2023). Authorization and privacy preservation in cloud-based distributed system using blockchain technology and anonymous digital ring signature. *Health Services and Outcomes Research Methodology*, vol.23, issue 2, pp.227–240.

[20] Liu, J., Fan, Y., Sun, R., Liu, L., Wu, C., and Mumtaz, S. (2023). Blockchain-aided privacy-preserving medical data sharing scheme for e-healthcare system. *IEEE Internet of Things Journal*, DOI: 10.1109/JIOT.2023.3287636.

[21] Ali, S., Abdullah, Armand, T. P. T., *et al.* (2023). Metaverse in healthcare integrated with explainable AI and blockchain: enabling immersiveness ensuring trust, and providing patient data security. *Sensors 2023*, vol.23, issue 2, p.565. https://doi.org/10.3390/s23020565

[22] Hannah, S., Deepa, A. J., Chooralil, S. V., *et al.* (2022). Blockchain-based deep learning to process IoT data acquisition in cognitive data. *BioMedical Research International*, vol.2022, p.5038851–5038857.

[23] Hazratifard, M., Gebali, F., and Mamun, M. (2022). Using machine learning for dynamic authentication in telehealth: a tutorial. *Sensors (Basel, Switzerland)*, vol.22, issue 19, p.7655.

[24] Mhamdi, H., Ayadi, M., Ksibi, A., Al-Rasheed, A., Soufiene, B. O., and Hedi, S. (2022). SEMRAchain: a secure electronic medical record based on blockchain technology. *Electronics (Basel)*, vol.11, issue 21, p.3617.

[25] Ghosh, S., Bindu, P. R., Chitra, B. L., and Deeksha Rani, B. N. (2022). A novel blockchain-based patient health record management system. *NeuroQuantology*, vol.20, issue 16, p.3336.

[26] Zaman, U., Imran, Mehmood, F., Iqbal, N., Kim, J., and Ibrahim, M. (2022). Towards secure and intelligent internet of health things: a survey of enabling technologies and applications. *Electronics (Basel)*, vol.11, issue 12, p.1893.

[27] Deebak, B. D., Memon, F. H., Cheng, X., *et al.* (2022). Seamless privacy-preservation and authentication framework for IoT-enabled smart eHealth systems. *Healthcare Analytics*, vol.3, DOI:10.1016/j.health.2023.100192

[28] Dubey, A., and Verma, A. S. (2022). Effective Remote Healthcare and Telemedicine Approaches for Improving Digital Healthcare Systems.

[29] Geetanjali, R. M., Rajendra, A., Pramod, K. S., Nidhi, K., Vinod, K., and Sanjay, K. Y. (2022). Applications of artificial intelligence, blockchain, and internet-of-things in management of chronic disease. *Cognitive Intelligence and Big Data in Healthcare*. https://doi.org/10.1002/9781119771982.ch13

[30] Tolba, A., and Al-Makhadmeh, Z. (2021). Predictive data analysis approach for securing medical data in smart grid healthcare systems. *Future Generation Computer Systems*, vol.117, pp.87–96.

[31] Srivastava, S., Singh, S. V., Singh, R. B., and Shukla, H. K. (2021). Digital transformation of healthcare: a blockchain study. *IJISET – International Journal of Innovative Science, Engineering & Technology*, vol.8, issue 5, pp. 414–425

[32] Renugadevi, N., Saravanan, S., Naga Sudha, C. M., and Tripathi P. (2021). IoT-enabled applications and other techniques to combat COVID-19. In: Kautish, S., Peng, SL., Obaid, A.J. (eds) *Computational Intelligence Techniques for Combating COVID-19. EAI/Springer Innovations in Communication and Computing*. Springer, Cham. https://doi.org/10.1007/978-3-030-68936-0_7

[33] Jennath, H. S., Anoop, V. S., and Asharaf, S. (2020). Blockchain for healthcare: securing patient data and enabling trusted artificial intelligence. *International Journal of Interactive Multimedia and Artificial Intelligence*, vol.6, issue 3, pp 15–23.

[34] Shuwandy, M. L., Zaidan, B. B., Zaidan, A. A., *et al.* (2020). mHealth authentication approach-based 3D touchscreen and microphone sensors for real-time remote healthcare monitoring system: comprehensive review, open issues, and methodological aspects. *Computer Science Review*, vol.38, DOI: 10.1016/j.cosrev.2020.100300

[35] Zhuang, Y., Lincoln, R. S., Yin-Wu, C., Zon-Yin, S., Jeffrey, J.P.T., and Chi-Ren, S. (2020). A patient-centric health information exchange framework using blockchain technology. *IEEE Journal of Biomedical and Health Informatics*, vol.24, issue 8, pp. 2169–2176.

[36] Ullah, H. S., and Arjomand, A. N. (2020). Blockchain in Healthcare and Medicine: A Contemporary Research of Applications, Challenges, and Future Perspectives. arXiv:2004.06795

[37] Hang, L., Choi, E., and Kim, D. H. (2019). A novel EMR integrity management based on a medical blockchain platform in hospital. *Electronics,* vol.8, p.467.

[38] Adeniyi, E. A., Ogundokun, R. O., and Awotunde, J. B. (2021). IoMT-based wearable body sensors network healthcare monitoring system. *IoT in Healthcare and Ambient Assisted Living*, vol.933, pp.103–121.

[39] Tripathy, S. S., Imoize, A. L., Rath, M., *et al.* (2022). A novel edge-computing-based framework for an intelligent smart healthcare system in smart cities. *Sustainability*, vol.15, issue 1, p.735.

[40] Awotunde, J. B., Sisodia, D. S., Ayodele, P. A., Ogundokun, R. O., and Chouhan, V. S. (2022, October). Diagnosis expert system on breast cancer using fuzzy logic and clustering technique. In *International Conference on Information Systems and Management Science* (pp. 589–601).Springer International Publishing,Cham.

[41] Kumar, R., Wang, W., Kumar, J., Yang, T., Khan, A., Ali, W., and Ali, I. (2021). Integration of blockchain and AI for secure data sharing and detection of CT images for hospitals. *Computerized Medical Imaging and Graphics*, vol.87, p.101812.

[42] Kibria, M. G., Nguyen, K., Villardi, G. P., Zhao, O., Ishizu, K., and Kojima, F. (2018). Big data analytics, machine learning, and artificial intelligence in next-generation wireless networks. *IEEE Access*, vol.6, pp.32328–32338.

[43] Kusherdianti, N., Ariswati, H. G., Wisana, I. D. G. H., *et al.* (2023, April). Analysis of finite impulse response (FIR) filter to reduce motion artifacts of heart rate signal based on photoplethysmography. In *Proceeding of the 3rd International Conference on Electronics, Biomedical Engineering, and*

Health Informatics: ICEBEHI 2022, 5–6 October, Surabaya, Indonesia (pp. 657–680). Springer Nature Singapore, Singapore.

[44] Andrew, J., Isravel, D. P., Sagayam, K. M., Bhushan, B., Sei, Y., and Eunice, J. (2023). Blockchain for healthcare systems: architecture, security challenges, trends and future directions. *Journal of Network and Computer Applications*. https://doi.org/10.1016/j.jnca.2023.103633

[45] Ramasamy, L. K., Khan, F., Imoize, A. L., Ogbebor, J. O., Kadry, S., and Rho, S. (2021). Blockchain-based wireless sensor networks for malicious node detection: a survey. *IEEE Access*, vol.9, pp.128765–128785.

[46] Kumar, R. L., Wang, Y., Poongodi, T., and Imoize, A. L. (eds). (2021). *Internet of Things, Artificial Intelligence and Blockchain Technology*. Springer, Cham.

[47] Awotunde, J. B., Folorunsho, O., Mustapha, I. O., Olusanya, O. O., Akanbi, M. B., and Abiodun, K. M. (2023). An enhanced internet of things enabled type-2 fuzzy logic for healthcare system applications. In *Recent Trends on Type-2 Fuzzy Logic Systems: Theory, Methodology and Applications* (pp. 133–151). Springer International Publishing, Cham.

[48] Suzuki, S., and Murai, J. (2017). Blockchain as an audit-able communication channel. *Proceedings – International Computer Software Application Conference*, vol.2, pp.516–522. https://doi.org/10.1109/ COMPSAC.2017.72.

[49] Xu, J. J. (2016). Are blockchains immune to all malicious attacks? *Finance Innovation*, vol.2, issue 1, pp.1–9. https://doi.org/10.1186/S40854-016-0046-5, 2016 21.

[50] Imoize, A. L., Odeyemi, S. D., and Adebisi, J. A. (2020). Development of a low-cost wireless bee-hive temperature and sound monitoring system. *Indonesian Journal of Electrical Engineering and Informatics (IJEEI)*, vol.8, issue 3, pp.476–485.

[51] Azaria, A., Ekblaw, A., Vieira, T., and Lippman, A. (2016). MedRec: using blockchain for medical data access and permission management. In *Proceedings – 2nd International Conference Open Big Data, (OBD)*, pp. 25–30. https://doi.org/10.1109/OBD.2016.11.

[52] Haleem, A., Javaid, M., Singh, R.P., Suman, R., and Rab, S. (2021). Blockchain technology applications in healthcare: an overview. *International Journal of Intelligent Networks*, vol.2, pp.130–139.

[53] Wenhua, Z., Qamar, F., Abdali, T.-A.N., Hassan, R., Jafri, S. T. A., and Nguyen, Q. N. (2023). Blockchain technology: security issues, healthcare applications, challenges and future trends. *Electronics 2023*, vol.12, issue 3. https://doi.org/10.3390/electronics12030546

[54] Paul, M., Maglaras, L., Ferrag, M. A., and Almomani, I. (2023). Digitization of healthcare sector: a study on privacy and security concerns. *ICT Express*. https://doi.org/10.1016/j.icte.2023.02.007

[55] Dmitry, K. (2023). Blockchain in Healthcare. https://ndlabs.dev/blockchain-in-healthcare (Accessed June 29, 2023).

[56] Javed, I. T., Alharbi, F., Bellaj, B., Margaria, T., Crespi, N., and Qureshi, K. N. (2021). Health-ID: a blockchain-based decentralized identity

management for remote healthcare. *Healthcare Basel*, vol.9, issue 6. doi: 10.3390/healthcare9060712.

[57] Porsdam Mann, S., Savulescu, J., Ravaud, P., and Benchoufi, M. (2020). Blockchain, consent and prosent for medical research. *Journal of Medical Ethics*, vol.47, issue 4, pp.244–250. doi:10.1136/medethics-2019-105963

[58] Maslove, D. M., Klein, J., Brohman, K., and Martin, P. (2018). Using blockchain technology to manage clinical trials data: a proof-of-concept study. *JMIR Medical Information*, vol.6, issue 4. doi:10.2196/11949.

[59] Hang, L., Chen, C., Zhang, L., and Yang, J. (2022). Blockchain for applications of clinical trials: taxonomy, challenges, and future directions. *IET Communications*, vol.16, issue 20, pp.2371–2393. https://doi.org/10.1049/cmu2.12488

[60] Zakari, N., Al-Razgan, M., Alsaadi, A., *et al.* (2022). Blockchain technology in the pharmaceutical industry: a systematic review. *Peer Journal of Computer Science*, vol.8, doi:10.7717/peerj-cs.840.

[61] Chirag (2022). How Blockchain Technology is Transforming the Insurance Industry. https://appinventiv.com/blog/blockchain-transforming-the-insurance-industry/ (Accessed June 29, 2023).

[62] Ahmad, R. W., Salah, K., Jayaraman, R., Yaqoob, I., Ellahham, S., and Omar, M. (2021). The role of blockchain technology in telehealth and telemedicine. *International Journal of Medical Informatics*, vol.148, https://doi.org/10.1016/j.ijmedinf.2021.104399.

[63] Shuaib, M., Alam, S., Alam, M. S., and Nasir, M. S. (2021). Compliance with HIPAA and GDPR in blockchain-based electronic health record. DOI:10.1016/j.matpr.2021.03.059

[64] Shi, S., He, D., Li, L., Kumar, N., Khan, M.K., and Choo, K. R. (2020). Applications of blockchain in ensuring the security and privacy of electronic health record systems: a survey. *Computer Security*, vol.97, doi:10.1016/j.cose.2020.101966.

[65] Han, H., Shiwakoti, R. K., Jarvis, R., Mordi, C., and Botchie, D. (2023). Accounting and auditing with blockchain technology and artificial intelligence: a literature review. *International Journal of Accounting Information Systems*, vol.48, https://doi.org/10.1016/j.accinf.2022.100598.

[66] Biswas, S., Sharif, K., Li, F., *et al.* (2020). Interoperability and Synchronization Management of Blockchain-Based Decentralized e-Health Systems. doi:10.1109/TEM.2020.2989779

[67] Alajlan, R., Alhumam, N., Frikha, M. (2023). Cybersecurity for blockchain-based IoT systems: a review. *Applications Science*, vol.13, issue 7432. https://doi.org/10.3390/app13137432

[68] Kiania, K, Jameii, S. M., and Rahmani, A. M. (2023). Blockchain-based privacy and security preserving in electronic health: a systematic review. *Multimedia Tools Applications*, vol.17, pp.1–27. doi:10.1007/s11042-023-14488-w.

[69] Alansari, S. (2020). A Blockchain-Based Approach for Secure, Transparent and Accountable Personal Data Sharing. https://www.researchgate.net/publication/350174991_A_blockchain-based_approach_for_secure_transparent_and_accountable_personal_data_sharing

[70] Maesa, D., Mori, P., and Ricci, L. (2019). A blockchain based approach for the definition of auditable Access Control systems. *Computers & Security*, vol.84, 10.1016/j.cose.2019.03.016.

[71] Bazel, M. A., Mohammed, F., and Ahmed, M. (2021, August). Blockchain technology in healthcare big data management: benefits, applications and challenges. In *2021 1st International Conference on Emerging Smart Technologies and Applications (eSmarTA)* (pp. 1–8). IEEE.

[72] Rai, B. K. (2023). PcBEHR: patient-controlled blockchain enabled electronic health records for healthcare 4.0. *Health Services and Outcomes Research Methodology*, vol.23, issue 1, pp.80–102.

[73] Bruland, P., Doods, J., Brix, T., Dugas, M., and Storck, M. (2018). Connecting healthcare and clinical research: workflow optimizations through seamless integration of EHR, pseudonymization services and EDC systems. *International Journal of Medical Informatics*, vol.119, pp.103–108.

[74] Elemento, O., Leslie, C., Lundin, J., and Tourassi, G. (2021). Artificial intelligence in cancer research, diagnosis and therapy. *Nature Reviews Cancer*, vol.21, issue 12, pp.747–752.

[75] Sigalov, K., Ye, X., König, M., *et al.* (2021). Automated payment and contract management in the construction industry by integrating building information modeling and blockchain-based smart contracts. *Applied Sciences*, vol.11, issue 16, p.7653.

[76] Al-Janabi, S., Al-Shourbaji, I., Shojafar, M., and Shamshirband, S. (2017). Survey of main challenges (security and privacy) in wireless body area networks for healthcare applications. *Egyptian Informatics Journal*, vol.18, issue 2, pp.113–122.

[77] Koutsouvelis, V., Shiaeles, S., Ghita, B., and Bendiab, G. (2020, June). Detection of insider threats using artificial intelligence and visualisation. In *2020 6th IEEE Conference on Network Softwarization (NetSoft)* (pp. 437–443). IEEE.

[78] Alfa, A. A., Alhassan, J. K., Olaniyi, O. M., and Olalere, M. (2021). Blockchain technology in IoT systems: current trends, methodology, problems, applications, and future directions. *Journal of Reliable Intelligent Environments*, vol.7, issue 2, pp.115–143.

Chapter 6

Artificial intelligence and blockchain-assisted projects and synergies for telehealth systems

Solomon Chiekezi Nwaneri[1] *and Hannah Chimere Ugo*[2]

Telehealth systems have continued to play vital roles in improving access to medical care. With the increased deployment of telehealth, congestion and waiting times in hospitals have reportedly reduced. The centralized nature of conventional telehealth systems poses security threats to patients' records and often restricts them from taking charge of their data. In order to address these concerns, blockchain technology and artificial intelligence (AI) can be harnessed for enhanced security, flexibility, transparency, and provenness in telehealth. This chapter discusses AI and blockchain technology-enabled projects' synergies for telehealth systems. Related studies on using AI and blockchain technology in telehealth systems were reviewed. The chapter revealed tools and approaches for creating synergies between AI and blockchain technology. Selected AI and blockchain-enabled projects in telehealth specifically, MedCredits, MedChain, BlockHeal, and MyHealthMyData were lucidly presented. Strengthening the synergies between AI and blockchain technology in telehealth will significantly engender the trust of patients and clinicians. The future holds great prospects for revolutionizing the practice of telehealth.

6.1 Introduction

Telehealth systems are designed to provide medical services over a long distance to diverse patients who may not have physical contact with their physicians [1]. Many telehealth services are now offered to patients, such as virtual consultations, remote monitoring, automated payments, and online pharmacy services [2]. Telehealth, among other benefits, has helped reduce waiting times and other inconveniences that patients suffering from various diseases face while physically trying to access medical services in hospitals. The use of telehealth to deliver healthcare services has significantly increased after the COVID-19 pandemic [3]. Since a greater

[1]Department of Biomedical Engineering, Faculty of Engineering, University of Lagos, Nigeria
[2]Department of Biomedical Engineering, College of Engineering, Afe Babalola University, Nigeria

emphasis has been placed on harnessing available digital technologies to provide remote healthcare services, exploiting existing technologies to enhance the efficiency and effectiveness of telehealth systems is imperative. Artificial Intelligence (AI) and blockchain technology are vital to delivering quality telehealth services. AI and blockchain-enabled technology projects are crucial to today's telehealth systems, with great prospects for future telehealth projects.

Blockchain comprises a series of blocks with complete and accurate transaction records [4,5]. Each block $B_{i>0}$ is linked to a single preceding block B_{i-1} by a hash function $H(B_{i-1})$ [6]. It performs data generation and updates using consistency algorithms. In addition, blockchain makes use of encrypted data to ensure that transmitted data is protected [7]. The information in blockchain databases cannot be edited or deleted once created [8]. Thus, it is considered to be secure.

The application of blockchain technology in cryptocurrency is well known as it transparently records various transactions between parties. Blockchain, as a distributed database solution, keeps increasing the list of data records confirmed by the nodes participating in it [9]. Blockchain technology is reputed for keeping persistent and transparent logs of data [10,11].

The overarching problems of overcentralization and data breaches in telehealth systems can be overcome by the distributed nature of blockchain technology required to effectively manage health records [12,13]. Blockchain technology is reputed to provide an immutable data-sharing technique between individual parties without a central server, thus protecting data [14].

Furthermore, blockchain technology has led to significant improvements in the security of patient consent management in modern electronic health records (EHRs). Patients can now effectively manage their records and track those who accessed patients' electronic records [15]. Ordinarily, in insecure telehealth systems, there are obvious threats to the privacy of patients' EHRs containing sensitive information that cybercriminals could hijack [16].

With the adoption of blockchain technology, these threats could be largely reduced. In telehealth systems, blockchain technology has enhanced the security of payment systems through automation and the removal of third-party servers. Thus, reducing failure points could lead to data breaches. A few examples of blockchain projects in telehealth systems include MedicalChain, Symptomatic platform, Docademic system, Robomed, and DocCoin projects [17].

AI applications in healthcare have improved clinical decision-making, especially in disease detection, owing to its ability to mimic the human brain. AI techniques such as neural networks, decision trees, random forests, support vector machines, XGBoost, and many others have shown useful applications in the diagnosis and management of various diseases such as diabetes mellitus, chronic kidney disease, breast cancer, cervical cancer, stroke, and many other diseases [18,19]. The combination of AI with other technologies, such as the Internet of Things (IoT), has enhanced the performance of traditional medical systems [20]. However, AI projects face teething challenges leading to high failure rates. Some factors responsible for high failure rates in AI projects include unrealistic expectations, project complexity, low budget, lack of expertise, and lack of transparency [21]. For a successful synergy to be established between AI and blockchain-enabled projects in telehealth systems, these challenges ought to be addressed.

Although the synergy between AI and blockchain technology projects has not been fully explored, the potential benefits of this synergy are immense. AI is known to improve the intelligence of blockchain applications and thereby reduce errors caused by human influence [22].

There is a growing need to harness the numerous advantages of AI and blockchain technology in creating sustainable and secure telehealth systems [15]. This technology would overcome several limitations of traditional telehealth systems. While there are genuine concerns about potential threats, such as model poisoning with fake data introduction, the benefits of this synergy will far outweigh the risks [23]. Blockchain provides the data infrastructure that specifies the engagement rules, while AI processes the data and optimizes the rules [24]. This chapter focuses on creating synergies between AI and blockchain technology in telehealth systems.

6.1.1 Key contributions of the chapter

The significant contributions of this chapter are as follows:

1. It highlights the benefits and prospects of synergy between AI and blockchain technology in telehealth systems and presents various applications of this synergy.
2. Identification of major knowledge gaps after an extensive review of related studies to extend the frontiers of knowledge.
3. The provision of various applications of AI and blockchain technology in telehealth.

6.1.2 Chapter organization

Section 6.2 presents the related works on AI and blockchain-enabled projects and their applications in telehealth systems. Section 6.3 describes the methodology of the study. In Section 6.4, the main focus is the application of AI and blockchain technology in telehealth. Section 6.5 discusses selected AI–blockchain projects for telehealth systems. Lessons learned are highlighted in Section 6.6. Section 6.7 summarizes the entire chapter and contains future directions of the research for AI and blockchain applications in telehealth.

6.2 Related work

The application of blockchain technology in medicine and healthcare and the challenges and prospects were reviewed by Siyal *et al.* [25]. The authors did not conduct empirical research but rather did a literature review of existing research on blockchain technology in healthcare. The study recommended that future research should focus on developing blockchain-based solutions for healthcare that can address the challenges faced by the industry.

In another study by Guo *et al.* [26], a blockchain attribute-based encryption (ABE) scheme with multi-authority for medical on-demand in telemedicine systems was proposed. The proposed scheme is based on ABE, which allows for fine-grained access control to encrypted data. The scheme uses blockchain to maintain a tamperproof record of encrypted data and access control policies. The ABE allows for fine-grained access control to encrypted data. The scheme also uses a multi-authority architecture to improve scalability and security, improving security against several attacks, including collusion, chosen ciphertext, and key extraction attacks.

Furthermore, in [27], a novel probabilistic model-based authentication and authorization framework for blockchain-enabled IoT networks was developed. The proposed framework consists of three main components: a lightweight authentication protocol based on the elliptic curve cryptography, a blockchain-based authorization system, and a lightweight access control mechanism. The lightweight authentication protocol was used to authenticate IoT devices and users. The blockchain-based authorization system was used to manage access to resources in the IoT network. The lightweight access control mechanism was used to control access to data in the IoT network. However, the framework was only evaluated in a simulation study and implemented only in a small-scale IoT network.

Blockchain technology enhanced the performance of three telehealth services Hasan *et al.* [28]: teleconsultation and drug administration. They proposed a private blockchain-based telehealth system that uses smart contracts to register users and manage telehealth transactions. The smart contracts were programmed to ensure that only authorized users can access data and that all transactions are recorded in an immutable ledger. The system also uses off-chain storage systems to store large-size digital content, such as images and audio and video recordings of telehealth service sessions. This was done to improve the system's performance and reduce the cost of storing data on the blockchain. The authors recommended further developing and testing the proposed system in a real-world environment.

Accordingly, [29] proposed an IoT with a cloud-based clinical decision support system for predicting and observing disease. The proposed framework consists of three main components: a patient side, a cloud server, and a blockchain network. The patient side collects data from the patient's medical devices and sends it to the cloud server. The cloud server stores the data and uses it to train a neural network classifier for predicting diseases and their severity level. The blockchain network stores the patient's medical records and the results of the neural network classifier. The proposed framework was evaluated using a dataset of 700 patients. The suggested model is tested using a variety of classifiers.

While [30] reviewed blockchain technology, its architecture, existing applications, and integration with other technologies, as well as openings in numerous clinical research and healthcare fields, they found that blockchain technology can potentially improve data security, privacy, interoperability, and transparency in healthcare. Also, [17] performed a systematic review to determine the viability of using blockchain technology for telehealth. The study revealed numerous blockchain-based telehealth applications. Although no "silver bullet" exists in this sector, the authors' review offers some interesting starting ideas. These features include access to medical data, processing of medical services, reporting of epidemiology, diagnostic support, and treatment support.

Also, Shi *et al.* [3] constructed a blockchain-based user authentication scheme for better efficiency and security in the telehealth environment. They proposed a blockchain-based user authentication scheme integrating access control and physical unclonable function. The scheme uses a permissioned blockchain to store the user's identity information and access. The authors evaluated the security and performance of their proposed scheme. They recommended implementing the proposed scheme in real-world telehealth systems to provide better efficiency and security. How blockchain technology can be integrated with AI in cardiovascular medicine as well as other healthcare applications of blockchain technology was studied in [31].

The convergence of AI with blockchain was investigated in [32], by reviewing various applications of AI approaches to secure data and transactions in blockchain implementations. Also, [33] developed an integrated IoT-based AI with a blockchain technology platform for the prediction of COVID-19 disease. In [34], various AI and robotics-assisted telehealth applications during COVID-19 were studied with suggestions for an alternative AI-assisted telehealth framework (Table 6.1).

Table 6.1 Related works

Author(s) and publication date	**Objectives, methodology, and limitations of the study**	**Findings and recommendations**
Siyal *et al.* [25]	This study reviews the current state of the art in applying blockchain technology in medicine and healthcare	The authors found that blockchain technology has the potential to revolutionize healthcare by improving data security, interoperability, and privacy
Guo *et al.* [26]	They proposed a new blockchain-based attribute-based encryption (ABE) scheme with multi-authority for medical on-demand (MoD) in telemedicine systems. The scheme uses a blockchain to maintain a tamperproof record of encrypted data and access control policies	The results of the simulation show that the proposed scheme is efficient and can be used to support a large number of users and transactions. Future research should focus on deploying the proposed scheme in a real-world system and evaluating its performance in a practical setting
Tahir *et al.* [27]	This study presented a novel probabilistic model-based authentication and authorization framework for blockchain-enabled IoT networks	The simulation results showed that the proposed framework provides high security for IoT networks. It is also lightweight and efficient in terms of computational resources

(Continues)

Table 6.1 *(Continued)*

Author(s) and publication date	Objectives, methodology, and limitations of the study	Findings and recommendations
Hasan *et al.* [28]	The authors proposed a private blockchain-based telehealth system that uses a smart contract to register users and manage telehealth transactions	The results showed that the system could successfully automate the execution of teleconsultation, drug administration, and medical testing using blockchain technology
Alabdulatif *et al.* [35]	The study investigated the potential of artificial intelligence and blockchain technology to improve the safety of decision-making in e-health. The authors adopted support vector machine and multilayered perceptron classifiers as the algorithms	Multilayered perceptron had better performance based on the values of their false positive and false negative rates. The authors recommended that future studies should focus on developing more efficient and effective algorithms that can be used in blockchain-based e-health systems
Fatoum *et al.* [30]	The authors reviewed blockchain technology, its architecture, existing applications, integration with other technologies, and openings in numerous fields of clinical research and healthcare	The authors found that blockchain technology improves data security, privacy, interoperability, and transparency in healthcare and healthcare ecosystems
Hameed *et al.* [29]	The study proposed an IoT with a cloud-based clinical decision support system for disease prediction	The neural network classifier achieved an accuracy of 98.98% in predicting diseases and their severity level than other classifiers
Bawany *et al.* [36]	The authors created an efficient telehealth framework BlockHeal, which unifies all crucial healthcare services under a single platform and ensures a fully trusted environment. The technique applied involves an analysis of the shortcomings and significant barriers to the widespread adoption of the existing telehealth systems. The suggested framework solves the drawbacks and involves all healthcare system stakeholders, creating a unified platform to provide real, secure, and timely healthcare facilities	The proposed framework was evaluated using a simulation study. The results showed that the framework improved the security, efficiency, and accessibility of healthcare services. The authors recommend that further research should focus on developing and deploying the framework in real-world settings

(Continues)

Table 6.1 (*Continued*)

Author(s) and publication date	**Objectives, methodology, and limitations of the study**	**Findings and recommendations**
Pap and Oniga [37]	The objective of this study was to provide an overview of various technologies employed in specific healthcare applications, ranging from remote patient monitoring in the field of telemedicine to the use of AI in medical imaging. The authors thoroughly analyzed the literature on merging artificial intelligence-related e-health technologies. For the limitation, the authors noted that many challenges must be addressed before these technologies can be widely adopted, including issues related to data privacy and security, regulatory barriers, and ethical concerns	The authors discovered that by enhancing patient outcomes, cutting costs, and expanding access to care, convergent technologies have the potential to change healthcare. The authors recommended that policymakers and healthcare providers work together to develop policies and guidelines that promote the responsible use of these technologies while protecting patient privacy and ensuring equitable access to care
Koshechkin *et al.* [17]	The authors evaluated the viability of using blockchain technology for telemedicine by conducting a systematic review	Several blockchain applications were found to be viable for telemedicine application

6.3 Methodology

This study used a mixed approach consisting of a targeted literature review on several relevant studies relating to AI and blockchain technology-enabled projects in telehealth systems as well as proposing suitable algorithms and models. We searched important keywords related to the topic, which include "artificial intelligence and blockchain," "artificial intelligence and telehealth," "artificial intelligence in telehealth," and "artificial intelligence-blockchain projects for telehealth systems." The search was done on the following electronic databases; Google Scholar, PubMed, ScienceDirect, and IEEE Xplore Library. The carefully reviewed papers consist of research articles, conference papers, and books published between 2017 and 2023. The papers were screened to ensure that only recent papers on AI and blockchain technology were selected. Papers not directly related to the title were excluded.

The flowchart for the methodology adopted for the study is shown in Figure 6.1.

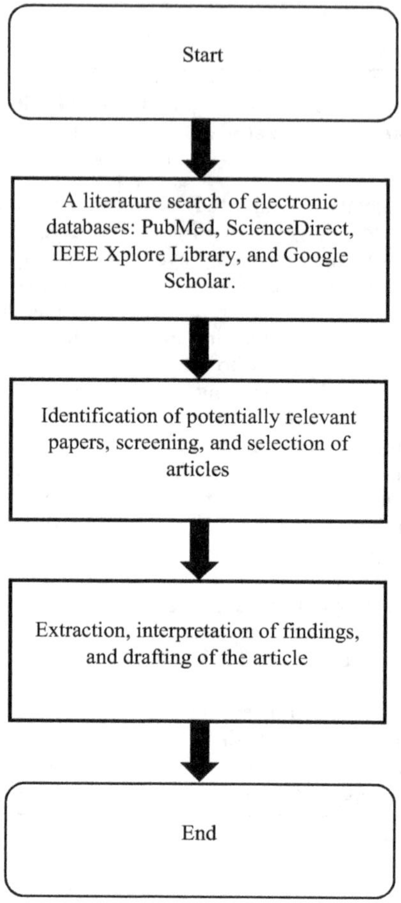

Figure 6.1 Study methodology flowchart

6.4 Applications of artificial intelligence and blockchain technology in telehealth

In this section, the various applications of AI and blockchain technology to telehealth projects using various architectures were discussed. The common architecture often used for AI–blockchain-based projects is the hyper ledger fabric architecture, a modular collaborative platform that consists of several layers. The overall goal of integrating blockchain technology into telehealth systems is to improve decentralization, making it possible for customers to take charge of their data securely. AI can use blockchain-based data in pattern generation and decision-making. Blockchain technology provides smart contracts. A smart contract consists of scripts written in blockchain that facilitate agreement implementation [38].

A variety of AI models, such as deep learning, neural networks, random forest, XGboost, and several others can be used to train secure and trusted blockchain-based

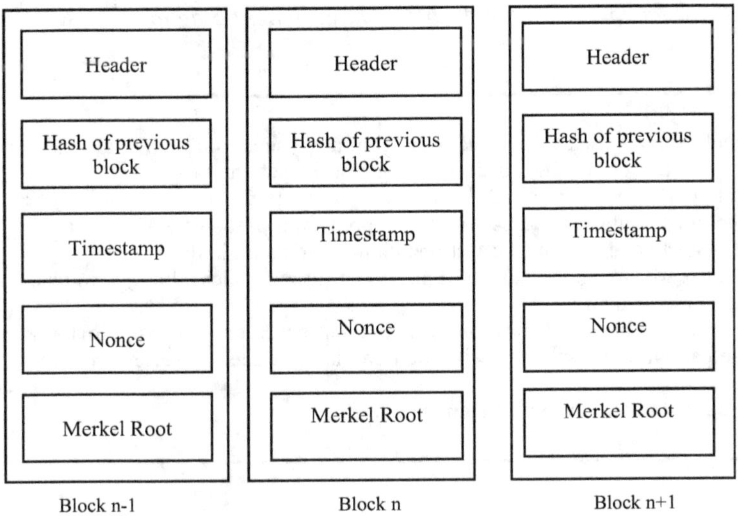

Figure 6.2 Blockchain structure

data. There are several applications of AI and blockchain in telehealth. Figure 6.2 shows the basic structure of blockchain. A typical block consists of a header, hash of previous blocks, timestamp, nonce, and market root.

6.4.1 AI–blockchain model for medical image analysis in telehealth systems

Medical images are necessary for the diagnosis of certain health conditions which are accompanied by tumors. When such images are taken, they are processed and interpreted by a radiologist either in hardcopy or in softcopy via electronic means. In telehealth systems, medical images can be transmitted in real-time or later through electronic means for clinical interpretation by radiologists. The use of AI to assist clinicians in medical diagnosis is well-reported. However, the adoption of blockchain technology in medical imaging is still in its early stages. The implementation of AI blockchain technology-enabled projects in teleradiology will provide a secure platform for AI-supported diagnosis of medical images and give the patient access to the test results, which could be used to seek a second opinion from other AI-supported telehealth systems within the distributed blockchain-enabled network. Blockchain provides opportunities to enable the storage and distribution of medical images [39] (Table 6.2).

6.4.2 Integrated blockchain and artificial intelligence chatbots synergies for telehealth projects

Chatbots are also called conversational assistants as they can mimic an intelligent human conversation [40]. AI support assistants play vital roles in modern telehealth systems as they provide a medium for patients to communicate and extract answers

Table 6.2 Algorithm steps for AI–blockchain patient diagnosis via telehealth system

1.	Start
2.	Patient receives medical consultation from a physician through a telehealth system
3.	Physician prescribes diagnostic imaging test for patient
4.	Patient undergoes prescribed diagnostic imaging test
5.	Radiologist analyzes images with the support of a pretrained AI model
6.	Radiologist sends diagnostic test results to patients digitally
7.	Patient sends imaging results to a physician through telehealth system using a decentralized blockchain
8.	Physician prescribes medication to the patient based on diagnostic imaging results
9.	If the patient is not satisfied with the treatment, he seeks a second opinion
10.	Else
11.	The patient continues with treatment
12.	End

concerning their health conditions using human language [41]. Communication between chatbots and patients is usually automated, leading to improved customer service [42]. Blockchain-enabled chatbots have been developed in other sectors, such as finance and healthcare. Typical examples include BONIK and Brokerbot, which have been used for various purposes, including financial transactions [43,44]. Chatbots can serve various purposes in telehealth systems, such as scheduling patient appointments, taking patient histories, and disease prediction [45]. There are a number of AI chatbot projects in healthcare. In [46], an AI-powered chatbot, Alleviate, was developed for a telehealth system to support patients suffering from mental health disorders. However, Alleviate's designers did not leverage the many benefits of blockchain technology. With the synergy of AI and blockchain technology, more secure chatbots can be used to communicate with patients taking advantage of the tamperproof nature of blockchain technology devoid of data manipulation or alteration [47]. The basic architecture of a typical chatbot consists of the user interface application that enables the user to interact with the chatbot. The chatbot has a response generation module that responds to the user after receiving the user's information. A chatbot can employ a dialogue manager to extract useful information from the knowledge base to answer user queries. Figure 6.3 shows the block diagram of an AI–blockchain chatbot for telehealth systems.

The integration of payment services into chatbots is rising [48]. Hence, payment systems can be fortified with blockchain technology.

6.4.3 AI–blockchain-based electronic health records projects

EHRs of patients in telehealth clinics, when integrated with AI and blockchain technology, ensure the privacy of patients' records. EHRs are generally preferred to paper-based records, particularly in telehealth practice. However, the problem

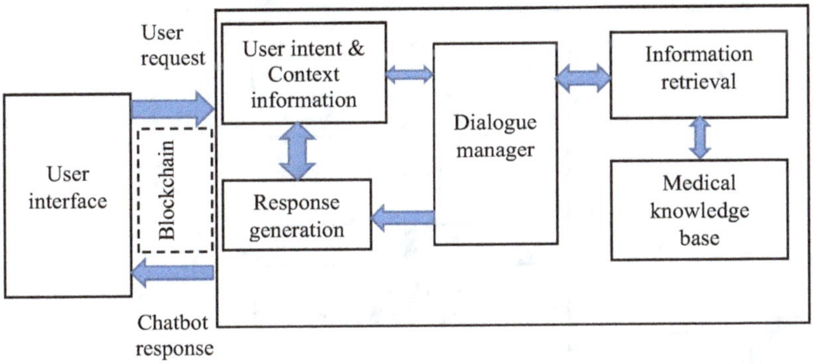

Figure 6.3 AI–blockchain-enabled chatbot for telehealth system

of the security of patient's health records is a major concern for various stakeholders, including hospital administrators and patients. AI has been combined with blockchain to provide access and help to analyze patients' medical history. The records are stored using the Interplanetary File System (IPFS) and linked to blockchain [11].

The key implementation stages for AI and blockchain-based EHRs include the development of: the front-end user interface, Ethereum decentralized app (DApp), in the IPFS for storing files, blockchain backend, the machine learning model, and the integration of the various modules as shown in the flowchart in Figure 6.1. The front-end user interface is developed to provide a platform for patients and healthcare providers to interact with the system. Ethereum is a decentralized network based on peer-to-peer technology and designed to enable smart contracts, which are commands capable of transactions with blockchain [49]. Ethereum works as a global network of computers designed to create, manage, and run "DApps," making it possible for users to enter into agreements and execute transactions directly [50]. Figure 6.4 shows the flowchart for AI-blockchain-based EHRs.

6.5 Artificial intelligence–blockchain enabled projects and synergies for telehealth: prospects and challenges

Synergies between AI and blockchain technology hold great promise for the future of telehealth systems. Global applications of AI and blockchain technology have witnessed massive growth. There are varieties of ways to create these synergies. While AI will serve as a tool for decision support, blockchain technology will provide a more secure, transparent, and tamperproof platform for sharing patient data and a secure payment system. With this synergy, cryptocurrencies can be used to pay bills for telehealth services. Thus, it makes expanded payment options for telehealth services possible. The impact of this synergy would lead to increased deployment of both technologies in many telehealth systems worldwide. There are

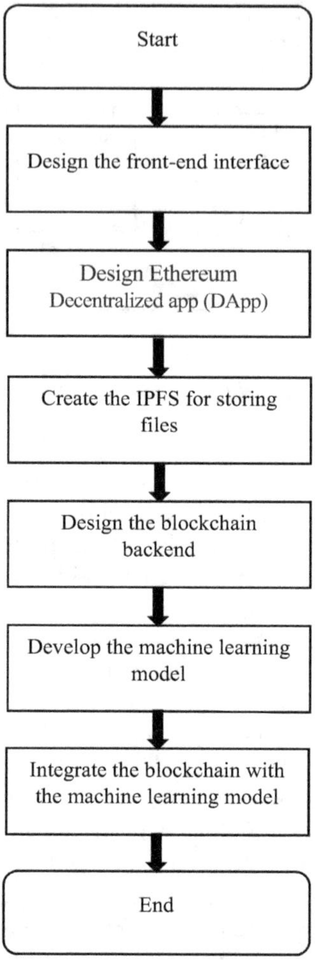

Figure 6.4 Flowchart for AI–blockchain-based electronic health records

some barriers to the effective synergy between AI and blockchain technology-enabled projects in telehealth [51]. Given that each AI and blockchain has its limitations and challenges, combining both technologies will likely give rise to various bottlenecks.

AI and blockchain technology are intricately complex. The complexity makes creating effective synergy between them difficult while implementing telehealth systems [52]. AI models are often seen as black boxes that are difficult to be understood and interpreted by clinicians. Similarly, there is a general lack of understanding about blockchain technology among healthcare practitioners. Therefore, innovative strategies must be adopted to create effective synergy between both technologies in telehealth systems.

While there is a great demand for experts with sufficient expertise in design and programming skills to execute AI and blockchain technology projects in telehealth, there is still a huge AI shortage of qualified experts to handle this demanding task. There are incidences of project failure of AI and blockchain projects, which could be mitigated by strategic planning, adequate training of manpower, and collaborative partnerships.

6.6 Selected AI–blockchain projects for telehealth systems

6.6.1 MyHealthMyData

MyHealthMyData (MHMD) is a project sponsored by the European Union and established to provide secure distributed network connections between healthcare organizations and patients. It takes advantage of emerging technologies such as blockchain to provide decentralized records. MHMD uses public blockchain to help individuals manage and control their data based on strict protection conditions [53].

6.6.2 MedCredits

MedCredits is a peer-to-peer network that provides telehealth services to dermatology patients by connecting them directly to physicians using a secure Ethereum-based system [15]. Since the development of MedCredits by Product Edge in 2016, MedCredits has transformed the practice of teledermatology by providing a decentralized platform for patients to receive specialized medical care and make payments for the services through a secure platform. The MedCredits network uses the MEDX token, which is known for providing a mechanism for physicians to be verified to ensure that only licensed physicians can treat patients [54].

6.6.3 MedicalChain

This refers to a blockchain-based EHRs system that utilizes two distinct decentralized networks, namely, blockchain and peer-to-peer networks, to link various healthcare providers and corporate organizations in the healthcare sector. MedChain solves the privacy problem in conventional EHRs [55]. Through MedChain, patients' information is stored in a secure blockchain network and accessed when required. The MedChain network comprises two kinds of peer nodes: super peers designed specifically for large organizations and edge peers designed for small organizations [56]. Designed with distributed data technologies, it uses a private permissioned blockchain [57]. MedChain adopts timed-based smart contracts for regulating transactions and managing access to EHRs using advanced encryption techniques [58]. Integration of MedChain with AI will potentially enhance the analysis of patients' health records.

6.6.4 BlockHeal

The BlockHeal framework is a blockchain technology-enabled telehealth platform designed to provide a wide range of services. The integration of various services of

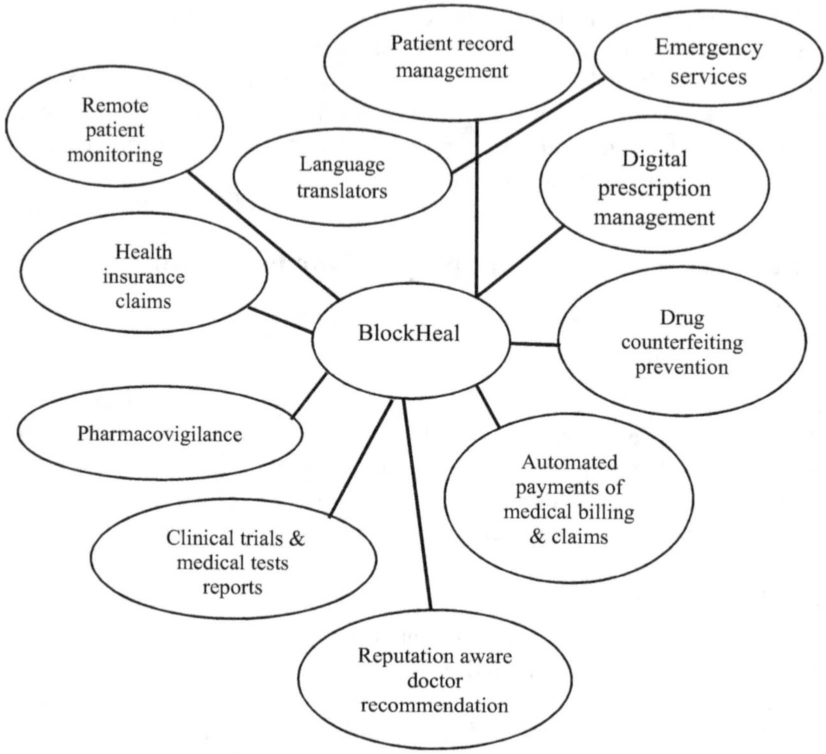

Figure 6.5 Components of the BlockHeal framework

the healthcare sector using transparent, trusted, and tamperproof blockchain technology is the overall goal of the BlockHeal framework. It achieves this using 11 various DApps. Figure 6.5 shows the various components of the BlockHeal framework.

The framework is managed by the central health regulatory authority [36]. The performance of the BlockHeal framework could be enhanced with the deployment of AI in several sectors. In the areas of pharmacovigilance, AI has been shown to optimize pharmacovigilance processes leading to improved monitoring and response to drug adverse reactions [59]. AI has been used widely in disease diagnostics. The integration of AI with BlockHeal has the potential to offer decision support to doctors handling various diseases. More secure personalized predictive modeling can be achieved by combining AI with blockchain technology.

6.7 Lessons learned

Some lessons have been learned from this study. First is the need to leverage AI and blockchain technology in developing modern telehealth systems. It is obvious that despite their challenges, these technologies will enhance the operational efficiency and security of telehealth systems. We learned about the various applications of AI and blockchain technology in telehealth systems and developed an algorithm for AI-blockchain patient diagnosis via a telehealth system. We learned to design AI chatbots and how they can be integrated with blockchain technology in telehealth systems. Identified major challenges of AI and blockchain technology project implementation and suggested solutions, including strategic planning, adequate training of manpower, and collaborative partnerships among stakeholders.

6.8 Conclusions and future scope

AI and blockchain technology should be harnessed to advance healthcare. The chapter reviewed related studies on using AI and highlighted the applications of AI and blockchain technology in telehealth systems. The application of AI and blockchain technology in the interpretation and transmission of digital medical images was highlighted. This chapter also explained the integration of blockchain into AI chatbots for telehealth services in the scheduling of patient appointments, taking of patient history, and disease prediction stressing the role of blockchain in ensuring increased security. The synergy between AI and blockchain technology in designing and managing EHRs also showed positive results. While the synergy between AI and blockchain technology in telehealth has not been fully explored, the future holds great prospects for revolutionizing telehealth practice. The impact of this synergy would lead to the deployment of both technologies in many telehealth systems worldwide. With several studies currently ongoing, the future applications of AI and blockchain technology in telehealth practice will be more prominent and widespread. The more public blockchain network infrastructure will be created. With recent advances in explainable AI research, there is likely to be increased transparency in the deployment of AI and blockchain models in telehealth. Therefore, increased user confidence reduces possible risks.

References

[1] S. Nwaneri and R. Oladele, Telemedicine System for the Diagnosis and Management of Invasive Fungal Infections in Nigeria. *Journal of Clinical Sciences*, vol. 20, no. 1, pp. 35–39, 2023.

[2] I. Yaqoob, K. Salah, R. Jayaraman, and Y. Al-Hammadi, Blockchain for Healthcare Data Management: Opportunities, Challenges, and Future Recommendations. *Neural Computing and Applications*, vol. 34, pp. 1–16, 2021.

[3] S. Shi, M. Luo, Y. Wen, L. Wang, and B. He, A Blockchain-Based User Authentication Scheme with Access Control for Telehealth Systems. *Security and Communication Networks*, vol. 2022, no. 1, pp. 1–18, 2020. Available: https://www.hindawi.com/journals/scn/2022/6735003/ [Accessed May 26, 2023].

[4] C. Lin, D. He, X. Huang, M. K. Khan, and K. K. R. Choo, DCAP: A Secure and Efficient Decentralized Conditional Anonymous Payment System based on Blockchain. *IEEE Transactions on Information Forensics Security*, vol. 15, pp. 2440–2452, 2020.

[5] P. Tagde, S. Tagde, T. Bhattacharya, *et al*., Blockchain and Artificial Intelligence Technology in e-Health. *Environmental Science and Pollution Research,* vol. 28, pp. 52810–52831, 2021. https://doi.org/10.1007/s11356-021-16223-0

[6] F. Knirsch, A. Unterweger, and D. Engel, Implementing a Blockchain from Scratch: Why, How, and What We Learned. *EURASIP Journal on Information Security*, vol. 2, pp. 1–14, 2019. https://doi.org/10.1186/s13635-019-0085-3.

[7] B. Wu, Y. Pi, and J. Chen, Privacy Protection of Medical Service Data Based on Blockchain and Artificial Intelligence in the Era of Smart Medical Care. *Wireless Communications and Mobile Computing*, 2022. Available: https://www.hindawi.com/journals/wcmc/2022/5295801/ [Accessed July 7, 2023]

[8] D.V. Dimitrov, Blockchain Applications for Healthcare Data Management. *Healthcare Informatics Research*, vol. 25, no. 1, pp. 51–56, 2019.

[9] J. Yli-Huumo, D. Ko, S. Choi, S. Park, and K. Smolander, Where is Current Research on Blockchain Technology?—A Systematic Review, *PLoS ONE*, vol. 11, no. 10, p. e0163477, 2016.

[10] V. Hassija, V. Chamola, V. Gupta, and G. S. S. Chalapathi, A Framework for Secure Vehicular Network Using Advanced Blockchain, In: *2020 International Wireless Communications and Mobile Computing (IWCMC)*, Limassol, Cyprus: IEEE, pp. 1260–1265, 2020. doi:10.1109/IWCMC48107.2020.9148201.

[11] V. Chamola, A. Goyal, P. Sharma, *et al.,* Artificial Intelligence-Assisted Blockchain-Based Framework for Smart and Secure EMR Management. *Neural Computing and Applications*, vol. 14, pp. 1–14, 2022. https://doi.org/10.1007/s00521-022-07087-7.

[12] A.F. da Conceição, F.S.C. da Silva, V. Rocha, A. Locoro, and J.M. Barguil, Eletronic Health Records Using Blockchain Technology, arXiv preprint arXiv:1804.10078, 2018. Available: https://arxiv.org/pdf/1804.10078.pdf [Accessed July 10, 2023].

[13] A. Dubovitskaya, Z. Xu, S. Ryu, M. Schumacher, and F. Wang, Secure and Trustable Electronic Medical Records Sharing Using Blockchain, In: *AMIA Annual Symposium Proceedings*, American Medical Informatics Association, p. 650, 2017.

[14] S. Shi, D. He, L. Li, N. Kumar, M. K. Khan, and K. R. Choo, Applications of Blockchain in Ensuring the Security and Privacy of Electronic Health Record Systems: A Survey, *Computers & Security*, vol. 97, p. 101966, 2020. https://doi.org/10.1016/j.cose.2020.101966.

[15] R. W. Ahmad, K. Salah, R. Jayaraman, I. Yaqoob, S. Ellahham, and M. Omar, The Role of Blockchain Technology in Telehealth and Telemedicine. *International Journal of Medical Informatics*, vol. 148, p. 104399, 2021. https://doi.org/10.1016/j.ijmedinf.2021.104399.

[16] R. Luna, E. Rhine, M. Myhra, R. Sullivan, and C. S. Kruse, Cyber Threats to Health Information Systems: A Systematic Review, *Technology and Health Care*, vol. 24, no. 1, pp. 1–9, 2016.

[17] K. Koshechkin, G. Lebedev, G. Radzievsky, R. Seepold, and N. M. Martinez, Blockchain Technology Projects to Provide Telemedical Services: Systematic Review. *Journal of Medical Internet Research*, vol. 23, no. 8, p. e17475, 2021. doi:10.2196/17475.

[18] J. B. Awotunde, A. L. Imoize, O. B. Ayoade, *et al.*, An Enhanced Hyper-Parameter Optimization of a Convolutional Neural Network Model for Leukemia Cancer Diagnosis in a Smart Healthcare System. *Sensors*, vol. 22, no. 24, p. 9689, 2022.

[19] J. B. Awotunde, A. L. Imoize, D. P. Salako, and Y. Farhaoui, An Enhanced Medical Diagnosis System for Malaria and Typhoid Fever Using Genetic Neuro-Fuzzy System, In: *Artificial Intelligence and SmartEnvironment: ICAISE'2022*, Cham: Springer International Publishing, pp. 173–183, 2023.

[20] S. Vyas, S. Shabaz, M., Pandit, L. R. Parvathy, and I. Ofori, Integration of Artificial Intelligence and Blockchain Technology in Healthcare and Agriculture. *Journal of Food Quality*, vol. 2022, pp. 1–11, 2022. https://doi.org/10.1155/2022/4228448.

[21] J. Westenberger, K. Schuler, and D. Schlegel, Failure of AI Projects: Understanding the Critical Factors. *Procedia Computer Science*, vol. 196, pp. 69–76, 2022.

[22] Z. Zhang, X. Song, L. Liu, J. Yin, Y. Wang, and D. Lan, Recent Advances in Blockchain and Artificial Intelligence Integration: Feasibility Analysis, Research Issues, Applications, Challenges, and Future Work. *Security and Communications Networks*, vol. 2021, p. 9991535, 2021. Available: https://www.hindawi.com/journals/scn/2021/9991535/ Retrived July 4, 2023.

[23] D. Połap, G. Srivastava, A. Jolfaei, and R. M. Parizi, Blockchain Technology and Neural Networks for the Internet of Medical Things, In: *IEEE INFOCOM 2020—IEEE Conference on Computer Communications Workshops (INFOCOM WKSHPS)*, Toronto, ON, Canada: IEEE, pp. 508–513, 2020. doi:10.1109/INFOCOMWKSHPS 50562.2020.9162735.

[24] P. Singh, Z. Elmi, Y. Lau, M. Borowska-Stefańska, S. Wiśniewski, and M. A. Dulebenets, Blockchain and AI Technology Convergence: Applications in Transportation Systems. *Vehicular Communications*, vol. 38, p. 100521, 2022. https://doi.org/10.1016/j.vehcom.2022.100521.

[25] A. A. Siyal, A. Z. Junejo, M. Zawish, K. Ahmed, A. Khalil, and G. Soursou, Applications of Blockchain Technology in Medicine and Healthcare: Challenges and Future Perspectives. *Cryptography*, vol. 3, no. 1, p. 3, 2019. https://doi.org/10.3390/cryptography3010003.

[26] R. Guo, H. Shi, D. Zheng, C. Jing, C. Zhuang, and Z. Wang, Flexible and Efficient Blockchain-Based ABE Scheme with Multi-Authority for Medical on Demand in Telemedicine System. *IEEE Access*, vol. 7, pp. 88012–88025, 2019. https://doi.org/10.1109/ACCESS.2019.2925625.

[27] M. Tahir, M. Sardaraz, S. Muhammad, and M. Saud Khan, A Lightweight Authentication and Authorization Framework for Blockchain-Enabled IoT Network in Health-Informatics. *Sustainability*, vol. 12, no. 17, p. 6960, 2020. https://doi.org/10.3390/su12176960.

[28] H. R. Hasan, K. Salah, R. Jayaraman, I. Yaqoob, M. Omar, and S. Ellahham, Blockchain-Enabled Telehealth Services Using Smart Contracts. *IEEE Access*, vol. 9, pp. 151944–151959, 2021. https://doi.org/10.1109/ACCESS.2021.3126025.

[29] K. Hameed, I. S. Bajwa, N. Sarwar, W. Anwar, Z. Mushtaq, and T. Rashid, Integration of 5G and Blockchain Technologies in Smart Telemedicine Using IoT. *Journal of Healthcare Engineering*, vol. 2021, pp. 1–18, 2021. https://doi.org/10.1155/2021/8814364.

[30] H. Fatoum, S. Hanna, J. D. Halamka, D. C. Sicker, P. Spangenberg, and S. K. Hashmi, Blockchain Integration with Digital Technology and the Future of Health Care Ecosystems: Systematic Review. *Journal of Medical Internet Research*, vol. 23, no. 11, p. e19846, 2021. https://doi.org/10.2196/19846.

[31] H. Krittanawong, M. Aydar, H. H. Virk, *et al.*, Artificial Intelligence-Powered Blockchains for Cardiovascular Medicine, *Canadian Journal of Cardiology*, vol. 38, no. 2, pp. 185–195, 2022. https://doi.org/10.1016/j.cjca.2021.11.011.

[32] J. K. Dhaniya, AI-Blockchain Convergence: Realigning Synergies for Connected Organizations, 2023. Available: https://www.academia.edu/44718511/AI_Blockchain_Convergence_Realigning_synergies_for_connected_organizations [Accessed May 22, 2023].

[33] K. A. Kumar, V. K. Reddy, and A. Narmada, An Integration of AI, Blockchain and IoT Technologies for Combating Covid-19, In: N. Marriwala, C.C. Tripathi, S. Jain, S. Mathapathi (eds), *Emergent Converging Technologies and Biomedical Systems. Lecture Notes in Electrical Engineering*, vol. 841, Singapore: Springer, 2022. https://doi.org/10.1007/978-981-16-8774-7_15.

[34] S. Bhaskar, S. Bradley, S. Sakhamuri, *et al.*, Designing Futuristic Telemedicine Using Artificial Intelligence and Robotics in the COVID-19 Era. *Frontiers in Public Health,* vol. 2, no. 8, p. 556789, 2020. doi:10.3389/fpubh.2020.556789.

[35] A. Alabdulatif, M. Al Asqah, T. Moulahi, and S. Zidi, Leveraging Artificial Intelligence in Blockchain-Based E-Health for Safer Decision Making Framework. *Applied Sciences,* vol. 13, no. 2, p. 1035, 2023. https://doi.org/10.3390/app13021035.

[36] N. Z. Bawany, T. Qamar, H. Tariq, and S. Adnan, Integrating Healthcare Services Using Blockchain-Based Telehealth Framework. *IEEE Access* vol. 10, pp. 36505–36517, 2022. https://doi.org/10.1109/ACCESS.2022.3161944.

[37] I. A. Pap and S. Oniga, A Review of Converging Technologies in eHealth Pertaining to Artificial Intelligence. *International Journal of Environmental*

Research and Public Health, vol. 19, no. 18, p. 11413, 2022. https://doi.org/10.3390/ijerph191811413.

[38] Q. Xia, E. B. Sifah, K. O. Asamoah, J. Gao, X. Du, and M. Guizani, MeDShare: Trust-Less Medical Data Sharing among Cloud Service Providers via Blockchain. *IEEE Access*, vol. 5, pp. 14757–14767, 2017. doi:10.1109/ACCESS.2017.2730843.

[39] M. P. McBee and C. Wilcox, Blockchain Technology: Principles and Applications in Medical Imaging. *Journal of Digital Imaging*, vol. 33, pp. 726–734, 2020. https://doi.org/10.1007/s10278-019-00310-3.

[40] W. Villegas-Ch, A. Arias-Navarrete, and X. Palacios-Pacheco, Proposal of an Architecture for the Integration of a Chatbot with Artificial Intelligence in a Smart Campus for the Improvement of Learning. *Sustainability*, vol. 12, no.4, p. 1500, 2020. Available: https://www.mdpi.com/2071-1050/12/4/1500 Retrieved June 19, 2023.

[41] N. S. Vasileiou, M. V. Maglogiannis, and G. Ilias, The Health ChatBots in Telemedicine: Intelligent Dialog System for Remote Support. *Journal of Healthcare Engineering*, vol. 2022, p. 4876512, 2022. https://doi.org/10.1155/2022/4876512.

[42] S. D'souza, D. Nazareth, C. Vaz, and M. Shetty, Blockchain and AI in Pharmaceutical Supply Chain, In: Proceedings of the International Conference on Smart Data Intelligence (ICSMDI 2021), 2021. Available at SSRN: https://ssrn.com/abstract=3852034 or http://dx.doi.org/10.2139/ssrn.3852034.

[43] M. S. I. Bhuiyan, A. Razzak, M. S. Ferdous, M. J. M. Chowdhury, M. A. Hoque, and S. Tarkoma, BONIK: A Blockchain Empowered Chatbot for Financial Transactions, In: *2020 IEEE 19th International Conference on Trust, Security and Privacy in Computing and Communications (TrustCom)*, Guangzhou, China: IEEE, pp. 1079–1088, 2020. doi:10.1109/TrustCom50675.2020.00143.

[44] M. Lee, L. Frank, and W. IJsselsteijn, Brokerbot: A Cryptocurrency Chatbot in the Social-technical Gap of Trust. *Computer Supported Cooperative Work,* vol. 30, pp. 79–117, 2021. https://doi.org/10.1007/s10606-021-09392-6.

[45] F.O. Chete and P. Oviawe, A Conversational Artificial Intelligence Chatbot to Deliver Telehealth Information on Covid-19. *NIPES Journal of Science and Technology Research*, vol. 4, no. 3, pp. 110–119, 2022.

[46] K. Roy, V. Khanddelwal, R. Goswami, N. Dolbir, J. Malekar, and A. Sheth, Demo Alleviate: Demonstrating Artificial Intelligence Enabled Virtual Assistance for Telehealth: The Mental Health Case. *The Thirty-Seventh AAAI Conference on Artificial Intelligence*, pp. 16479–16480. Available: https://arxiv.org/abs/2304.00025 Retrieved July 8, 2023.

[47] R. Sapra and P. Dhaliwal, A Blockchain Solution for the Privacy of Patients' Medical Data, In: P.Kumar, Y.Kumar, M. A. Tawhid (Eds.), *Intelligent Data-Centric Systems, Machine Learning, Big Data, and IoT for Medical*

Informatics, San Diego, CA, USA:Academic Press, pp. 327–347, 2021. https://www.sciencedirect.com/science/article/pii/B9780128217771000252.

[48] E. Adamopoulou and L. Moussiades, An Overview of Chatbot Technology, In: I. Maglogiannis, L. Iliadis, and E. Pimenidis. (eds.), *AIAI 2020, IFIP AICT, IFIP International Federation for Information Processing 2020*, vol. 584, Switzerland: Springer Nature Switzerland AG 2020, pp. 373–383, 2020.

[49] F. K. Nishi, M. Shams-E-Mofiz, M. M. Khan, *et al*., Electronic Healthcare Data Record Security Using Blockchain and Smart Contract. *Journal of Sensors*, vol. 2022, no. 13, pp. 1–22, 2022. Available: https://www.hindawi.com/journals/js/2022/7299185/ Retrieved June 20, 2023.

[50] T. Fatokun, A. Nag, and S. Sharma, Towards a Blockchain Assisted Patient Owned System for Electronic Health Records. *Electronics*, vol. 10, no. 5, p. 580, 2021. Available: https://www.mdpi.com/2079-9292/10/5/580 Retrieved June 20, 2023.

[51] I. Yaqoob, K. Salah, R. Jayaraman, and Y. Al-Hammadi, Blockchain for Healthcare Data Management: Opportunities, Challenges, and Future Recommendations. *Neural Computing and Applications*, vol. 34, pp. 11475–11490, 2022. https://doi.org/10.1007/s00521-020-05519-w.

[52] B. Xing and T. Marwala, The Synergy of Blockchain and Artificial Intelligence, 2018. Available at SSRN: https://ssrn.com/abstract=3225357 [Accessed October 31, 2023].

[53] E. Morley-Fletcher, MHMD: My Health, MyData, EDBT/ICDT Workshops. Available: http://www.myhealthmydata.eu/wp-content/uploads/2018/05/EuroPro_paper_04.pdf [Accessed June 28, 2023].

[54] J.M. Todaro, Overview of MedCredits, 2020. Available online at: http://medcredits.io/team/ [Accessed June 28, 2023].

[55] H. L. Gururaj, B. Goutham, V. Janhavi, K. C. Suhas, M. N. Manu, Medchain: Securing Electronic Medical Records with a Peer to Peer Networks and Distributed File System, In: P.K. Singh, G. Veselov, V. Vyatkin, A. Pljonkin, J.M. Dodero, Y. Kumar (eds.), *Futuristic Trends in Network and Communication Technologies, FTNCT 2020. Communications in Computer and Information Science*, vol. 1395, Singapore: Springer, 2021. https://doi.org/10.1007/978-981-16-1480-4_1.

[56] B. Shen, J. Guo, and Y. Yang, MedChain: Efficient Healthcare Data Sharing via Blockchain. *Applied Science*, vol. 9, no. 6, p. 1207, 2019. Available: https://www.mdpi.com/2076-3417/9/6/1207 Retrieved June 20, 2023.

[57] J. R. Troncoso-Pastoriza, J. L. Raisaro, L. Gasser, B. Ford, and J. Hubaux, MedChain: Accountable and Auditable Data Sharing in Distributed Medical Scenarios, In: *2019 AMIA Informatics Summit*, San Francisco, CA, USA, March 25–28, 2019. Available: https://infoscience.epfl.ch/record/301750 Retrieved June 21, 2023.

[58] E. Y. Daraghmi, Y.-A. Daraghmi, and S.-M. Yuan, MedChain: A Design of Blockchain-Based System for Medical Records Access and Permissions

Management. *IEEE Access*, vol. 7, pp. 164595–164613, 2019. doi:10.1109/ACCESS.2019.2952942.

[59] M. Salas, J. Petracek, P. Yalamanchili, *et al.,* The Use of Artificial Intelligence in Pharmacovigilance: A Systematic Review of the Literature. *Pharmaceutical Medicine*, vol. 36, no. 5, pp. 295–306, 2022. doi:10.1007/s40290-022-00441-z.

Chapter 7

Recent advances in AI and blockchain technology in modern telehealth systems

Nne Rena Saturday[1], Kingsley Theophilus Igulu[2] and Promise Elechi[3]

The modernization of medicine is becoming inevitable worldwide, especially with the outbreak of COVID-19, and that has led to the adoption of viable technologies to deliver effective and efficient telehealth systems. This chapter highlights how telehealth is delivered and the remarkable enhancement of telehealth using artificial intelligence (AI) and blockchain technologies. The chapter explores the relevant AI models such as deep learning, machine learning, Internet of Things and others used to deliver healthcare remotely. In addition, the security aspect for medicine, data ownership and data privacy using blockchain in healthcare delivery is presented. Finally, the chapter highlights the recent advancement in these technologies such as RapidAI, ProvChain, extreme data privacy and application layer security.

7.1 Introduction

Healthcare delivery has changed globally in the form of telehealth systems. Telehealth is a technological process that bridges demographic and time constraints [1], enabling delivery of health and health-related services which include health information services, medical care, provider education, patient education and self-care through the use of telecommunication and digital communication technologies [2]. This has expanded health services especially as it affects homebound aged individuals. This system has successfully been accepted by different specialties in medicine, and they are listed as psychiatry, dentistry, COVID-19 consultation and dermatology [3–7]. The World Health Organization (WHO) records that the number of aged people is fast increasing with 1 billion individuals above 60 years in 2020, 1.4 billion by 2030, and will be twice in number by 2050 [8]. Researchers have delved into this area with extensive reviews that have birthed terminologies

[1]Department of Computer Science, Rivers State University, Nigeria
[2]Department of Computer Science, Kenule Beeson Saro-Wiwa Polytechnic, Nigeria
[3]Department of Electrical and Electronics Engineering, Rivers State University, Nigeria

that border around healthcare services such as telehealth, telemedicine, tele dentistry, remote activity monitoring, health coaching systems, telenursing, health information technology, decision support systems, telecare, remote care programs, structured telephone and telephone only support [9]. Interestingly, the traditional healthcare structure has long since been considered to be reviewed due to the technological innovations, epidemic shift and demographic shift in order to deliver health services; the outbreak of COVID-19 has fast-tracked these innovations that have changed the dynamics of healthcare delivery. The use of digital solutions is inevitable as there are increase of complex health conditions which require specialists that are somewhat limited. This technological shift will likely continue as it enhances growth in this sector and post-epidemic recovery. The United Nations Conference on Trade and Development's major focus on the global policy initiative was on the promotion of e-health applications and telehealth, including training of health personnel and manufacturing of medical equipment and consumables [10]. Also, WHO clearly outlined that digital health should be a core part of the priorities of health and should benefit the masses in a way that is ethical, secured and safe, reliable, equitable and sustainable; its development should include the principle of transparency, scalability, privacy, replicability, accessibility, interoperability, security and confidentiality in its global strategy on digital health overarching principles for health innovation, 2020 [11]. Consequently, these cannot be achieved without recent technologies and innovations like blockchain and artificial intelligence (AI). Thus, telehealth is viewed as a medium that can handle the constraints of cost, access and quality of healthcare services. A greater part of telehealth borders in the back-office transmission of health diagnostic data and reports from one location to another for the medical specialist interpretation and synchronous monitoring of intensive care unit data [12]. It has been globally accepted as a resourceful alternative for physical consultations and the management of severe diseases and is equally very useful in the prevention of COVID-19 transmission.

7.1.1 Key contributions of the chapter

The following are the significant contributions of this chapter:

1. This chapter explores the recent advancements in technology based on the telehealth system.
2. The chapter highlights the specific application of AI in the telehealth system and how it has transformed the delivery of healthcare.
3. The chapter exposes the applicability of the blockchain technology in telehealth system and its corresponding impact.
4. The chapter discusses possible innovations with these technologies in the telehealth system.

7.1.2 Chapter organization

Section 7.2 presents the related works in effectiveness of AI and blockchain technology in the telehealth system. It discusses the key elements of telehealth systems.

Section 7.3 discusses AI and the healthcare industry, highlighting the application of AI in specific areas of healthcare and how it has significantly impacted the processes. Section 7.4 discusses blockchain technology and the telehealth system, highlighting how this technology has transformed the security and privacy of data in the telehealth system. Section 7.5 discusses the AI models adopted in the telehealth system, and Section 7.6 discusses the application of blockchain security in the telehealth system. Section 7.7 highlights the recent advances in the technological telehealth system. Section 7.8 highlights future considerations on application of AI and blockchain technology in the telehealth system and concludes the chapter.

7.2 Key elements of telehealth services

7.2.1 Web services

Telehealth as initially described is the use of information and communication technologies in the medical industry for delivery of healthcare services and other medical practices. A wide range of technologies are adopted in the delivery of healthcare, public health and health education in a virtual mode. The web infrastructure facilitates the process of healthcare-related services. Cloud storage is a very significant web service in telehealth. It is a cloud computing representation of storing digital data on distant servers that can be accessed through the internet. Usually, the physical infrastructure is hosted by companies like IBM, Amazon Web Services, Microsoft and Google. This technology presents telehealth as a time saver for healthcare establishments by offering user-friendly and safe access to medical records to patients and medical personnel from any location via the internet. This has helped to reduce crowded hospital and clinics as well as rate of infection. Some of its services are eClinicalWorks, Cloud DX, Epic Systems, IBM Merge iConnect, GE Health Cloud, Novarad etc.

7.2.2 Support platforms

These are application tools that enable real-time interaction between the medical personnel and the patient, access to EMR (electronic medical records) etc. There are wide range of these applications used by patients and clinicians such as MyChart application, Epic EMR, Haiku for mobile phones, Cantu for tablets, InTouch Health, VSee and Zoom for healthcare these platforms are being housed by varying devices in order to connect with the internet of things (IoT). The list of support platforms in this chapter is not exhaustive.

7.2.3 Mobile broadband communications

One of the fundamental technical components of telehealth system is a broadband connection. Lack of a broadband connection has an extensive impact on the implementation of telehealth systems as well as hinder patients access to the healthcare. This has helped to facilitate delivery of healthcare by supporting the role of the medical personnel in decision support and serving as a hub for medical information on the web. Also, it has served as a tool in learning for continuing education.

7.3 AI and healthcare industry

AI has taken a toll on several fields of research, and healthcare is not an exception even though it has been there for over a decade. The demand for healthcare services is fast increasing, and as such, there exist a limited number of medical personnel especially physicians. There is high positive expectation that AI can offer improved applications at all levels of healthcare delivery from diagnosis to treatment of patients [13]. There are substantial evidences that AI seems to be performing better than human in several tasks such as analysis of medical images, correlation of symptoms and biomarkers in EMR with the characteristics and prognosis of the disease [14]. In addition, Google DeepMind and IBM Watson have proved that AI is able to beat humans in certain tasks like Go and chess. Presently, these innovations from Google and IBM are being used in medical-related applications such as medical image diagnostics, medical mobile assistant, patient deterioration prediction and drug discovery, advanced cancer modeling and management of diabetes, respectively [15]. Interestingly, there are different aspects of healthcare that highlights the application of AI and how it has transformed these areas, and also Figure 7.1 captures significant variables in healthcare.

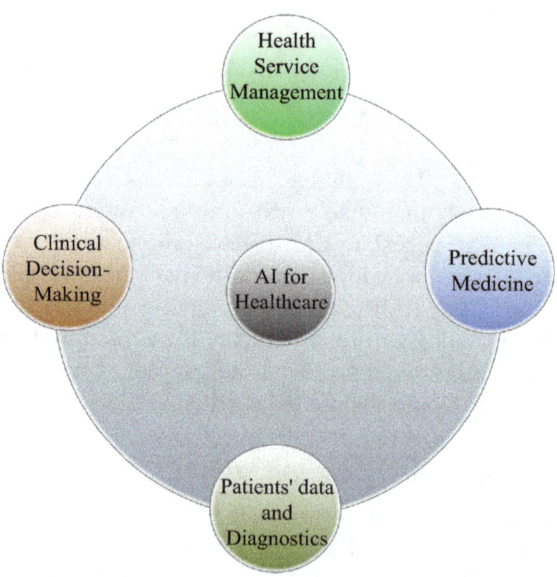

Figure 7.1 Significant variables for AI in healthcare

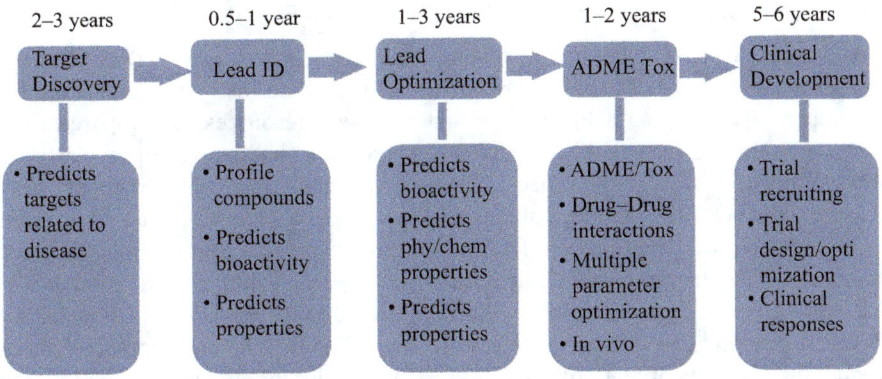

Figure 7.2 Machine learning opportunities within the small molecule drug discovery and development process.

7.3.1 The process of drug discovery

Drug discovery involves different aspect that certify a drug to be accepted and ubiquitous in the market. The first aspect deals with drug molecule identification and development, and it possibly takes a period of over 10 years with approval and marketing inclusive as illustrated in Figure 7.2. Within this period, if there is any failure, it hugely impacts on the process financially. Obviously, the process is challenging and quite inefficient. However, techniques in AI are being adopted to enhance the process for better results; from support vector machine, neural network and random forest to deep learning (DL) [16].

7.3.2 Property and activity prediction of drug

This aspect of drug development is very crucial because it deals with the identification of drug molecules and its behavior in the human body. Also, machine learning techniques are being adopted to evaluate biological activity, absorption, distribution, metabolism, excretion characteristics, as well as physicochemical properties of drug molecules. There are machine-readable libraries that store information on drug molecules which are used to generate machine learning models for drug discovery. An illustration will be that convolutional neural networks are used to generate footprints of these molecules from huge set of molecular graphs, which in turn give details of each molecule at the atomic level. These footprints are further used to predict the characteristics of a particular molecule. DeepTox is a DL model that measures the toxicity effects of compound comprising drug molecules. Deep learning applications in drug discovery also include generation of chemical structures, which is a molecular design of protein with specific functions or binding and so many applications like autoencoders. In recent times, the use of AI applications for drug discovery and development tilts toward DL approaches.

7.3.3 The process for clinical trials

Clinical trials are procedures in which newly manufactured drugs are tried on patients in order to observe the effect and how well it will work on them. The procedure has been reportedly usurping a lot of time and monetary resources as compared to its success rate. In this regard, AI is adopted to handle the challenge of these wastes by introducing automation in the process especially the data monitoring procedure since AI can handle very large amount of data and can produce accurate results. According to [17,18], the third serial report of the biopharma value chain on AI impacts, it has proven to reduce the time for a clinical trial cycle as well as improve the productivity and clinical development results. Furthermore, application of AI models and advanced analytics to predict real-world data (RWD) will assist researchers to expand their understanding of diseases, identify appropriate patients, significant investigators and develop unconventional study designs. RWD are scientific and research information which are obtained by biopharma businesses from a large number of sources and are unable to use the data. Also, using AI algorithms, clinical trial data can be cleansed, collated, coded, saved and maintained. In addition, capturing the data electronically can ameliorate the aspect of human error in the collection of data as well as hitch-free system integration [19].

7.3.4 Clinical intelligent systems for patients' care

The application of AI in healthcare has enhanced maternal care in different ways. AI models are used to predict whether pregnant mothers would encounter measurable risks during delivery based on electronic health-related data. The use of digital technology has increased patients' entry to regular and high nursing intensity within the duration of pregnancy, thus reducing the risk of developing serious maternal medical conditions. To reduce the tasks of medical personnel, robots that function based on AI algorithms assist patients, such as exoskeleton robots that assist paralyzed patients to learn how to use their feet and become independent [20]. Another application of robots is the bionic limbs that is attached to a patient's muscles with sensors and covered with bionic skin. It is reported to be more accurate and responsive than human body parts. Robots are also able to help in surgeries and rehabilitation. Robotic-assisted surgery is applied in cardiothoracic, urological, orthopedic, colorectal, maxillofacial, neurosurgery and in general [21].

AI algorithms are used for intelligent clinical decision-making support systems (CDSS). This is a very critical and sensitive aspect of medical practice. These algorithms also assist in data analysis with other AI learning tools in research using electronic health records (EHRs). These EHRs are used to generate viable real-time information for medical professionals, health system administrators, health policymakers using AI-assisted analysis tools. This is possible by linking the EHR to other sources such as pharmacovigilance surveillance systems, biomedical research databases, pathology laboratories, genome sequencing databases, insurance claims and data from IoT devices (e.g., heart rate monitor), thus generating big data. Due to the rise in cost of healthcare, AI-assisted CDSS is inevitable [22,23]. AI technologies are the most applied technology in the field of medical classification and quality of patients' care [24].

Health service management is a significant aspect of AI technique applications in healthcare. It enables an all-inclusive health services management that supports administrators, nurses, doctors and other medical personnel in their work. Particularly, it can provide medical professionals with consistent real-time updates of medical information via several sources such as textbooks, journals and clinical practices [25]. This specific application became more effective and significant during the outbreak of COVID-19, where exchange of information was crucial in order to manage the spread of the pandemic globally [26]. This has cumulatively enhanced healthcare services in the following ways: (i). prompt access to data by medical personnel when needed, (ii). nurses can ascertain better patients' safety when giving medications and (iii). patients are constantly informed and involved in their care process by communicating with the medical teams assigned to them within their hospital stays. In addition, AI predictive algorithms are used to optimize logistic processes such as medical equipment and drug supply in time; as well as AI applications serve as a support in the training of personnel in health services. Another important contribution of AI in healthcare is handling the snag of data redundancy in EHRs by prediction of the presence of multiple data across clinics and hospitals, merging patient representation, scanning for outliers, benchmarking data for service delivery thereby fostering transparency, carrying out clinical tests on data and future models' improvement for prediction of diagnostic test and analysis [27].

7.4 Blockchain and healthcare industry

The information communication and computation technology has its advancement on the general-purpose technology which one of them is the blockchain technology. Blockchain technology has been in use for over a decade. It has the capacity to create records across several digital devices of a process or an activity, or many computers of an activity or a process without any retroactive alteration. A blockchain is a unique type of database, based on its design as it has read-only-once feature [28]. Its immutability feature makes it highly restricted from an intruder or authorized user to fake the network thereby making it very reliable [29]. Its structure is decentralized and distributed in blocks and can offer a fast and reliable real-time transaction. In the blockchain network, transactions and processes are transparent to all eligible users in the network. To describe the blockchain technology further, it is a time series block of data that are connected and has a chain structure formation with an encrypted security technique. Its features include validation and storage of data, distribution of a similar algorithm that generates and updates data, secure data transfer and authentication technique, automatic code scripting which forms a new computing structure and distributed infrastructure connected with smart contract [30], and Figure 7.3 shows its architecture. This technology is not used only in cryptocurrencies but has also been adopted in other areas of endeavor such as healthcare, transportation system in a smart cities, big data, industry, security and privacy, IoT. It has been applied in healthcare based on its key principles, which are anonymity, decentralization, auditability and persistence.

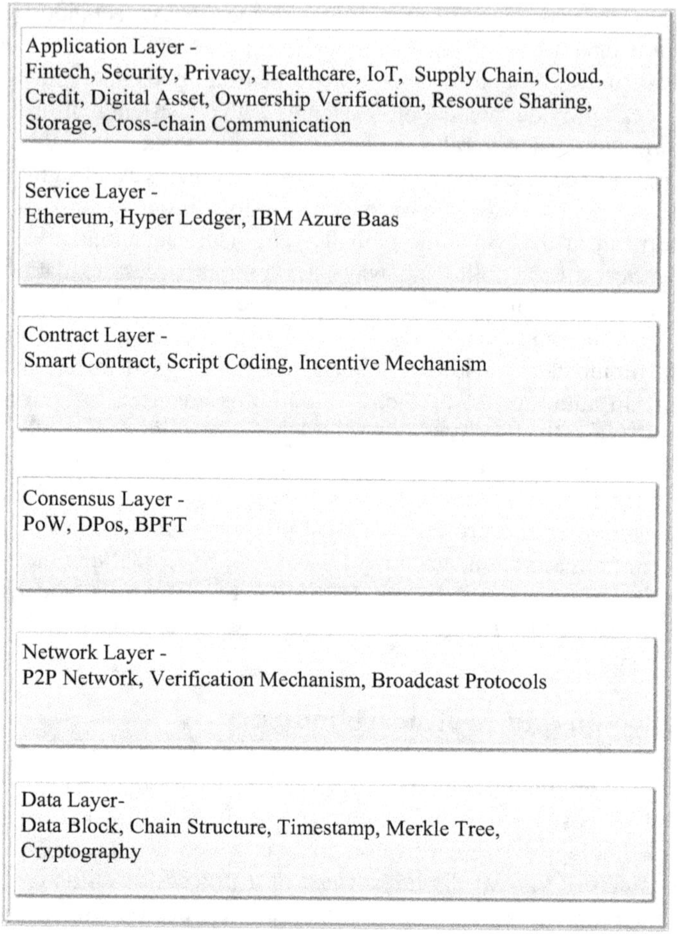

Figure 7.3 Architecture of blockchain technology

Blockchain technology has transformed healthcare delivery as it serves as a digital exchange and allows the patient to have control of his/her information. Also, smart contracts can be used for payment and insurance automatically, and this is cost-effective. The healthcare industry is benefiting from the BCT due to its structure and implementation by offering a secured transmission of patients' medical and clinical data as well as secured storage of the data that are also distributed. There is transparency in the audit process of clinical trials, and the system is usually patient centric. A secure and immutable control management system is achievable with BCT in the healthcare system.

There are specific areas in telehealth system or remote healthcare system that blockchain technology has made very effective. The suitability of any medicine to a disease is usually confirmed through the process of clinical trials as well as the side effects of that medicine. Challenges that surround this process are being curbed by adopting the blockchain technology. Usually, patients are recruited and failure to recruit them on time; i.e., within the stipulated time could lead to complicated statistical records, waste of time and waste of funds [31]. Blockchain offers a peer-to-peer system with external transaction auditing, secured data support and patients' privacy. These provide suitable innovative model in clinical trials. Transactions are validated by recruited patients as well as enabled public auditing since the system is decentralized.

Blockchain technology has enhanced telehealth and telemedicine in a significant way especially since the outbreak of COVID-19. Its decentralized management structure has enabled delivery of remote healthcare services and thereby curbing the spread of chronic diseases. It has also enhanced authenticity of legitimate users, management of device identity on the network, preserve anonymous patients and automated payment of bills.

7.5 AI models adopted in telehealth system

7.5.1 Deep learning

DL is a robust AI technique that offers a wide range of uses in the healthcare services. This section will highlight some of the specific models and frameworks that are viable in healthcare. Predictive models are very important because they enable predictions of disease diagnostics, thereby averting the cost of delay in diagnostics and treatment. It helps to reveal medical information in a big data which in turn helps in clinical decision-making. The unique attributes of representation and recognition in DL make it very vital in handling issues with healthcare. However, the following models are mostly adopted when dealing with resolving healthcare issues with DL:

Deep belief network (DBN): It has a one-directional connection at two layers on the top of layers. Each subnetwork has hidden layers that serve as a visible layer for the next layer. It is used for drug combination prediction and also appropriate for detection of type 1 diabetes. DBN supports supervised and unsupervised learning. This model is computationally expensive due to it initialization process during the training of the model.

Generative adversarial network: This is generally used for generating realistic images. Also, it is applied in the generation of synthetic brain CTs, reconstruction of natural images from brain activity and medical imaging platform. Its architecture is made up of two networks – the generator and the discriminator, which competes at the training phase. It is an appropriate method for training classifiers using semi-supervised learning. It is very hard to generate discrete data and hard to train (for example, text).

Convolution neural network: This is used for high-dimensional image analysis. It is made up of convolutional filters that transforms 2D to 3D image. Its applications include abnormal heart sound detection, radiology and myocardial infarction detection. It requires large labeled data for classification; however, it provides excellent performance for 2D data, and learning of the model is fast.

Deep neural network: This enables complex nonlinear relationship due to having more than two layers. It is applied for heart sound recognition, phonocardiography etc. The training process is important as the error propagates backward to the previous layers and becomes very little. The model learning process is quite slow; however, it is generally used with great accuracy.

Recurrent neural network: This is a type of neural network architecture that has recurrent connections between hidden states. These connections are used to identify relationships between the inputs over time. It has the capacity to model time dependencies and learning sequences. It serves well for health services that involves modeling of varying clinical data over a period. It provides a very good accuracy in character and speech recognition as well as natural language processing tasks. Its applications include detection of heart failure, classification of lung abnormalities, and requires large datasets. Gradient vanishing is usually associated with this model.

7.5.2 Machine learning

Classification: This machine learning algorithm enables medical experts to determine and label the type of disease or medical condition that is being handled.

Clustering: This is a machine learning algorithm that enables the grouping of similar health conditions in order to analyze the patterns and conduct future research.

Logistic regression: This is a machine learning model used for prediction of an outcome from two possible outcomes. It also shows the importance of each variable as it relates to the outcome. In addition, it is used for medical diagnostics, adjustment of behavioral plans, treating patients who are at risks etc. It has a binary nature that makes it easy to implement and has become one of the most prominent machine learning algorithms in healthcare.

Support vector machine: It is usually used for classification problems on incomplete datasets with missing values. It identifies samples of classes by the further away the points are from the y-axis; they belong to the classes, respectively. They can be used for drug development, image and text segmentation, and medication adherence prediction.

Artificial neural network: Oftentimes, it is referred to as the most humanized machine learning algorithm. It basically filters incoming information that is on set parameters and often requires minimal human interaction during training. It is used for medical imaging in radiology; it is also used for text and speech recognition.

7.5.3 Internet of Things

The IoT has advanced largely as technology is embraced in all aspects of life. Its nomenclature changes as it relates to the context in which it is being applied. In the domain of healthcare, its nomenclature is internet of medical things (IoMT), which is also termed healthcare IoT. It is simply described as the combination of medical devices and software applications that offer extensive medical services which are connected to a healthcare system. Currently, IoMT is being adopted massively by its ubiquitous potential applications. This is a result of high rise of mobile devices equipped with near field communication readers, which enables them to communicate with IT systems. Medical organizations, interested innovators etc., are getting ready to leverage on the IoMT tools that will lessen the burden laden on healthcare systems and delivery. This dynamic technology is applied in different healthcare services such as transmitting health information via wearables between medical professionals and remote patients, patients' monitoring from a remote location, medical orders tracking etc.

Interestingly, the outbreak of COVID-19 pandemic has stirred up the use of some already existing innovations surrounding this technology that are beneficial to healthcare delivery. The internet-compliant thermometers (smart thermometers) that are able to screen high fever. It became useful to detect potential COVID-19 carriers all over the USA.

Kinsa, a health technology company in the USA, launched this unique thermometer to track common flu. However, at the emergence of the pandemic, over a million of the products were deployed to different homes in the cities of the USA. The thermometer transmits readings promptly to the company via a mobile application. The data are used to generate day-to-day maps displaying the regions experiencing high fever and thus identifying dangerous spots of the pandemic, and these interactive maps have been certified to be accurate in the predictions of the spread of flu in the US [32].

Further useful innovations with this technology are the Wanda Quick Touch (IoT buttons) developed to maintain excellent cleaning routine standards, thereby reducing the number of hospital-acquired infections. Its functionality ensures prompt alerts on sanitation and maintenance issues that may likely put the safety of the public at risk. It has a unique feature of independence and so can be stuck on any given surface. They are installed in some hospitals in Canada and are powered by DC batteries.

Telemedicine is one of the benefits of IoMT technology, which facilitates patient monitoring remotely, also referred to as telehealth. This solved a lot of challenges posed by the emergence of COVID-19 pandemic. Four significant technologies linked to IoT that impacted the resistance against COVID-19 are the smart wearables, medical drones, mobile apps and medical robots.

7.6 Blockchain security in telehealth systems

7.6.1 Data ownership

Massive data are generated daily in the internet space via IoT and other sources, which are utilized in different fields of endeavor. In the healthcare sector, patients' records are critical and sensitive to the process of healthcare services and so authentic patients' data are required as well as the integrity of the data. Data ownership refers to the individual who is responsible for and in control of the quality of the data. In other words, it is defined as a complete control over data, including its rights and privileges. However, there seems not to be a standard definition for data ownership but have been defined based on the focus of this chapter. The advancement of technology has raised large generation of big data and so poses a challenge of security and privacy, sharing of data etc. Thus, one of the unique features in blockchain technology allows the owner of a health data to maintain the privacy of the data. A third party can access a patient's data only on the consent policy of the patient, and this is made possible by the smart contracts feature found in blockchain technology. Blockchain has a flexibility feature that enables the owner of data to share and still be in control of the data so that only legitimate users can access it based on its terms and conditions already set.

7.6.2 Data privacy

Patients' data that include medical information, health insurance, patients' prescriptions etc. are sensitive and are stored in EHRs with the recent innovation of digitalization. It requires some level of security essentially because it is an important asset in the field of healthcare. Privacy of data refers to the confidentiality of data, whether it is digital or non-digital. Most EHRs are resident on a central server; thus, deployments attract privacy and security issues. Blockchain offers a feature that handles these inherited issues since it is built based on two important mathematical concepts – hashes and cryptography. This technology stores data as an immutable ledger, which is then replicated and shared on all networks in a delegated manner from a central control. Furthermore, it can create a mechanism that manages access control to the EHRs stored on cloud. Smart contracts implemented with blockchain would ease the process of consent for data access by doctors.

7.7 Recent advances in telehealth systems

7.7.1 RapidAI

This is one of the healthcare innovations based on AI that has revolutionized healthcare delivery and services. It enables medical personnel to treat patients at a reduced time frame with a significant patient improvement. With RapidAI, accurate clinical diagnostic and transfer decisions are faster. It also enhances the connection and communication of a medical team responsible for a patient's healthcare. Furthermore, it is at the forefront of handling vascular and neurovascular conditions using AI.

7.7.2 ProvChain

A blockchain architecture that collects and verifies data provenance from cloud by attaching the data provenance into a blockchain transaction. This innovation operates in three stages as follows: provenance data collection, provenance data storage and validation of data provenance. Data provenance is the tracing of the record of data to its original source as well as the details of its transition to the current repository. ProvChain offers features such as tamperproof provenance, user privacy and reliability of access to data with less overhead for the applications in cloud storage.

7.7.3 TempChain

TempChain is simply a temporary blockchain that is created for the purpose of ensuring security of data and transactions via an open channel. In the delivery of healthcare services over the diverse networks and technologies, patients' data are sensitive, and it is important to ensure data privacy and confidentiality. This innovation is proposed to handle sharing of health data and hence improving security and privacy. To achieve the purpose of the scheme, data sharing is done by mapping properties of the required data, requesting blockchain and sharing with the requester temporary blockchain only. This is efficiently curbing the interception of hackers and attackers.

7.7.4 TrailChain

This is a unique blockchain framework that watermarks a trusted trade and generates a trail for the purpose of tracking the data ownership, which spans across multiple decentralized marketplaces. This innovation possesses good features such as mechanisms for detecting unauthorized data reselling inside and on all marketplaces. Also, there is an opportunity for fair resell payment sharing format that considers all data owners for resell revenue sharing. It poses to have a good performance metrics on execution time, throughput, execution gas costs and latency.

7.8 Conclusions and research direction

The TrailChain innovation can be applied in the healthcare sector in the circumstances of a patient receiving services from multiple health personnel in different domains. This can also be useful when referrals are made on a patient based on critical conditions and the need for specialized expertise. This is a good research direction that should be considered. Also, more applications that integrate AI and blockchain for telehealth will provide a stable virtual health system as these technologies have the features for expansion of varying usefulness. Technology adoption is on the high rise in healthcare services and delivery. This chapter has x-rayed the different uses and the efficiency it has offered in the healthcare sector. The innovations captured here are not exhaustive, and some are underway. The use of AI and blockchain technology poses to ameliorate the delivery of healthcare and its service costs, especially at this era of global economy downturn. Blockchain technology is very important in telehealth as it protects the privacy of patients' details and maintains security over the internet. Telehealth is a key solution for bridging the gap for remote population even as mobile broadband is on the increase; it is curbing the issue of access to healthcare and overcoming mobility issues. It has also minimized the spread of infectious and communicable diseases especially with the outbreak of COVID-19. AI methods and algorithms are quite inexhaustible. They possess the capacity to develop robust solutions that can extensively enhance the telehealth system globally.

References

[1] C. Scott Kruse, P. Karem, K. Shifflett, L. Vegi, K. Ravi, and M. Brooks, (2018). Evaluating barriers to adopting telemedicine worldwide: a systematic review. *J Telemed Telecare*, 24(1), 4–12.

[2] NEJM Catalyst, (2018). What is telehealth? *NEJM Catal,* 4(1).

[3] S. N. Gajarawala and J. N. Pelkowski, (2021). Telehealth benefits and barriers. *J Nurse Pract,* 17(2), 218–221

[4] N.D. Jampani, R. Nutalapati, B.S. Dontula, and R. Boyapati, (2011). Applications of teledentistry: a literature review and update. *J Int Soc Prev Community Dent*, 1(2), 37–44.

[5] S. Malhotra, S. Chakrabarti, and R. Shah, (2013). Telepsychiatry: promise, potential, and challenges. *Indian J Psychiatry*, 55(1), 3–11.

[6] J. Zhang, Q. H. Chua, X. M. Shen, J. A. Viseikumaran, T. Teoh, and N. G. Tan, (2022). A systematic implementation of telemedicine in Singapore's COVID-19 community recovery facilities. *Telemed J E Health,* 28(11), 1587–1594.

[7] P. Elsner, (2020). Teledermatology in the times of COVID-19 – a systematic review. *J Dtsch Dermatol Ges*, 18(8), 841–845.

[8] Ageing and health. World Health Organization. 2021. URL: https://www.who.int/news-room/fact-sheets/detail/ageing-and-health.

[9] Y. Zhang, J. S. P. Leuk, and W. P. Teo, (2023). Domains, feasibility, effectiveness, cost and acceptability of telehealth in aging care: scoping review of systematic reviews. *JMIR Aging*, 6, e40460. https://aging.jmir.org/2023/1/e40460 (Accessed on May 31, 2023).

[10] United Nations, 2022. Entrepreneurship and Innovation in the New Health Economy. *United Nations Publications*. https://shop.un.org/ (Accessed by June 2, 2023)

[11] WHO, (2021). *Global Strategy on Digital Health 2020–2025.* https://www.who.int/docs/default-source/documents/ gs4dhdaa2a9f352b0445bafbc79-ca799dce4d.pdf (Accessed by June 3, 2023).

[12] K. A. Alawy and I. A. Moonesar, (2023). Perspective: Telehealth – beyond legislation and regulation. *SAGE Open Med*, 11, 1–12. journals.sagepub.com/home/smo (Accessed by June 3, 2023).

[13] A. Bohr and K. Memarzadeh, (2020). *Artificial Intelligence in Healthcare.* Elsevier. https://doi.org/10.1016/B978-0-12-818438-7.00002-2.

[14] D. D. Miller and E. W. Brown, (2018) Artificial intelligence in medical practice: the question to the answer? *Am J Med 2018*, 131(2), 129–133.

[15] D. A. Hashimoto, G. Rosman, D. Rus, and O. R. Meireles, (2018). Artificial intelligence in surgery: promises and perils. *Ann Surg 2018*, 268, 70–76.

[16] H. C. S. Chan, H. Shan, T. Dahoun, H. Vogel, and S. Yuan, (2019). Advancing drug discovery via artificial intelligence. *Trends Pharm Sci*, 40 (8), 592–604.

[17] D. C. Angus, (2020). Randomized clinical trials of artificial intelligence. *JAMA*, 323(11), 1043–1045.

[18] E. Lee, (2021). How do we build trust in machine learning models? *Available at SSRN3822437.*

[19] I. Mayorga-Ruiz, A. Jiménez-Pastor, B. Fos-Guarinos, R. López-González, F. García-Castro and Á. Alberich-Bayarri, (2019). The role of AI in clinical trials. In E. Ranschaert, S. Morozov, and P. Algra. (eds.) *Artificial Intelligence in Medical Imaging* (pp. 231–243). Springer, Cham. Switzerland. https://doi.org/10.1007/978-3-319-94878-2_16

[20] D. Shi, W. Zhang, W. Zhang and X. Ding, (2019). A review on lower limb rehabilitation exoskeleton robots. *Chinese J Mech Eng*, 32(1), 1–11.

[21] T. M. Connelly, Z. Malik, R. Sehgal, G. Byrnes, J. C. Coffey and C. Peirce, (2020). The 100 most influential manuscripts in robotic surgery: a bibliometric analysis. *J Robot Surg*. 14(1), 155–165.

[22] T. Lysaght, H. Y. Lim, V. Xafis and K. Y. Ngiam, (2019). AI-assisted decision-making in healthcare. The application of an ethics framework for big data in health and research. *Springer*, 11, 299–314.

[23] S. Secinaro, D. Calandra, A. Secinaro, V. Muthurangu and P. Biancone, (2021). The role of intelligence in healthcare: a structured literature review. *BMC Med Inf Dec Making*, 21:125, https://doi.org/10.1186/s12911-021-01488

[24] Y. Guo, Z. Hao, S. Zhao, J. Gong and F. Yang, (2020). Artificial intelligence in health care: bibliometric analysis. *J Med Internet Res*, 22(7).

[25] B. X. Tran, G. T. Vu, G. H. Ha, *et al.* (2019). Global evolution of research in artificial intelligence in health and medicine: a bibliometric study. *J Clin Med.*, 8(3), 360.

[26] A. A. Hussain, O. Bouachir, F. Al-Turjman and M. Aloqaily, (2020). AI techniques for COVID-19. *IEEE Access*, 8, 128776–128795.

[27] B. Shickel, P. J. Tighe, A. Bihorac and P. Rashidi, (2018). Deep EHR: a survey of recent advances in deep learning techniques for electronic health record (EHR) analysis. *IEEE J Biomed Health Inform.*, 22(5), 1589–604.

[28] P. S. Aithal, A. Aithal and E. Dias, (2021). Blockchain technology – current status and future research opportunities in various areas of healthcare industry. *Int J Health Sci Pharm (IJHSP)*, 5(1), 130–150. DOI: https://doi.org/10.5281/zenodo.5105896

[29] I. Faria, (2019) Trust, reputation and ambiguous freedoms: Financial institutions and subversive libertarians navigating blockchain, markets, and regulation. *J Cult Econ*, 12, 119–132.

[30] A. K. Kibet, D. G. Bayyou and R. A. Esquivel, (2019). Blockchain: its structure, principles, applications and foreseen issues. *J Emerg Technol Innov Res.*, 6(4), 515–526.

[31] O. Choudhury, N. Fairoza, I. Sylla and A. Das, (2020). A blockchain framework for managing and monitoring data in multi-site clinical trials. *IBM Res, arXiv*:1902.03975v1

[32] D. G. Mcneil, Jr., Can smart thermometers track the spread of the Coronavirus? *The New York Times*, Mar. 2020. [Online]. Available: https://www.nytimes.com/2020/03/18/health/coronavirusfever-thermometer%s.html

Chapter 8

Architectural design criteria for AI and blockchain technology in telehealth systems

Emeka Ogbuju[1,2], *Abubakar Aliyu*[1], *Chinecherem Umezuruike*[3] and *Francisca Oladipo*[4]

Telehealth systems have become increasingly popular due to their potential to improve the accessibility of healthcare services through effective remote quality care provision. However, the need to provide architectural design criteria that would integrate artificial intelligence (AI) and blockchain technology exists. In this chapter, we explore the integration of AI and blockchain technology into the telehealth system. While AI techniques employ machine learning algorithms to analyze patient data with the utmost confidentiality in real time, blockchain technology improves data security and integrity and makes data sharing transparent. To achieve these, we discuss the implementation of four design criteria such as the development of secure blockchain networks, the use of smart contracts to automate the processing of transactions, the development of user-friendly interfaces to facilitate control of patient data, and the consideration of ethical and legal issues in the overall system design framework. The implementation of this framework following key design considerations with an algorithm is simulated in the results.

8.1 Introduction

In recent years, significant attention has been given to telehealth systems because of their potential to improve the accessibility and efficiency of healthcare services. These systems enable the remote provision of quality care. They allow patients to consult with healthcare professionals, monitor their health conditions, and receive medical advice from the comfort of their homes or remote locations [1]. Their convenience has made them a preferred option, especially in situations where in-person visits are challenging or not feasible.

[1]Department of Computer Science, Faculty of Science, Federal University Lokoja, Nigeria
[2]Department of Computer Science, School of Computing, Miva Open University, Nigeria
[3]Department of Software Engineering, College of Computing and Communication Studies, Bowen University, Nigeria
[4]Department of Computer Science, Faculty of Computing and Applied Science, Thomas Adewumi University, Nigeria

The generation of large datasets evident in the telehealth system leaves it with some challenges, such as compliance with ethical regulations as well as data privacy and security, data interoperability, and integration and exchange with other healthcare infrastructures. However, artificial intelligence (AI) techniques, such as machine learning (ML) algorithms, can analyze massive amounts of patient data in real time to aid diagnosis, treatment planning, and personalized healthcare delivery [2].

In line with this, Esteva *et al.* [3] stated that ML algorithms can process diverse data types, including electronic health records (EHRs), medical images, wearable device data, and patient-reported information. On the other hand, Rajkomar *et al.* [4] noted that telehealth systems can provide real-time monitoring, early detection of health deterioration, prediction of disease progression, and personalized treatment recommendations by leveraging ML techniques. Furthermore, while the capabilities of AI/telehealth systems abound, Kuo *et al.* [5] noted that blockchain technology offers robust data security, integrity, and transparent sharing by addressing concerns related to privacy, data breaches, and interoperability. It is, therefore, apparent that the integration of these technologies can significantly enhance the capabilities and trustworthiness of telehealth systems. So, the integration of ML algorithms and blockchain technology has become essential to overcome some challenges in the telehealth domain and enhance overall effectiveness.

The importance of this integration cannot be overemphasized. First, federated learning enables training ML models on distributed datasets without sharing sensitive patient information [6]. AI algorithms can employ encryption and de-identification methods to anonymize patient data while preserving its utility for analysis and research [7]. AI builds trust and fosters the widespread adoption of telehealth systems by safeguarding patient privacy. So, the confidentiality and privacy of patient data is assured.

Second, blockchain technology can provide a decentralized and immutable ledger that enhances the security and integrity of patient data in telehealth systems. Yue *et al.* [8] opined that blockchain ensures that data remains tamper-proof and verifiable by leveraging cryptographic techniques and distributed consensus algorithms. Each transaction or interaction within the telehealth system would be recorded as a block in the chain, creating an audit trail that can be traced and verified. This feature mitigates the risk of unauthorized access, data manipulation, and fraud. So, the data security and integrity are enhanced thereby bolstering the overall trustworthiness of the system [9].

Third, blockchain-based solutions enable patients to have ownership and control over their data and would only grant access permissions to healthcare providers as needed [10]. The decentralized nature of blockchain ensures that data sharing occurs with the patient's consent and maintains a transparent record of every access or modification, promoting accountability and auditability [11]. In essence, transparent data sharing and traceability are put in place.

Following the overarching importance of this technology integration, the need to articulate and propose standard architectural design criteria for this purpose becomes critical. This is because system designers in this domain may require specialized skill sets to assemble the essential components of these systems to solve specific problems in telehealth.

8.1.1 Key contributions of the chapter

The following are the significant contributions of this chapter:

1. The chapter reviewed relevant research on the application of blockchain and ML algorithms in telehealth systems and set the stage for the integration of both technologies.
2. The provision of four significant design criteria and other key design considerations for integrating AI/ML algorithms and blockchain technology into the telehealth system.
3. A proposed architectural framework that best implements the design criteria for effective operations in the telehealth domain.
4. A suggested algorithm for practical implementation/simulation of the integration task.
5. Demonstration of standard measurement and evaluation standards for integration AI/blockchain with a programming language.
6. A valuable insight into the ongoing development of digital healthcare technologies through the exploration of the applications of both ML algorithms and blockchain technology in telemedicine.

8.1.2 Chapter organization

Section 8.2 presents the related works on the various types and aspects of ML and blockchain technology applications in telemedicine systems and sets the stage for their integration. Section 8.3 presents the architectural design using the design science research (DSR) methodology, which provides the guide for the application of the design criteria in the architectural framework. Section 8.4 presents the result and discussion of the proposed architectural design with a basis for its integration into the telehealth system and gives a guided algorithm/pseudo-code for practical simulation/implementation. Section 8.5 concludes the chapter with future directions.

8.2 Related work

Both blockchain technology and AI/ML algorithms have been extensively applied in telemedicine. These applications have yielded good results in supporting the capabilities of telehealth systems. While this practice persists, the need to rethink and restructure the use of these technologies together deserves to be filled. The related works in this section show that leveraging the data analytic capabilities of ML algorithms and the security features of blockchain technology will provide a more robust and effective telemedicine system.

8.2.1 Blockchain technology in telemedicine

The security of medical records is of utmost importance to both patients and healthcare professionals. Telehealth is a valuable solution in remote areas with limited access to healthcare services. The use of technology, such as drones, has facilitated the delivery of medical supplies to these areas [12]. AI has also played a significant role in telehealth, enabling remote medical surgeries and enhancing patient monitoring and diagnosis. AI's ability to analyze health data has led to more accurate predictions and diagnoses, ultimately reducing mortality rates in remote regions [13,14]. These advancements in telehealth and the integration of AI have revolutionized healthcare delivery and improved patient health in underserved areas.

In addition to the advancements in AI, blockchain technology has emerged as another innovative solution for medical record management. The application of blockchain in healthcare aims to improve communication and bridge gaps in sharing medical data, ultimately creating a global health space [15]. As a decentralized digital ledger, blockchain securely stores and manages transactional data among participating peers. Once recorded, the information becomes immutable, and the use of cryptographic verification ensures data consistency [16,17].

There are four main types of blockchain technology: private, public, hybrid, and consortium. Based on the literature, the hybrid blockchain has been identified as particularly applicable in the healthcare sector. Hybrid blockchain technology combines private and public blockchain features, creating a system where organizations have control over access to specific data while allowing some data to be publicly accessible. In a hybrid blockchain, transactions and records are not fully public but can be verified through smart contracts when necessary. This ensures that confidential information remains within the network while allowing verification. A secure smart health monitoring system enabled by blockchain technology has been demonstrated to effectively protect medical data from various attacks during evaluation [18].

Toshtemirov *et al.* [19] showed the telemedicine market's explosive growth, particularly during the COVID-19 pandemic, and emphasized how blockchain technology can handle problems, including data breaches, privacy concerns, bogus medications, and individualized care. Blockchain's decentralized architecture guarantees secure user authentication and upholds the confidentiality and integrity of patient data. It is a safe and efficient platform for telemedicine applications. It has the potential to transform healthcare data sharing and management. The benefits of engaging blockchain in telehealth promise a secure data interchange, improved data administration and transparency, and automatic self-custody of personal health data.

Hussien *et al.* [20] conducted a comprehensive study on a telemedicine system using blockchain technology. Their objective was to develop a secure data exchange platform on mobile terminals for telemedicine applications. Koshechkin *et al.* [21] conducted a study examining the gap between the healthcare sector and blockchain technologies and the significant impact of blockchain on the sector. Using bibliometric analysis, they analyzed datasets, locations, keywords, and citations related to blockchain technology in healthcare to identify trends. The study focused on security and privacy aspects, evaluating case studies of telecare medical information systems and e-health. Also, Hasan *et al.* [22] systematically reviewed the feasibility of using blockchain technology in telemedicine applications. The review concludes that blockchain technology holds potential for integration into telemedicine and healthcare, enabling activities such as managing medical data and supporting diagnostic and therapeutic procedures.

Ahmad *et al.* [23] presented a pioneering blockchain-based telehealth solution. They aimed to enhance remote healthcare services by ensuring the traceability, integrity, and availability of telehealth transactions and records. Using smart contracts on a private Ethereum blockchain, the authors establish a secure and accountable communication network for participants. They propose a system design encompassing teleconsultation, drug administration, and medical testing scenarios. Off-chain storage systems like the cloud are integrated, allowing recorded video calls and medical test results to be stored and accessed. The solution leverages blockchain technology to protect privacy, scalability, and compatibility with various blockchain platforms. The authors highlighted the system's flexibility, extending its applicability beyond COVID-19 for remote healthcare services. The comprehensive approach and insightful findings contribute to advancing decentralized telehealth solutions, benefiting both patients and healthcare providers.

Likewise, La Valle *et al.* [24] conducted a study examining the role of blockchain technology in telehealth and telemedicine systems. Their research aimed to enhance information security, privacy, operational transparency, health records immutability, and fraud detection. The authors emphasized the significant role of blockchain in providing secure and decentralized remote healthcare services. The findings indicated that blockchain technology improves telehealth and telemedicine by offering a tamper-proof, traceable, and reliable platform. It enables accurate verification of physician credentials, fraud detection in insurance claims, and secure transmission of health data. The study underscored the need for further research to address challenges and promote the general adoption of blockchain technology in telemedicine systems.

8.2.2 Machine learning applications in telemedicine

ML has significant potential to transform telehealth, enabling more efficient and accurate healthcare services. ML algorithms have been used to analyze patient data, including medical records, imaging scans, and sensor readings, to assist in diagnosing diseases or conditions. By leveraging large datasets, ML models learn patterns and make predictions, helping healthcare professionals make more informed decisions. Dahiya *et al.* [25] in their work examined the use of telehealth in promoting a diagnosis of youths with developmental crises. Most of the studies examined used a method called store and forward as well as videoconferencing in real time. The stakeholders reported high satisfaction and diagnostic agreement between face-to-face and remote methods were recorded. Also, Cui *et al.* [26] reviewed the use of telehealth technologies to facilitate diagnosis. The technologies reviewed were live videoconferencing, asynchronous video observations, retrospective video analysis, mobile and web applications, and online websites and phone interviews. They believed that there is a high prospect of the use of these technologies in facilitating diagnosis.

In remote monitoring of patients, ML algorithms have been seen to monitor patients remotely by analyzing real-time data from wearable devices [27], such as heart rate monitors, glucose monitors, and activity trackers. This helps in the early detection of abnormalities and the prediction of health deterioration, allowing for timely interventions. Bidsorkhi [27] in their work came up with a smart face mask (SFM), a wearable device to monitor human respiration on real-time bases. The systematic review used SFMs with electrical, electromechanical, and sensing properties. The result showed remarkable durability and fast response time.

Vodrahalli *et al.* [28] proposed TrueImage, an automated ML pipeline to address the photo quality issue in telehealth systems. Their approach involved three stages: semantic segmentation, feature generation, and a computationally light-weight quality classifier. To capture aspects like blur, lighting conditions, and zoom, the authors curated datasets from Google Images, Stanford Health Care, and additional data they collected. The dataset consisted of 362 images split into training and testing sets. The TrueImage algorithm was trained using a Gaussian mixture model. Evaluation of the algorithm demonstrated its performance, resulting in the generation of four labels: good/poor quality, blurry/not blurry, good/poor lighting, and good/poor zoom or crop. In the first scenario, the algorithm successfully rejected approximately 50% of poor-quality images while retaining around 80% of good-quality images. In the second scenario, the algorithm achieved a higher retention rate for good-quality images, with over 95% being retained, but at the cost of only rejecting around 10% of poor-quality images.

Molina *et al.* [29] developed an integrated open-source EHR system to address challenges in epilepsy diagnostic services. The system manages patients' personal, clinical, and electroencephalogram (EEG) data while automatically identifying abnormal EEG signals. They used a multilayer perceptron on a dataset of 100 children with suspected epilepsy, selecting 32 features. The EEG signals were acquired using the BWII-EEG device, and the software BWAnalysis was used for data collection. Each EEG test was reviewed by a pediatric neurologist, who identified and registered epileptiform abnormalities such as spikes, poly-spikes, and spikes with slow waves. The EEG signals were segmented into one-second windows containing 200 samples, enabling efficient signal processing within 3 min. The model achieved a precision of 85.10%, a recall of 97.16%, and an accuracy of 99.92% during evaluation.

Cascella *et al.* [30] conducted a study where they developed ML models to predict the need for remote consultations in cancer pain management. They collected data from 158 patients participating in a telemedicine-based program. The study utilized four ML algorithms: random forest (RF), gradient boosting machine, artificial neural network (ANN), and the LASSO-RIDGE algorithm. The dataset included 13 variables related to demographics, social factors, clinical information, and therapy. The authors performed preprocessing and exploratory data analysis on the dataset. To optimize the classifiers and evaluate their performance, repeated cross-validation was employed to determine the best hyperparameters. The dataset was split into a training set (80%) and a testing set (20%) for evaluation purposes. The authors also conducted simulations to assess the risk of multiple remote consultations for specific patient groups. Simulated odds ratios were calculated based on approximately 500 simulations performed 150 times. The odds ratios and 95% credibility intervals (95% CIs) were calculated for each patient group. The model's performance was evaluated. The training set showed an accuracy of approximately

95% for ANN and 98% for RF. However, when tested on the independent test set, the RF model achieved the highest accuracy at 70%.

Shah *et al.* [31] proposed a ML-based system to predict and categorize future values of vital signs for cardiovascular and chronic respiratory diseases. The authors used regression techniques, specifically linear regression and higher degree polynomial regression to forecast vital sign values for the next 1–3 min. Support vector machine, naive Bayes, and decision tree were also used to evaluate the overall health of patients based on the predicted vital sign values. The dataset was obtained from the University of Queensland, where vital signs were recorded at intervals of 10 ms, resulting in a total of 10 million samples of biomedical readings. The dataset was divided into separate files for cardiovascular and chronic respiratory diseases. The result shows that linear regression performed high in predicting vital signs for cardiovascular disease within 60 s and polynomial regression models performed well in forecasting vital signs within 3 min.

In their study, Hussain *et al.* [32] introduced a supervised learning approach known as learning to rank, which aimed to prioritize patients who displayed a high susceptibility to symptoms related to chronic disease. The researchers utilized seven datasets obtained from the UCI repository: breast cancer, breast cancer in Wisconsin, diabetes, heart disease, hepatitis, liver disorders, and lung cancer. To preprocess the data, demographic and categorical attributes were eliminated, and a vector space model representation was constructed. The authors examined three list-wise ranking algorithms to achieve the desired ranking: LambdaMART, Coordinate Ascent, and AdaRank. By evaluating the performance of the models, it was determined that LambdaMART outperformed AdaRank and Coordinate Ascent in selecting more suitable patients based on the mean average precision criterion and generating patient lists according to the Normalized Discounted Cumulative Gain criterion.

Reinforcement learning is a great advancement in the area of AI [33]. Teaching AI agents through trial and error is anticipated to make additional advancements. AI systems may become increasingly capable and autonomous as a result of innovations in the fields of multi-agent reinforcement learning. Other areas of advancement are explainable AI. XAI [34,35] increase the transparency and understandability of AI algorithms by supplying justifications for their choices and deeds. The adoption of AI systems is improved by advancements in XAI, especially in crucial industries like healthcare. Imoize *et al.* [36] addressed the challenges of applying AI with the XAI, which involves combining ML with XAI. This makes it possible to explain how AI works and provide suggestions. The work focused on medical decision support systems, which are computer applications that assist doctors in making patient decisions in real time, helping improve patient safety and care, especially for long-term illnesses. Also, generative models like GANs (generative adversarial networks) and VAEs (variational autoencoders) are being utilized more and more to produce synthetic data, realistic content (pictures, videos, and text), and help with tasks like data augmentation and creativity, and they fell into the category of generative AI. Generative AI has been applied in the area of drug discovery and development [37].

A smart telehealth system with a deep learning-based algorithm was developed by [38]. The system was designed to manage foot ulcers and diabetic retinopathy. The researchers utilized the CNN algorithm for implementation. The system comprises modules that rely on knowledge to classify severity level, provide clinical decision support, detect foot ulcer, and screen their boundaries in real time. The system usability scale was used to measure the usability of the system in terms of performance, and a score of 88.5% was obtained, which shows that the system has good system usability but not exceptional system usability.

Research on the application of ML and deep learning technology for the virtual diagnosis of diseases in telemedicine was carried out by [39]. The paper used a dataset from the Good Doctor website in 2018–19. The study used the ML model to extract symptom keywords and a deep learning model for disease/symptom classification. The SERVQUAL and the BERT model were used. The BERT model was able to achieve an accuracy of 96.29%.

8.2.3 Related work on the integration of blockchain and AI algorithms in telemedicine

The literature reviewed highlights the potential of blockchain technology in the telemedicine domain. It emphasizes the benefits of blockchain in ensuring secure data sharing and improving healthcare services. The findings indicate that blockchain technology can enhance the security and privacy of telemedicine transactions and medical records. The papers show the possibility of a decentralized architecture, secure user authentication, and data integrity. However, the literature acknowledges challenges that need to be addressed for the widespread adoption of blockchain in healthcare. These challenges include scalability, storage capacity, interoperability, and standardization. The reviews also provided insights into various ML applications in telehealth, remote patient monitoring, and predicting patient health status. Again, a common gap identified is the need for the development of ML-enabled predictive analytic systems as well as the integration of ML algorithms in telehealth. Further research is needed to overcome these challenges and ensure the seamless integration of blockchain technology and AI in telehealth systems. This chapter provides part of this research by proposing architectural design criteria for the integration of AI and blockchain technologies.

8.3 Architectural design

The architectural design in this chapter followed the DSR methodology. The DSR is a systematic paradigm that focuses on creating artifacts in the form of a construct, representation, or technique for problem-solving through creative innovations in technical domains [40]. Following the guidelines of the DSR, we created a framework that shows the integration of AI and blockchain in telehealth keeping in mind the application of the design criteria. We used relevant literature on the integration of these technologies to construct the design and described the various components and their interactions.

8.4 Results and discussions

The result of this chapter is a proposed architectural framework that incorporates some design criteria for the integration of AI/blockchain. The criteria are outlined in Section 8.4.1, while the framework is presented in Section 8.4.2. The rest of the subsections discussed the implementation details of the architecture in line with the design criteria and relevant considerations.

8.4.1 Design criteria for AI and blockchain integration

Four design criteria must be implemented to ensure effective integration. These criteria are listed below as follows:

1. development of secure blockchain networks,
2. use of smart contracts to automate the processing of transactions,
3. development of user-friendly interfaces to facilitate control of patient data, and
4. consideration of ethical and legal issues in the overall system design framework.

The application of these criteria in the integration process of AI and blockchain would bring the importance of these technologies to bare in finding solutions to different problems in telehealth.

First, the implementation of a consensus mechanism for ensuring robustness and resilience against cyber threats is the focus of criteria one. This is because the design of secure blockchain networks involves implementing cryptographic algorithms, consensus mechanisms, and secure communication protocols to protect against cyber threats such as hacking, data breaches, and denial-of-service attacks [41]. Techniques such as proof-of-work (PoW), proof-of-stake (PoS), and practical Byzantine fault tolerance can be employed to achieve consensus among network participants, and this would help in preventing malicious activities and maintaining the accuracy of the distributed ledger [42]. This may be referred to as smart security, and it should be the first layer of the architecture. Traditional protocols for detecting malicious nodes often rely on centralized routing procedures, which present challenges such as the irreversibility of original information, hindrance in reproduction and verification of execution, and increased complexities. Ramasamy *et al.* [43] explored blockchain integration to create Blockchain-based Wireless Sensor Networks for identifying malicious nodes.

Second, the implementation of smart contracts to automate transaction processing and reduce administrative burden becomes the focus of criterion two. Smart contracts are self-executing programs stored on the blockchain. They enable the automation and validation of transactions in telehealth systems. The application of smart contracts ensures that payment processes, insurance claims, and data exchange between different stakeholders would be streamlined and executed with transparency and efficiency [44]. Huckle *et al.* [45] noted that this would eliminate the need for intermediaries and manual intervention in transaction processing and also reduce administrative overhead with an improvement in the efficiency of the system.

Third, the focus of criteria three is the implementation of user-friendly interfaces for patient data control and seamless interaction. User-friendly interfaces in telehealth systems are essential to empower patients in managing their health data effectively. Intuitive and accessible interfaces should provide patients with granular control over their data, including consent management, data sharing preferences, and the ability to track data access and usage. User interfaces should be designed with simplicity and accessibility in mind. The interfaces should be easy to navigate, visually appealing, and compatible with various devices and assistive technologies [46]. This may be referred to as smart user interfaces, and it may be placed in the third layer of the architecture where it is directly accessible to the user.

Finally, the focus of criteria four is the implementation of ethical considerations in the system design framework by adhering to privacy regulations and healthcare standards. While this is not a layer in the architectural framework, it is woven into the overall system design. The design of telehealth systems should prioritize ethical considerations, privacy protection, and respect for patients' data ownership rights. There are many privacy regulations, such as General Data Protection Regulation or Health Insurance Portability and Accountability Act as noted in [47]. As a part of the entire system, ethical frameworks should be established to guide the collection, storage, and use of patient data to ensure transparency, informed consent, and compliance with ethical standards. Telehealth systems must comply with relevant regulatory requirements and healthcare standards to ensure the delivery of safe and high-quality care by ensuring compliance with standards and interoperability frameworks to enable seamless data exchange and integration across different healthcare systems and providers.

8.4.2 Framework design

The framework presented in this section depicts the architectural structure of the integration following the presented design criteria (Figure 8.1).

The telehealth data stack is the main component of the architecture around the three blockchain technology layers. As the main stack of the architecture, it holds the data (electronic medical records) upon which the ML algorithms may act for predictive insights. There are several user interfaces (A, B, and C) for different functions of the user/developer. The smart contract layer controls the administration of the telehealth stack as well as the secured blockchain network layer, which holds the communication protocols, consensus mechanisms, and cryptographic algorithms.

8.4.3 Design considerations for implementation

Abreast of the design criteria for the integration, the following are key design considerations that can help to ensure the successful implementation and operation of such an integrated system:

1. Security and privacy: Telehealth systems deal with sensitive patient data, making security and privacy paramount. Blockchain can provide a decentralized and

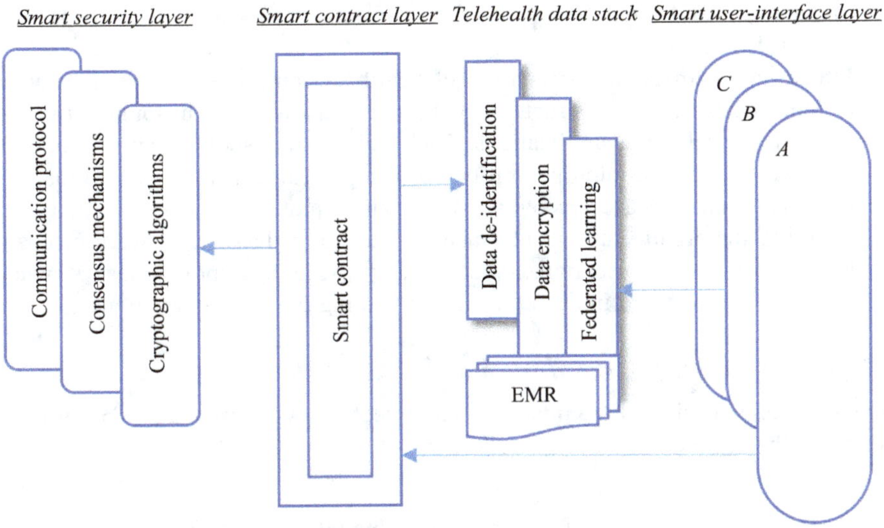

Figure 8.1 AI/blockchain integration architecture in telehealth system

immutable ledger that enhances data security and integrity. AI can be used for tasks like anomaly detection and access control to strengthen security measures.

2. Scalability and performance: Telehealth systems must be capable of handling a large volume of data and concurrent users. The architecture should be designed to ensure scalability and high performance, allowing for seamless and real-time interactions. AI algorithms should be optimized to process data efficiently, and blockchain solutions should consider scalability mechanisms such as sharding or off-chain transactions.
3. Interoperability: The architectural design should follow widely accepted standards and protocols to ensure smooth integration with existing healthcare systems and interoperability across different telehealth platforms. AI models and blockchain protocols should be compatible with industry standards to facilitate seamless data exchange.
4. Real-time analytics: AI algorithms can provide real-time insights and analytics by processing large datasets generated during telehealth consultations. The architecture should support the integration of AI models that can extract valuable information, such as predictive analytics, decision support systems, and personalized recommendations.
5. Consensus mechanisms: In blockchain-based telehealth systems, selecting an appropriate consensus mechanism is crucial. Considerations such as transaction speed, energy efficiency, and governance requirements should guide the choice of consensus algorithms, such as PoW, PoS, or delegated PoS.
6. User experience: The architecture should prioritize a user-centric design that enhances the experience of both healthcare providers and patients. AI can be leveraged to improve user interfaces, natural language processing for voice

interactions, and intelligent routing to connect patients with the right healthcare professionals.

7. Integration with legacy systems: Telehealth systems need to integrate with existing healthcare infrastructure, including EHR systems, hospital networks, and other healthcare applications. The architecture should support smooth integration and data interoperability, ensuring a seamless flow of information.
8. Continuity and disaster recovery: To ensure uninterrupted service and data integrity, the architecture should incorporate robust disaster recovery mechanisms. Blockchain's decentralized nature can provide inherent redundancy, while AI algorithms can aid in detecting and mitigating potential disruptions.

8.4.4 Algorithm for the design

For a systematic design of the integration architecture, we present an algorithm that can guide the architectural design as follows:

1. Identify system requirements:
   - (i) Define the goals and objectives of the telehealth system.
   - (ii) Identify the specific AI and blockchain functionalities required.
   - (iii) Consider regulatory and compliance requirements.

2. Understand existing infrastructure:
   - (i) Evaluate the current telehealth system architecture and infrastructure.
   - (ii) Identify strengths, weaknesses, and potential areas for improvement.
   - (iii) Assess the compatibility of existing systems with AI and blockchain integration.

3. Determine AI use cases:
   - (i) Identify specific AI use cases that can enhance telehealth operations.
   - (ii) Examples include real-time analytics, anomaly detection, and decision support.
   - (iii) Prioritize AI functionalities based on their potential impact and feasibility.

4. Determine blockchain use cases:
   - (i) Identify specific use cases where blockchain technology can bring value.
   - (ii) Consider data security, privacy, interoperability, and auditability.
   - (iii) Determine the appropriate level of decentralization required.

5. Define system architecture:
   - (i) Design a high-level system architecture that incorporates AI and blockchain components.
   - (ii) Consider scalability, performance, interoperability, and security.
   - (iii) Define the interaction among AI algorithms, blockchain nodes, and telehealth components.

6. Select AI technologies:
   - (i) Choose appropriate AI technologies, algorithms, and models for the identified use cases.

   (ii) Consider factors like real-time processing, data privacy, and model explainability.
   (iii) Determine whether local processing or cloud-based solutions are more suitable.

7. Select blockchain technologies:
   (i) Choose the appropriate blockchain platform (e.g., Ethereum, Hyperledger) based on use case requirements.
   (ii) Determine the consensus mechanism (e.g., PoW, PoS) that aligns with scalability and security needs.
   (iii) Consider privacy-enhancing technologies (e.g., zero-knowledge proofs) if required.
8. Define data management strategy:
   (i) Establish a data management strategy that ensures data integrity, security, and compliance.
   (ii) Determine how data will be stored, encrypted, and shared within the telehealth system.
   (iii) Consider methods for secure data exchange between AI algorithms and the blockchain.
9. Address ethical and regulatory considerations:
   (i) Ensure the architectural design adheres to ethical guidelines and regulatory requirements.
   (ii) Incorporate mechanisms for transparency, fairness, and accountability of AI algorithms.
   (iii) Implement privacy controls to protect patient data and comply with relevant regulations.
10. Prototype, test, and iterate:
   (i) Develop a prototype of the telehealth system architecture.
   (ii) Test the integration of AI and blockchain components, ensuring functionality and performance.
   (iii) Gather feedback from stakeholders and iterate on the design as needed.
11. Deploy and monitor:
   (i) Deploy the telehealth system architecture in a controlled environment.
   (ii) Monitor system performance, security, and user experience.
   (iii) Continuously evaluate and optimize the architecture based on real-world usage and feedback.

8.4.5 The pseudo-code for practical simulation

In this section, we provide the pseudo-code of 12 main functions that may implement the algorithm as follows:

1. DefineSystemRequirements():
   (i) Define system goals, objectives, and regulatory requirements.
   (ii) Identify AI and blockchain functionalities needed.

2. UnderstandExistingInfrastructure():
   (i) Evaluate current telehealth system architecture and infrastructure.
   (ii) Identify strengths, weaknesses, and areas for improvement.

3. DetermineAIUseCases():
   (i) Identify AI use cases to enhance telehealth operations.
   (ii) Prioritize functionalities based on impact and feasibility.

4. DetermineBlockchainUseCases():
   (i) Identify blockchain use cases for data security, privacy, and interoperability.
   (ii) Determine the appropriate level of decentralization.

5. DefineSystemArchitecture():
   (i) Design high-level system architecture with AI and blockchain components.
   (ii) Consider scalability, performance, interoperability, and security.

6. SelectAITechnologies():
   (i) Choose appropriate AI technologies, algorithms, and models.
   (ii) Consider real-time processing, privacy, and explainability.

7. SelectBlockchainTechnologies():
   (i) Choose a suitable blockchain platform (e.g., Ethereum, Hyperledger).
   (ii) Determine consensus mechanisms and privacy-enhancing technologies.

8. DefineDataManagementStrategy():
   (i) Establish a strategy for data integrity, security, and compliance.
   (ii) Determine data storage, encryption, and sharing mechanisms.

9. AddressEthicalAndRegulatoryConsiderations():
   (i) Ensure adherence to ethical guidelines and regulatory requirements.
   (ii) Implement transparency, fairness, and privacy controls.

10. PerformCostBenefitAnalysis():
    (i) Assess the costs and benefits of architectural design choices.
    (ii) Consider implementation complexity, infrastructure, and maintenance costs.

11. PrototypeTestAndIterate():
    (i) Develop a prototype of the telehealth system architecture.
    (ii) Test AI and blockchain integration for functionality and performance.
    (iii) Gather feedback and iterate on the design.

12. DeployAndMonitor():
    (i) Deploy telehealth system architecture in a controlled environment.
    (ii) Monitor system performance, security, and user experience.
    (iii) Continuously evaluate and optimize the architecture.

A general implementation of the pseudo-code in line with the general structure of the algorithm is provided in Listing 8.1. The actual requirement details of each system design may be filled under a specific integration task.

```
def define_system_requirements():
# Implementation logic for defining system requirements def under-
stand_existing_infrastructure():
# Implementation logic for understanding existing infrastructure def deter-
mine_ai_use_cases():
# Implementation logic for determining AI use cases def determine_-
blockchain_use_cases(): # Implementation logic for determining
Blockchain use cases def define_system_architecture():
# Implementation logic for defining system architecture def select_ai_-
technologies(use_cases):
selected_technologies = [] for use_case in use_cases:
if use_case == "Real-time Analytics":
selected_technologies.append("Machine Learning algorithms")
selected_technologies.append("Stream processing frameworks")
elif use_case == "Anomaly Detection":
selected_technologies.append("Statistical modeling techniques")
selected_technologies.append("Deep learning algorithms")
elif use_case == "Decision Support":
selected_technologies.append("Expert systems")
selected_technologies.append("Natural Language Processing (NLP)")
# Add more use cases and corresponding AI technologies as needed
return selected_technologies
def select_blockchain_technologies():
# Implementation logic for selecting Blockchain technologies
def define_data_management_strategy():
# Implementation logic for defining data management strategy
def address_ethical_and_regulatory_considerations():
# Implementation logic for addressing ethical and regulatory considerations
def perform_cost_benefit_analysis():
# Implementation logic for performing cost-benefit analysis
def prototype_test_and_iterate():
# Implementation logic for prototyping, testing, and iteration
def deploy_and_monitor():
# Implementation logic for deploying and monitoring the system
# Main function to initiate the algorithm
def main()
define_system_requirements()
understand_existing_infrastructure()
determine_ai_use_cases()
determine_blockchain_use_cases()
define_system_architecture()
ai_use_cases = ["Real-time Analytics", "Anomaly Detection"]
```

```
selected_ai_technologies = select_ai_technologies(ai_use_cases)
select_blockchain_technologies()
define_data_management_strategy()
address_ethical_and_regulatory_considerations()
perform_cost_benefit_analysis()
prototype_test_and_iterate()
deploy_and_monitor()

    # Run the algorithm
    main()
```

Listing 8.1: Pseudo-simulation

8.4.6 Evaluation of the algorithm

The algorithm may be measured using six indices such as

1. Accuracy: It measures the percentage of correct predictions made by the algorithm.
2. Execution time: This metric measures the time taken by the algorithm to complete its execution.
3. Memory usage: Measure the algorithm's memory usage, such as the amount of RAM or disk space required during execution. Monitoring memory usage helps identify potential performance issues and scalability concerns.
4. Scalability: Evaluate the algorithm's scalability by measuring its performance with varying input sizes or workloads. This helps assess how the algorithm handles larger datasets or increased user demands.
5. Resource utilization: Assess the algorithm's utilization of system resources, such as CPU usage or network bandwidth. Monitoring resource consumption helps identify potential bottlenecks and optimize the algorithm's efficiency.
6. User satisfaction: Collect feedback from users or stakeholders regarding their experience with the algorithm or the telehealth system as a whole.

An example code with these indices for the evaluation is presented in Listing 8.2 in the Python programming language.

Execution Time

```
import time
start_time = time.time()
# Run the algorithm
# ...
end_time = time.time()
execution_time = end_time - start_time
```

```
print("Execution Time:", execution_time)
```

Accuracy

```
from sklearn.metrics import accuracy_score
# True labels
true_labels = [1, 0, 1, 1, 0]
# Predicted labels
predicted_labels = [1, 1, 1, 0, 0]
accuracy = accuracy_score(true_labels, predicted_labels)
print("Accuracy:", accuracy)
```

Scalability

```
import time
def algorithm(input):
# Implementation logic for the algorithm
# Define different input sizes or workloads
input_sizes = [100, 1000, 10000, 100000]
execution_times = []
for size in input_sizes:
# Generate input data with the given size
input_data = generate_input(size)
# Measure the execution time of the algorithm
start_time = time.time()
algorithm(input_data)
end_time = time.time()
# Calculate the execution time
execution_time = end_time - start_time
execution_times.append(execution_time)

# Print the execution times for each input size
for i, size in enumerate(input_sizes):
print(f"Execution time for input size {size}: {execution_times[i]} seconds")
```

Graph

```
import matplotlib.pyplot as plt
# Evaluation metrics
metrics = ['Accuracy', 'Execution Time', 'Scalability', 'Resource Usage', 'User Feedback']
scores = [0.85, 6.2, 8.5, 7.3, 4.7]
# Create a bar chart
plt.bar(metrics, scores)
plt.xlabel('Metrics')
plt.ylabel('Scores')
plt.title('Algorithm Performance Evaluation')
plt.show()
```

Listing 8.2: Simulated evaluation code

The output of the code is given in Figure 8.2.

Evaluating these metrics allows for a comprehensive assessment of the algorithm's performance. It helps identify strengths, weaknesses, and areas for optimization or refinement. These metrics collectively provide a holistic view of how well the algorithm meets the desired objectives and user expectations.

- Accuracy measures the proportion of correct predictions made by the algorithm. It is particularly relevant for classification tasks. A higher accuracy indicates that the algorithm is making more correct predictions, while a lower accuracy suggests that the algorithm is less reliable. Accuracy is a fundamental metric for evaluating the effectiveness of a classification algorithm.
- Execution time measures the time taken by the algorithm to complete its execution. It reflects the efficiency and speed of the algorithm's computations. A shorter execution time is generally desirable as it indicates faster processing and responsiveness. However, it's important to note that execution time can vary based on factors such as input size, algorithm complexity, hardware resources, and implementation optimizations.
- Scalability refers to how well the algorithm performs as the input size or workload increases. A scalable algorithm maintains or improves its performance as the problem size grows. In the context of scalability, it's important to assess how execution time, resource usage, or other performance metrics change with increasing input sizes. A highly scalable algorithm will exhibit consistent or improved performance even with larger datasets or higher workloads.
- Resource usage measures the consumption of system resources, such as CPU, memory, or disk space, by the algorithm during execution. Monitoring resource

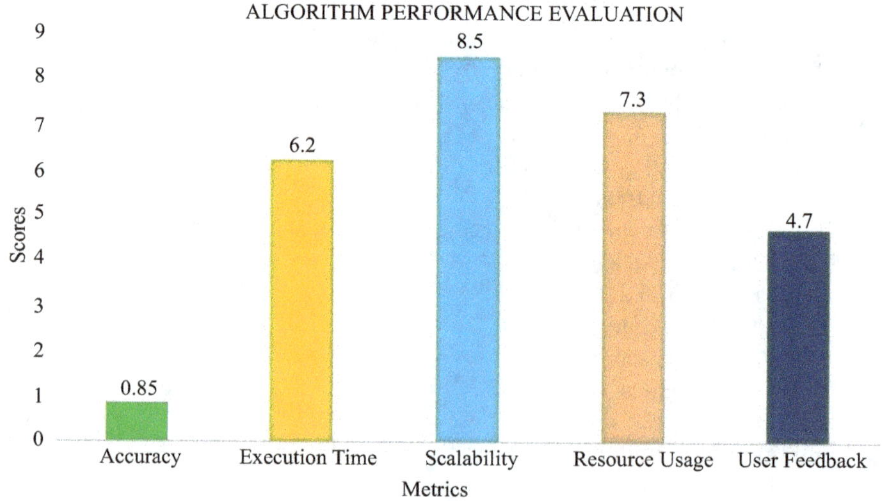

Figure 8.2 Evaluation result

usage helps identify whether the algorithm is utilizing resources efficiently or if it requires excessive computational or memory resources. Optimizing resource usage is crucial for efficient algorithm performance, especially when dealing with large-scale or resource-constrained environments.

- User feedback encompasses the opinions, satisfaction levels, and experiences of users or stakeholders interacting with the algorithm or the telehealth system as a whole. User feedback can be collected through surveys, interviews, or user testing sessions. It provides valuable insights into the algorithm's usability, user experience, and perceived effectiveness. User feedback helps identify areas of improvement and guides future enhancements of the algorithm or system.

8.5 Conclusions and future scope

This chapter proposed four main design criteria and shows how they could be used in the architectural design framework to integrate AI and blockchain in telehealth. Also, for practical implementations, other key design considerations have been discussed alongside an extensive algorithm that may be used. While these criteria may not be exhaustive, the chapter had shown at a high level that some challenges in the telehealth domain may be solved through the application of the framework in developing health solutions. The suggested algorithm/pseudo-code has been implemented using Python programming, and evaluation results have been explained. Future work would focus on demonstrating this framework with a live telehealth system and showcasing the application of the presented criteria.

Acknowledgment

The authors acknowledge the invaluable contributions of the reviewers/editors of this chapter.

References

[1] R. L. Bashshur, J. D. Howell, and E. A. Krupinski, "The empirical foundations of telemedicine interventions in primary care," *Telemedicine and e-Health*, vol. 26, no. 5, pp. 551–568, 2020.

[2] E. J. Topol, "High-performance medicine: The convergence of human and artificial intelligence," *Nature Medicine*, vol. 25, no. 1, pp. 44–56, 2019.

[3] A. Esteva, A. Robicquet, B. Ramsundar, *et al.*, "A guide to deep learning in healthcare," *Nature Medicine*, vol. 25, no. 1, pp. 24–29, 2019.

[4] A. Rajkomar, E. Oren, K. Chen, *et al.*, "Scalable and accurate deep learning with electronic health records," *npj Digital Medicine*, vol. 2, no. 18, pp. 1–10, 2018. https://doi.org/10.1038/s41746-018-0029-1

[5] T. T. Kuo, H. E. Kim, and L. Ohno-Machado, "Blockchain distributed ledger technologies for biomedical and health care applications," *Journal of the American Medical Informatics Association*, vol. 27, no. 11, pp. 1760–1763, 2020.

[6] Q. Yang, Y. Liu, T. Chen, and Y. Tong, "Federated machine learning: Concept and applications," *ACM Transactions on Intelligent Systems and Technology*, vol. 10, no. 2, pp. 1–19, 2019.

[7] S. Choi, S. Kim, and T. Kim, "Multi-view deep learning for consistent semantic interpretation of heterogeneous clinical measures," *Journal of Biomedical Informatics*, vol. 82, pp. 112–123, 2018.

[8] X. Yue, H. Wang, D. Jin, M. Li, and W. Jiang, "Blockchain-based data storage: A survey," *IEEE Transactions on Services Computing*, vol. 13, no. 3, pp. 498–513, 2020.

[9] A. Ekblaw, A. Azaria, J. D. Halamka, and A. Lippman, "A case study for blockchain in healthcare: "MedRec" prototype for electronic health records and medical research data," in *Proceedings of IEEE Open & Big Data Conference*, Vol. 13, p. 13, Aug. 2016.

[10] M. Mettler, "Blockchain technology in healthcare: The revolution starts here," in *2016 IEEE 18th International Conference on e-Health Networking, Applications, and Services (Healthcom)*, pp. 1–3, Sep. 2016.

[11] Reuters. (2021, December 16). Uganda tests drones to speed up delivery of HIV medicine. Retrieved from https://www.reuters.com/world/africa/uganda-tests-drones-speed-up-delivery-hiv-medicine-2021-12-16/

[12] A. R. El-Sherif, M. El Sherif, R. Atta, and K. Shaalan, "Telehealth and artificial intelligence insights into healthcare during the COVID-19 pandemic," *Journal of Personalized Medicine*, vol. 10, no. 2, p. 385, 2022. [Online]. Available: doi:10.3390/jpm10020385.

[13] M. Ali, M. J. Haider, and Z. Akhtar, "A systematic literature review of artificial intelligence in the healthcare sector: Benefits, challenges, methodologies, and functionalities," *Journal of Innovation & Knowledge*, 2023. Retrieved from https://www.sciencedirect.com/science/article/pii/S2444569X2300029X

[14] A. Ali, N. Rehman, S. A. Choudhary, and S. Anwar, "AI's ability to analyze health data has led to more accurate predictions and diagnoses, ultimately contributing to a reduction in mortality rates in remote regions," in *2023 IEEE 16th International Conference on Software Testing, Verification and Validation Workshops (ICSTW)*, 2023, pp. 377–382.

[15] C. Crosby, P. Pattanayak, S. Verma, and V. Kalyanaraman, "Blockchain technology: Beyond bitcoin," *Applied Innovation*, vol. 2, no. 6–10, pp. 71, 2016.

[16] A. A. Vazirani, O. O'Donoghue, D. Brindley, and E. Meinert, "Implementing blockchains for efficient health care: Systematic review," *Journal of Medical Internet Research*, vol. 21, no. 2, p. e12439, 2019.

[17] S. Vazirani, "Blockchain, as a decentralized digital ledger, securely stores and manages transactional data among participating peers. Once recorded, the information becomes immutable, and the use of cryptographic

verification ensures data consistency," in *2019 IEEE International Conference on Blockchain and Cryptocurrency (ICBC)*, 2019, pp. 1–2.

[18] A. Takyar (n.d.). Blockchain in telemedicine. Retrieved from https://www.leewayhertz.com/blockchain-in-telemedicine/

[19] A. Toshtemirov, G. Mihuba, and M. J. Shundi, "Using blockchain technology for the design of telemedicine system based on mobile terminal," *International Journal of Emergency Technology and Engineering Research*, vol. 6, no. 12, pp. 12–19, 2018.

[20] H. M. Hussien, S. M. Yasin, N. I. Udzir, M. I. H. Ninggal, and S. Salman, "Blockchain technology in the healthcare industry: Trends and opportunities," *Journal of Industrial Information Integration*, vol. 22, p. 100217, 2021. doi:10.1016/j.jii.2021.100217.

[21] K. Koshechkin, G. Lebedev, G. Radzievsky, R. Seepold, and N. Martinez, "Blockchain technology projects to provide telemedical services: Systematic review," *Journal of Medical Internet Research*, vol. 23, no. 8, pp. e17475, 2021. doi:10.2196/17475.

[22] H. R. Hasan, K. Salah, R. Jayaraman, I. Yaqoob, M. Omar, and S. Ellahham, "Blockchain-enabled telehealth services using smart contracts," *IEEE Access*, vol. 9, pp. 151944–151959, 2021.

[23] R. W. Ahmad, K. Salah, R. Jayaraman, I. Yaqoob, S. Ellahham, and M. Omar, "The role of blockchain technology in telehealth and telemedicine," *International Journal of Medical Informatics*, vol. 148, p. 104399, 2021.

[24] C. La Valle, E. Johnston, and H. Tager-Flusberg, "A systematic review of the use of telehealth to facilitate a diagnosis for children with developmental concerns," *Research in Developmental Disabilities*, vol. 127, p 104269, 2022.

[25] A. V. Dahiya, J. R. Bertollo, C. G. McDonnell, and A. Scarpa, "Remote telehealth assessments for autism spectrum disorder," in *Neural Engineering Techniques for Autism Spectrum Disorder*, 2023, doi:10.1016/B978-0-12-824421-0.00008-4.

[26] J. Cui, H. Du, and X. Wu, "Data analysis of physical recovery and injury prevention in sports teaching based on wearable devices," *Preventive Medicine*, 2023, doi:10.1016/j.ypmed.2023.107589.

[27] H. C. Bidsorkhi, N. Faramarzi, B. Ali, *et al.*, "Wearable Graphene-based smart face mask for Real-Time human respiration monitoring," *Materials & Design*, vol. 230, p. 111970, 2023.

[28] K. Vodrahalli, R. Daneshjou, R. A. Novoa, A. Chiou, J. M. Ko, and J. Zou, "TrueImage: A machine learning algorithm to improve the quality of telehealth photos," in *Pacific Symposium on Biocomputing*, 2021, pp. 220–231, 2020.

[29] E. Molina, C. E. Sarmiento Torres, R. Salazar-Cabrera, D. M. López, and R. Vargas-Cañas, "Intelligent telehealth system to support epilepsy diagnosis," *Journal of Multidisciplinary Healthcare*, vol. 13, pp. 433–445, 2020.

[30] M. Cascella, S. Coluccia, F. Monaco, *et al.*, "Different machine learning approaches for implementing telehealth-based cancer pain management strategies," *Journal of Clinical Medicine*, vol. 11, no. 18, p. 5484, 2022.

[31] W. Shah, M. Aleem, M. A. Iqbal, *et al.*, "A machine-learning-based system for prediction of cardiovascular and chronic respiratory diseases," *Journal of Healthcare Engineering*, vol. 2021, pp. 1–17, 2021.

[32] S. Hussain, H. Afzal, M. R. Mufti, A. Khan, A. A. Khan, and F. E. Amin, "A methodology to rank the patients prone to chronic diseases in telehealth," *Journal of Medical Imaging and Health Informatics*, vol. 9, no. 3, pp. 418–425, 2019.

[33] M. Kim, J. S. Kim, and C. W. Ahn, "Evolving population method for real-time reinforcement learning," *Expert Systems with Applications*, pp. 120493, 2023, doi:https://doi.org/10.1016/j.eswa.

[34] S. Rajpal, A. Rajpal, M. Agarwal, *et al.*, "XAI-CNVMarker: Explainable AI-based copy number variant biomarker discovery for breast cancer subtypes," *Biomedical Signal Processing and Control*, vol. 84, 104979, 2023. doi:10.1016/j.bspc.2023.104979.

[35] M. Arashapour, "AI explainability framework for environmental management research," *Journal of Environmental Management*, vol. 342, pp. 118149, 2023, doi.org/10.1016/j.jenvman.2023.118149.

[36] A. L. Imoize, P. A. Gbadega, H. I. Obakhena, D. O. Irabor, K. V. N. Kavitha, and C. Chakraborty, "Artificial intelligence-enabled internet of medical things for COVID-19 pandemic data management," in *Explainable Artificial Intelligence in Medical Decision Support Systems*, 2022, pp. 357–380.

[37] X. Zeng, F. Wang, Y. Luo, *et al.*, "Deep generative molecular design reshapes drug discovery," *Cell Reports Medicine*, vol. 100794, 2022.

[38] I. Wijesinghe, C. Gamage, I. Perera, and C. Chitraranjan, "A smart telemedicine system with deep learning to manage diabetic retinopathy and foot ulcers," In *2019 Moratuwa Engineering Research Conference*, pp. 686–691, 2019.

[39] F. Hao and K. Zheng, "Online disease identification and diagnosis and treatment based on machine learning technology," *Journal of Healthcare Engineering*, vol. 2022, no. 1, pp. 1–7, 2022

[40] G. Bisandu, "Design science research," in *Encyclopedia of Management Theory*, SAGE Publications, 2016, pp. 1–4. doi:10.4135/9781452276090.n2.

[41] J. Bonneau, A. Miller, J. Clark, A. Narayanan, J. A. Kroll, and E. W. Felten, "Research perspectives and challenges for bitcoin and cryptocurrencies," *IEEE Security & Privacy*, vol. 13, no. 4, pp. 98–103, 2015.

[42] S. Bano, S. Zawoad, M. S. Rahman, and S. Hassan Choudhury, "Towards blockchain-enabled healthcare systems: A systematic review," in *2017 IEEE 19th International Conference on e-Health Networking, Applications and Services (Healthcom)*, 2017.

[43] L. K. Ramasamy, F. K. KP, A. L. Imoize, J. O. Ogbebor, S. Kadry, and S. Rho, "Blockchain-based wireless sensor networks for malicious node detection: A survey," *IEEE Access*, vol. 9, pp. 128765–128785, 2021.

[44] N. Kshetri, "Can blockchain strengthen the Internet of Things?," *IT Professional*, vol. 19, no. 4, pp. 68–72, 2017.

[45] S. Huckle, R. Bhattacharya, and M. White, "Internet of things, blockchain, and shared economy applications," *Procedia Computer Science*, vol. 98, pp. 461–466, 2016.

[46] A. J. Bokolo, "Use of telemedicine and virtual care for remote treatment in response to COVID-19 pandemic," *Journal of Medical Systems*, vol. 44, no. 7, p. 132, 2020.

[47] T.-F. Lee, I.-P. Chang, G.-J. Su, "Compliance with HIPAA and GDPR in certificateless-based authenticated key agreement using extended chaotic maps," *Electronics*, vol. 12, no. 5, pp. 1108, 2023. https://doi.org/10.3390/electronics12051108.

Chapter 9

Addressing computational complexity issues in telehealth systems using artificial intelligence and blockchain technology

Friday Udeji[1], *Agbotiname Lucky Imoize*[2], *K. V. N. Kavitha*[3], *Vinoth Babu Kumaravelu*[4] *and Samarendra Nath Sur*[5]

The integration of artificial intelligence (AI) and blockchain technology in telehealth systems holds great potential for transforming healthcare delivery. This chapter explores the architecture, functionality, and key applications of AI and blockchain in telehealth systems. We begin by highlighting the increasing utilization of telehealth services, particularly during the COVID-19 pandemic, and the advantages they offer, such as convenience, cost savings, and improved patient insights. The chapter also outlines the challenges and research gaps in telehealth systems, including privacy concerns, efficient data processing, regulatory compliance, and the urgency associated with resolving the ensuing computational issues arising from the use of telehealth systems. The proposed solution involves leveraging AI-based algorithms for the analysis of complex patient data, leading to improved outcomes, reduced costs, and enhanced decision-making for healthcare providers. Additionally, the chapter delves into the integration of blockchain technology to guarantee data security, privacy, interoperability, and addressing concerns related to data integrity and access control while AI systems are more tailored toward remote patient monitoring, accurate diagnosis, treatment planning, patient engagement, and chronic disease management. Furthermore, the chapter discusses the implications of recent research findings in telehealth care, emphasizing the ethical considerations of bias in AI algorithms and the importance of

[1]Department of Mechanical Engineering, Faculty of Engineering, Ambrose Alli University, Nigeria
[2]Department of Electrical and Electronics Engineering, Faculty of Engineering, University of Lagos, Nigeria
[3]School of Electronics Engineering, Vellore Institute of Technology, India
[4]Department of Communication Engineering, School of Electronics Engineering, Vellore Institute of Technology, India
[5]Department of Electronics and Communication Engineering, Sikkim Manipal Institute of Technology, Sikkim Manipal University, India

transparency and accountability. Also, in this chapter, regulatory compliance is identified as a critical factor, and the need for careful integration of AI and blockchain technologies within existing healthcare frameworks is highlighted. Finally, future research directions focusing on addressing scalability challenges, improving interoperability, developing user-friendly interfaces, and enhancing the usability of AI and blockchain-empowered telehealth systems are presented.

9.1 Introduction

Telehealth, a transformative healthcare approach leveraging advanced technologies to improve access, reduce costs, and improve the quality of care, has witnessed a remarkable surge in adoption and utilization over the past decade [1–3]. With advancements in technology and the advent of high-speed Internet connectivity, telehealth has emerged as a transformative approach to delivering healthcare services. From the advent of voice-only systems to the revolutionary integration of live video-conferencing and broadband Internet capabilities, telehealth has evolved into a pivotal solution, delivering accessible, and efficient care [4]. It offers a range of benefits, including enhanced accessibility, improved patient outcomes, and reduced healthcare costs [5,6]. However, the successful implementation of telehealth systems is not without challenges. For instance, amidst the growing utilization of telehealth systems, computational complexity has emerged as a critical challenge that demands attention [3,7]. The sheer volume of healthcare data generated and processed by telehealth platforms, coupled with the need for real-time analysis and decision-making, has placed substantial computational burdens on existing infrastructure. These complexities encompass issues such as data processing, storage, analysis, and the need for efficient and scalable algorithms.

Although the unprecedented impact of the COVID-19 pandemic catapulted telehealth into the forefront, driving exponential growth and offering a lifeline for both healthcare providers and patients seeking safer and more convenient alternatives to traditional in-person care, there is a need for a thorough investigation of the computational issues associated with telehealth systems and the development of suitable solutions for clinical adoption [8–11]. The objective of this chapter is to explore the integration of artificial intelligence (AI) and blockchain technologies as empowering models to address these computational complexity issues in telehealth systems. By harnessing the capabilities of AI, such as machine learning (ML) and natural language processing (NLP), and leveraging the secure and transparent nature of blockchain, we aim to overcome the computational hurdles and unlock the full potential of telehealth systems.

Through our exploration of the potential synergies between AI and blockchain, we propose solutions to overcome the computational complexity challenges present in telehealth systems, unlocking the full potential of this transformative approach to healthcare delivery. This research thus enhances experimentation, and collaborative efforts among healthcare professionals, and technologists while helping policymakers pave the way for the widespread adoption and seamless integration of AI and blockchain technologies in telehealth, ushering in novel healthcare provisions that are accessible, efficient, and patient-centric.

The implementation of blockchain technology offers an innovative solution to address the computational complexity challenges faced by telehealth systems [12]. By harnessing the decentralized and immutable nature of blockchain, we can ensure secure storage, sharing, and access of healthcare data by authorized parties. The transparency and traceability provided by blockchain significantly enhance data integrity, privacy, and security within telehealth systems. Additionally, blockchain-based smart contracts have the potential to automate and streamline administrative processes, effectively reducing inefficiencies and enhancing the overall workflow of telehealth platforms [13]. The fusion of AI and telehealth presents vast opportunities and promises exceptional outcomes. AI algorithms play a vital role in automating data processing tasks, facilitating the analysis of medical images, detecting patterns in patient data, and providing invaluable decision support to healthcare providers [14]. With the utilization of ML techniques, telehealth systems are empowered to deliver more accurate diagnoses and personalized treatment plans through predictive analytics [15]. Furthermore, NLP algorithms facilitate efficient and precise communication between patients and healthcare providers, enabling effective remote consultations.

9.1.1 Key contributions of the chapter

In this chapter, we aim to address the computational complexity issues in telehealth systems by leveraging the integration of AI and blockchain technologies. The key contributions of this chapter can be summarized as follows:

- Comprehensive overview of telehealth systems: We provide an overview of the growing importance of telehealth systems in healthcare. By examining the historical progression from voice-only systems to the incorporation of live video-conferencing and broadband connectivity, we establish the foundation for understanding the transformative potential of telehealth.
- Identification of computational complexity challenges: We highlight the challenges associated with computational complexity in telehealth systems. The exponential growth in healthcare data and the need for real-time processing and analysis place significant burdens on existing infrastructure. We delve into the complexities of data processing, storage, analysis, and the demand for efficient and scalable algorithms.
- Integration of AI and blockchain: We investigate the synergies between AI and blockchain in tackling computational complexity in telehealth systems. By combining the data processing capabilities of AI with the secure and transparent framework of blockchain, we can create robust telehealth solutions. We provide examples and case studies showcasing successful integrations of AI and blockchain in improving telehealth system performance and efficiency.
- Recommendations and future directions: Based on our findings, we present practical recommendations for addressing computational complexity in telehealth systems using AI and blockchain. We discuss potential solutions,

technological advancements, and research directions to enhance the integration of AI and blockchain in telehealth. We highlight the significance of continued exploration and innovation in this field to unlock the full potential of telehealth systems.

9.1.2 Chapter organization

In Section 9.1, the introduction provides an overview of the importance of telehealth systems and the computational complexity challenges they face. It highlights the contributions of using AI and blockchain to address these challenges. Section 9.2 reviews related work in computational complexity, AI applications, and blockchain in healthcare. Section 9.3 presents the materials, methods, and experimental design used to tackle computational complexity in telehealth systems using AI and blockchain. In Section 9.4, the results and discussions of applying AI and blockchain are presented, analyzing their impact on system performance. Finally, Section 9.5 concludes the chapter, by summarizing the key findings, discussing implications, and identifying future research directions.

9.2 Related work

Telehealth has roots in early experiments and developments in telecommunication technologies [16]. The concept of telehealth gained traction in the twentieth century with the advent of video conferencing and tele-physician coverage across multiple sites [17]. These technological advancements laid the foundation for modern telehealth practices. The first instances of telemedicine can be traced back to the late nineteenth century when physicians used telegraphy to provide medical consultations remotely [18]. In recent times, telehealth systems have emerged as a significant advancement in modern healthcare, leveraging technology to provide remote medical services and consultations [19]. These systems enable healthcare professionals to deliver care to patients who are geographically distant, ensuring access to quality healthcare regardless of location. However, the successful implementation of telehealth systems requires addressing computational complexity issues, including data processing, storage, and analysis.

Telehealth systems encompass a range of technologies and applications that facilitate remote healthcare delivery making them more complicated to develop and manage. With the rise of robust wireless connection technologies like the 6G, telehealth enables healthcare providers to communicate, diagnose, monitor, and treat patients remotely using various tools, such as video conferencing, remote monitoring devices, and secure messaging platforms [10], [20]. As a modern technology contributing to clinical practices, telehealth technology leads to improved access to healthcare. Specifically, telehealth systems break down geographical barriers, allowing patients in remote or underserved areas to access healthcare services [21–23]. This is particularly crucial for individuals with limited mobility, chronic illnesses, or those living in rural areas with limited access to specialized healthcare facilities. Second, they provide financial cost and time savings measures by eliminating the need for in-person visits thereby reducing travel costs and time commitments for both patients and healthcare providers [24]. Clinically, they enhance patient monitoring and chronic disease management. With telehealth systems, the possibility of continuous monitoring of the vital signs of patients is achieved even in the physical absence of the doctors allowing healthcare providers to remotely track and manage chronic conditions [25]. This leads to more proactive and personalized care, reducing the risk of complications and hospital readmissions.

According to [13], a vulnerable legacy system in the network can potentially serve as an entry point for attackers, allowing them to exploit vulnerabilities and gain unauthorized access. This not only puts patient data at risk of being stolen but also poses a threat to the integrity and functionality of telehealth processes. They recommended implementing a private blockchain-based solution to overcome the limitations of current telehealth systems, as telehealth has gained significant traction during the COVID-19 pandemic. By utilizing blockchain technology, physicians and medical care providers can remotely care for patients and monitor their symptoms with enhanced transparency, immutability, traceability, security, and trustworthiness [26]. The proposed solution specifically focuses on enhancing teleconsultation, drug administration, and medical testing services through blockchain integration.

Any leaks or breaches of patient data may lead to major ramifications for medical institutions, especially in the contemporary context where the security of personally identifiable information is heavily monitored, as emphasized by [27]. These worrying statistics revealed that about 30% of the questioned participants reported times when patient data at their clinics had been compromised as a direct consequence of telemedicine interactions. Such findings underscore the significant dangers linked with telehealth and give insight into the probable gaps within the system. In particular, it stresses the importance to address computation problems and build adequate data security processes to reduce the threat of data leaks and maintain patient information. Misdiagnosis has been seen in organizations as a result of low picture or video quality [7]. This problem derives in part from the last one: video-conferencing software often decreases visual quality to insure a seamless session. However, difficulties might emerge as a result of congested servers or communication channels. Greater comfort, the possibility to cut clinical overhead expenses, and even new insight into the lives of patients have been mentioned as significant advantages of the telemedicine revolution, as stated by [28]. According to their intriguing approach, the height of the COVID-19 epidemic witnessed a dramatic shift in the way doctors and patients interacted, with telemedicine accounting for 50%–80% of medical appointments, a tremendous leap from the preceding 1%. This disruptive trend underlined the advantages of telemedicine, providing patients with enhanced comfort while lessening the financial load on healthcare organizations. Furthermore, it provided healthcare practitioners with unique insights into the daily lives of their patients, allowing a more extensive awareness of their healthcare needs and enabling tailored treatment approaches.

Oyebiyi *et al.* [29] explored various approaches and algorithms in areas such as ML methods and procedures used in health systems. They examined the significance and relevance of 73 selected chapters after excusing some articles based on specific criteria. Their review also included a quantitative analysis of feature extraction methods, showing a geometric approach as the most prominent at 36%, followed by the local method at 27%. Additionally, they made useful highlights on the use of different architectures, such as convolutional neural network (CNN), restricted Boltzmann machine, auto-encoder, deep belief network, and unspecified architectures, for addressing challenges in health systems [29].

9.3 Computation and telehealth systems

Computation serves as the backbone of telehealth systems, enabling essential functions such as processing and analyzing patient data, facilitating communication between healthcare providers and patients, securely storing and managing patient information, and harnessing the power of AI for improved diagnostics and remote monitoring. As telehealth continues to evolve and expand, the demand for efficient computation becomes even more significant. One of the primary applications of computation in telehealth lies in processing and analyzing patient data. Telehealth systems collect vast amounts of data, including medical histories, symptoms, and test results. Computation plays a vital role in processing this data to generate accurate diagnoses and treatment recommendations. Additionally, it enables the analysis of medical images, such as X-rays, MRIs, and ultrasounds, aiding in disease detection, injury assessment, and treatment monitoring.

Furthermore, computation facilitates seamless communication between healthcare providers and patients in telehealth systems. Videoconferencing and other communication technologies rely on computational processes to transmit and receive video and audio data, ensuring effective remote consultations. Computation also plays a role in speech recognition, enabling transcription of patient interviews, report generation, and device control within telehealth systems.

Secure storage and management of patient data is another critical aspect of telehealth systems. Computation is utilized to encrypt patient data, protecting it from unauthorized access and ensuring confidentiality. Additionally, computation enables the creation and management of databases for efficient organization and retrieval of patient records, contributing to streamlined workflows and accurate data management. The advent of AI-powered applications has brought transformative capabilities to telehealth systems. Computation is pivotal in developing and deploying these AI applications, which encompass disease diagnosis, treatment recommendations, and remote patient monitoring. By leveraging computation, telehealth systems can harness the potential of ML algorithms to continuously improve healthcare outcomes.

9.3.1 Computational issues in telehealth systems

Telehealth systems have revolutionized healthcare delivery, but they also present unique computational challenges that need to be addressed. Among the plethora of challenges faced by telehealth systems, computational complexity challenges are

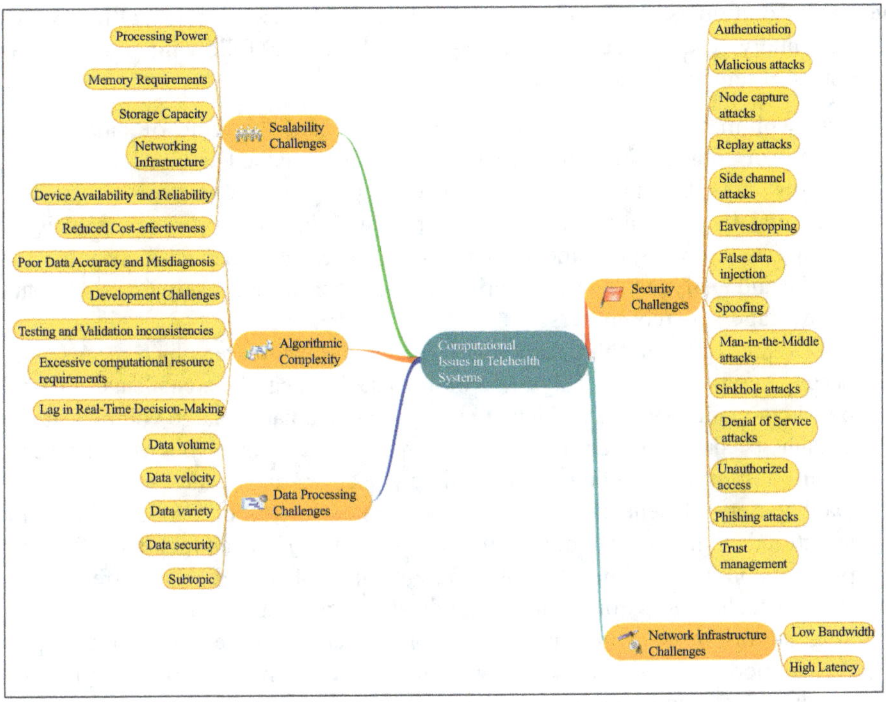

Figure 9.1 A map of the computational issues in telehealth systems

the most common due to the volume and nature of healthcare data involved. These challenges encompass various aspects, including data processing, network infrastructure, security, and scalability. In this section, we delve into these computational issues on a technical level, discussing their causes and implications. Figure 9.1 shows a map of the common computational issues in the telehealth systems which are further discussed subsequently.

9.3.2 Data processing challenges in telehealth systems

One of the primary computational challenges in telehealth is the processing of vast amounts of medical data [30]. Telehealth systems generate a wealth of data from diverse sources, including wearable sensors, medical devices, and patient records. Managing and analyzing this data in a timely manner can be a significant hurdle. For decades, telehealth systems employed traditional computing approaches that relied on centralized servers for data processing. However, this approach has often led to performance bottlenecks and latency due to the large volume of data transmitted and processed. To address this, distributed computing models, such as cloud computing and edge computing, have been introduced. Cloud computing leverages remote servers to process data, while edge computing brings computation closer to the data source, reducing latency and enhancing real-time analysis capabilities but even this solution is still not enough for large-scale use of telehealth systems. Fundamentally, these processing issues arise from the following crucial characteristics of telehealth data:

1. Data volume: Telehealth systems generate a large volume of data from a variety of sources, including wearable sensors, medical devices, and patient records. This data can be terabytes or even petabytes in size, which can be a challenge to store and process. The sheer volume of data requires efficient storage and processing mechanisms to ensure that telehealth systems can handle and analyze the data effectively. These sizes can already be problematic for average supercomputers.
2. Data velocity: Telehealth data is often generated in real-time, which means that it needs to be processed quickly to be of any use. This can be a challenge for traditional computing systems, which are not designed to handle large volumes of data at high speeds. Real-time monitoring, diagnostics, and interventions in telehealth require fast data processing to enable timely decision-making and responses.
3. Data variety: Telehealth data can come in a variety of formats, including structured, semi-structured, and unstructured data. This can make it difficult to process and analyze the data, as different types of data require different processing techniques. For example, medical images may require image processing algorithms, while patient records may require NLP techniques. Accommodating the diverse formats and extracting meaningful insights from the data pose computational challenges.
4. Data security: Telehealth data is often sensitive and confidential, so it is important to protect it from unauthorized access. This can be a challenge, as telehealth systems often connect to the Internet, which can make them vulnerable to cyberattacks. Ensuring data security through robust encryption, secure communication protocols, and access control mechanisms is crucial to maintaining patient trust and complying with privacy regulations such as Health Insurance Portability and Accountability Act (HIPAA).

9.3.2.1 Traditional approaches to addressing issues with data processing

Traditionally, telehealth systems have used centralized computing approaches to process data. This means that all the data is collected and processed on a central server. While this approach can be effective for small-scale telehealth systems, it can become a challenge for large-scale systems. The centralized processing of data can lead to performance bottlenecks and latency issues, especially when dealing with the significant volume of data transmitted and processed.

1. Distributed computing approaches: To address the challenges of data processing in telehealth, distributed computing approaches have been introduced. These approaches distribute the data processing load across multiple servers, improving performance and reducing latency.
2. Cloud computing: Cloud computing is a model of computing where data and applications are stored and processed on remote servers. This approach can be

effective for telehealth systems as it allows for scalability and flexibility. By leveraging remote servers, cloud computing enables telehealth systems to handle the large volume of data efficiently. However, it is important to consider the costs associated with cloud computing and address concerns related to data security and privacy when adopting this approach.

3. Edge computing: Edge computing is a model of computing where data and applications are processed closer to the data source. In telehealth, this means processing data at or near the point of generation, such as wearable devices or local servers. Edge computing reduces latency and enhances the performance of real-time applications in telehealth systems. By bringing computation closer to the data source, edge computing enables faster response times, which is crucial for real-time monitoring and decision-making. However, managing and coordinating distributed edge computing resources can be more complex compared to traditional centralized approaches, and data security concerns must be addressed.

9.3.3 Algorithmic complexity in telehealth systems

Algorithmic complexity poses computational challenges in telehealth and telemedicine systems. As these systems evolve, the algorithms used to process data are becoming increasingly complex. The complexity arises from the need to consider a wide range of factors, including the extensive overview of the medical history of patients, their current symptoms, test results, and other relevant data. However, the growing complexity of these algorithms brings about several computational issues that need to be addressed. The challenges of algorithmic complexity result in:

1. Poor data accuracy and misdiagnosis: Another potential barrier to effective telehealth practice is the accuracy of data transmission. A study investigating the accuracy of physical function measurements revealed that Internet bandwidth affects the validity and reliability of fine motor task measurements. This can result in healthcare practitioners making clinical treatment decisions and recommendations based on potentially inaccurate patient data if they are ignorant of differences in technological systems. Fortunately, data accuracy is regulated by the Digital Imaging and Communications in Medicine format, which is an international gold standard for medical images and associated information. This provides clear standards for the acceptable format quality for medical images and data required for clinical use and the associated interpretations [31].
2. Development challenges: Designing and developing complex algorithms for telehealth and telemedicine systems can be a daunting task. The algorithms must account for various factors, analyze multiple data sources, and incorporate sophisticated decision-making processes. Developing such algorithms requires domain expertise, collaboration between healthcare professionals and technologists, and a deep understanding of the specific medical context. The complexity involved in translating medical knowledge and requirements into algorithmic models adds to the development challenges.

3. Testing and validation inconsistencies: Verifying and validating complex algorithms in telehealth systems pose significant computational hurdles. Thorough testing is essential to ensure the accuracy, reliability, and safety of the algorithms. However, testing complex algorithms becomes more intricate due to the large number of possible inputs and the intricate relationships between variables. Exhaustively testing all possible scenarios can be computationally expensive and time-consuming. Moreover, the potential risks associated with algorithmic errors, such as misdiagnosis or incorrect treatment recommendations, necessitate rigorous testing and validation procedures.
4. Excessive computational resource requirements: Complex algorithms often require substantial computational resources to process and analyze data efficiently. As telehealth systems generate large volumes of diverse data, including medical records, diagnostic images, sensor data, and real-time streaming data, the algorithms must handle these inputs effectively. Resource-intensive operations like data preprocessing, feature extraction, ML, and predictive modeling demand significant computational power and memory. Ensuring that telehealth systems have adequate computational resources to handle the algorithmic complexity is crucial to maintaining system performance and responsiveness.
5. Lag in real-time decision-making: Many telehealth and telemedicine applications require real-time decision-making to support timely and accurate healthcare interventions. For example, during a video consultation, the system may need to process live data streams, analyze symptoms, and provide immediate recommendations or interventions. The complex algorithms involved in real-time decision-making must be optimized for efficiency to ensure that the processing time remains within acceptable limits. High algorithmic complexity can introduce delays and affect the ability of the system to deliver timely care, compromising diagnostic effectiveness and accuracy [32].

9.3.4 Network infrastructure challenges in telehealth systems

Telehealth systems heavily rely on network infrastructure to facilitate the seamless transmission of data between healthcare providers and patients. However, inadequate network bandwidth, connectivity issues, and limited coverage in remote areas can hinder the efficient operation of telehealth systems. In the past, conventional Internet protocols and network architectures were used for data transmission. As technology evolved, advancements, such as 5G networks and satellite communications, have emerged to address these challenges. 5G networks offer faster speeds, lower latency, and greater capacity, enabling real-time video consultations and remote monitoring with improved quality and reliability. Satellite communications provide connectivity to remote and underserved areas, expanding access to telehealth services. In remote areas (where telehealth is most needed), poor network reception is often still a major challenge and is experienced in two modes:

1. Low bandwidth: Telehealth and telemedicine systems require high-speed Internet connections to transmit data effectively. The bandwidth refers to the

amount of data that can be transmitted over a network connection within a given time. In areas with poor Internet connectivity, limited bandwidth can impede the transmission of large medical data files, real-time video consultations, and remote monitoring. To address bandwidth limitations, several strategies and technologies have been employed including:

(i) Internet service provider (ISP) upgrades: Collaboration with Internet service providers (ISPs) and telecommunication companies to improve the infrastructure and connectivity in underserved areas. ISP upgrades are characterized by expanded broadband coverage, increased network capacity, and improved network stability.

(ii) Data compression and optimization: Implementing data compression techniques to reduce the size of transmitted data without significant loss of quality. This can help maximize the utilization of available bandwidth and ensure efficient data transmission.

(iii) Prioritization and quality of service (QoS): Implementing QoS mechanisms to prioritize telehealth traffic over other noncritical Internet traffic. This ensures that telehealth data receive higher priority, reducing the risk of delays and ensuring a reliable connection.

2. High latency: In telehealth and telemedicine systems, latency can be a significant problem, as it can delay the delivery of care and disrupt real-time interactions between healthcare providers and patients. To address latency challenges, several approaches have been employed:

(i) Improved network technologies: The evolution of network technologies, such as 5G, has significantly reduced latency compared to previous generations. 5G networks offer faster speeds, lower latency, and greater capacity, enabling real-time video consultations, remote monitoring, and interactive telehealth applications with improved quality and reliability.

(ii) Edge computing: By deploying computing resources closer to the network edge, edge computing reduces the physical distance that data needs to travel, thereby minimizing latency. This approach brings data processing capabilities closer to the patient, enabling real-time analysis and faster response times in telehealth systems.

(iii) Content delivery networks (CDNs): CDNs consist of distributed servers strategically placed across various locations. They cache and deliver content, including telehealth applications and data, from the server nearest to the location of the target user. By reducing the distance data needs to travel, CDNs can minimize latency and enhance the overall performance of telehealth systems.

(iv) QoS management: Implementing QoS mechanisms to prioritize time-sensitive telehealth data traffic and ensure timely delivery. QoS management can involve traffic shaping, packet prioritization, and network optimization techniques to minimize latency and ensure a smooth user experience.

9.3.5 Security challenges in telehealth systems

The sensitive nature of medical data necessitates robust security measures in telehealth systems. Protecting patient privacy, ensuring data confidentiality, and preventing unauthorized access are critical concerns [33]. Despite these advancements, telehealth systems face various security challenges that can compromise the confidentiality, integrity, and availability of medical data.

In the past, telehealth systems primarily relied on encryption techniques, firewalls, and virtual private networks to safeguard data during transmission and storage. However, emerging technologies, such as blockchain, have introduced new possibilities for enhancing security in telehealth. The decentralized and immutable nature of blockchain provides a transparent and tamper-proof framework for storing and sharing medical data. It offers enhanced data integrity, and control, mitigating privacy leakage concerns and security vulnerabilities. Common security challenges associated with telehealth include:

1. Authentication: Strong authentication mechanisms are crucial in telehealth systems to ensure the secure computation and transmission of data. Authenticating devices and users prevents unauthorized access and maintains the integrity of the system.
2. Malicious attacks: Malicious attacks exploit vulnerabilities in telehealth systems by injecting malicious code or compromising smart devices. These attacks can lead to unauthorized access, data breaches, or system compromise, posing significant risks to patient privacy and safety.
3. Node capture attacks: In telehealth systems, smart devices are deployed in different locations as part of IoT applications. However, adversaries can capture or replace these devices with malicious ones, gaining unauthorized access to the network. This physical attack makes it challenging to distinguish between genuine and false nodes, compromising the security of the system.
4. Replay attacks: Adversaries can intercept and later replay messages in telehealth systems, leading to unauthorized access and manipulation of data. In an IoT environment, attackers can compromise smart devices and send data as authorized nodes, compromising the integrity of the telehealth system.
5. Side-channel attacks: Side-channel attacks exploit information leakage from devices to extract sensitive data, such as encryption keys. As telehealth systems rely on encryption techniques to protect data, side-channel attacks pose a threat to the confidentiality of patient information.
6. Eavesdropping: Eavesdropping attacks occur when attackers intercept and access data transmitted between devices in an insecure communication channel. This compromises patient privacy and confidentiality, as adversaries can obtain sensitive medical information.
7. False data injection: Telehealth systems rely on sensors and smart devices deployed in various locations to collect environmental and patient data. Attackers can capture or manipulate data and inject false information into the network, leading to incorrect diagnoses, improper treatment decisions, and compromised patient safety.

8. Spoofing: Spoofing attacks involve attackers gaining unauthorized access to smart devices or nodes and masquerading as legitimate entities. By transmitting false messages and commands, attackers can manipulate telehealth data and disrupt the operation of the system, compromising patient care.
9. Man-in-the-middle (MITM) attacks: MITM attacks occur when attackers intercept and manipulate communication between two parties without their knowledge. In telehealth systems, MITM attacks can compromise the confidentiality and integrity of patient data, leading to unauthorized access or manipulation.
10. Sinkhole attacks: Sinkhole attacks target the routing protocols used in telehealth systems, causing network traffic to be routed through compromised or malicious nodes. These attacks disrupt network performance and can lead to unauthorized access to sensitive data.
11. Denial of service (DoS) attacks: DoS attacks aim to overwhelm telehealth systems by flooding them with a large volume of traffic, rendering them unavailable or causing significant performance degradation. Such attacks impact patient care by disrupting the availability and functionality of telehealth services.
12. Unauthorized access: Attackers target resource-constrained devices connected to telehealth systems to gain unauthorized access to the network. Compromised gateways or captured credentials can lead to unauthorized access to patient information and compromise the integrity and security of the system.
13. Phishing attacks: Phishing attacks target users of telehealth systems by sending false messages or emails, tricking them into revealing important information. These attacks compromise user privacy, lead to unauthorized access, and facilitate other types of cyber threats.
14. Trust management: Trust management is a challenging task in telehealth systems, where information is shared among decentralized nodes. Establishing trust models and ensuring the integrity and authenticity of data exchanged among nodes is essential to prevent malicious behavior.

9.3.6 Scalability challenges in telehealth systems

Scalability is a key consideration in telehealth systems as they need to accommodate increasing numbers of users, handle growing data volumes, and support a wide range of healthcare services. As a result of the complexities of telehealth systems, any attempt to increase the scale of operation presents an immediate computational issue. Historically, telehealth systems faced scalability challenges primarily due to hardware limitations and capacity constraints. The hardware used in telehealth and telemedicine systems, including servers, networking equipment, and computing devices, has played a crucial role in determining the scalability of these systems. The following are some of the impacts of hardware limitations on scalability:

1. Power: Telehealth systems require significant processing power to handle complex medical data processing tasks, real-time video consultations, and data

analytics. Limited processing power can become a bottleneck, restricting the ability of telehealth systems to handle a large number of concurrent users and process data efficiently. As the user base grows and more data is generated, the processing capabilities of the hardware may reach their limits, hindering system scalability.

2. Memory requirements: Telehealth systems often deal with large volumes of medical data, including patient records, diagnostic images, and sensor data. Storing and accessing this data quickly and efficiently requires sufficient memory capacity. Inadequate memory resources can lead to slower data retrieval, increased latency, and reduced system performance. This can be especially problematic when handling a large number of concurrent users or performing resource-intensive tasks like real-time data analysis or image processing.
3. Storage capacity: The storage capacity of hardware infrastructure is critical for telehealth systems, as they generate and accumulate vast amounts of medical data over time. Insufficient storage capacity can limit the ability of the system to store and manage patient records, medical images, and other essential data. This can hinder the scalability of the system, particularly when faced with increasing data volumes or the need to retain data for extended periods.
4. Networking infrastructure: The networking infrastructure, including routers, switches, and network interfaces, plays a crucial role in facilitating data transmission and communication in telehealth systems. Limited networking capacity or outdated networking equipment can result in bandwidth limitations, slower data transfer rates, and increased latency. These factors can negatively impact the scalability of telehealth systems, particularly when dealing with real-time video consultations or transmitting large medical data files.
5. Device availability and reliability: The availability and reliability of hardware devices used in telehealth systems are crucial for seamless operation and scalability. Hardware failures or limited availability of devices can disrupt the system, impact user experience, and hinder scalability. Reliable hardware components and redundancy measures are essential to ensure system uptime and accommodate increasing user demands.
6. Reduced cost-effectiveness: Computational complexity directly impacts the cost-effectiveness of telehealth systems. Complex data processing and storage requirements may necessitate expensive hardware infrastructure and high-speed network connectivity.

Managing computational resources efficiently and leveraging cost-effective technologies can help mitigate the ensuing financial implications of these computational challenges. However, with the advent of cloud computing and virtualization technologies, scalability challenges related to hardware limitations have been alleviated to a considerable extent. Cloud-based telehealth solutions offer the flexibility to scale resources up or down based on demand, eliminating the need to invest in costly hardware infrastructure upfront. Cloud providers can dynamically allocate computing resources, storage, and networking capabilities of the system to match the scalability requirements. This scalability-as-a-service model ensures efficient resource utilization and accommodates a larger user base without being constrained by the limitations of individual hardware components.

9.4 Architecture and functionality of AI and blockchain-empowered telehealth systems

A plethora of advantages are associated with the merging of AI and ML methods with telehealth technologies. This convergence promises to change healthcare delivery and enhance patient outcomes. In this section, we highlight various critical use cases where AI and ML are efficiently applied in telehealth systems such as the provision of remote monitoring, diagnosis, treatment planning, patient engagement, and chronic illness management. Although useful as indicated by the direct use of AI in telehealth systems, AI and blockchain integration provides better telehealth service reach and efficiency by eradicating the computational issues involved in the use of telehealth systems. Common use of AI and ML systems in telehealth industries are seen as follows:

1. Telemonitoring: One prominent utilization of AI and ML in telehealth systems is remote patient monitoring. These technologies allow healthcare practitioners to observe the vital signs of patients and detect possible health risks at an early stage. By accessing data such as blood pressure, pulse rate, respiration rate, blood oxygen level, weight, and body temperature, AI algorithms give insights and trigger alarms for further medical treatment. This feature allows quicker treatments, improves patient results, and decreases the need for in-person visits. Additionally, gadgets that automatically send data to telehealth systems or patient input into the system at regular intervals allow smooth and efficient monitoring.
2. Diagnosis: AI and ML assist in accurate diagnosis by supporting healthcare practitioners in examining medical data remotely. Image analysis, such as X-rays, CT scans, and diagnostic test data, is a prominent utilization of AI in telehealth systems. Patients safely transmit their photos to a server, and AI algorithms deliver insights and suggestions based on symptoms and medical history. These AI-driven diagnostics enable healthcare practitioners in making quicker and more accurate diagnoses, especially when access to specialist expertise is hindered. Cloud-based solutions provide scalability, safe storage, and speedy exchange of diagnostic data, boosting the diagnostic capabilities of telehealth systems.
3. Treatment plans: AI and ML algorithms allow the generation of tailored treatment plans in telehealth systems. By assessing unique patient preferences, treatment kinds, and geography, AI systems deliver tailored solutions for the best care. ML algorithms examine huge volumes of patient data, including medical history and treatment results, to discover the most effective therapy choices. This tailored strategy enhances treatment results, patient satisfaction, and adherence to treatment programs. The integration of AI in telehealth

systems boosts the efficiency of treatment planning and empowers healthcare clinicians with data-driven insights for better decision-making.

4. Patient engagement: AI technologies promote patient participation in telehealth systems by giving reminders for appointments, medication adherence, and follow-up treatment. AI-powered chatbots play a significant role in patient engagement, providing rapid replies to frequent enquiries and giving helpful information [34]. These automated solutions boost accessibility, allow simple communication, and guarantee patients remain informed and actively engage in their treatment. By boosting patient interaction, AI-driven telehealth solutions strengthen the patient-provider connection, increase patient happiness, and contribute to better treatment results.
5. Chronic disease therapy: AI and ML approaches enable the treatment of chronic illnesses, a prevalent healthcare concern globally. Telehealth apps employ AI capabilities to give personalized treatment regimens, reminders, and progress monitoring for patients with illnesses including diabetes, hypertension, and heart disease. ML algorithms examine patient data to forecast outcomes, including the possibility of developing illnesses. This enables early treatments and individualized medicines, boosting patient self-management, and saving healthcare expenditures. AI-driven chronic illness management in telehealth systems allows patients to actively engage in their treatment, improves patient outcomes, and decreases the strain on healthcare resources.

9.4.1 AI and computational issues in telehealth systems

In addressing computational issues, AI and ML frameworks can be used to address problems involving:

1. Scalability: AI can help telehealth systems grow successfully by forecasting user demand, improving resource allocation, and boosting system performance. Specific approaches include:
2. Machine learning algorithms: Algorithms, such as regression, time series analysis, and deep learning models, may be applied to examine previous usage trends and anticipate future demand for telehealth services. These models may aid in resource planning, infrastructure scalability, and ensuring adequate computing resources are accessible when required.
3. Reinforcement learning: Reinforcement learning methods may be used to improve resource allocation dynamically. By continually learning from system feedback and user interactions, AI agents may alter resource allocation depending on real-time demand, enhancing the performance and responsiveness of the system.
4. Cloud computing and virtualization: Leveraging cloud-based infrastructure and virtualization technology enables telehealth systems to grow resources on demand. AI may be used to automate resource provisioning and orchestration, allowing effective allocation of computing resources depending on workload needs.

5. Real-time data processing: AI algorithms may be applied to process and interpret real-time patient data effectively. Specific approaches include as follows:
6. Stream processing: Stream processing frameworks, such as Apache Kafka or Apache Flink, may be used to manage continuous streams of data in real time. AI algorithms may be embedded into these frameworks to conduct real-time analytics, anomaly detection, and decision-making on streaming patient data.
7. Edge computing and edge AI: By installing AI algorithms directly on edge devices (e.g., wearables or IoT devices), real-time data processing may be handled locally, lowering latency and minimizing the strain on the central healthcare system. Edge AI approaches, such as federated learning or edge inference, allow real-time analysis and decision-making at the edge while preserving data privacy and security.
8. Complex event processing (CEP): CEP approaches, paired with AI algorithms, may find and analyze patterns, correlations, and anomalies in real-time patient data. CEP engines may constantly monitor patient data streams, generate alerts for crucial events, and give decision assistance to healthcare practitioners.
9. Data security and privacy: AI can contribute to strengthening data security and privacy in telehealth systems. Specific approaches include:
10. Anomaly detection: AI-based anomaly detection approaches, such as unsupervised learning or deep learning models, may uncover odd patterns or behaviors that suggest possible security breaches or illegal access to patient data. These algorithms continually analyze system records, network traffic, and user behaviors to identify and mitigate security risks.
11. Privacy-preserving techniques: Homomorphic encryption, secure multi-party computing, or differential privacy approaches may be utilized to safeguard patient data while doing calculations. These approaches allow data analysis without disclosing sensitive information, guaranteeing privacy compliance in telehealth systems.
12. Integration of multiple data sources: AI approaches may simplify the integration and harmonization of varied data sources in telehealth systems. Specific approaches include:
13. NLP: NLP algorithms may be applied to extract structured information from unstructured healthcare data, such as medical reports, clinical notes, or patient-generated language. NLP approaches may aid in data standards, semantic interoperability, and ontology mapping, allowing smooth integration of disparate data sources.
14. Data integration frameworks: AI-driven data integration frameworks, such as Apache Spark or Google Cloud Data Fusion, may be deployed to automate the integration of disparate data sources. These frameworks can perform data transformation, cleaning, and standardization, assuring data consistency and interoperability among telehealth systems.
15. Real-time analytics and decision support: AI can deliver real-time analytics and decision support capabilities in telehealth systems. Specific approaches include:

16. Deep learning models: Deep learning designs, such as CNNs or recurrent neural networks, may scan real-time medical imagery, sensor data, or patient records to give immediate insights and help in diagnostic or treatment decision-making.
17. Explainable AI: Utilizing explainable AI models, such as rule-based systems or transparent ML algorithms, may deliver interpretable information to healthcare professionals. This enables them to understand and validate AI-driven recommendations, enhancing trust and facilitating clinical decision-making.
18. Clinical decision support systems: AI-powered clinical decision support systems can leverage electronic health records (EHRs), medical guidelines, and patient data to provide personalized treatment recommendations, alert healthcare providers about potential drug interactions or contraindications, and support evidence-based care [35].

9.4.2 Addressing the security issues in telehealth systems

Addressing the security challenges in telehealth systems requires a comprehensive approach that includes robust encryption algorithms, secure communication protocols, access control mechanisms, intrusion detection systems, user education, and adherence to security best practices. Regular security audits and updates are essential to maintaining the integrity, confidentiality, and availability of telehealth systems and safeguarding patient information. These solutions lead to more complex systems and increase the cost of telehealth systems. Thus, better security measures are required to efficiently curb the emergence of these different security breaches while maintaining simplicity of design and operation.

Emerging as a promising solution for various industries, blockchain technology has changed the way security and contract execution have been carried out in various applications including in telehealth systems. The decentralized and distributed nature of blockchain along with the ability to ensure data integrity and security making it well suited for applications in the healthcare sector [36]. In a blockchain network, nodes are interconnected in a mesh-like topology. Each node possesses a private key and a public key, serving distinct purposes. The public key functions as a unique address used for message encryption within the network, while the private key enables the signing of transactions and decryption of received messages from other nodes.

9.4.3 Architecture and functionality of blockchain in telehealth systems

Based on their intended use, blockchain networks can be categorized into two types: public (permissionless) and private (permissioned). The public blockchain allows anyone to participate in the network and validate transactions, while the private blockchain restricts access to a select group of authorized participants. In this section, we explore the implications of blockchain architecture and functionality that can address the privacy concerns of patients, uphold medical confidentiality, as well as enhance the efficiency and security of telehealth systems.

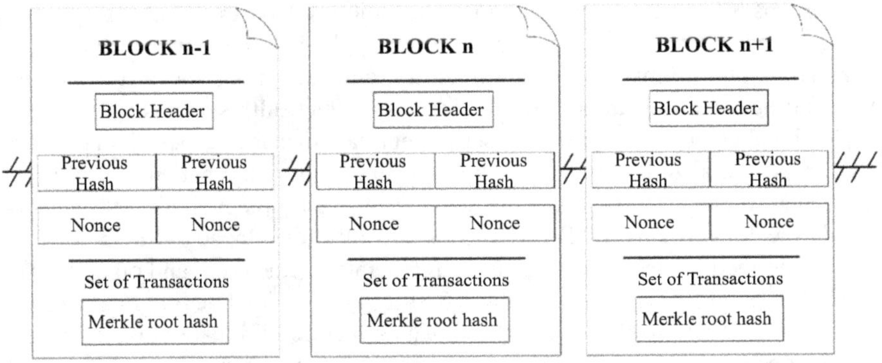

Figure 9.2 A typical blockchain block

Figure 9.2 shows a typical blockchain block which symbolizes the basic building component of a decentralized and immutable ledger system. It acts as a container for crucial information and transactions, encapsulating the basic concepts of transparency, security, and trust across many businesses. At a core level, a typical blockchain block has many critical components. The block header serves a significant function since it incorporates essential metadata and cryptographic information. This comprises the unique identity or hash assigned to the block, timestamp, and a nonce value needed in the mining process to verify and secure the block. The timestamp inside the block header represents the exact instant that the block is added to the network. This chronology maintains the proper sequencing of blocks, producing an immutable historical record of transactions and occurrences. Embedded inside the block structure is the Merkle root hash, which works as a condensed representation of all the transactions included within the block. This cryptographic hash maintains the integrity and tamper-resistance of the transactional data while giving a verifiable confirmation of the contents of the block.

A typical blockchain block comprises a collection of transactions particular to the sector it serves. In the context of telehealth systems, these transactions may represent patient medical records, diagnostic information, treatment plans, or other healthcare-related data. Each transaction inside the block is securely recorded, timestamped, and connected to the prior block, producing an unalterable chain of trust.

To ensure the immutability and security of the blockchain, consensus techniques are deployed. These procedures guarantee that all participating nodes in the network agree on the authenticity and sequence of transactions inside each block. Common consensus algorithms in blockchain networks include proof-of-work, proof-of-stake, and practical Byzantine fault tolerance, among others. Moreover, the distributed nature of a typical blockchain block indicates that it lives on numerous nodes throughout the network. This decentralization removes the need for a central authority and strengthens the robustness and fault tolerance of the blockchain system.

In terms of security, cryptographic techniques like the SHA-256 hashing algorithm and elliptic curve cryptography are applied inside a typical blockchain block. These algorithms enable data integrity, authentication, and privacy protection, securing sensitive patient information inside telehealth systems [37].

The blockchain structure comprises patient data managed blockchain contracts stored in decentralized storage. The key players such as the patients, health providers, and medical technicians access the E-health records and frameworks through local gateways. EHRs managers are also developed to help sort and organize the medical records, diagnoses, treatments, medication, and other relevant information about the patients. Figure 9.3 shows the various degree of interaction and access available to the key players. This structure eliminates to a significant level the occurrence of system privacy breaches and the security challenges covered in Section 9.3.5.

Besides the use of AI systems to manage the computation of AI and blockchain technologies to address the computational issues of telehealth systems, the wide adoption of large language models across different industries and now in healthcare shows the possibilities that AI and blockchain present to the health sector.

Blockchain technology: Implementing blockchain-based solutions may boost data security and integrity in telehealth systems. The tamper-resistant characteristics of blockchain, paired with AI algorithms for consensus procedures and smart contract execution, may enable safe storage, sharing, and access control of medical data.

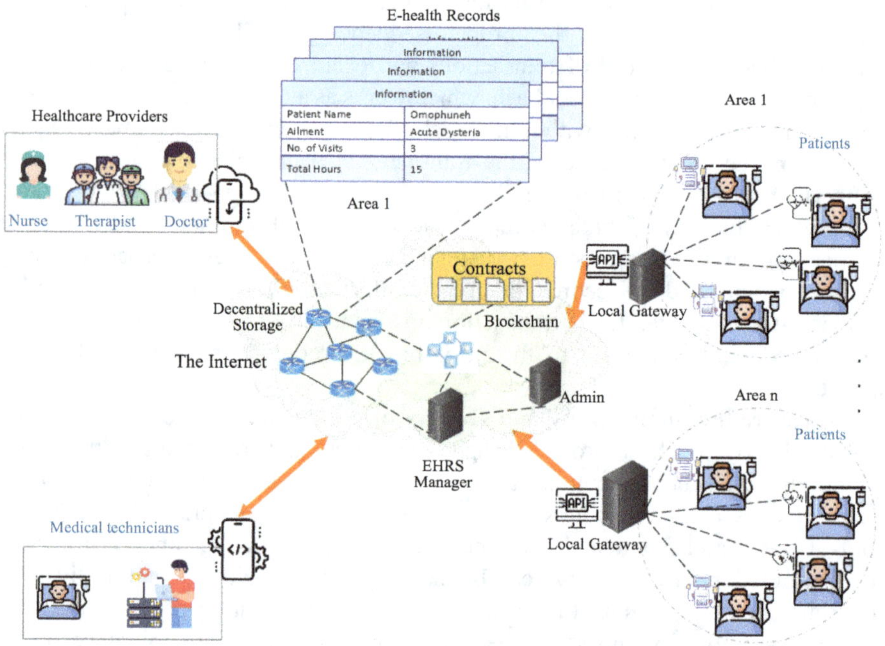

Figure 9.3 Blockchain solution architecture for telehealth systems

9.4.4 Limitations of blockchain and AI models in telehealth systems

Ethical concerns: The integration of AI models in telehealth systems brings ethical concerns that need to be addressed to enable responsible and trustworthy usage of these technologies. One significant problem is the possible bias in algorithmic decision-making. AI models are trained on historical data, which may include biases relating to race, gender, or socioeconomic aspects. If these prejudices are not addressed, they might result in unjust treatment or discrepancies in healthcare results. It is necessary to establish techniques to uncover and minimize bias in AI systems via thorough data pretreatment, algorithm design, and continual monitoring.

Transparency and accountability are also key ethical factors. AI models generally function as dark boxes, making it tough to comprehend their decision-making processes. In the context of telehealth systems, where choices affect patient care, it is vital to maintain openness by constructing explainable AI models. Patients and healthcare practitioners should have insights into how AI models arrive at their suggestions or conclusions. This increases trust, facilitates improved cooperation, and allows for informed decision-making.

Regulatory compliance: Telehealth systems are subject to several rules, including data protection and privacy legislation. For instance, in the United States, the HIPAA specifies rules for the privacy and security of protected health information. When incorporating blockchain technology and AI models into telehealth systems, compliance with these rules becomes crucial.

The immutability and decentralization of blockchain might offer issues in satisfying regulatory obligations. For example, securing the right to be forgotten or the capacity to amend or remove particular patient data might be problematic in a blockchain context. Organizations need to carefully analyze how blockchain fits inside the regulatory framework and adopt suitable methods to maintain compliance. This may use anonymization techniques, consent management systems, or encryption approaches to secure sensitive data while harnessing the advantages of blockchain and AI.

Adoption and integration: Integrating blockchain and AI technologies into current telehealth infrastructure may be a challenging process that needs careful planning and resource allocation. Organizations need to invest in qualified employees, such as data scientists and blockchain specialists, who can traverse the technological complexity and assure effective adoption.

Adopting blockchain and AI technologies may also require infrastructure upgrades to support the increased computational requirements and storage capacity. This might require investing in secure and scalable blockchain networks, strong data storage systems, and high-performance computer resources.

Moreover, the integration of these technologies needs change management techniques to enable a seamless transition and acceptability by stakeholders. Healthcare practitioners and patients may need education and training to comprehend the advantages and functions of blockchain and AI models in telehealth systems. Collaboration with stakeholders, including IT teams, healthcare professionals, and patients, is vital to identify requirements, resolve concerns, and align the technology deployment with the aims and values of the healthcare organization.

9.4.5 *Trends and global adoption of telehealth systems*

There has been an increasing reliance on telehealth services which has been accompanied by a surge in the number of telehealth users across many countries. In the United States alone, there has been an escalating demand for telehealth systems since the COVID-19 pandemic leading to a consequent need for enhanced computational techniques to address the challenges posed by the increasing number of users [38].

Table 9.1 reveals a significant increase in the number of telehealth-eligible beneficiaries in recent years. Notably, the 0–64 age group experienced a staggering 55% surge in telehealth-eligible beneficiaries between 2019 and 2021. This remarkable growth can be attributed to the global COVID-19 pandemic, which has compelled individuals to seek healthcare remotely due to limitations in accessing in-person medical consultations. The COVID-19 pandemic has acted as a catalyst for the widespread adoption of telehealth services [39]. The necessity to minimize in-person interactions and adhere to social distancing measures has further emphasized the importance of remote healthcare. As a result, telehealth systems have become a vital tool in ensuring continued access to medical care, especially for patients in

Table 9.1 Number of telehealth users in the United States

Age of benefactors	Race of benefactors	Enrolled candidates	Eligible candidates
0–64	American Indian/Alaska Native	645,297	496,446
0–64	Asian/Pacific Islander	1,196,506	863,318
0–64	Black/African American	10,336,644	7,862,715
0–64	Hispanic	5,714,449	4,310,685
0–64	Non-Hispanic White	37,389,942	28,920,973
65–74	American Indian/Alaska Native	969,245	746,257
65–74	Asian/Pacific Islander	7,007,612	4,758,900
65–74	Black/African American	16,404,022	12,108,140
65–74	Hispanic	12,821,984	8,436,616
65–74	Non-Hispanic White	173,250,759	133,346,018
75–84	American Indian/Alaska Native	595,322	488,958
75–84	Asian/Pacific Islander	425,3215	3,225,112
75–84	Black/African American	7,859,298	6,420,476
75–84	Hispanic	6,647,731	4,887,565
75–84	Non-Hispanic White	109,587,108	92,840,293
85 and over	American Indian/Alaska Native	209,812	174,962
85 and over	Asian/Pacific Islander	2,032,394	1,581,586
85 and over	Black/African American	3,211,954	2,674,003
85 and over	Hispanic	2,915,528	2,239,554
85 and over	Non-Hispanic White	46,272,496	40,462,454

the 0–64 age group. However, this increased reliance on telehealth services has introduced new challenges for telehealth systems, particularly in terms of computational power. The processing and transmission of vast amounts of patient data necessitate robust computational infrastructure to ensure accurate diagnoses, secure data storage, and efficient communication between healthcare providers and patients.

One promising avenue for enhancing computational capabilities in telehealth systems is the integration of AI algorithms. By leveraging AI, telehealth systems can harness advanced data analytics, image analysis, speech recognition, and ML to provide accurate diagnoses, personalized treatment recommendations, and remote patient monitoring [40]. Moreover, the integration of blockchain technology also offers additional benefits in terms of data security, privacy, and interoperability within telehealth systems. Blockchain can enhance data integrity and confidentiality while addressing concerns related to patient data protection and privacy regulations.

Table 9.1 reveals a significant increase in the number of telehealth-eligible beneficiaries in recent years. Notably, the 0–64 age group experienced a staggering 55% surge in telehealth-eligible beneficiaries between 2019 and 2021. This remarkable growth can be attributed to the global COVID-19 pandemic, which has compelled individuals to seek healthcare remotely due to limitations in accessing in-person medical consultations.

In Figures 9.4 and 9.5 a decline in the initial surge of people using telehealth services as presented by [38] has gradually reduced however still above the initial level it was at the zenith of the COVID-19 pandemic.

While Figure 9.6 presents a plot of the number of users who enrolled for telehealth services to those who benefited from the service from 2020 to 2022, Figure 9.7 is a bar chart that shows the yearly telehealth service count and the various telehealth types such as live audio/video, remote patient monitoring, store and forward, and other telehealth services. It can be seen that there were more registrations in 2020 and concurrently more beneficiaries than in 2021 and 2022.

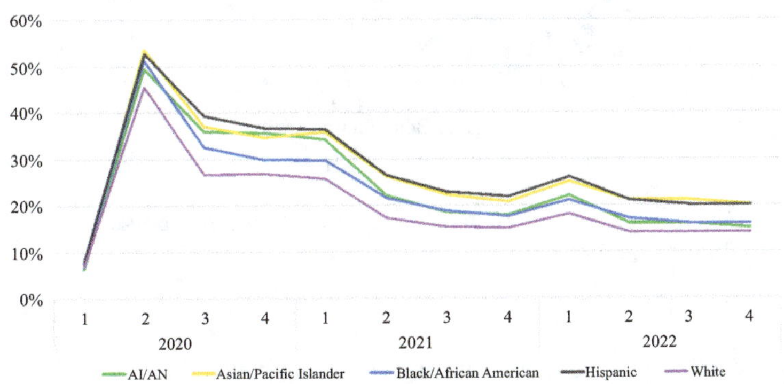

Figure 9.4 Percentage of medicare users with a telehealth service by quarter: by race/ethnicity

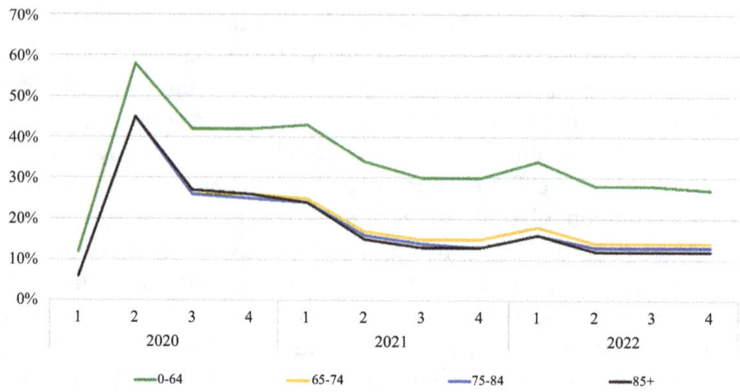

Figure 9.5 Percentage of medicare users with a telehealth service by quarter: by race/ethnicity

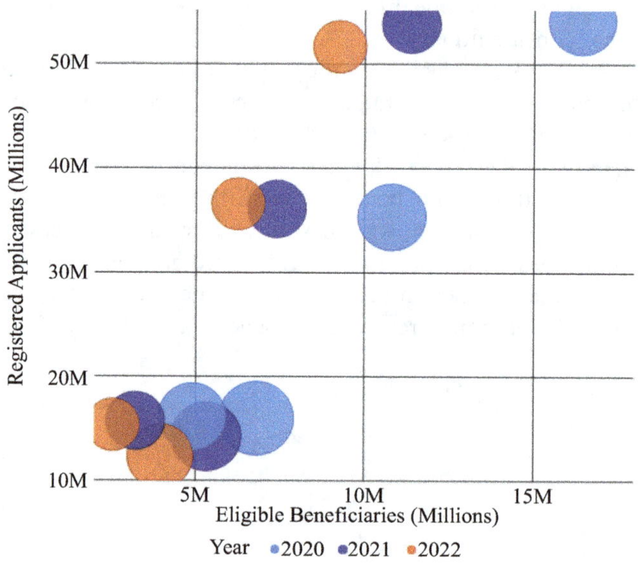

Figure 9.6 Number of registered telehealth users to actual beneficiaries from 2020 to 2022

Despite the decline in enrolment values as seen in Figures 9.4 and 9.5, Figure 9.7 shows that more services have been especially in live audio/video and remote patient monitoring has been on the increase.

Evidently, the COVID-19 pandemic has acted as a catalyst for the widespread adoption of telehealth services. The necessity to minimize in-person interactions and

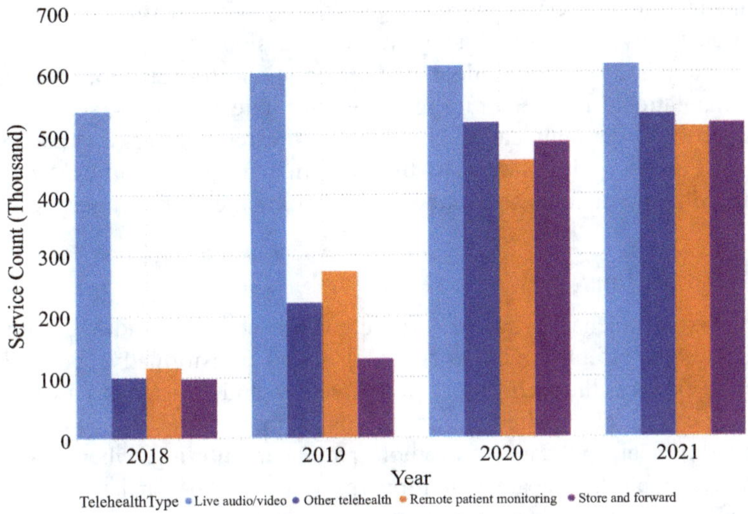

Figure 9.7 Service count for various telehealth types from 2018 to 2021

Table 9.2 Number of telehealth users in the United States

Year	Type	Service count (thousands)
2018	Live audio/video	537
	Remote patient monitoring	115
	Store and forward	97
	Other telehealth	99
2019	Live audio/video	599
	Remote patient monitoring	273
	Store and forward	129
	Other telehealth	221
2020	Live audio/video	610
	Remote patient monitoring	454
	Store and forward	484
	Other telehealth	516
2021	Live audio/video	612
	Remote patient monitoring	509
	Store and forward	515
	Other telehealth	530

adhere to social distancing measures has further emphasized the importance of remote healthcare. As a result, telehealth systems have become a vital tool in ensuring continued access to medical care, especially for patients in the 0–64 age group.

However, this increased reliance on telehealth services as shown in Table 9.2 indicating the rising number of people subscribing to telehealth services introduces new challenges for the effective running of the systems, particularly in terms of computational power. The processing and transmission of vast amounts of patient high-resolution imagery and videos and other telehealth data forms necessitate robust computational infrastructure to ensure accurate diagnoses, secure data storage, and efficient communication between healthcare providers and patients. The strain placed on telehealth systems by the surge in demand has highlighted the need for enhanced computational techniques to overcome these challenges.

9.4.6 Discussions

In the context of telehealth systems, the convergence of AI and ML with blockchain technology offers numerous advantages and transformative potential [41]. This section explores the architecture, functionality, and critical use cases where AI and ML are effectively applied in telehealth systems.

One prominent application is remote patient monitoring, where AI and ML technologies enable healthcare practitioners to observe the vital signs of patients remotely. By analyzing data such as blood pressure, pulse rate, respiration rate, and more, AI algorithms provide insights and trigger alarms for timely medical treatment. This remote monitoring feature improves patient outcomes, reduces the need for in-person visits, and enhances the efficiency of telehealth systems.

Another important use case is AI-assisted diagnosis, where healthcare practitioners can examine medical data remotely with the support of AI and ML. Image analysis, such as X-rays, CT scans, and diagnostic test data, benefits from AI algorithms that provide insights and suggestions based on symptoms and medical history. This enables quicker and more accurate diagnoses, particularly in situations where access to specialist expertise is limited. Cloud-based solutions facilitate the scalability, secure storage, and rapid exchange of diagnostic data, enhancing the diagnostic capabilities of telehealth systems.

AI and ML algorithms also contribute to the generation of tailored treatment plans in telehealth systems. By considering individual patient preferences, treatment types, and geographic factors, AI systems deliver customized solutions for optimal care. These algorithms analyze large volumes of patient data, including medical history and treatment outcomes, to identify the most effective therapy choices. This personalized approach improves treatment outcomes, patient satisfaction, and adherence to treatment programs, ultimately empowering healthcare clinicians with data-driven insights for better decision-making.

AI technologies play a significant role in patient engagement within telehealth systems. Through features like reminders for appointments, medication adherence, and follow-up treatments, AI-powered chatbots and automated solutions enhance patient participation and communication. Patients receive rapid responses to common inquiries, enabling easy access to information and active engagement in their treatment. By strengthening the patient-provider connection, AI-driven telehealth solutions improve patient satisfaction and contribute to better treatment outcomes.

Chronic disease therapy is another area where AI and ML have a positive impact on telehealth systems. These technologies facilitate personalized treatment regimens, reminders, and progress monitoring for patients with chronic illnesses such as diabetes, hypertension, and heart disease. ML algorithms analyze patient data to predict outcomes and identify the risk of developing related conditions. This enables early interventions, individualized treatments, and improved patient self-management, resulting in better health outcomes and reduced healthcare costs.

While AI and ML bring significant benefits to telehealth systems, there are several challenges and limitations to consider. Ethical considerations, such as bias in algorithmic decision-making and ensuring transparency and accountability, require careful attention. Regulatory compliance, particularly regarding data protection and privacy laws, needs to be addressed when integrating these technologies. Adoption and integration of AI and blockchain technologies into existing telehealth infrastructure can be complex and require investment in resources and change management processes. Additionally, the scalability of blockchain and computational issues in managing large volumes of data and real-time analytics pose challenges that need to be overcome.

This study finds significance and thus justification for the transformative potential of integrating AI and blockchain models in telehealth systems as presented in it. The concepts and strategies covered in this chapter in addressing the common computational issues experienced in telehealth systems offer improved patient outcomes and reduced healthcare costs. The chapter also explores various applications, including remote patient monitoring, diagnosis, treatment planning, and chronic disease management, backed by real-world examples and research insights. Although challenges, such as ethical concerns and infrastructure requirements, are acknowledged, the chapter also emphasizes that careful planning and continuous assessment can overcome these weaknesses and strengthen the overall justification for adopting these technologies in telehealth.

9.4.7 Lessons learned

The integration of AI and blockchain technologies into telehealth systems presents a transformative potential in addressing the challenges posed by the increasing reliance on telehealth services. As discussed in Section 9.1, the exponential growth in telehealth usage during the COVID-19 pandemic has emphasized the need for effective solutions to handle the rising computational complexity of telehealth systems. The insights and recommendations provided in Sections 9.3 and 9.4 have shed light on the advantages of AI and blockchain in remote patient monitoring, accurate diagnosis, personalized treatment planning, patient engagement, and chronic disease management.

Lesson one: To overcome computational challenges, and achieve robust infrastructure and real-time analytics capabilities, efficient integration of AI and blockchain in telehealth systems can substantially influence the scalability and efficiency of medical services.

Lesson two: By leveraging AI algorithms, telehealth systems can efficiently process and analyze large datasets, enabling remote patient monitoring and accurate diagnoses, ultimately minimizing the need for in-person visits and ensuring timely medical treatment.

Lesson three: The decentralized and tamper-resistant nature of blockchain technology enhances data security and privacy, addressing critical concerns related to patient information protection and ensuring compliance with regulatory obligations.

Lesson four: AI-driven telehealth solutions can be used to generate personalized treatment plans by analyzing patient data, leading to more effective therapy choices and improved patient adherence to treatment programs.

Lesson five: Ethical considerations, such as bias in AI algorithms and transparency in decision-making, require careful attention to ensure responsible and trustworthy usage of these technologies in telehealth.

Lesson six: Regulatory compliance and collaboration with stakeholders, including IT teams, healthcare professionals, and patients, are vital to the successful integration of AI and blockchain technologies in telehealth.

9.5 Conclusion and future scope

The COVID-19 pandemic has accelerated the adoption and utilization of telehealth services, offering a safer and more convenient alternative to traditional in-person care. The exponential growth in telehealth use since the pandemic has highlighted the need for effective solutions to address the rising computational complexity in telehealth systems. This chapter has demonstrated how AI and blockchain technologies can play a pivotal role in solving these challenges.

Telehealth systems are faced with increasing demands for remote patient monitoring, accurate diagnosis, personalized treatment planning, patient engagement, and chronic disease management. The sheer volume of patient data and the need for real-time analytics pose significant computational challenges. However, AI algorithms have shown promise in efficiently processing and analyzing large datasets, enabling remote monitoring, accurate diagnoses, and personalized treatment plans. By leveraging AI capabilities, telehealth systems can improve patient outcomes, reduce healthcare costs, and enhance overall healthcare delivery efficiency.

Furthermore, the integration of blockchain technology in telehealth systems addresses critical concerns regarding data integrity, privacy, and security. With a decentralized and tamper-resistant nature, blockchain provides a robust framework for secure storage, sharing, and access control of medical data. By leveraging blockchain, telehealth systems can ensure the privacy of patient information, maintain data integrity, and facilitate interoperability among various healthcare systems.

Looking ahead, there are still areas for further research and development in the field of AI and blockchain in telehealth. Ethical considerations, such as bias in AI algorithms and transparency in decision-making, need to be addressed to ensure responsible and trustworthy usage of these technologies. Regulatory compliance and the integration of AI and blockchain into existing healthcare frameworks require careful planning and collaboration among stakeholders.

Future research should focus on enhancing interoperability, developing user-friendly interfaces, and improving the usability of AI and blockchain-empowered telehealth systems. Finally, addressing scalability and computational challenges will be crucial in enabling seamless integration and efficient data processing.

References

[1] N. Z. Bawany, T. Qamar, H. Tariq, and S. Adnan, "Integrating Healthcare Services Using Blockchain-Based Telehealth Framework," *IEEE Access*, vol. 10, pp. 36505–36517, 2022, doi: 10.1109/ACCESS.2022.3161944.

[2] T. Russell, N. Gillespie, N. Hartley, D. Theodoros, A. Hill, and L. Gray, "Exploring the Predictors of Home Telehealth Uptake by Elderly Australian Healthcare Consumers," *J. Telemed. Telecare*, vol. 21, no. 8, pp. 485–489, 2015, doi: 10.1177/1357633X15606264.

[3] J. Li and L. S. Wilson, "Telehealth Trends and the Challenge for Infrastructure," *Telemed. e-Health*, vol. 19, no. 10, pp. 772–779, Oct. 2013, doi: 10.1089/tmj.2012.0324.

[4] B. P. Ng, C. Park, C. L. Silverman, D. O. Eckhoff, J. C. Guest, and D. A. Díaz, "Accessibility and Utilisation of Telehealth Services among Older Adults During COVID-19 Pandemic in the United States," *Health Soc. Care Community*, vol. 30, no. 5, 2022, doi:10.1111/hsc.13709.

[5] D. V. Gunasekeran, R. M. W. W. Tseng, Y.-C. Tham, and T. Y. Wong, "Applications of Digital Health for Public Health Responses to COVID-19: A Systematic Scoping Review of Artificial Intelligence, Telehealth and Related Technologies," *npj Digit. Med.*, vol. 4, no. 1, p. 40, 2021, doi: 10.1038/s41746-021-00412-9.

[6] S. S. Tripathy, A. L. Imoize, M. Rath, *et al.*, "A Novel Edge-Computing-Based Framework for an Intelligent Smart Healthcare System in Smart Cities," *Sustainability*, vol. 15, no. 1, p. 735, 2022, doi: 10.3390/su15010735.

[7] S. N. Gajarawala and J. N. Pelkowski, "Telehealth Benefits and Barriers," *J. Nurse Pract.*, vol. 17, no. 2, pp. 218–221, 2021, doi: 10.1016/j.nurpra.2020.09.013.

[8] B. Clipper, "The Influence of the COVID-19 Pandemic on Technology," *Nurse Lead.*, vol. 18, no. 5, pp. 500–503, 2020, doi: 10.1016/j.mnl.2020.06.008.

[9] D. M. El-Sherif, M. Abouzid, M. T. Elzarif, A. A. Ahmed, A. Albakri, and M. M. Alshehri, "Telehealth and Artificial Intelligence Insights into Healthcare during the COVID-19 Pandemic," *Healthcare*, vol. 10, no. 2, p. 385, 2022, doi: 10.3390/healthcare10020385.

[10] A. Haleem and M. Javaid, "Medical 4.0 and Its Role in Healthcare During COVID-19 Pandemic: A Review," *J. Ind. Integr. Manag.*, vol. 5, no. 4, pp. 531–545, 2020, doi: 10.1142/S2424862220300045.

[11] S. Sattar and R. Kuperman, "Telehealth in Pediatric Epilepsy Care: A Rapid Transition during the COVID-19 Pandemic," *Epilepsy Behav.*, vol. 111, p. 107282, 2020, doi: 10.1016/j.yebeh.2020.107282.

[12] A. L. Imoize, D. O. Irabor, P. A. Gbadega, and C. Chakraborty, "Blockchain Technology for Secure COVID-19 Pandemic Data Handling," in *Smart Health Technologies for the COVID-19 Pandemic: Internet of Medical Things Perspectives*, Institution of Engineering and Technology, 2022, pp. 141–179. doi: 10.1049/PBHE042E_ch6.

[13] H. R. Hasan, K. Salah, R. Jayaraman, I. Yaqoob, M. Omar, and S. Ellahham, "Blockchain-Enabled Telehealth Services Using Smart Contracts," *IEEE Access*, vol. 9, pp. 151944–151959, 2021, doi: 10.1109/ACCESS.2021.3126025.

[14] C.-Y. Chen, H.-H. Huang, C.-Y. Wu, L.-T. Kuo, S.-Y. Shih, and P. Lai, "Telehealth Data-Derived Visual Analytics for Health Informatics Applications in Coordinated Care of Patients with Multiple Comorbidities," in *2022 IEEE Biomedical Circuits and Systems Conference (BioCAS)*, IEEE, 2022, pp. 444–447. doi: 10.1109/BioCAS54905.2022.9948673.

[15] J. B. Awotunde, A. L. Imoize, D. P. Salako, and Y. Farhaoui, "An Enhanced Medical Diagnosis System for Malaria and Typhoid Fever Using Genetic Neuro-Fuzzy System," In *The International Conference on Artificial Intelligence and Smart Environment 2022*, pp. 173–183, Cham: Springer International Publishing. doi: 10.1007/978-3-031-26254-8_25.

[16] S.-T. Cheung, R. F. Davies, K. Smith, R. Marsh, H. Sherrard, and W. J. Keon, "The Ottawa Telehealth Project," *Telemed. J.*, vol. 4, no. 3, pp. 259–266, 1998, doi: 10.1089/tmj.1.1998.4.259.

[17] O. Zur, "Telehealth and the Technology for Delivering Care," in *Boundaries in Psychotherapy: Ethical and Clinical Explorations.*, Washington, DC: American Psychological Association, 2007, pp. 133–146. doi: 10.1037/11563-008.

[18] S. Gogia, "Rationale, History, and Basics of Telehealth," in *Fundamentals of Telemedicine and Telehealth*, Elsevier, 2020, pp. 11–34. doi: 10.1016/B978-0-12-814309-4.00002-1.

[19] S. Tuli, S. Tuli, G. Wander, *et al.*, "Next Generation Technologies for Smart Healthcare: Challenges, Vision, Model, Trends and Future Directions," *Internet Technol. Lett.*, vol. 3, no. 2, p. e145, 2020, doi: 10.1002/itl2.145.

[20] A. L. Imoize, V. E. Balas, V. K. Solanki, C.-C. Lee, and M. S. Obaidat (eds.). (2023). *Handbook of Security and Privacy of AI-Enabled Healthcare Systems and Internet of Medical Things* (1st ed.). CRC Press. https://doi.org/10.1201/9781003370321

[21] M. J. Ackerman, R. Filart, L. P. Burgess, I. Lee, and R. K. Poropatich, "Developing Next-Generation Telehealth Tools and Technologies: Patients, Systems, and Data Perspectives," *Telemed. e-Health*, vol. 16, no. 1, pp. 93–95, 2010, doi: 10.1089/tmj.2009.0153.

[22] Z. Agha, C. R. Weir, and Y. Chen, "Usability of Telehealth Technologies," *Int. J. Telemed. Appl.*, vol. 2013, pp. 1–2, 2013, doi: 10.1155/2013/834514.

[23] S. M. A. Ullah, M. M. Islam, S. Mahmud, S. Nooruddin, S. M. T. U. Raju, and M. R. Haque, "Scalable Telehealth Services to Combat Novel Coronavirus (COVID-19) Pandemic," *SN Comput. Sci.*, vol. 2, no. 1, p. 18, 2021, doi: 10.1007/s42979-020-00401-x.

[24] S. M. Finkelstein, S. M. Speedie, and S. Potthoff, "Home Telehealth Improves Clinical Outcomes at Lower Cost for Home Healthcare," *Telemed. e-Health*, vol. 12, no. 2, pp. 128–136, 2006, doi: 10.1089/tmj.2006.12.128.

[25] H. Miner, K. Koenig, and K. J. Bozic, "Value-based Healthcare: Not Going Anywhere—Why Orthopaedic Surgeons Will Continue Using Telehealth in a Post-COVID-19 World," *Clin. Orthop. Relat. Res.*, vol. 478, no. 12, pp. 2717–2719, 2020, doi: 10.1097/CORR.0000000000001561.

[26] R. W. Ahmad, K. Salah, R. Jayaraman, I. Yaqoob, S. Ellahham, and M. Omar, "The Role of Blockchain Technology in Telehealth and Telemedicine," *Int. J. Med. Inform.*, vol. 148, p. 104399, Apr. 2021, doi: 10.1016/J.IJMEDINF. 2021.104399.

[27] A. Haleem, M. Javaid, R. P. Singh, and R. Suman, "Telemedicine for Healthcare: Capabilities, Features, Barriers, and Applications," *Sensors Int.*, vol. 2, p. 100117, 2021, doi: 10.1016/j.sintl.2021.100117.

[28] R. Lisa and F. Lawrence, "The Pitfalls of Telehealth — And How to Avoid Them," *Harvard Business Review*, 2020. https://hbr.org/2020/11/the-pitfalls-of-telehealth-and-how-to-avoid-them (accessed Jul. 17, 2023).

[29] O. G. Oyebiyi, A. Abayomi-Alli, O. 'Tale Arogundade, A. Qazi, A. L. Imoize, and J. B. Awotunde, "A Systematic Literature Review on Human Ear Biometrics: Approaches, Algorithms, and Trend in the Last Decade," *Information*, vol. 14, no. 3, p. 192, 2023, doi: 10.3390/info14030192.

[30] K. V. N. Kavitha, S. Ashok, A. L. Imoize, *et al.*, "On the Use of Wavelet Domain and Machine Learning for the Analysis of Epileptic Seizure Detection from EEG Signals," *J. Healthc. Eng.*, vol. 2022, pp. 1–16, 2022, doi: 10.1155/2022/8928021.

[31] M. Acharya, M. M. Ali, C. J. Hayes, C. A. Bogulski, E. F. Magann, and H. Eswaran, "Trends in Telehealth Visits During Pregnancy, 2018 to 2021," *JAMA Netw. Open*, vol. 6, no. 4, p. e236630, 2023, doi: 10.1001/jamanetworkopen.2023.6630.

[32] J. B. Awotunde, A. L. Imoize, O. B. Ayoade, *et al.*, "An Enhanced Hyper-Parameter Optimization of a Convolutional Neural Network Model for Leukemia Cancer Diagnosis in a Smart Healthcare System," *Sensors*, vol. 22, no. 24, p. 9689, 2022, doi: 10.3390/s22249689.

[33] Y. Sei, A. Ohsuga, and A. L. Imoize, "Statistical Test with Differential Privacy for Medical Decision Support Systems," in *Explainable Artificial Intelligence in Medical Decision Support Systems*, Institution of Engineering and Technology, 2022, pp. 401–433. doi: 10.1049/PBHE050E_ch15.

[34] A. T. Rufai, K. F. Dukor, O. M. Ageh, and A. L. Imoize, "XAI Robot-Assisted Surgeries in Future Medical Decision Support Systems," in *Explainable Artificial Intelligence in Medical Decision Support Systems*,

Institution of Engineering and Technology, 2022, pp. 167–195. doi: 10.1049/PBHE050E_ch6.

[35] O. B. Ayoade, T. O. Oladele, A. L. Imoize, *et al.*, "Explainable Artificial Intelligence (XAI) in Medical Decision Systems (MDSSs): Healthcare Systems Perspective," in *Explainable Artificial Intelligence in Medical Decision Support Systems*, Institution of Engineering and Technology, 2022, pp. 1–43. doi: 10.1049/PBHE050E_ch1.

[36] R. L. Kumar, Y. Wang, T. Poongodi, and A. L. Imoize, *Internet of Things, Artificial Intelligence and Blockchain Technology*. Cham: Springer International Publishing, 2021. doi: 10.1007/978-3-030-74150-1.

[37] O. C. Abikoye, E. T. Oladipupo, A. L. Imoize, J. B. Awotunde, C.-C. Lee, and C.-T. Li, "Securing Critical User Information over the Internet of Medical Things Platforms Using a Hybrid Cryptography Scheme," *Futur. Internet*, vol. 15, no. 3, p. 99, 2023, doi: 10.3390/fi15030099.

[38] Centres Medicare & Services Medicaid, "Medicare Telehealth Trends Report," 2023. [Online]. Available: https://data.cms.gov/summary-statistics-on-use-and-payments/medicare-service-type-reports/medicare-telehealth-trends

[39] A. L. Imoize, P. A. Gbadega, H. I. Obakhena, D. O. Irabor, K. V. N. Kavitha, and C. Chakraborty, "Artificial Intelligence-Enabled Internet of Medical Things for COVID-19 Pandemic Data Management," in *Explainable Artificial Intelligence in Medical Decision Support Systems*, Institution of Engineering and Technology, 2022, pp. 357–380. doi: 10.1049/PBHE050E_ch13.

[40] A. L. Imoize, J. Hemanth, D.-T. Do, and S. N. Sur (eds.), *Explainable Artificial Intelligence in Medical Decision Support Systems*. Institution of Engineering and Technology, 2022. doi:10.1049/PBHE050E.

[41] L. K. Ramasamy, F. Khan K. P., A. L. Imoize, J. O. Ogbebor, S. Kadry, and S. Rho, "Blockchain-Based Wireless Sensor Networks for Malicious Node Detection: A Survey," *IEEE Access*, vol. 9, pp. 128765–128785, 2021, doi: 10.1109/ACCESS.2021.3111923.

Chapter 10

Examining the potential issues and risks associated with the integration of AI and blockchain technology in telehealth systems

Abidemi Emmanuel Adeniyi[1], Peace Busola Falola[2], Joseph Bamidele Awotunde[3], Rasheed Gbenga Jimoh[4], Solomon Olalekan Akinola[5] and Agbotiname Lucky Imoize[6]

There has been significant improvement in telehealth with the development of blockchain and artificial intelligence (AI) technologies in recent years. AI enables intelligent decision-making and automation in healthcare, while blockchain offers decentralized and secure data management. However, the integration of these technologies introduces a set of challenges and risks that need to be carefully addressed. The interoperability and integration of AI and blockchain within telehealth systems present technical challenges. AI algorithms require a large amount of data, which may be stored on distributed blockchain networks. Ensuring seamless interaction between AI models and blockchain infrastructure poses data access, sharing, and computation challenges. AI-driven diagnosis and treatment decisions may lead to errors or biases, requiring transparent accountability and liability framework. Blockchain's immutability raises questions about the right to be forgotten and data privacy regulations, as personal health information stored on the blockchain may be challenging to delete or modify. The cybersecurity risks associated with integrating AI and blockchain cannot be overlooked because blockchain decentralized nature provides robust security against data tempering. However, vulnerabilities in smart contracts or AI algorithms could be exploited. Moreover, the vast amount of data exchanged in telehealth systems creates

[1]Department of Computer Science, Bowen University, Nigeria
[2]Department of Computer Sciences, Faculty of Pure and Applied Sciences, Precious Cornerstone University, Nigeria
[3]Department of Computer Science, Faculty of Information and Communication Sciences, University of Ilorin, Nigeria
[4]Department of Computer Sciences, Faculty of Communication and Information Sciences, University of Ilorin, Nigeria
[5]Department of Computer Science, Faculty of Sciences, University of Ibadan, Nigeria
[6]Department of Electrical and Electronics Engineering, Faculty of Engineering, University of Lagos, Nigeria

opportunities for data breaches and unauthorized access. To mitigate these issues and risks, stakeholders in telehealth systems must collaborate to develop robust technical standards, governance mechanisms, and regulatory frameworks. Transparent and explainable AI models, privacy-preserving mechanisms, and secure blockchain protocols should be designed and implemented. Interdisciplinary research involving healthcare, technology, law, and ethics experts is crucial to address the challenges and maximize the advantages of incorporating AI and blockchain in telehealth systems. While integrating AI and blockchain technology systems offers numerous benefits, it also presents a range of potential issues and risks. By acknowledging and addressing these challenges, stakeholders can harness the transformative power of AI and blockchain technologies to create more efficient, secure, and ethical telehealth systems.

10.1 Introduction

Telehealth, which encompasses the delivery of healthcare services remotely via technology, has sparked a proportion of attraction in latest years because of its capability to increase accessibility to healthcare, lower costs, and improve patient outcomes [1]. Because of the fast improvements in artificial intelligence (AI) and blockchain technology, there is growing attention in research on their incorporation into telehealth systems. Telemedicine and virtual medical services are the technological advances in healthcare that enable “recovery from afar” [2]. It often consists of primarily using cellphone conversations, video, and message services such as electronic mail, medical messaging platforms, and smartphone applications to monitor patients’ various phytosociological signs and symptoms [3]. The use of audiovisual technologies like smart devices, portal apps, computing devices, and live calling to assist clinicians in diagnosing, evaluating, treating, monitoring, and advising patients digitally in telehealth has been of great help. Electronic health records and telemedicine are the most developed areas in the healthcare sector. Much of this expansion may be ascribed to its advantages, which include less travel, fewer missed appointments, and reduced wait periods. It enables the management of medical information costs, ease, and accessibility. Previous research indicates [4–6] that telemedicine lowers costs and increases patient access to care.

Furthermore, because the welfare of the medical staff is the cornerstone of a functional health system, delivering healthcare virtually could reduce the chance of medical personnel becoming infected [6]. Furthermore, Awotunde *et al.* [6] found that patients report enhanced accessibility and dialog, better medication adherence, and overall excellent experience with telehealth-related services.

Telehealth allows medical workers to monitor patients virtually, identify, and manage patients while also reducing patient accessibility and employee constraints, extending technology abilities, and lowering the possibility of doctors, employees, or patients being exposed to the COVID-19 virus. Furthermore, telemedicine uses electronic data and telecommunication technology to assist patients in handling their illnesses by improving personal care and facilitating

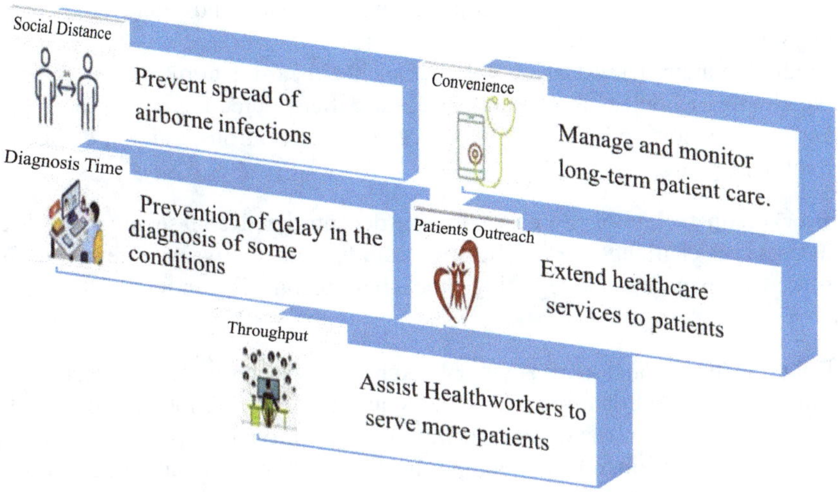

Figure 10.1 The importance of telemedicine and telehealth in healthcare services

educational access and assistance services. [7–10]. The key advantages of current telemedicine platforms are emphasized in Figure 10.1, which demonstrates that online medical facilities can effectively prevent the transmission of pandemic environmental infections. Furthermore, incorporating blockchain technology into current telehealth and telemedicine platforms can open up a plethora of possibilities for safe healthcare digitization, involving effectively establishing the source of medical information, the credibility of people looking for patient information, managing the characteristics of devices used for virtual patient tracking equipment, preserving patient confidentiality, and automating payment deal.

Because of the fast improvements in AI and Blockchain technology, there is rising attention to examining their incorporation into telehealth systems. This chapter examines the background and rationale for integrating AI and blockchain technology in telehealth systems.

AI has emerged as a transformative technology in healthcare, offering the potential for improved diagnostics, personalized treatment, and efficient healthcare delivery. In telehealth, AI can play a vital role in various aspects, such as

1. Remote diagnostics: AI techniques can analyze medical data, including images, laboratory results, and patient history, to assist in diagnosing conditions remotely. This can enable faster and more accurate diagnoses, particularly in underdeveloped places with limited access to specialized healthcare.
2. Virtual assistants: AI-powered chatbots or virtual assistants can interact with patients, answer their queries, and provide basic healthcare information,

reducing the burden on healthcare professionals and enhancing patient engagement.

3. Predictive analytics: Massive volumes of healthcare data may be analyzed by AI systems to detect trends and forecast patient outcomes. This can help in early detection of diseases, proactive interventions, and personalized treatment plans.

Blockchain technology, known for its decentralized and secure nature, can address several challenges in telehealth, including data privacy, interoperability, and trust. Key benefits of integrating blockchain technology in telehealth systems include:

1. Data security and privacy: Blockchain can provide a secure and immutable patient data record, guaranteeing that delicate medical information is protected from unauthorized access. Additionally, patients can have authority over their information and the ability to provide authorization for its use, enhancing privacy.
2. Interoperability: Blockchain's decentralized nature enables seamless sharing and integration of healthcare data across different providers and systems. This can facilitate better coordination of care, reduce duplication of tests, and enable a comprehensive view of a patient's medical history.
3. Trust and transparency: By utilizing blockchain, telehealth systems can establish trust among stakeholders, including patients, healthcare providers, and payers. Transactions recorded on the blockchain are transparent, traceable, and tamper-proof, ensuring data integrity and reducing fraudulent activities.

The combination of AI and Blockchain technology in telehealth systems holds immense potential to revolutionize healthcare delivery. Nevertheless, examining and comprehending the possible issues and risks related to this integration is critical to ensure its successful implementation and address any challenges. This study explores the potential issues and risks of integrating AI and blockchain technology in telehealth systems. Figure 10.2 shows the potential risk involved in incorporating AI and blockchain technology in telehealth.

10.1.1 Important achievements made by the chapter

This chapter made the resulting notable contributions:

1. The chapter systematically identifies and explores the challenges and risks that may arise from integrating AI and blockchain technology in telehealth systems.
2. The chapter addresses the potential issues related to data quality and reliability in AI and blockchain-powered telehealth systems, and
3. It provides valuable insights for researchers, healthcare providers, policymakers, and developers working in the field, contributing to advancing knowledge and guiding the development of robust and secure telehealth systems.

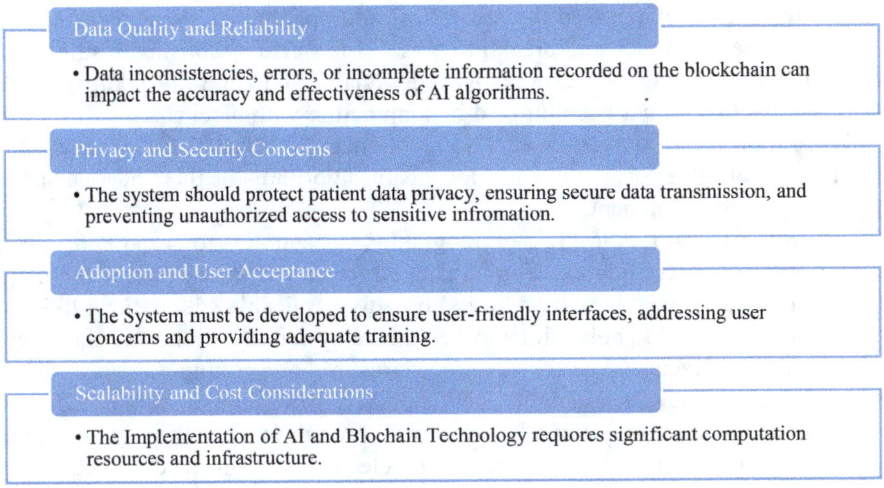

Figure 10.2 An overview of potential issues and risks of AI and blockchain integration in telehealth

10.1.2 Chapter organization

Section 10.2 includes relevant articles on the possible hazards involved with incorporating AI and blockchain technology in telehealth. Section 10.3 examines data privacy concerns in AI and blockchain integration. Section 10.4 discusses the analysis of security measures and encryption techniques. Section 10.5 presents the encryption techniques in AI and blockchain integration. Section 10.6 discusses the privacy-preserving blockchain mechanisms. The regular security audits and compliance are discussed in Section 10.7, and considerations of data protection regulations and compliance are presented in Section 10.8. Section 10.9 discusses the trust and transparency potential risk of the integration of AI and blockchain technology, while the proposed strategies for addressing identified issues and risks are presented in Section 10.10. Finally, Section 10.11 gives the conclusion with future directions.

10.2 Related work

The author in [11] described how blockchain technology has expanded at a quick speed over the previous decade. Because of its security and privacy advantages, it quickly found use in various sectors after being introduced as the foundation of cryptocurrencies like Bitcoin. Blockchain has been utilized in healthcare for several resolutions, such as protected data logging, transactions, and smart contract management. A lot of effort has gone into making blockchain intelligent, including the integration of AI to integrate the greatest qualities of both technologies.

The research encompassed the theoretical and operational elements of blockchain and AI technologies and breakthroughs. AI has also established a solid fundamental understanding of the domains individually and carefully addressed the different ways that AI has been utilized in conjunction with blockchain to drive the healthcare industry. The assessment also mentioned the issues these systems continue to confront due to the AI and blockchain algorithms at their heart and the scope of future development.

According to authors in [12], cryptography, decentralization, and consensus, assuring transaction confidence offers a data structure like blockchain technology with intrinsic safety qualities. It addresses broadly applicable solicitations like the Internet of things (IoT) applications in healthcare systems. Its inherent characteristics, such as contracts and consensus procedures, provide cutting-edge benefits in terms of data privacy, accessibility, and honesty. The authors also noted how security concerns are progressively discovered through extensive study and rapid growth. Modern medical records are stored electronically instead of old paper storage systems. However, technology's "trust-less" safety was readily misconstrued, hampering the safety distinctions between open and closed blockchains. The aforementioned benefits and drawbacks prompted the authors to conduct a thorough investigation into the application of blockchain technology. By comparing and assessing current safety measures, this study concentrated on healthcare safety challenges using modern technologies like AI-based models and blockchain. It also investigated and characterized the many safety assaults and issues associated with the use of blockchain technology in healthcare sectors.

The author in [13] emphasized how advances in AI have permitted, facilitated, and expedited the growth of telehealth. The primary goal of telehealth is to surmount difficulties caused by time or geography restrictions in the provision of high-value treatment. The ultimate objective is to distribute and simplify high-quality, high-value care rather than replace it. However, many constraints and problems, notably legislative and technological, persist. Excellent practice recommendations are an example of adapting regulations governing data interchange, reimbursement growth, and significant ethical difficulties. Critical challenges like data confidentiality, safety, and governance, bias induced by AI, the black box aspect of some AI/ML techniques, and the influence of AI technologies/techniques on health inequalities and injustices are among the latter. Variations in telehealth access and usage were always recognized, but they were emphasized during the COVID-19 epidemic. Recognizing this barrier resulted in the developing and quickly expanding subject of electronic determinants of health, which include variables such as digital competence, access to AI/technology, and community infrastructure such as WiFi/broadband Internet access.

In their chapter, Verma *et al.* [14] emphasized how telemedicine is a novel way to improve distant healthcare access via telecommunications and current information technology. This strategy has made communicating easier for patients and healthcare practitioners while providing convenience and devotion. It ensured the transmission of sensitive information and its safeguarding from one site to another. According to the authors, people in remote areas of the nation seek treatment at public health clinics (PHCs). An individual cannot manage a large group of people. India assigned one patient to a doctor in PHCs. As a result, they proposed developing an autonomous T-health monitoring framework. Actual therapy delivery always involves physical professional interaction, the degree of which changes depending on the ailment. Information and communication technologies can be used in telehealth to tackle the dilemma of need in comparison to the availability of healthcare services. An AI-based model might assist in solving this issue by developing methods that correspond to the availability of doctors with the necessary clinical knowledge to the requirement for such competence in the nearby neighborhood. AI can help to reduce these problems by facilitating human or virtual contacts and resolving obstacles like clinician availability and scheduling. AI will help to increase clinical procedure knowledge. Deep learning has been proposed to reduce difficulty and improve output accuracy in automated feature descriptions. The novel era of medical care heavily relies on applying various AI-based models that are advantageous in the field and rely on accessible data. The study is expected to aid academics in generating novel concepts for enhancing healthcare in the context of deep learning.

Clinical databases, especially those comprising large data, have significant security issues, according to Krittanawong *et al.* [15]. The accessible, dispersed, and distributed ledger known as the blockchain technology that powers cryptocurrencies safely stores transactions without requiring third-party verification. Decentralized blockchain networks provide a safe, functional route for clinical study, and practice data in healthcare. The authors highlighted current breakthroughs in blockchain technological advances, their application with AI-based models in heart attack care, and potential future approaches. They began by reviewing the fundamental underlying ideas of this technological advances and contextualizing them within the framework of existing popular apps. They next explored particular cardiovascular care and research applications like high-throughput in clinical trials, wearable sensors, and DNA sequencing. They then assessed the present barriers to effective implementation as well as potential directions. They also summarized, and they also outlined the medical applications that may be achieved by merging distributed blockchain computing platforms (for data safety) with AI computing (for data analytics). Blockchain integration could offer clinically significant projections, contribute to improving analytical methods, and offer virtual tools in clinical practice by utilizing high-performance computing and AI able to handle massive and quickly growing medical databases safely. The scientists found that combining AI and blockchain methodologies synergistically magnifies the capabilities of both methodologies, allowing for the development of fresh results to deliver accurate cardiovascular treatment.

According to Ahmad *et al.* [10], telehealth and telemedicine systems seek to provide virtual medical care services to reduce the transmission of COVID-9. They can also help with the handling of precious medical care resources hospitals have to handle the enormous number of COVID-19 casualties. But many of the telehealth and telemedicine technologies in use today are focused on meeting the needs of various patients and helping healthcare professionals. However, fail to meet offering the required safety and confidentiality, functional openness, confidentiality of health records, and tracking to detect thefts involving patients' insurance claims and medical qualification. As a result, their research looked into the prospective advantages and problems of blockchain technology in the telehealth and telemedicine industries. It investigated blockchain technology's critical role in ensuring information safety and confidentiality, operational transparency, the immutability of health data, and traceability to identify theft connected to victims' insurance claims and medical credentials. One of the issues mentioned was the security flaws of smart contracts. The authors found that blockchain technology may enhance healthcare systems generally by providing Telemedicine with relevant devices and sensors in a dependable, identifiable, decentralized, trustful, tamper-proof, and safe manner. It allowed medical practitioners to precisely recognize scams involving physician degrees and medical testing kits widely used for residence-based diagnosis. It was found that the application of blockchain in healthcare systems, in general, is in its infancy.

The author in [16] emphasized how the usage of blockchain technology in medical care is rapidly growing and has a big influence on the sector. The disparity between the medical industry and blockchain technology was examined in their study by examining prior actions. In order to determine the trend of blockchain technology in healthcare, a bibliometric study of the dispersion of datasets, places, key phrases, and references was performed. In terms of safety and confidentiality, remote care medicine data systems and e-health cases were also examined and evaluated. This research looked at possible future obstacles, such as blockchain size, database capacity, worldwide connectivity, and laws. The motives for using blockchain technology in the medical business were underlined in this study. Possibilities in health data collection and exchange, clinical studies, the drug industry, big information, AI, fifth generation (5G) ultrasonic equipment, safety, and confidentiality.

The concurrent development of numerous electronic and telecommunications technologies in 2020, according to [17], has presented an unparalleled chance for ophthalmology to adjust to novel paradigms of treatment employing telehealth backed by digital breakthroughs. AI, 5G communications networks, and the IoT are among the digital advancements that have created an interconnected ecosystem with the potential to build novel models of eye care that meet the struggles of COVID-19 and beyond. Ophthalmology has prospered in a few of these fields, partly thanks to its numerous image-based research.

Telehealth and AI offer synchronized answers to the problems that ophthalmologists and healthcare professionals face throughout the earth. This research looked at how nations throughout the earth have used electronic advancements to treat diabetic retinopathy, retinopathy of prematurity, age-related macular degeneration, glaucoma, refractive error correction, cataract, and other anterior segment problems. The research outlined nations' electronic plans and explored technology that may progressively join ophthalmologists' clinical workflows and processes.

Furthermore, when governments throughout the earth began a sequence of rising prevention and abatement efforts during the COVID-19 pandemic, global eye care service delivery has been greatly disrupted. The quick adoption of certain telemedicine and electronic invention amid the pandemic is also explored as ophthalmology services adjust and develop a "new normal." Finally, the obstacles of validation and clinical application are discussed, in addition to future options recommended.

The author in [18] examined how aging populations and an increasing number of chronic, curable illnesses are contributing to a global shortage of ophthalmic care providers. Virtual and robotic systems are guaranteed to expand the scope and capability of healthcare measures while also easing the strain on healthcare services by offering reliable, customized, quick, and economical services. However, considerable obstacles remain. In order to ensure patient safety, confidence in electronic services, data protection, medicolegal concerns, and digital exclusion, service design must be planned ahead of time. The authors investigated the effects and obstacles that patients and doctors face when incorporating AI and telemedicine into ophthalmic care and how they may shape its future trajectory. The authors also examined how technological innovations, like the emergence of AI and telemedicine, have transformed the face of the healthcare system, especially during the COVID-19 pandemic hastening the incorporation of new technologies into clinical practice. They investigated the effects and obstacles that patients and physicians face when incorporating AI and telemedicine into ophthalmic care, and how they may affect its development.

During COVID-19, author [19] presented how various academics have recently focused on novel innovations to enhance healthcare systems for the enhancement of smart healthcare workflow. Blockchain technology can fight pandemics by allowing distributed healthcare data interchange, protecting users' confidentiality, strengthening data, and allowing dependable data administration throughout epidemic control. Furthermore, AI delivers sophisticated computer-assisted solutions for efficient treatments, prospective breakout prediction, and medication production by assessing a victim's medical pictures and signs produced by coronavirus. Integrating blockchain and AI might change the present healthcare environment by democratizing and streamlining clinical operations.

The author in [20] described how, with the introduction of the "Smart Healthcare" era, a slew of innovative technology has offered fresh perspectives to severe illness treatment. For example, intelligent wearable technology encourages individuals to live better lifestyles and delivers a constant movement of medical data for illness detection and management by vigorously collecting physiological characteristics and measuring metabolic status. However, determining how to collect and analyze data to reach the definitive aim of resolving severe illness care concerning the standard of living, patient results, and confidentiality is a pressing problem that must be addressed. According to scientists, AI can deliver creative concepts for illness diagnosis and therapy by assessing a patient's physiological data via wearable devices. Furthermore, blockchain could enhance healthcare services by enabling decentralized data exchange, safeguarding user confidentiality, empowering data, and assuring data management dependability. Incorporating AI, blockchain, and wearable technology has the potential to improve existing chronic illness care approaches by shifting from a hospital-centered to a patient-centered paradigm. The authors theoretically showed a patient-centric technological architecture founded on AI, blockchain, and wearable technology in this study. Then they went on to investigate the implementation of these interconnected technologies in severe illness management. Finally, the flaws of this novel approach were examined, as well as future research options.

The author in [21] recognized and investigated some of the possible domains of the healthcare business that might profit from the utilization of blockchain technology concepts in their work. This research also aimed to examine the present implementation issues of blockchain technology in healthcare industry services. Through thorough analysis, the authors discovered the up-to-date state of blockchain use in multiple sectors of the healthcare sector. The ideal status, the knowledge gap around blockchain technology utilization in many healthcare industries, and the identification of various realistic research objectives for the future. The authors found that the technology aids in the augmentation of excellent solutions in the medical field, and many study objectives are offered to do additional studies for patient happiness and convenience.

The author in [22] described how, over the last 20 years, the advancement and adoption of more advanced linked technology has expedited the growth of telemedicine. The authors proceeded to state that in rheumatology, e-health involvements are used in a variety of ways telemedicine has various benefits, including improved availability of healthcare and individualized and continual patient tracking. According to the study, various restrictions remain to be addressed, such as data safety, constitutional issues, repayment methods, availability, and the incorporation of suggestions into tool development.

According to Hameed *et al.* [23], the Internet of Health Things (IoHT) is used in healthcare in a variety of ways. The latest IoHT incorporates health-related items such as detectors and virtually monitored medical equipment to evaluate and administer a patient's record to give the patient wiser and more efficient health diagnostics. To project and track the severity of illnesses using 5G services and blockchain technology, the authors proposed an IoT with a cloud-based system for clinical decision-making in the present study. A blockchain is a safe mechanism for keeping and disseminating information due to its openness. They propose using patient-connected medical equipment to collect patient data, which would then be stored in an Internet server along with related medical records. The use of blockchain with 5G technology enables the safe movement of patient data at a quick pace with a short reaction time. The suggested model was verified using several classifiers. To find the best classification for the dataset, the effectiveness of various algorithms was assessed by comparing the results, with an accuracy of 98.98% for the NN. Additionally, the NN was created for the dataset so that it could predict the results of the class of unstructured datasets. Contrary to other classifiers, the trained NN predicted and cleverly displayed the results with higher accuracy.

In their study, Shen *et al.* [24] discussed how the COVID-19 crisis in the year 2020 crossed with the growth and maturity of several computerized technologies such as the IoT with next-generation 5G networks, AI that utilizes deep learning, big data analytics, and blockchain and robotic technology, emanating in a new chance for the advancement of telemedicine. The authors also noted that telemedicine systems based on digital technology have been established in numerous nations. It has been incorporated into the clinical workflow using four different techniques: "many to one" mode, "one to many" mode, "consultation" mode, and "practical operation" mode. It has also demonstrated that it is feasible, valuable, and efficient for spreading epidemiological data. This enables direct links between medical professionals or patients across distances, reducing the risk of disease transmission, improving the quality of victim care, and sparing healthcare costs. The authors understood the potential advantages of signifying telemedicine in the setting of a significant health catastrophe by examining studies investigating the utilization of technological advances in telemedicine applications.

Author [25] noted the utilization of AI in healthcare contexts to analyze difficult and large data and provide outputs without man interaction is becoming more widely acknowledged. Nevertheless, this technique can potentially improve diagnostic and treatment procedures. There may be hurdles and mistakes due to numerous safety issues. The authors studied AI in healthcare and its implications for security to offer light on such potential and difficulties. This study found that secure layout, security stores, secure fail, and procedural safeguards are critical techniques for providing safer technology through AI, while expenses, dangers, and unknown should be considered for all conceivable technological systems. To build and execute safer AI technologies in the medical industry, it is also advised that comprehensive regulations and rules be created and shared with all stakeholders.

According to Chamola *et al.* [9], the shortage of assets to deal with the COVID-19 pandemic, along with the concern about overcrowded healthcare systems, has driven a large number of nations into a part or total lockdown. Countless erroneous reports, disinformation, and unwarranted coronavirus anxieties have been shared daily since the COVID-19 epidemic. Concerning such activities, the writers drew on various credible sources to thoroughly examine the important features of the COVID-19 epidemic. This study emphasized the consequence of the COVID-19 outbreak on the world's economy and immediate health concerns. The authors also looked into how COVID-19 may be lessened by using technologies like the IoT, unmanned aerial vehicles, blockchain, AI, and 5G, among others.

The author in [26] investigated and classified the positive and negative aspects of using blockchain technology in a healthcare system. PubMed, CINAHL, IEEE, Springer, and ScienceDirect databases were examined with keywords relating to blockchain, healthcare, benefits, and dangers. Eight blockchain advantages were categorized as either patient-related or organizational-related, and their threats were classified into three categories: organizational threats and technological threats. The authors concluded that blockchain is a workable technology that could improve the system for disseminating and storing healthcare data because of its distributed nature, indestructibility, transparency, and transparency. However, many healthcare firms are still hesitant to embrace blockchain technology due to difficulties like safety and permission issues, compatibility problems, and a lack of technical capabilities in blockchain technology.

The author in [27] discussed how blockchain in healthcare applications necessitates a vigorous safety and confidentiality process for excellent verification, interoperability, and medical record sharing. Blockchain technology in the healthcare business has significantly increased attention recently. This research was reviewed to significantly assess and describe the study setting of existing technologies. The study methodically examined three available databases for all relevant research publications on blockchain in healthcare applications. The final papers for evaluation were reviewed in five ways: (1) the year of release, (2) the country of origin of the authors, (3) the publisher or journal, (4) the reason for using blockchain in health systems and the accompanying contributions, and (5) the sorts of problems and offered solutions. This research also highlighted motives, open problems, and ideas for applying blockchain technology in the healthcare industry. The study added to the body of knowledge by thoroughly examining viable options and highlighting research shortcomings. As a result of a thorough discussion on the relevance of blockchain and its incorporation into different healthcare apps, researchers and developers were presented with appealing potential to continue to create decentralized healthcare applications.

According to Onik *et al.* [28], the primary problem in disseminating EHRs for patient-centered research, market analysis, medical inquiry, mining health data, and other purposes is the confidentiality of data. Handling vast amounts of data while protecting patients' confidentiality has always been a difficulty for researchers. Alternatively, blockchain technology has helped solve a few issues by offering a secure and distributed platform. However, the authors addressed how data processing, slow communication, and other issues plague present EHR administration systems and trustless collaboration in gathering data, storage, and delivery. As a result, the present concerns of healthcare data confidentiality and existing and prospective rules in this area were explored in this study. This research also includes a critique of the architecture, current difficulties, and potential reach of blockchain technology for properly managing confidentiality and medical data in the present and future. The chapter highlighted a few blockchain ideas that argued for additional study opportunities in healthcare, big data, and blockchain.

According to Thesmar *et al.* [29], combining healthcare claims data with extra datasets provides enormous and extensive sources of information. The dimensionality and intricacy of these coupled datasets might make typical statistical studies difficult to handle. Recent advances in AI have resulted in algorithms and systems that may acquire and identify intricate trends from such data. AI has previously been effectively used for such mixed datasets, with applications ranging from enhancing the insurance claim processing pipeline to minimizing estimate biases in retrospective research. Nonetheless, the writers highlighted that there is still IoT more that can be done. The discovery of intricate trends within high-dimensional datasets may lead to the discovery of novel illness start predictors or a more proactive provision of individualized preventative treatments. According to the authors, while there are dangers and obstacles involved with the deployment of AI, they are not insurmountable. As with the emergence of any new technology, we must be cautious and accountable as we progressively employ AI technologies in healthcare.

Author [30] stated that their work aimed to spark discussion about the use of cutting-edge technologies and their ability to promote the advancement of pan-Canadian monitoring and surveillance activities related to environmental impacts on health and the health system. Its main goal was to present an overview of novel technologies and their existing applications in the environment and healthcare. The chapter initially described the present applications of technologies at the interface of public health and the environment, including AI, blockchain, and the IoT. It also defined each of the aforementioned technologies, as well as a synopsis of their existing uses and a discussion of the problems that may be encountered while implementing them.

In their chapter, the author [31] discussed the possible breadth of use of AI approaches within the telehealth sector. Given observations regarding recent improvements, these strategies concentrated on clinical requirements and gave some insight into present trends. On the backbone of specialist knowledge, the authors discovered examples of telehealth developments employing AI to assist or enhance virtual healthcare delivery from recent research. The findings from the instances were combined to give a summary of current trends in the projected significance of AI in telehealth. Two important focal points for relevant current directions have been identified. The first was to raise the level of medical practice and service delivery, and the other was to create and support innovative models of care. For demonstration reasons, instances from each emphasis area have been chosen. The authors stated that widespread usage will need additional development of underpinning algorithms and technique validation. As AI-enabled telehealth spreads, several critical social and moral problems must be tackled more broadly in the health system.

According to Rabah [32], blockchain automated data authentication abilities, specifically, can resolve many of the trust challenges associated with obtaining data from diverse sources. Applications of the technology in healthcare showed potential for addressing difficulties such as data dissemination in EHR and countrywide interoperability. The application of blockchain in healthcare is projected to reshape the ecosystem in infinite ways, benefiting patients and advancing procedures, results, safety, and prices. Therefore, by placing patients at the center of medical environments and enhancing the safety and scalability of healthcare data, blockchain technology has the potential to transform the provision of healthcare services. This technology is projected to create a new paradigm for health information exchanges by improving electronic medical data's efficiency, disintermediation, and security. One of blockchain technology's main characteristics that makes it an obvious choice for supply chains across sectors is its unchanging, time-stamped, tamper-proof record available to all or preapproved parties. The authors of this article walk through how blockchain might help with patient care management efficiency, safety, and confidentiality.

The above literature review gives adequate works in the area of blockchain and AI in the medical section. Therefore, there is a need to summarize the related work to identify various literature gaps and give future research direction. Section 10.2.1 presents the summary of related works in a tabular form.

10.2.1 Summary of related works

Table 10.1 gives the summary of related works stating the methodology, result, and gap or future direction of the literature reviewed.

Table 10.1 Related work

Author	Methodology	Result	Gap/future direction
Kumar [33]	AI and blockchain were both employed	Great work has been carried out to make blockchain smart, with artificial intelligence (AI) integration to integrate the most advantageous aspects of the two technologies	There are challenges still encountered by the systems that they acquire from the AI and blockchain algorithms that power them
Wenhua [12]	Blockchain technology was employed	Blockchain technology provided without third-party assurances, a decentralized solution to trustless situations between distrusting parties is proposed	Different security attacks and challenges when applying blockchain technology were identified to be handled in research work
Verma *et al.* [14]	A deep learning framework was employed	The framework aided in the accessibility and planning of clinicians. AI has also helped to increase clinical process knowledge	The security of the system was not ascertained
Ahmad *et al.* [10]	Blockchain technology was employed	Blockchain technology improved telehealth and telemedicine services	One of the challenges was the safety vulnerabilities of smart contracts
Xie *et al.* [20]	AI, blockchain, and wearable technologies were used to create a patient-centric technological framework	Current chronic illness treatment approaches were improved by shifting from a hospital-centered to a patient-centered one	There were shortcomings to the new paradigm
Krittanawong *et al.* [15]	Blockchain and AI were both employed	The combination of AI and blockchain methodologies increased the capabilities of both technologies, resulting in unique solutions to	The limitation(s) were not stated

(Continues)

Table 10.1 (*Continued*)

Author	Methodology	Result	Gap/future direction
		the goal of delivering precision cardiovascular treatment	
Hussien *et al.* [16]	Blockchain was employed	The motivations for employing blockchain technology in the healthcare industry were highlighted	Future issues might include storage space and flexibility, blockchain size, global interoperability, and standardization
Ramessur *et al.* [18]	The authors explored the impact and challenges facing patients and clinicians in integrating AI and telemedicine into ophthalmic care—and how they could affect its course	Technological advances revolutionized the face of healthcare through the rise of artificial intelligence (AI) and telemedicine	There were impacts and challenges facing patients and clinicians in integrating AI and telemedicine into ophthalmic care
Jabarulla and Lee [19]	A decentralized, patient-centric healthcare framework based on blockchain and AI to mitigate COVID-19 challenges was proposed	Significant applications of integrated blockchain and AI technologies to augment existing public healthcare strategies for tackling COVID-19 were gotten	Challenges and implications for future research within a patient-centric paradigm were identified
Aithal *et al.* [21]	Blockchain technology was employed	Blockchain technology facilitates the improvement of quality services in the healthcare sector	Challenges of blockchain technology in healthcare industry services were identified
Song *et al.*, [22]	Neither blockchain nor AI was employed in telemedicine for rheumatology	Telemedicine offered several advantages, in specific by enabling admission to healthcare and providing personalized and continuous patient monitoring	Limitations such as data safety, legal challenges, repayment method, accessibility, as well as the application of recommendations in the development of the tools were identified
Hameed *et al.* [23]	Blockchain and 5G technology and neural network classifier were employed	The proposed model was validated by employing different classifiers. The efficiency of several classifiers was evaluated by examining the values to determine the optimal classifier for the dataset. The	The security of the system was not ascertained

(*Continues*)

Table 10.1 (Continued)

Author	Methodology	Result	Gap/future direction
		accuracy of the NN classifier was 98.98%	
Onik *et al.* [28]	Blockchain technology was employed	The work presented a few blockchain solutions that were recommended for upcoming blockchain, big data, and healthcare research possibilities	AI was not incorporated into the systems
Kuziemsky *et al.* [31]	AI was employed	The applicability of AI to telehealth was positive	Further developments of underlying algorithms and verification of methods will be necessary for widespread use
Thesmar *et al.* [29]	AI was employed	AI has already been applied successfully to such integrated datasets, with applications ranging from enhancing the insurance claim processing pipeline to minimizing estimating flaws in past research	There are hazards and obstacles involved with the usage of artificial intelligence

10.3 Examination of data privacy concerns in AI and blockchain integration

Both telemedicine practitioners and patients are concerned about data safety [34]. External invasion of personal medical data is a problem that cannot be avoided in platforms where medical data are housed on or sent from an Internet-accessible computer [34]. Although there are techniques to limit this danger, it will continue to be an issue until intriguing innovations are developed [34]. Hackers' cybersecurity danger has long been known to the media. However, as telemedicine application grows, so do worries about data safety and privacy.

Ongoing spikes in security intrusions and digital monitoring underline the need for increased confidentiality and safety, especially concerning users' personal information [35]. Data privacy is a crucial barrier to further advancement of machine learning and AI breakthroughs [36]. Data confidentiality generally means that the data should only be used or exploited for authorized reasons. Data confidentiality is the ability of people to influence how their data is gathered and utilized [37]. Data confidentiality or information protection is a subset of data safety that deals with data management following permission, notification, and regulatory obligations. If data is utilized for purposes that were not intended, we might claim there has been a breach of privacy or an infringement of data confidentiality [38]. So, how can the primary impediment posed by data privacy be overcome? This is where blockchain and AI will come into play to secure data privacy while not hindering data analysis efficiency.

Blockchain and distributed ledger technologies can secure user data in novel ways via distributed authentication and other confidentiality measures [39]. Such platforms may offer users more freedom by giving them access to resources that let them control and own their data. AI creates new opportunities to augment datasets, strengthen platforms and user safety, and allow better analytical models [40].

In the current era of information, AI and blockchain technologies are increasingly being applied across various domains, with data security and privacy protection emerging as pressing issues to be addressed [33]. Blockchain technology is a new distributed ledger technology that employs consensus algorithms, such as proof of stake [41], to maintain on-chain data and encrypt transaction data through cryptography. Despite its transparency and openness, the exposure of sensitive data on the blockchain poses challenges to data confidentiality and safety [42]. Various data protection technologies, such as zero-knowledge proof (ZKP), ring signature, homomorphic encryption, and secure multiparty computing, have been suggested to enhance data privacy in the blockchain [43]. Among them, homomorphic encryption can be applied to data. However, ZKP and ring signatures are limited to user anonymity rather than data confidentiality.

For AI, the process of training models is contingent upon the availability of data, which serves as the fundamental basis for contemporary deep learning [44]. In certain domains, the data under analysis may contain confidential personal information, such as medical prescription data [45]. Among the challenges posed by AI is ensuring the prevention of personal data leakage. Privacy data encompass various types of information, such as personal assets, medical records, and behavioral patterns. The potential harm to users resulting from the exploitation of their private data by malicious actors has garnered the interest of scholars in both academic and industrial settings [46]. Machine learning commonly employs various privacy protection techniques, such as secure multiparty computation and homomorphic encryption. Some of the highlights of the data privacy concerns in integrating AI and blockchain into telehealth are discussed below.

10.3.1 Patient confidentiality

AI algorithms and blockchain ledgers store and process sensitive patient data, such as medical records and personal information [47]. Ensuring patient confidentiality becomes crucial to prevent unauthorized access and protect patient privacy [48]. This is truer than ever in this age of fast-evolving information technology. The interests of the patient and the practitioner are served by patient privacy. It protects patient data from being misused. It is also at the highest advantage of physicians. Both confidentiality and data security bring significant societal advantages. The major reason for safeguarding personal confidentiality is to defend persons' interests [49]. However, it is crucial to underline that secrecy has societal value since it enables challenging activities to be carried out in a way that protects people's dignity, such as studies and public health chores. Additionally, health research may benefit people by making it easier for them to get a grasp on cutting-edge treatments, improved testing, and more effective ways to stay healthy and get care. However, encryption techniques and access controls must be implemented to safeguard patient data [50].

10.3.2 Identity protection

Blockchain's immutable nature may pose challenges in protecting patient identities [12]. Public blockchain networks can expose patient identities when transactional data are linked to personally identifiable information. Privacy-enhancing technologies like ZKPs or private/permission blockchains can address this concern [50].

10.3.3 Consent management

Integrating AI and blockchain introduces complexities in managing patient consent [51]. Patients ought to have access to their data, including the option to provide and rescind consent. Smart contracts on blockchain can facilitate transparent and auditable consent management [52].

10.3.4 Data breaches

AI and blockchain systems are not immune to data breaches, and healthcare consequences can be severe. Robust security measures, including encryption, data anonymization, and intrusion detection, are necessary to mitigate the risk of breaches [12].

10.3.5 Data ownership and control

Blockchain's decentralized nature challenges traditional data ownership models. Patients, healthcare providers, and other stakeholders need clarity on who owns and controls the data. Governance frameworks and smart contracts can define data ownership and access rights [53].

10.4 Analysis of security measures and encryption techniques

The incorporation of AI and blockchain technology in telehealth offers numerous advantages but raises concerns regarding data security and privacy. The following focuses on analyzing the security measures and encryption techniques used in the integration of AI and blockchain in telehealth to ensure data protection.

10.4.1 Security measures in AI and blockchain integration

10.4.1.1 Access controls

Access control describes the process of regulating who can access or use resources within a computing environment. It is a safety concept used by companies to reduce risks by restricting entry to a resource or location (The Importance of Access Control Systems in Healthcare Organizations, 2022). Implementing robust access controls ensures that only approved individuals can gain entry to sensitive healthcare data. Role-based access control (RBAC) restricts network access based on the functions of individuals within an organization. RBAC and multifactor authentication can be employed to strengthen access management.

10.4.1.2 Secure data transmission

Encryption protocols, such as Transport Layer Security, safeguard data during transmission among AI systems, blockchain nodes, and telehealth platforms [44]. Secure communication channels prevent unauthorized interception and tampering of data.

10.4.1.3 Intrusion detection and prevention

Intrusion detection systems (IDSs) and intrusion prevention systems evaluate network activity and detect potential security breaches. Real-time threat detection and response mechanisms help prevent unauthorized access and protect sensitive data.

10.4.1.4 Secure application development

Following secure coding practices and conducting regular security audits ensure that AI and blockchain applications are free from vulnerabilities. Regular software updates and patches mitigate the risk of exploitation by malicious actors.

10.5 Encryption techniques in AI and blockchain integration

Here, the encryption techniques in AI and blockchain integration these include end-to-end encryption, homomorphic encryption, and encrypting data at rest.

10.5.1 End-to-end encryption

End-to-end encryption protects data throughout its lifecycle, ensuring confidentiality between sender and recipient. This technique prevents unauthorized access to sensitive healthcare information, even if intercepted during transmission [54].

10.5.2 Homomorphic encryption

Homomorphic encryption enables the processing of encrypted material without decoding it [55]. This technique enables privacy-preserving AI analysis on encrypted healthcare data, ensuring data confidentiality.

10.5.3 Data encryption at rest

Encrypting data at rest, such as storing medical records on the blockchain or AI systems, prevents unauthorized access in case of breaches. Strong encryption algorithms, like Advanced Encryption Standard, protect data integrity and confidentiality [56].

10.5.4 Differential privacy

Differential privacy techniques add noise or randomness to aggregated data to protect individual privacy. Privacy-preserving AI algorithms, such as federated learning or secure multiparty computation, ensure privacy without compromising data utility [57].

10.6 Privacy-preserving blockchain mechanisms

10.6.1 Private/permissioned blockchains

Private or permission blockchains limit participation to trusted entities, enhancing data privacy. Access controls and consensus mechanisms within the blockchain ensure the confidentiality and integrity of healthcare data [58].

10.6.2 Off-chain data storage

Storing sensitive healthcare data off-chain and utilizing blockchain for data references or proofs ensures data privacy. Hashing or encryption techniques can be used to maintain data integrity and privacy while maintaining a verifiable record on the blockchain [59].

10.6.3 Zero-knowledge proofs

ZKPs allow verification of information without revealing the underlying data, ensuring privacy. ZKPs can be used to authenticate identities or validate transactions without exposing sensitive healthcare information [60].

10.7 Regular security audits and compliance

10.7.1 Penetration testing

Regular penetration testing identifies vulnerabilities and weaknesses in AI and blockchain systems [61]. This proactive approach helps address security issues before they are exploited.

10.7.2 Compliance with regulatory standards

Adhering to healthcare data protection regulations, such as the Health Insurance Portability and Accountability Act (HIPAA), ensures compliance and safeguards Top of Form.

10.8 Consideration of data protection regulations and compliance

The incorporation of AI and blockchain technology in telehealth systems brings significant benefits but requires careful consideration of data protection regulations and compliance. This section examines the key aspects and considerations related to data protection regulations and compliance when integrating AI and blockchain in telehealth systems.

10.8.1 Understanding data protection regulations

10.8.1.1 General data protection regulation

General data protection regulation (GDPR) defines rules for the processing and protection of private data within the European Union and the European Economic Area. Compliance involves obtaining explicit user consent, ensuring data minimization, providing data subject rights, and implementing appropriate security measures.

10.8.1.2 Health Insurance Portability and Accountability Act

HIPAA regulates the use, disclosure, and safeguarding of protected health information (PHI) in the United States [62]. Compliance includes ensuring the privacy, credibility, and accessibility of PHI, as well as the implementation of administrative, physical, and technical measures and adherence to privacy standards.

10.8.2 Key considerations for compliance in AI and blockchain integration

10.8.2.1 Consent management

Consent plays a vital role in data processing. Telehealth systems must ensure transparent and informed consent from patients for data collection, storage, and analysis. Consent management mechanisms should be implemented, allowing users to provide, modify, or withdraw consent as per regulatory requirements.

10.8.2.2 Data minimization

Adhering to the principle of data minimization helps limit personal data gathering and archiving to what is necessary for the intended purpose. Telehealth systems should assess and minimize the amount of personal data stored, reducing the risk associated with data breaches or misuse [63].

10.8.2.3 Security measures

Implementing appropriate security measures is crucial for compliance with data protection regulations. This includes encryption of sensitive data, access controls, regular security audits, IDSs, and incident response plans.

10.8.2.4 Anonymization and pseudonymization

Anonymizing or pseudonymizing patient data reduces the risk of reidentification and enhances privacy. AI and blockchain systems should employ differential privacy, tokenization, or hashing techniques to protect patient identities [64].

10.8.2.5 Data transfers and international compliance

Transferring personal data across borders may require additional safeguards and compliance with specific regulations. Telehealth systems should assess the necessity of cross-border data transfers and ensure compliance with relevant regulations, such as the EU–US Privacy Shield or Standard Contractual Clauses.

10.8.2.6 Data breach response and notification

Establishing incident response protocols and notification procedures is essential to comply with data breach requirements. Telehealth systems should have plans in place to promptly detect, respond to, and notify individuals and regulatory authorities in case of a data breach.

10.9 Trust and transparency potential risk of integration of AI and blockchain technology

The incorporation of AI and blockchain in telehealth systems presents unique challenges related to trust and transparency [64]. Trust is crucial in healthcare settings, and the use of emerging technologies can raise concerns among patients, healthcare professionals, and other stakeholders. The challenges related to trust and transparency are listed around each technology circle as displayed in Figure 10.3.

Data privacy and security: Trust is closely linked to the confidentiality and safety of patient data. When AI algorithms and patient health data are saved on a blockchain, ensuring the data's confidentiality, integrity, and availability becomes

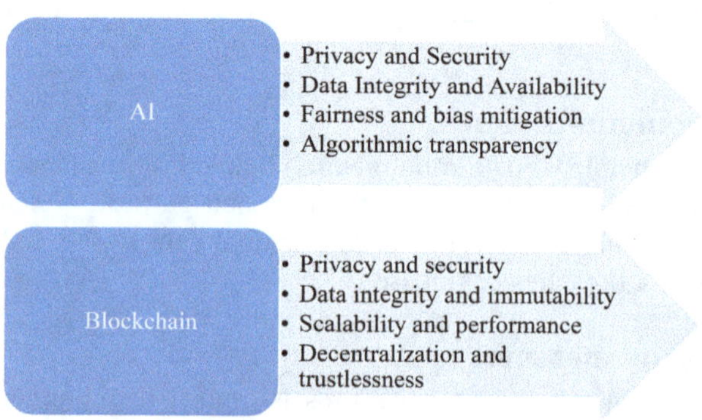

Figure 10.3 Challenges of AI and blockchain trust and transparency in telehealth

Table 10.2 Data privacy and security challenges

Challenges	Description
Confidentiality	Protecting patient data from unauthorized and maintaining privacy
Data integrity	Ensuring the accuracy and consistency of patient data stored on the blockchain
Data availability	Ensuring that patient data is accessible to authorized entities when needed

Table 10.3 Algorithmic transparency challenges

Challenges	Description
Explainability	Ensuring that AI algorithms used in telehealth systems are explainable and understandable to healthcare professionals and patients
Interpretability	Providing insights into how AI algorithms arrive at specific outcomes or recommendations
Fairness and bias	Mitigating biases in AI algorithms to guarantee just and equal results for all patient categories

paramount. Blockchain's distributed nature and cryptographic techniques can enhance security, but concerns may arise regarding unauthorized access, data breaches, or vulnerabilities in the technology. Demonstrating robust privacy measures, implementing encryption protocols, and complying with data protection regulations can help establish trust. Table 10.2 displays the challenges of data privacy and security with a description.

Algorithmic transparency: AI algorithms in telehealth systems require transparency to foster trust [65]. Healthcare professionals and patients need to understand how algorithms make decisions and the factors influencing those decisions. However, some AI algorithms, such as deep learning models, can be considered "black boxes" as their decision-making processes are complex and not easily explainable. Efforts to develop explainable AI (XAI) techniques and methods to interpret and explain AI algorithms can enhance transparency and build trust. Table 10.3 displays the algorithmic transparency challenges.

1. Bias and fairness: Inadvertent biases in training data can be perpetuated by AI systems, potentially leading to discriminatory consequences in healthcare. Bias can arise due to skewed data, underrepresenting certain groups, or inherent biases in the algorithms [66]. Fairness and mitigating bias require transparency in the data collection process, algorithm design, and ongoing monitoring [67]. Transparency reports and audits can help address concerns about bias and demonstrate a commitment to fairness.
2. Trust in decentralized systems: Blockchain technology is built on the principles of decentralization and trustlessness [68]. While this enhances security and

immutability, it may also challenge trust in traditional healthcare settings where centralized authorities and governance structures are the norm. Building trust in decentralized systems involves educating stakeholders about the benefits, security measures, and consensus mechanisms of blockchain. Clear communication and demonstrating the advantages of decentralization can help overcome initial skepticism.

3. Stakeholder engagement and inclusion: Engaging stakeholders, including healthcare professionals, patients, policymakers, and regulatory bodies, is essential for building trust and ensuring transparency. Including stakeholders during the selection procedure, soliciting feedback, and addressing their concerns can foster a sense of ownership and trust in the integration of AI and blockchain [69]. Transparent communication about the objectives, benefits, risks, and safeguards associated with the technologies is critical to maintaining trust.
4. Ethical considerations: Trust is closely tied to legitimate considerations in the utilization of AI and blockchain in telehealth. Ethical frameworks, guidelines, and codes of conduct can provide a basis for ensuring transparent and responsible use of these technologies [70]. Clearly articulating ethical principles, addressing potential conflicts of interest, and incorporating ethical considerations into the design and implementation of AI and blockchain systems can help build trust and ensure transparency. Figure 10.3 displays the challenges of AI and blockchain trust and transparency in telehealth.

10.9.1 Evaluation of blockchain governance models in telehealth

Blockchain technology holds immense potential for revolutionizing the healthcare industry, particularly in the domain of telehealth [71]. Evaluating different blockchain governance models in telehealth becomes crucial to ensure the successful integration of blockchain in telehealth systems. The various factors include decision-making processes, consensus mechanisms, participation levels, and scalability. Table 10.4 shows the evaluation models.

Several factors should be considered when evaluating blockchain governance models for telehealth systems. Table 10.5 displays the evaluation description of the blockchain governance model.

10.9.2 Mechanisms for auditing and verifying AI algorithms for telehealth systems

AI has gained significant attention and adoption in the healthcare industry, particularly in telehealth systems [72]. These systems leverage AI algorithms to analyze patient data, provide diagnoses, offer treatment recommendations, and facilitate remote monitoring [73]. However, as AI algorithms become more complex and critical in healthcare decision-making, ensuring transparency, fairness, and reliability becomes crucial. Table 10.6 provides the mechanism for auditing AI algorithms in telehealth systems.

Table 10.4 Blockchain evaluation governance models

Governance model	Decision-making	Consensus mechanism	Participation	Scalability
Centralized	Controlled by a single entity	Typically relies on a trusted third-party consensus	Limited to the controlling entity	Limited scalability due to reliance on a central authority
Consortium	Joint decision-making among consortium members	Consensus mechanism vary	Limited to consortium members	Scalability depends on the consensus mechanism and network design
Decentralized	Decisions made through community consensus mechanisms	The consensus mechanism enables trust and agreement among participant	Open participation to any network participant	Scalability can be challenging due to the need for consensus among all participants

Table 10.5 Evaluation factors of the blockchain model

Evaluation	Description
Security	Assess the security measures and protocols employed by each governance model to assure the privacy, honesty, and accessibility of patient data
Privacy	Evaluate the governance model approaches to data privacy and compliance with relevant regulations to protect patient information
Transparency	Examine the transparency mechanism in place, including the visibility of decision-making processes and accountability of participants
Flexibility and innovation	Consider the governance models' ability to adapt to evolving telehealth needs and integrate new technologies or features
Stakeholder engagement	Evaluate the models' inclusiveness, stakeholder involvement, and mechanisms for addressing concerns and feedback from healthcare professionals, patients, and regulators

Table 10.6 AI algorithm mechanism for telehealth systems

Mechanism	Description
Transparency	Assessing the algorithm's transparency and explainability
Algorithmic bias	Identifying and mitigating bias in the algorithm's decision-making
Privacy and security	Ensuring compliance with privacy regulations and data security measures
Data integrity	Validating the integrity and quality of data used by the algorithm

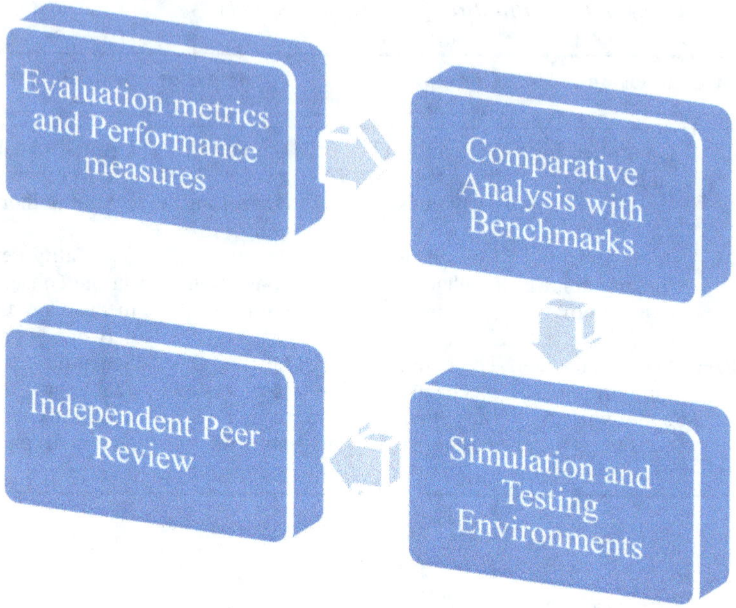

Figure 10.4 Framework for verifying AI algorithms in telehealth systems

The table above outlines the mechanisms for auditing AI algorithms in telehealth systems, including transparency, algorithmic bias, privacy and security, and data integrity. Each mechanism represents an area of focus when conducting audits of AI algorithms to ensure their trustworthiness and compliance. Figure 10.4 depicts a framework for verifying AI algorithms in telehealth systems.

The framework illustrates the various components involved in the verification process, such as evaluation metrics and performance measures, comparative analysis with benchmarks, simulation and testing environments, and independent peer review.

10.9.3 Components of potential risks of integration of AI and blockchain in telehealth systems

The integration framework components include data collection, data privacy, AI algorithms, smart contracts, interoperability, governance, scalability, and continuous monitoring. The table below shows the components of integration. Table 10.7 displays the components of potential risks of AI and blockchain.

The risks associated with AI and blockchain integration in telehealth systems are categorized into five main areas: privacy and security, ethical and legal, technical, governance, and adoption and user acceptance. Figure 10.5

Table 10.7 Potential risks of AI and blockchain integration

Component	Description
Data collection	Collecting patient data from various sources, including wearables and electronic health record systems
Data privacy	Ensuring confidentiality and compliance with privacy regulations
AI algorithms	Developing and implementing AI algorithms for analysis and decision-making
Smart contracts	Utilizing smart contracts for automation and execution of predefined rules
Interoperability	Enabling seamless data exchange between different systems and stakeholders
Governance	Establishing governance mechanisms and regulatory compliance
Scalability	Addressing scalability challenges to handle large volumes of data
Continuous monitoring	Monitoring and evaluating system performance and making improvements

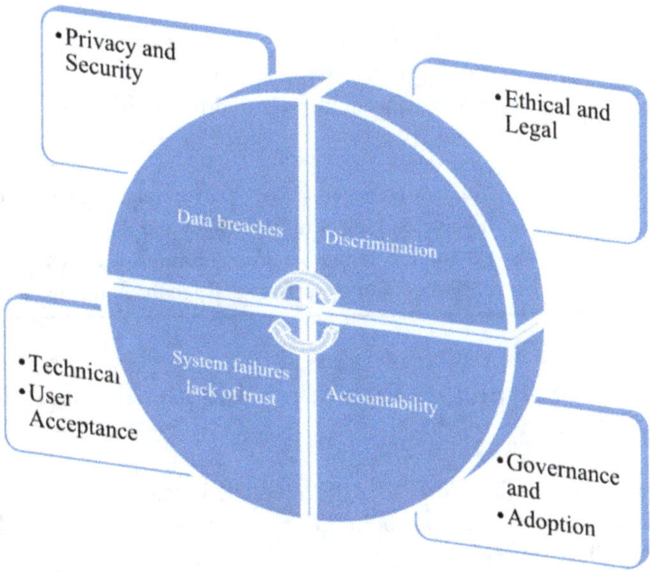

Figure 10.5 Potential risk of AI and blockchain integration in telehealth

displays the potential risk of the integration of AI and blockchain in telehealth systems.

The figure represents the risks of AI and Blockchain integration in telehealth systems. It illustrates the different risk categories and their interconnectedness within the integration framework.

Table 10.8 Proposed strategies for addressing issues and risks

Risk category	Proposed strategies
Privacy and security	• Implement robust data encryption techniques • Utilize secure access control mechanisms • Update and repair security flaws regularly • Perform security reviews and penetration tests • Comply with privacy regulations and adopt privacy-enhancing technologies
Ethical and legal	• Implement transparent and unbiased AI algorithms • Conduct regular audits and assessments for algorithmic biases • Establish guidelines for ethical issues and decision-making • Stay informed about legal and regulatory requirements
Technical	• Test and validate AI algorithms for accuracy and reliability • Implement fail-safe mechanisms and redundancy systems • Establish interoperability standards and protocols • Continuously monitor system performance and address technical issues
Governance	• Establish a clear governance framework • Promote transparency and accountability • Involve stakeholders from different domains • Regularly review and update governance policies and procedures
Adoption and user acceptance	• Conduct comprehensive user training and education programs • Involve end-users in the design and development process • Communicate the benefits and improvements in patient care • Provide ongoing support and feedback mechanisms

10.10 Proposed strategies for addressing identified issues and risks

The proposed strategies for addressing the identified issues and risks are categorized based on the risk categories, including privacy and security to adoption and user acceptance. The strategies are outlined in Table 10.8 for the specific solutions that may be put in place to reduce the hazards connected with integrating AI and blockchain technology in telehealth systems.

10.11 Conclusions and future scope

The integration of AI and blockchain technology in telehealth systems holds significant promise for enhancing healthcare delivery and improving patient outcomes. It does, however, introduce significant hazards that must be properly addressed to guarantee the safe and appropriate adoption of new technologies. The potential risks identified in this chapter include privacy and security risks that require robust measures to protect patient information. Ethical and legal risks call for unbiased and transparent AI algorithms and adherence to relevant regulations. Technical risks demand accurate algorithms, reliable systems, and interoperability. Governance risks necessitate clear frameworks and accountability mechanisms. Finally, adoption and user acceptance risks require targeted user training and education to build trust and overcome resistance.

Stakeholders must implement strategies and mechanisms to mitigate these risks, ensuring the safe and responsible integration of AI and blockchain in telehealth systems. Regular monitoring, evaluation, and continuous improvement are essential to address emerging risks and maintain the integrity of these integrated systems. Ultimately, by proactively addressing the potential risks, the integration of AI and blockchain in telehealth systems can realize its full potential in revolutionizing healthcare delivery, improving patient care, and advancing the field of medicine.

This chapter contributes to identifying and categorizing potential hazards connected with the incorporation of AI and blockchain in telehealth systems. The study also contributes to proposing strategies for addressing the identified risks and providing valuable insights into how healthcare stakeholders can mitigate the potential challenges.

The future study of this chapter should conduct a longitudinal study to track the risks and their evolution over time as AI and blockchain technologies advance and become more prevalent in telehealth systems. Future studies can also perform quantitative risk assessments to evaluate the likelihood and impact of different risks associated with AI and blockchain integration. Finally, future studies can explore innovative mechanisms and technologies to enhance trust and transparency in AI and blockchain integration and investigate the role of explainability, interpretability, and auditing mechanisms in building trust and addressing concerns related to algorithmic decisions and data integrity.

Acknowledgment

The authors appreciate the chapter editor for the privilege to contribute to this book.

References

[1] Romanovs, A., Sultanovs, E., Buss, E., Merkuryev, Y., and Majore, G. (2021, April). Challenges and solutions for resilient telemedicine services. In *2020 IEEE 8th Workshop on Advances in Information, Electronic and Electrical Engineering (AIEEE)* (pp. 1–7). IEEE.

[2] Leite, H., Hodgkinson, I. R., and Gruber, T. (2020). New development: 'Healing at a distance'—telemedicine and COVID-19. *Public Money & Manage*. 40(6):483–485. doi:10.1080/09540962.2020.1748855.

[3] Imoize, A. L., Gbadega, P. A., Obakhena, H. I., Irabor, D. O., Kavitha, K. V. N., and Chakraborty, C. (2022). Artificial Intelligence-enabled Internet of Medical

Things for COVID-19 pandemic data management. *Explainable Artificial Intelligence in Medical Decision Support Systems*, 357–380.

[4] Vidal-Alaball, J., Acosta-Roja, R., Pastor, N., *et al.* (2020). Telemedicine in the face of the COVID-19 pandemic. *Atención Primaria.* 52(6):418–422. doi:10.1016/j.aprim.2020.04.003.

[5] Wright, J. H., and Caudill, R. (2020). Remote treatment delivery in response to the COVID-19 pandemic. *Psychother Psychosom.* 89(3):1. doi:10.1159/000507376.

[6] Awotunde, J. B., Imoize, A. L., Ayoade, O. B., *et al.* (2022). An enhanced hyper-parameter optimization of a convolutional neural network model for leukemia cancer diagnosis in a smart healthcare system. *Sensors*, 22(24), 9689.

[7] Ramasamy, L. K., KP, F. K., Imoize, A. L., Ogbebor, J. O., Kadry, S., and Rho, S. (2021). Blockchain-based wireless sensor networks for malicious node detection: A survey. *IEEE Access*, 9, 128765–128785.

[8] Ayoade, O. B., Oladele, T. O., Imoize, A. L., *et al.* (2022). Explainable artificial intelligence (XAI) in medical decision systems (MDSSs): Healthcare systems perspective. The Institute of Engineering Technology (IET).

[9] Chamola, V., Hassija, V., Gupta, V., and Guizani, M. (2020). A comprehensive review of the COVID-19 pandemic and the role of IoT, drones, AI, blockchain, and 5G in managing its impact. *IEEE Access*, 8, 90225–90265, doi:10.1109/ACCESS.2020.2992341.

[10] Ahmad, R. W., Salah, K., Jayaraman, R., Yaqoob, I., Ellahham, S., and Omar, M. (2021). The role of blockchain technology in telehealth and telemedicine. *International Journal of Medical Informatics*, 148, doi:10.1016/j.ijmedinf.2021.104399.

[11] Yaqoob, I., Salah, K., Jayaraman, R., and Al-Hammadi, Y. (2022). Blockchain for healthcare data management: Opportunities, challenges, and future recommendations. *Neural Computing and Applications*, 34, 11475–11490. https://doi.org/10.1007/s00521-020-05519-w

[12] Wenhua, Z., Qamar, F., Abdali, T.-A.N., Hassan, R., Jafri, S.T.A., and Nguyen, Q. N. (2023). Blockchain technology: Security issues, healthcare applications, challenges and future trends. *Electronics (Switzerland).* 12(3).

[13] Efstathia, A. (2023). The rise of AI in telehealth. *Emerging Practices in Telehealth*, 183–207, https://doi.org/10.1016/B978-0-443-15980-0.00011-9.

[14] Verma, S., Malviya, R., Alam, M. A., and Tripathi, B. D. (2022). *Tele-Health Monitoring Using Artificial Intelligence Deep Learning Framework.* Wiley Online Library. https://doi.org/10.1002/9781119857983.ch7

[15] Krittanawong, C., Aydar, M., Virk, H. U. H., *et al.* (2022). Artificial intelligence-powered blockchains for cardiovascular medicine. *Canadian Journal of Cardiology*, 38(2), 185–195, https://doi.org/10.1016/j.cjca.2021.11.011.

[16] Hussien, H. M., Yasin, S. M., Udzir, N. I., Ninggal, M. I. H., and Salman, S. (2021). Blockchain technology in the healthcare industry: Trends and

opportunities. *Journal of Industrial Information Integration,* 22. https://doi.org/10.1016/j.jii.2021.100217.

[17] Ting, D. S. W. (2021). Digital technology, telemedicine and artificial intelligence in ophthalmology: A global perspective. *Progress in Retinal and Eye Research,* 82, https://doi.org/10.1016/j.preteyeres.2020.100900.

[18] Ramessur, R. B. M, Laxmi, R., Kilduff, C. L. S., *et al.* (2021). Impact and challenges of integrating artificial intelligence and telemedicine into clinical ophthalmology. *Asia-Pacific Journal of Ophthalmology*, 10(3), 317–327, DOI:10.1097/APO.0000000000000406

[19] Jabarulla, M. Y. and Lee, H.-N. (2021). A blockchain and artificial intelligence-based, patient-centric healthcare system for combating the COVID-19 pandemic: Opportunities and applications. *Healthcare*, 9(1019). https://doi.org/10.3390/healthcare9081019

[20] Xie, Y., Lu, L., Gao, F., *et al.* (2021). Integration of artificial intelligence, blockchain, and wearable technology for chronic disease management: A new paradigm in smart healthcare. *Current Medical Science*, 41, 1123–1133. https://doi.org/10.1007/s11596-021-2485-0

[21] Aithal, P. S., Aithal, A. and Dias, E. (2021). Blockchain technology – Current status and future research opportunities in various areas of healthcare industry. *International Journal of Health Sciences and Pharmacy (IJHSP)*, ISSN: 2581-6411, 5(1).

[22] Song, Y., Bernard, L., Jorgensen, C., Dusfour, G. and Pers, Y. (2021). The challenges of telemedicine in rheumatology. *Frontiers in Medicine, Sec. Rheumatology*, 8, https://doi.org/10.3389/fmed.2021.746219

[23] Hameed, K., Bajwa, I. S., Sarwar, N., Anwar, W., Mushtaq, Z., and Rashid, T. (2021). Integration of 5G and blockchain technologies in smart telemedicine using IoT. *Journal of Healthcare Engineering*, 2021, Article ID8814364, 1–18. https://doi.org/10.1155/2021/8814364

[24] Shen, Y., Chen, L., Yue, W., and Xu, H. (2021). Digital Technology-Based Telemedicine for the COVID-19 Pandemic. Frontiers in Medicine.

[25] Ellahham, S., Ellahham, N., and Simsekler, M. C. E. (2020). Application of artificial intelligence in the health care safety context: Opportunities and challenges. *American Journal of Medical Quality,* 35(4), 341–348. doi:10.1177/1062860619878515

[26] Abu-elezz, I., Hassan, A., Nazeemudeen, A., Househ, M., and Abd-alrazaq, A. (2020). The benefits and threats of blockchain technology in healthcare: A scoping review. *International Journal of Medical Informatics*, 142, https://doi.org/10.1016/j.ijmedinf.2020.104246.

[27] Hussien, H. M., Yasin, S. M., Udzir, S. N. I., Zaidan, A. A., and Zaidan, B. B. (2019). A systematic review for enabling of develop a blockchain technology in healthcare application: Taxonomy, substantially analysis, motivations, challenges, recommendations, and future direction. *Journal of Medical Systems*. 43(10) DOI: 10.1007/s10916-019-1445-8.

[28] Onik, M. H., Aich, S., Yang, J., Kim, C., and Kim, H. (2019). Blockchain in healthcare: Challenges and solutions. In *Advances in ubiquitous sensing*

applications for healthcare, Big Data Analytics for Intelligent Healthcare Management. pp. 197–226. https://doi.org/10.1016/B978-0-12-818146-1.00008-8.

[29] Thesmar, D., Sraer, D., Pinheiro, L., Dadson, N., Veliche, R., and Greenberg P. (2019). Combining the power of artificial intelligence with the richness of healthcare claims data: Opportunities and challenges. *PharmacoEconomics*. 10.1007/s40273-019-00777-6

[30] Bublitz, M. F., Oetomo, A., Sahu, K. S., *et al.* (2019). Disruptive technologies for environment and health research: An overview of artificial intelligence, blockchain, and internet of things. *International Journal of Environmental Research and Public Health,* 16(3847). https://doi.org/10.3390/ijerph16203847

[31] Kuziemsky, C., Maeder, A. J., John, O., *et al.* (2019). Role of artificial intelligence within the telehealth domain. *Yearbook of Medical Informatics,* 28(1), DOI:10.1055/s-0039-1677897

[32] Rabah, K. V. (2017). Challenges and Opportunities for Blockchain-Powered Healthcare Systems: A Review. *Mara Res. J. Med. Health Sci*, 1(1), 45–52.

[33] Kumar, R. L., Wang, Y., Poongodi, T., and Imoize, A. L. (eds.). (2021). *Internet of Things, Artificial Intelligence and Blockchain Technology*. Cham: Springer.

[34] Rosemol (2022). Data Security in Telemedicine: What You Need to Know. Accessed June 2023: https://www.cabotsolutions.com/data-security-in-telemedicine-what-you-need-to-know

[35] Heister S., and Yuthas K. (2022). *How Blockchain and AI Enable Personal Data Privacy and Support Cybersecurity*. Licensee IntechOpen. DOI:10.5772/intechopen.

[36] Singhar, S. S., Jena, D., and Sharma, S. (2020). Integrating machine learning with blockchain to ensure data privacy. In *2020 11th International Conference on Computing, Communication and Networking Technologies (ICCCNT)*, Kharagpur, India. pp. 1–6, DOI:10.1109/ICCCNT49239.2020.9225342.

[37] Adeniyi, A. E., Abiodun, K. M., Awotunde, J. B., Olagunju, M., Ojo, O. S., and Edet, N. P. (2023). Implementation of a block cipher algorithm for medical information security on cloud environment: Using modified advanced encryption standard approach. *Multimedia Tools and Applications*, 82, 20537–20551. https://doi.org/10.1007/s11042-023-14338-9

[38] Adeniyi, A. E., Misra, S., Daniel, E., and Bokolo Jr, A. (2022). Computational complexity of modified blowfish cryptographic algorithm on video data. *Algorithms*, 15(10), 373.

[39] Abiodun, K. M., Adeniyi, E. A., Awotunde, J. B., *et al.* (2022). Blockchain and internet of things in healthcare systems: Prospects, issues, and challenges. In *Digital Health Transformation with Blockchain and Artificial Intelligence* (pp. 1–22). Boca Raton, FL: CRC Press.

[40] Ndunagu, J. N., Jimoh, R. G., Chidiebere, U., and Opeoluwa, G. D. (2022, November). Enhanced open and distance learning using an artificial intelligence (AI)-powered chatbot: A conceptual framework. In *2022 5th*

Information Technology for Education and Development (ITED) (pp. 1–4). Piscataway, NJ: IEEE.

[41] Awotunde, J. B., Ogundokun, R. O., Misra, S., Adeniyi, E. A., and Sharma, M. M. (2021). Blockchain-based framework for secure transaction in mobile banking platform. In *Hybrid Intelligent Systems: 20th International Conference on Hybrid Intelligent Systems (HIS 2020), December 14–16, 2020* (pp. 525–534). Cham: Springer International Publishing.

[42] Long, Y, Chen, Y., Ren, W., Dou, H., and Xiong, N. N. (2020). Depet: A decentralized privacy preserving energy trading scheme for vehicular energy network via blockchain and k – Anonymity, *IEEE Access*, 8, 192587–192596.

[43] Awotunde, J. B., Jimoh, R. G., Folorunso, S. O., Adeniyi, E. A., Abiodun, K. M., and Banjo, O. O. (2021). Privacy and security concerns in IoT-based healthcare systems. In *The Fusion of Internet of Things, Artificial Intelligence, and Cloud Computing in Health Care* (pp. 105–134). Cham: Springer International Publishing.

[44] Dar, A. A., Alam, M. Z., Ahmad, A., Reegu, F. A., and Rahin, S. A. (2022). Blockchain framework for secure COVID-19 pandemic data handling and protection. *Computational Intelligence and Neuroscience*, 2022, 11. Article ID 7025485. https://doi.org/10.1155/2022/7025485.

[45] Li, X., Chen, T., Luo, X., and Yu, J. (2020). Characterizing erasable accounts in Ethereum, In *Proceedings of the Information Security Conference (ISC)*, Springer, pp. 352–371.

[46] Li, P., Su, J., and Wang, X. (2020). iTLS: Lightweight transport-layer security protocol for IoT with minimal latency and perfect forward secrecy. *IEEE Internet of Things Journal*. DOI:10.1109/JIOT.2020.2988126

[47] Tagde, P., Tagde, S., Bhattacharya, T., *et al.* (2021). Blockchain and artificial intelligence technology in e-Health. *Environmental Science and Pollution Research*, 38, 52810–52831. DOI:10.1007/s11356-021-16223-0.

[48] Rayhan, A. T. and Pamela, B. H. (2023). Patient Confidentiality. Accessed June, 2023: https://www.ncbi.nlm.nih.gov/books/NBK519540/

[49] Lord, N. (2020). Healthcare Cybersecurity: Tips for Securing Private Health Data. Accessed June, 2023: https://www.digitalguardian.com/blog/healthcare-cybersecurity-tips-securing-private-health-data

[50] Burleson, J., Korver, M., and Boneh, D. (2022). Privacy-Protecting Regulatory Solutions Using Zero-Knowledge Proofs: Full Paper. Accessed June, 2023: https://a16zcrypto.com/posts/article/privacy-protecting-regulatory-solutions-using-zero-knowledge-proofs-full-paper/

[51] Davagdorj, K., Bae, J. W., Pham, V. H., Theera-Umpon, N., and Ryu, K. H. (2021). Explainable artificial intelligence-based framework for non-communicable disease prediction. *IEEE Access*, 9, 123672–123688.

[52] Khan, S. N., Loukil, F., Ghedira-Guegan, C., Elhadj Benkhelifa E., and Anoud Bani-Hani, A. (2021). Blockchain smart contracts: Applications, challenges, and future trends. *Peer-to-Peer Networking and Application*, 14, 2901–2925. https://doi.org/10.1007/s12083-021-01127-0

[53] Liu, Y., Zhang, Y., Yang, Y., and Ma, Y. (2022) DOCS: A data ownership confirmation scheme for distributed data trading. *Systems*, 10(226), 1–16. https://doi.org/10.3390/ systems10060226.

[54] Buldakova, T.I., and Krivosheeva, D.A. (2022). Application of biosignals in the end-to-end encryption protocol for telemedicine systems. *Studies in Systems, Decision and Control book series (SSDC)*, 416, pp. 29–39.

[55] Othman, S.B., Almalki, F.A., Chakraborty, C., and Sakli, H. (2022). Privacy-preserving aware data aggregation for IoT-based healthcare with green computing technologies. *Computers and Electrical Engineering*, 101, https://doi.org/10.1016/j.compeleceng.2022.108025.

[56] Tawalbeh, L.A., and Saldamli, G. (2021). Reconsidering big data security and privacy in cloud and mobile cloud systems. *Journal of King Saud University – Computer and Information Sciences*, 33(7), 810–819, https://doi.org/10.1016/j.jksuci.2019.05.007.

[57] Mugunthan, V., Polychroniadou, A., Byrd, D., and Balch, T.H. (2019). SMPAI: Secure multi-party computation for federated learning. In *33rd Conference on Neural Information Processing Systems (NeurIPS 2019)*, Vancouver, Canada. pp 1–9.

[58] Bhushan, B., Sinha, P., Sagayam, K.M., and Andrew, J. (2021). Untangling blockchain technology: A survey on state of the art, security threats, privacy services, applications and future research directions. *Computers & Electrical Engineering*, 90. https://doi.org/10.1016/j.compeleceng.2020.106897.

[59] Dagher, G. G., Mohler, J., Milojkovic, M., and Praneeth Babu Marella, P. B. (2018). Ancile: Privacy-preserving framework for access control and interoperability of electronic health records using blockchain technology. *Sustainable Cities and Society*, 39, 283–297. https://doi.org/10.1016/j.scs.2018.02.014.

[60] Jones, M, Johnson, M, Shervey, M, Dudley, J. T., and Zimmerman, N. (2019). Privacy-preserving methods for feature engineering using blockchain: Review, evaluation, and proof of concept. *Journal of Medical Internet Research*, 21(8), doi:10.2196/13600.

[61] Awotunde, J. B., Imoize, A. L., Salako, D. P., and Farhaoui, Y. (2022, November). An enhanced medical diagnosis system for malaria and typhoid fever using genetic neuro-fuzzy system. In *The International Conference on Artificial Intelligence and Smart Environment* (pp. 173–183). Cham: Springer International Publishing.

[62] McGraw D. (2013). Building public trust in uses of Health Insurance Portability and Accountability Act de-identified data. *Journal of the American Medical Informatics Association*, 20(1), 29–34, https://doi.org/10.1136/amiajnl-2012-000936

[63] Arora, S., Yttri, J., and Nilse, W. (2014). Privacy and security in mobile health (mHealth) research. *Alcohol Research*, 36(1), 143–151

[64] Durneva, P., Cousins, K., and Chen, M. (2020). The current state of research, challenges, and future research directions of blockchain technology in patient care: Systematic review. *Journal Medical Internet Research*, 22(7), doi:10.2196/18619.

[65] Matheny, M. E., Whicher, D., and Israni, S. T. (2020). Artificial intelligence in health care: A report from the National Academy of Medicine. *JAMA*, 323 (6), 509–510.

[66] Mehrabi, N., Morstatter, F., Saxena, N., Lerman, K., and Galstyan, A. (2021). A survey on bias and fairness in machine learning. *ACM Computing Surveys (CSUR)*, 54(6), 1–35.

[67] Johnson, G. M. (2021). Algorithmic bias: On the implicit biases of social technology. *Synthese*, 198(10), 9941–9961.

[68] Sultana, M., Hossain, A., Laila, F., Taher, K. A., and Islam, M. N. (2020). Towards developing a secure medical image sharing system based on zero trust principles and blockchain technology. *BMC Medical Informatics and Decision Making*, 20(1), 1–10.

[69] Mackey, T. K., Shah, N., Miyachi, K., Short, J., and Clauson, K. (2019). A framework proposal for blockchain-based scientific publishing using shared governance. *Frontiers in Blockchain*, 2, 19.

[70] Tzafestas, S. G. (2018). Ethics and law in the internet of things world. *Smart Cities*, 1(1), 98–120.

[71] Ullah, H., Manickam, S., Obaidat, M., Laghari, S. U. A., and Uddin, M. (2023). Exploring the potential of metaverse technology in healthcare: Applications, challenges, and future directions. *IEEE Access*, 11, 69686–69707, 2023, doi: 10.1109/ACCESS.2023.3286696.

[72] Sharma, A., Pruthi, M., and Sageena, G. (2022). Adoption of telehealth technologies: An approach to improving healthcare system. *Translational Medicine Communications*, 7(1), 20.

[73] The Importance of Access Control Systems in Healthcare Organizations (2022). Accessed June, 2023: https://www.ertech.io/the-importance-of-access-control-systems-in-healthcare-organizations

Chapter 11

Artificial intelligence and Blockchain technology enabling cybersecurity in telehealth systems

Wasswa Shafik[1,2]

New technologies like artificial intelligence (AI) and Blockchain have significantly transformed the telehealth industry. AI can revolutionize healthcare, improving treatment outcomes, enabling personalized medicine, and electronic health record (EHRs) management systems. However, this trend also poses many cybersecurity risks, making telehealth systems an easy target for hackers. Data breaches in telehealth are most often caused by inadequate cybersecurity measures, insider threats, and third-party breaches, which cost economies heavily on the taxpayer's revenue per incident. Telehealth systems' most common types of cyberattacks include ransomware, phishing, and malware attacks. This chapter exhaustively presents various telehealth concerns triggered by cybersecurity from a universal telehealth system perspective, its vulnerability, and what the future could hold for telehealth systems at the facility, patients' level, and other stakeholders. Identifiable attacks and imperatives for telehealth systems, over 15 global significances for medical data, are demonstrated and presented. The effects of these attacks can be identically complex, like data leaks, system downtime, financial losses, and damage to a person's reputation. In order to deal with these risks, the study further demonstrates a privacy and security framework that telehealth organizations can adopt to ensure that privacy and security are attained amidst better quality of services using a multipronged cybersecurity strategy that includes regular risk assessments, adequate cybersecurity measures, employee training, and incident response plans. Lastly, highlight how Blockchain can store, secure, and share patient data, including Electronic Health Records (EMR) and medical research data.

11.1 Introduction

Telehealth is one of the most data-intensive sectors, with an increasing volume of medical records, clinical trials, and research data generated daily. Conversely, Blockchain can offer secure and efficient storage and sharing of sensitive medical

[1]School of Digital Science, Universiti Brunei Darussalam, Brunei
[2]Dig Connectivity Research Laboratory (DCRLab), Uganda

data, ensuring patient privacy and confidentiality [1]. Also, to transform telehealth, providing advanced data analysis tools to help doctors make more accurate diagnoses and better treatment decisions. Machine learning (ML) algorithms can analyze vast amounts of medical data, including medical records, imaging data, and laboratory test results, and identify patterns that would be difficult for humans to detect [2]. Artificial intelligence (AI) can also help in drug discovery by predicting drug efficacy and safety, reducing the time and cost of clinical trials.

Furthermore, Blockchain technology can provide secure and decentralized patient data storage, which authorized telehealth providers can access. As a result, patients can maintain control over their data and grant access to doctors, researchers, and other stakeholders as needed [3]. This development can facilitate more efficient medical data sharing, leading to better collaboration and improved patient outcomes. Additionally, Blockchain can help authenticate and verify medical records, ensuring their accuracy and integrity [4].

Telehealth systems' most common types of cyberattacks include ransomware, phishing, and malware attacks. However, this trend toward digitization also poses significant cybersecurity risks. Telehealth systems, including hospitals and clinics, have become prime targets for cyberattacks due to the sensitive and valuable patient data they hold [5]. Therefore, the question arises: are telehealth systems safe from cyber threats? These breaches occur for various reasons, such as inadequate cybersecurity measures, insider threats, and third-party breaches.

Furthermore, telehealth organizations frequently have outdated systems and software, making them an easy target for cybercriminals. As a result, the telehealth system is vulnerable to various types of cyberattacks, such as phishing attacks, ransomware attacks, and malware attacks [6]. Ransomware attacks are one of the most prevalent types of cyberattacks in telehealth systems, where cybercriminals encrypt patient data and demand a ransom to release it.

Cybercriminals also often use phishing attacks to get employees to click on a malicious link or download an attachment that contains malware. Another type of cyberattack is malware, in which cybercriminals infect the telehealth system with malware that can steal patient data or cause system downtime [7]. Cyberattacks on telehealth systems can have devastating consequences. Cyberattacks can lead to data breaches, compromising patient confidentiality and trust. Moreover, cyberattacks can cause system downtime, affecting patient care and hospital operations [8]. Furthermore, telehealth organizations may incur significant financial losses because of the cost of data recovery, legal fees, and reputational harm. Therefore, telehealth organizations must take a proactive, multilayered approach to improve cybersecurity in telehealth systems.

Telehealth organizations need regular risk assessments and implement suitable cybersecurity measures like firewalls, antivirus software, and data encryption. Secondly, telehealth organizations must provide cybersecurity awareness training to all employees to prevent insider threats and phishing attacks [9]. Thirdly, telehealth organizations must implement a cybersecurity incident response plan to mitigate the impact of cyberattacks. Adequate cybersecurity measures, regular risk assessments, employee training, and incident response plans ensure that patient data remains confidential and secure. With these safeguards in place, telehealth organizations can mitigate the impact of cyberattacks while preserving patient trust [10,11].

In today's digital world, cybercrime is a growing problem that affects people, businesses, and the government. It includes many illegal activities, such as identity theft, financial fraud, cyberbullying, cyberstalking, ransomware attacks, and more [12]. Cybercrime costs money and threatens personal and national security because hackers can get private information and stop essential services from working. The consensus about cybercrime is that it is everyone's job to stop it [13]. Governments, businesses, and individuals must work together to prevent and mitigate the impact of cybercrime. Governments can establish laws and regulations to prosecute cybercriminals and enforce cybersecurity standards [14]. Businesses can invest in cybersecurity measures to protect their assets and customers' data. Individuals can secure their online presence by using strong passwords, enabling two-factor authentication, and being cautious of suspicious emails or links [15].

11.1.1 Key contributions of the chapter

The subsequent are the imperative contributions of the chapter:

- Examines the vulnerability of the health sector as it relates to cybersecurity and cyberattacks in the broader medical sector.
- According to the detailed challenges telehealth faces, we propose a graphical privacy and security framework for the health industry.
- Since cybersecurity tends to have several traits or aspects, the study further provides significant elements and considerations of cybersecurity for healthcare.
- The study presents numerous attacks instigated by cyber attackers within telehealth infrastructure and data security threats.
- Demonstrate the main imperatives for refining cybersecurity in the telehealth industry.
- The study avails several future research trends for telehealth from cybersecurity perspectives.

11.1.2 Chapter organization

Section 11.2 provides an overview of Blockchain technology and AI as applied in telehealth systems. Section 11.3 demonstrates the limitation of the edge-cutting proposed model; the different stakeholders can utilize these limitations to solve the concern as far as telehealth is concerned and how the health sector is vulnerable when it comes to cybersecurity, including the sensitivity of patient data, inadequate cybersecurity measures, outdated systems and software, insider threats, third-party breach, lack of employee training, high-value targets, telehealth system complexity, and increasing use of technology. Section 11.4 presents significant aspects of cybersecurity for healthcare, like preclusion, alertness, and knowledge. Section 11.5 illustrates abundant attacks instigated by cybersecurity attackers have been provoked too, including malware, internet of things (IoT)-based attacks, AI-driven attacks, eavesdropping attacks, password attacks, cross-site scripting (XSS) attacks, distributed denial-of-service (DDoS) attacks, Domain Name System (DNS) tunneling, structured query language (SQL) injection, and phishing. Section 11.6 shows the main imperatives for refining cybersecurity in healthcare, like plans for responding to an incident, risk assessments, and real-world telehealth data breaches in tabular format depicting the date when the breach was done, the number of impacted people, and compromised items, and we precisely propose possible solutions. Section 11.7 demonstrates telehealth infrastructure and data security threats like insider threats, third-party breaches, physical security breaches, and data theft. Future telehealth cybersecurity aspects are presented in Section 11.8. Section 11.9 entails the lesson learned and future directions. Finally, the conclusion is presented in Section 11.10.

11.2 Overview of Blockchain technology and artificial intelligence in telehealth systems

11.2.1 Blockchain technology in healthcare

A distributed, secure, and transparent digital archive that can be used to record connections and information safely and tamper-proof. In the telehealth industry, Blockchain can transform how data is shared, stored, and accessed, particularly regarding raw data [16]. This data is critical for improving patient care, conducting medical research, and advancing telehealth technology. However, several challenges are associated with managing this data, including security concerns, data privacy, and interoperability issues [17]. Blockchain techs solve these challenges by providing a secure and distributed platform for sharing and storing telehealth information. With Blockchain, telehealth providers can securely store and share patient data tamper-proof, ensuring that the data is accurate, reliable, and accessible only to authorized parties. In telehealth applications, Blockchain expertise can improve patient care, clinical research, and telehealth supply chain management [18]. Blockchain can be used to develop electronic health records (EHRs) easily accessible to telehealth providers, patients, and other stakeholders. It can also be used to facilitate secure and transparent clinical trials, as well as to track the authenticity and quality of pharmaceuticals and medical devices [19].

Several key players are involved when it comes to stakeholders in ensuring the patient's quality of services. These include telehealth workers, patients, researchers, regulators, and technology companies. For example, telehealth benefactors provide patient data that is accurate, reliable, and accessible. In contrast, patients have the right to control their health data and determine who has access to it [20], particularly raw data, as illustrated in Figure 11.1. However, ensuring the patient quality of services requires collaboration among telehealth providers, patients, researchers, regulators, and technology companies. By working together, stakeholders can ensure that telehealth data is managed ethically, securely, and in compliance with regulatory requirements, ultimately improving patient care and advancing telehealth technology.

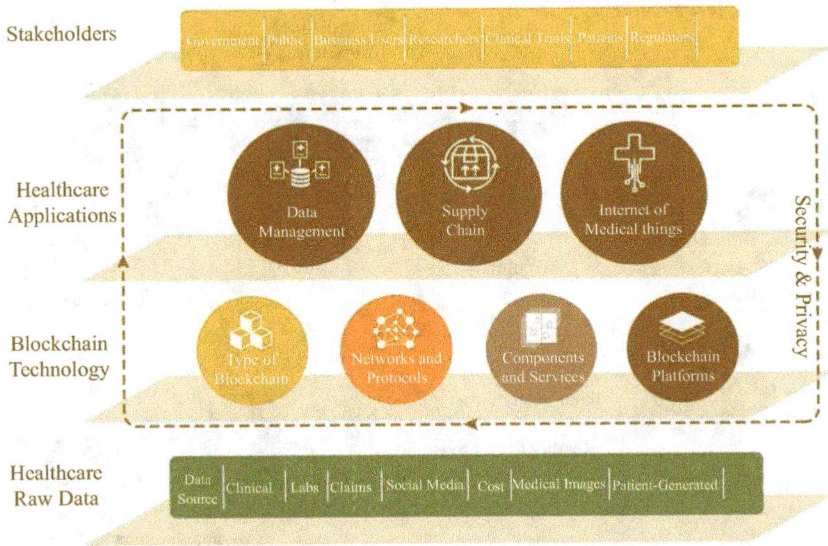

Figure 11.1 *Blockchain-centered telehealth application workflow; this approach mainly entails main layers, for instance, the data layer (telehealth system raw data); the current technology layers (Blockchain technology) that ensure security and privacy to both Blockchain layer; telehealth application and to different stakeholders [21]*

11.2.2 Artificial intelligence in telehealth systems

Disease diagnosis and management are among smart health's most promising AI applications. For example, in mobile health, AI algorithms can analyze large amounts of data, including medical images, laboratory results, and patient histories, to help telehealth professionals diagnose and manage diseases more accurately and efficiently [22]. One of the utmost mutual uses of AI in disease diagnosis and management is the analysis of medical images; an AI medical scenario is demonstrated in Figure 11.2.

Medical imaging techniques like CT scans, MRI, and X-rays scans generate vast amounts of data, and analyzing this data manually can be time-consuming and error-prone. AI algorithms can explore these images quickly and accurately, detecting even subtle changes that human observers might miss. For example, a mobile app can use AI to analyze a photo of a skin lesion and determine whether it is cancerous [24]. AI can also analyze patient data to predict the likelihood of developing certain diseases. For example, ML algorithms can analyze a patient's medical history, lifestyle factors, and genetic data to predict the possibility of growing conditions such as diabetes, heart disease, or cancer [25]. This development can enable telehealth professionals to recognize patients who are at high risk and take preventive measures.

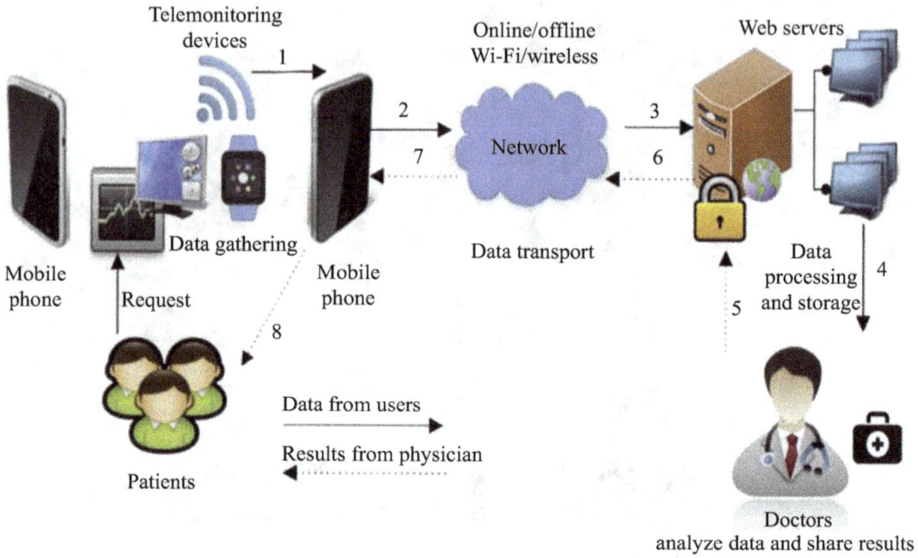

Figure 11.2 An AI medical support (telehealth); this diagram demonstrates how a patient can be given a medical service. A patient makes a request using the available internet of medical things like a smartphone. The data is gathered using telemonitoring devices, and the demand is transported either online or offline to the web server's data processing, which is done and stored to and from the doctors after analysis and results are transferred back to the web server that shares it via the network back to the patient [23].

In addition to disease diagnosis, AI can be applied to manage chronic conditions like diabetes, asthma, and hypertension. For example, mobile apps can use AI algorithms to analyze data from wearable devices, such as smartwatches and fitness trackers, to monitor patients' vital signs and detect changes in their condition [26]. This can enable telehealth professionals to intervene early and prevent complications. Other applications include medical chatbots, drug discovery, behavioral intervention, and remote patient monitoring [27].

Cybercrime and telehealth have different focuses but are interconnected through the lens of cybersecurity. For example, identity theft, cyberbullying, and ransomware attacks are all examples of cybercrime [28]. On the other hand, telehealth is about medical services and keeping track of patient data. Unfortunately, the telehealth sector is vulnerable to cyberattacks due to data sensitivity, leading to data breaches and system downtime [29]. To combat these threats, telehealth organizations must take a proactive approach to cybersecurity by conducting regular risk assessments, executing adequate cyberattack measures, employee training, and developing incident response plans [30].

11.3 Limitations and vulnerability of the traditional models used in healthcare systems

Cyberattacks can happen in the telehealth sector because of several things, such as sensitive patient data, outdated systems, insider threats, third-party breaches, lack of employee training, and high-value targets.

11.3.1 Limitations in the existing models

Several limitations exist in research, development, and implementation; possible approaches are demonstrated. Limited data availability in smart medical care can create significant privacy and security concerns. Smart medical care involves using various smart devices, such as wearables and sensors, to collect and transmit data about patients' health and medical conditions [31]. This data may include sensitive information such as medical diagnoses, medications, and personal identification information. If this data falls into the wrong hands, it can be used for malicious purposes such as identity theft, fraud, or blackmail. Additionally, if the data is not adequately secured, it can be vulnerable to hacking, cyberattacks, and other unauthorized access [32]. The limited data available in this context means there may be insufficient data to properly train ML models to detect and prevent privacy and security breaches. If the models are not adequately trained, they may be less effective in identifying and preventing such breaches, leaving patient data vulnerable [33].

There are a few strategies that can be used. First, telehealth organizations can work to gather more data on privacy and security breaches in smart medical care. This data can be used to train ML models to identify better and prevent these breaches [34]. Second, telehealth organizations can work to improve data-sharing practices, both internally and across organizations [35]. Finally, another strategy is to improve patient education and awareness around privacy and security issues in smart medical care. Patients should be aware of the risks and how to protect their data. In addition, they should be encouraged to participate in research initiatives designed to improve the privacy and security of smart medical care [24,36]. This can help ensure that patient data is properly secured and that privacy and security breaches are identified and addressed promptly.

Complex data structures in smart medical care can create security and privacy concerns in several ways. Smart device applications, such as wearables and sensors, can generate vast amounts of data about patients' health and medical conditions [25]. This data is often heterogeneous and unstructured, which makes it challenging to process and analyze. Additionally, this data may include sensitive information such as medical diagnoses, medications, and personal identification information, making it a valuable target for cyber attackers. Finally, the complexity of the data can make it challenging to develop machine-learning models that can effectively detect and prevent privacy and security breaches [37].

One approach is to improve the standardization and normalization of data structures. Standardizing the data makes it easier to analyze and process, which can improve the accuracy and reliability of ML models [38]. Additionally, standardization can help ensure that privacy and security protocols are consistently applied across different data types. Another approach is to use advanced techniques such as data encryption and differential privacy to protect patient data. Data encryption can be used to secure data while it is being transmitted or stored, which can help prevent unauthorized access [39]. Differential privacy is a technique that adds random noise to data to protect individual privacy while allowing the data to be analyzed. Finally, it is important to involve patients in the data collection and obtain their consent for data sharing and analysis [40]. Patients should be informed about the types of data being collected, how it will be used, and how it will be protected. This can help to build trust between patients and telehealth organizations, which is critical for the success of smart medical care initiatives.

A lack of standardization in smart medical care can create significant privacy and security concerns. Smart medical care involves using various smart devices, such as wearables and sensors, to collect and transmit data about patients' health and medical conditions. However, this data can be challenging to analyze and interpret without proper standardization and may be vulnerable to security breaches [41]. For instance, combining and analyzing data from different sources can be challenging if different devices use different data formats or protocols for transmitting data. Additionally, if the devices do not have consistent security protocols, they may be vulnerable to hacking, cyberattacks, and other unauthorized access. Lack of standardization can also make it challenging to develop ML models that can effectively detect and prevent privacy and security breaches [42]. Models may struggle to identify patterns in unstructured data or may be biased toward certain data types. This can lead to inaccurate or incomplete analyses, compromising patient privacy and security.

The diversity of systems in smart medical care can create security and privacy concerns. Various smart devices and systems can generate vast amount of data about patients' health and medical conditions [43]. However, these systems may not be compatible, leading to challenges in integrating data from different sources. This can make it difficult to analyze the data effectively and identify potential privacy and security risks. Furthermore, the diversity of systems also makes it more challenging to secure the data. Each system may have different security protocols, and if these protocols are incompatible or do not communicate, it may create vulnerabilities that can be exploited by hackers or other malicious actors [43]. One approach is to establish industry-wide standards for data formats and protocols. These standards can help ensure that data can be easily combined and analyzed across different devices and organizations [44].

Another approach is to use advanced technologies such as APIs and middleware to integrate data from different systems. APIs can provide a standardized interface for different methods to communicate with each other, enabling data sharing and analysis [45]. Middleware can provide a layer of abstraction that helps ensure that different systems can share without exposing vulnerabilities or sensitive data. This technology can help ensure data is not tampered with or corrupted and provide an audit trail for tracking data access and usage [46]. Patients should be informed about the types of data being collected, how it will be used, and how it will be protected. This can help build trust between patients and telehealth organizations, which is critical for smart medical care initiatives [47].

Adversarial attacks are a growing concern in smart medical care, as they can compromise the privacy and security of patients' data. Malicious attacks are a type of cyberattack that involves exploiting weaknesses in ML models, such as those used in smart medical care, to cause the model to make incorrect predictions or classifications [48]. This can be done by adding small amounts of noise or intentionally modifying the data inputs in a way the ML model cannot detect. Adversarial attacks can have severe consequences for smart medical care [49]. For example, an attacker could modify the data inputs to make a patient appear healthier than they are or to make a patient's medical condition appear less severe than it is. This could result in an incorrect diagnosis or treatment, potentially life-threatening for the patient [50]. Several strategies can be used. One approach uses ML models designed to be robust against adversarial attacks. These models incorporate techniques such as negative training, where the model is trained on data intentionally modified to simulate malicious attacks [51]. This can help improve the model's ability to detect and mitigate these attacks.

Another strategy is to use data encryption and access controls to protect patient data. Data encryption can be used to secure data while it is being transmitted or stored, which can help prevent unauthorized access [52]. Access controls can restrict access to sensitive data to only authorized personnel. It is also essential to use strong authentication and authorization mechanisms to prevent unauthorized access to medical devices and systems [53]. This condition can involve using two-factor authentication, biometric authentication, or other advanced security measures to ensure that only authorized personnel can access patient data. Strong security policies and procedures are essential, including regular security audits and vulnerability assessments [54]. In addition, regular training and awareness programs can help educate telehealth personnel about the risks of adversarial attacks and how to prevent them [55].

The black-box nature of some ML models makes it difficult to understand how they arrive at their conclusions. Limited interpretability in innovative medical care can cause privacy and security concerns because it can be challenging to know how ML models make patient health predictions or decisions [56]. However, these models can be complex and difficult to interpret, challenging the identification of potential privacy and security risks. It can also make it difficult to identify and correct errors or biases in ML models [57]. The best approach is to use ML models designed to be interpretable. These models are often more straightforward and transparent than traditional ML models, making it easier to understand how they make predictions or decisions [58].

Another strategy is using model-agnostic interpretability techniques, such as partial dependence plots or feature importance analysis, to understand how a model makes predictions. These techniques can help identify which features or factors are most important in the model's decision-making process, which can help identify potential biases or errors [59]. It is also essential to involve telehealth professionals and patients in developing and testing ML models. Including telehealth professionals and patients in the process makes it possible to ensure that the models are designed to meet their needs and are understandable and interpretable [60]. This can include data encryption, access controls, and regular security audits to identify and address vulnerabilities. Additionally, regular training and awareness programs can help educate telehealth personnel about the risks of limited interpretability and how to prevent privacy and security concerns [61].

Limited expertise in smart medical care can cause privacy and security concerns because telehealth professionals may not have the necessary knowledge. For illustration, telehealth professionals may not thoroughly understand data privacy regulations, such as the Health Insurance Portability and Accountability Act (HIPAA), or may not be familiar with best practices for securing medical devices and systems [62]. This can result in data breaches or other privacy and security incidents that put patient data at risk. One approach is to provide telehealth professionals with training and education on privacy and security best practices [63]. This can include training on data privacy regulations, like HIPAA, and securing medical devices and systems. It is also important to involve IT professionals and cybersecurity experts in developing and managing smart medical care systems. These experts can provide guidance on best practices for securing medical devices and systems and can help to identify and mitigate potential privacy and security risks [64].

Building and deploying effective models often requires significant computational resources, which may be a barrier for smaller telehealth organizations. High computational requirements in smart medical care can cause privacy and security concerns because they can lead to less secure computing environments, such as cloud computing [65]. If a telehealth organization does not have the computational resources to perform complex data analysis in-house, it may turn to cloud computing providers to perform these tasks. While cloud computing can provide the necessary computational power, it can also introduce additional privacy and security risks, such as data breaches or unauthorized access to patient data [66]. This can help reduce the need for high-performance computing resources and make it easier for telehealth organizations to analyze in-house data [67].

Cost can be a significant factor that causes privacy and security concerns in smart medical care. Telehealth organizations may have limited budgets for implementing privacy and security measures. As a result, they may be unable to invest the necessary resources and expertise to manage privacy and security risks effectively [68]. For example, telehealth organizations may not have the funds to purchase and maintain the latest cybersecurity technologies or to hire dedicated cybersecurity professionals to manage their intelligent medical care systems. This can lead to a lack of resources and expertise to manage privacy and security risks, increasing the risk of data breaches and other security incidents [69]. Several strategies can be used. One approach is prioritizing investments in privacy and security measures critical to protecting patient data [70]. This can include investing in technologies most effective at detecting and preventing security incidents, such as intrusion detection and prevention systems, and implementing strong access controls and user authentication mechanisms [71].

Telehealth data is often sensitive and confidential, making it challenging to share data across different organizations for research and model development. Data privacy concerns are a significant driver of privacy and security concerns in smart medical care [72]. Patient data is susceptible, and the risk of data breaches and unauthorized access can lead to significant patient harm, including identity theft, financial loss, and reputational damage. Data privacy concerns are exacerbated by the complexity of smart medical care systems, which can involve many interconnected devices and data sources, making it difficult to track and manage patient data across the system [73]. To address these issues, telehealth organizations must prioritize data privacy as a core component of their privacy and security strategies. This can involve implementing strong access controls and authentication mechanisms to limit access to patient data to authorized personnel and regularly auditing and monitoring patient data to detect and prevent unauthorized access [74]. Additionally, telehealth organizations can leverage encryption technologies to protect patient data at rest and in transit and implement data loss prevention mechanisms to detect and prevent data exfiltration [75].

Telehealth regulations can be complex and vary by country, making it challenging to develop models that comply with all relevant laws. Regulatory hurdles can create privacy and security concerns in smart medical care by creating ambiguity and confusion around compliance requirements, leading to non-compliance [76]. The complexity of regulatory frameworks and rapidly evolving technology and privacy risks can make it difficult for telehealth organizations to keep up with regulatory requirements and ensure that their privacy and security programs comply [77]. To address these challenges, telehealth organizations must prioritize compliance with regulatory requirements as a core component of their privacy and security strategies. This can involve investing in compliance management tools and technologies to track and manage compliance requirements, developing comprehensive policies and procedures aligned with regulatory requirements and industry best practices, and conducting regular risk assessments to identify areas of non-compliance and develop mitigation strategies [78]. Additionally, telehealth organizations can leverage external resources, such as consultants and auditors, to help navigate complex regulatory frameworks and ensure compliance with their privacy and security programs [14].

Models developed for one telehealth organization or system may not be effective when applied to another. Limited generalizability can create privacy and security concerns in smart medical care, potentially leading to biased or inaccurate diagnoses and treatment recommendations [79]. Telehealth-based ML models rely on large amounts of data to train and refine their algorithms. Still, if that data does not represent the broader population, the models may not generalize well to new patients [80]. This can result in inaccurate diagnoses and treatment recommendations, potentially harming patients and eroding trust in the telehealth system. Therefore, telehealth organizations must prioritize diversity and inclusivity in their data collection and modeling practices [81]. This can involve collecting data from diverse patients to ensure that the data used to train ML models represents the broader population. Also, telehealth organizations can work to mitigate bias in their data by implementing algorithms that identify and correct bias and by including diverse perspectives in developing and testing their models.

The nature of cyber threats is constantly evolving, which means models must be continually updated to remain effective. Cyber threats pose significant privacy and security concerns in smart medical care as the telehealth industry embraces digital technologies to improve patient care and outcomes [82]. Cyber attackers increasingly target telehealth organizations, seeking to steal valuable patient data and disrupt critical systems. To address these evolving cyber threats, telehealth organizations must implement robust cybersecurity measures and protocols to safeguard their digital assets and protect patient data [83].

Models that work well for small telehealth organizations may not be scalable to larger organizations with more complex systems and larger volumes of data. Limited scalability can cause significant privacy and security concerns in smart medical care, as it can impede the ability of the telehealth sector to effectively manage and secure patient data as their operations grow and expand [82]. Furthermore, as the volume of data and the number of connected devices and systems increases, the risk of privacy breaches and cyberattacks also increases, placing patient data at risk. To address these concerns, telehealth organizations must prioritize scalability and invest in systems and technologies to accommodate their growing needs [84]. This can involve adopting cloud-based solutions that offer flexible storage and computing capabilities and implementing scalable security protocols and controls that can adapt to changing threat landscapes.

Telehealth organizations must prioritize data privacy and security at every stage of the scalability process. This includes implementing access controls and data encryption to ensure that only authorized users can access sensitive patient data and conducting regular security audits and vulnerability assessments to identify potential weaknesses in systems and processes [85]. In addition, telehealth organizations must ensure their staff is appropriately trained in privacy and security best practices, such as recognizing phishing attempts and avoiding data breaches [86]. This can involve providing regular training sessions and resources and incentivizing employees to prioritize privacy and security in their day-to-day operations, as summarized in Table 11.1.

To ensure patient data remains confidential and secure, telehealth organizations must take proactive measures to improve cybersecurity, such as regular risk assessments, employee training, and incident response plans. Some identified instances include the following.

11.3.2 Sensitive patient data

Sensitive patient data can be used to determine an individual's name, date of birth, medical history, social security number, and information about their insurance. This data is precious to cybercriminals and can be used for identity theft, financial fraud, and other malicious activities [59]. The telehealth industry is especially vulnerable to cyberattacks because it stores sensitive patient information needed to provide medical care [60]. In addition, these systems are often connected and can

Table 11.1 A complete summary of artificial intelligence applications and their restrictions in smart health

Area	Application(s)	AI technology	Limitations
Forecasting pandemics or epidemics [87–89]	Explore the dynamic disease pattern	Long short-term memory networks	It makes learning more complex with the increase in search space dimension
		Feed-forward propagation neural networks	It necessitates multiple hidden layers, heightened for color images
		Multilayer perceptron	Time-consuming computations are complex, depend on the quality of the training, and are impulsive
		autoRegressive integrated moving average	Deprived performance for long-term forecasts, challenging to predict turning points, computationally expensive
	Virus and disease prediction	Polynomial neural network with corrective feedback, Deep neural networks	Computationally expensive, augmented training resources
	Yellow fever analysis	Multilayer perceptron neural network classifiers	Depends on the quality of the training
Forecasting pandemics or epidemics [87–89]	Swift diagnosis of TB defendants Detect TB bacillus	Tuberculosis-AI	Difficult to predict turning points
	Zika predictions	Deep neural networks	It involves massive data to perform better than other methods, affluent, no standard theory to select deep learning tools
	Seasonal influenza forecast	ML anonymized mobility map, ML feed-forward propagation neural network	Massive input and target set for the training processes

(Continues)

Table 11.1 (Continued)

Area	Application(s)	AI technology	Limitations
Personalized treatment [50,51]	Data interpretation, image analysis, anesthesia, and vasodilator care	Automated treatment planning, hybrid intelligent systems, fuzzy expert systems, evolutionary computational	Mysterious functioning of the network, hard regulating the appropriate network structures and hardware dependencies
Drug discovery [48,49,90,91]	Drug-target collaboration	Chem Mapper transfer learning	Model generalization, flexibility deficiency
	Physicochemical properties of trivial molecules determination	Estimation program interface suite	It needs massive data and computational possessions
Digital therapy [52,53]	Toxicity of radiation therapy, prediction of outcomes, radiotherapy	Radiomics	Standards are not turned out into optimum results, exertion of showing the problem to the system
Disease diagnosis [54–58]	Dermatological diseases, dementia, arial fibrillation, cancer	Unsupervised learning, neural networking, deep learning	Computationally affluent versus outdated algorithms

be accessed through the internet, which makes them vulnerable to cyberattacks. Data breaches can happen when there are not enough security measures, when systems and software are out of date, or when someone on the inside is a threat. This lets cybercriminals see sensitive information about patients.

The consequences of a data breach in the telehealth sector can be severe. Patients can suffer from identity, financial, and medical identity theft, resulting in reputational damage and a loss of trust in the telehealth organization. Furthermore, data recovery costs, legal fees, and fines for non-compliance with data protection regulations can result in significant financial losses for telehealth organizations [61]. Therefore, protecting sensitive patient data is crucial in the telehealth sector to ensure patient confidentiality and trust and to maintain the integrity of the telehealth system. Unfortunately, telehealth organizations store sensitive patient data, including medical history, personal information, and financial information, making them an appealing target for cybercriminals [62].

11.3.3 Inadequate cybersecurity measures

Inadequate cybersecurity measures mean insufficient effective ways to protect telehealth systems and patient information from cyber threats. Outdated software, weak passwords, networks that are not secure, and not encrypting patient data can all be signs of poor cybersecurity in telehealth [63]. Different kinds of cyberattacks, like ransomware, phishing, and malware, can happen because of these holes. Cybercriminals use ransomware to lock up patient data and demand a ransom to unlock it. Phishing attacks trick employees into clicking on a malicious link or downloading an attachment containing malware [64]. Malware attacks involve infecting the telehealth system with malware that can steal patient data or cause system downtime. Inadequate cybersecurity measures can seriously impact telehealth organizations, including data breaches, loss of patient trust, legal liabilities, and financial losses. To prevent insider threats and phishing attacks, telehealth organizations must also provide cybersecurity awareness training to all employees [65,66].

11.3.4 Outdated systems and software

In healthcare, using legacy technology that is no longer supported by the manufacturer or has not had security updates in a long time is called using outdated systems and software [67]. Cyberattacks are often more likely to happen on these systems because they do not have the latest security features and patches to fix holes. Many outdated systems remain in use because telehealth organizations cannot afford to replace them or are deemed too critical to be taken offline for upgrades [68]. Cybercriminals can take advantage of flaws in outdated telehealth systems and software to gain unauthorized access to patient data, install malware, or cause the system to go down. These risks are further compounded by using interconnected medical devices, which can also be susceptible to cyberattacks [69].

Furthermore, telehealth organizations may lack the resources or expertise to secure these systems, leaving them vulnerable to cyber threats [70]. To address the issue of outdated systems and software in healthcare, organizations must prioritize system upgrades and invest in newer technologies that are more secure and compliant with industry standards. In addition, regular patch management and security updates are essential to keep systems up-to-date and protect against emerging cyber threats. Telehealth organizations can also consider adopting cloud-based solutions or outsourcing their IT functions to manage service providers specializing in cybersecurity to improve their security posture [71].

11.3.5 Insider threats

Insider threats refer to the risk of a security breach caused by an organization's employees, contractors, or other insiders with authorized access to the organization's systems or data. Insider threats are a significant concern in the telehealth sector due to the sensitive patient data that telehealth organizations handle [72]. Employees, contractors, or other insiders may intentionally or unintentionally cause security breaches, such as stealing or leaking patient data, installing malware, or exploiting system vulnerabilities [73]. The motivations for insider threats may vary, including financial gain, personal grudges, or ignorance of security policies and procedures.

Insiders may also be coerced or tricked by external factors, such as cybercriminals, into conducting malicious activities [74]. To prevent and detect insider threats, telehealth organizations must implement robust cybersecurity measures such as access controls, monitoring systems, and employee training. Furthermore, organizations should have incident response plans in place to lessen the impact of insider threats if they occur. Employees with access to patient data can pose a significant cybersecurity threat, intentionally or unintentionally [92]. Disgruntled employees can steal or leak patient data, while unwitting employees can fall prey to phishing or other social engineering attacks.

11.3.6 Third-party breach

Third-party breaches are leaks of sensitive patient information caused by the actions of outside vendors or partners who have access to that information. Third-party vendors often help hospitals and clinics with things like medical billing and maintenance of medical equipment [93]. These third-party vendors may have access to patient data, making them a potential target for cybercriminals. One of the significant challenges in dealing with third-party breaches is the lack of control that telehealth organizations have over the cybersecurity practices of their vendors [75]. The security of the vendor's systems and software may not be up to the same standards as that of the telehealth society, making them an easy target for cyberattacks.

Third-party vendors may not have the same cybersecurity awareness and training as telehealth association employees [76]. To reduce the risk of third-party breaches, telehealth organizations must implement strict vendor management policies requiring vendors to adhere to the same cybersecurity standards as the telehealth organization. These policies may include regular security assessments of the vendor's systems and software and training on cybersecurity best practices for all vendors with access to patient data [77]. Telehealth organizations frequently use third-party vendors to provide billing and medical equipment services. These vendors may not have robust cybersecurity measures, making them a potential weak link in the telehealth organizations' security chain [94].

11.3.7 Lack of employee training

The term "lack of employee training in healthcare" refers to the situation in which telehealth employees are not adequately trained to recognize and respond to cybersecurity threats. Because they have not been qualified, they are vulnerable to cyberattacks like phishing, in which attackers send fake emails to employees to trick them into giving up sensitive information or downloading malware [14]. Employees can also cause security problems without meaning to by mishandling sensitive data or not following cybersecurity policies and procedures. For example, employees might forget to lock their computers, letting unauthorized people see confidential patient information [79]. This training should cover managing passwords, encrypting data, spotting phishing emails, and reporting strange behavior. In addition, employees should receive ongoing training and refresher courses to stay current with the latest threats and best practices [80]. By giving thorough and ongoing training, telehealth organizations can reduce the risk of insider attacks, improve their overall cybersecurity, and keep cybercriminals from accessing patient data.

11.3.8 High-value target

Telehealth systems are high-value targets for cybercriminals due to the sensitive and valuable patient data they hold. This data includes personal information such as name, address, and social security number, as well as medical information such as diagnosis, treatment, and prescription details [95]. This information can be sold on the dark web to identity thieves for financial fraud or blackmail. Moreover, patient data can be used for identity theft, where cybercriminals use the patient's identity to commit fraud, or credit cards, file fraudulent tax returns, or apply for loans [96]. In addition to patient data, telehealth systems contain valuable research and development data, which cybercriminals can steal for financial gain or use to create counterfeit drugs [97].

11.3.9 Telehealth system complexity

The complexity of the telehealth system increases its vulnerability to cyberattacks. This complexity results in multiple entry points for cybercriminals to access patient data, and it becomes challenging to secure every point of admission [81]. Moreover, telehealth systems often use multiple systems and applications to manage patient data, and the interoperability between these systems can create vulnerabilities [82]. For example, if one system is compromised, the attacker can access other systems that share data with the compromised system. In addition, telehealth organizations frequently rely on legacy systems not designed to deal with modern cybersecurity threats. These systems might have flaws that manufacturers or vendors have not addressed, making them attractive targets for cybercriminals [82,96].

11.3.10 Increasing use of technology

Technology is used increasingly in healthcare, opening new opportunities for patients and providers. EHRs, telemedicine, and mobile health (mHealth) applications are just a few examples of how technology has transformed the telehealth industry. However, this also means that telehealth systems are becoming more complex and interconnected, which increases the risk of cyberattacks. Cybercriminals have more ways to get in when more technology is used in telehealth [83]. This complexity is further compounded by the fact that telehealth organizations often use various systems and applications that may not be designed to work together seamlessly, creating vulnerabilities in the system. As a result, telehealth organizations must take extra precautions to ensure the security of their technology and the seamless integration of all applications and strategies [84,98].

11.4 Significant aspects of cybersecurity for healthcare

It is also imperative for the telehealth sector to prioritize cybersecurity in their overall risk management strategy, comply with relevant laws and regulations, and collaborate with other organizations and stakeholders to address cybersecurity threats and challenges in the telehealth sector.

11.4.1 Preclusion

Prevention is a critical aspect of cybersecurity in healthcare. To reduce the risk of cyberattacks, telehealth organizations must implement preventive measures. This includes conducting regular risk assessments to identify vulnerabilities and implementing adequate cybersecurity measures, such as firewalls, antivirus software, and data encryption [85]. Furthermore, telehealth organizations must implement an incident response plan when a cyberattack occurs to mitigate the impact.

11.4.2 Alertness

Alertness is an essential aspect of cybersecurity in healthcare. It refers to the ability of telehealth organizations to detect and respond to cybersecurity. Telehealth organizations should also conduct regular cybersecurity risk assessments to identify potential vulnerabilities and areas for improvement. This can include vulnerability scanning, penetration testing, and threat modeling to ensure robust and secure systems and processes [86]. In addition to taking technical measures, alertness also involves training employees on cybersecurity and best practices and encouraging a culture of security awareness. Employees should be prepared to recognize potential cyber threats, such as phishing emails or social engineering scams, and know how to respond appropriately [87].

11.4.3 Knowledge

Knowledge of telehealth and cybersecurity means understanding and being aware of possible cyber threats and how to stop them. It includes knowledge of the best practices for securing patient data and maintaining system security. Telehealth professionals and information technology staff must be trained and knowledgeable about cybersecurity measures such as firewalls, data encryption, and password management [88]. They should also be aware of the most common types of cyberattacks, such as phishing, ransomware, and malware, and how to identify and respond to them. A knowledgeable workforce can help telehealth organizations improve cybersecurity and protect patient data from cyber threats.

11.5 Numerous attacks instigated by attackers

Cyber attackers have been known to employ various attacks to compromise organizations' security, including telehealth systems, as demonstrated below.

11.5.1 Malware

In the telehealth sector, malware attacks are a common cybercrime with severe consequences, such as data theft or system shutdown. Ransomware attacks, for example, can encrypt an organization's data and make it useless until a ransom is paid, while phishing attacks can steal login credentials or personal information [89]. Telehealth organizations must ensure that all software is current and use antivirus and firewall software to reduce the risk of malware attacks.

11.5.2 IoT-based attacks

Increasingly, medical devices, like insulin pumps, pacemakers, and monitors, are being connected to the internet as part of the IoT. Nevertheless, this has also led to more cyberattacks in the telehealth industry that use IoT. Attackers can access these devices, control their operations, and steal sensitive patient data. IoT-based attacks can have bad results, like risking patient safety and privacy, stopping doctors from doing their jobs, or even killing someone [90]. To prevent IoT-based attacks, telehealth organizations must prioritize cybersecurity by executing strong authentication measures, monitoring network activity, and regularly updating their software and firmware [91]. They should also educate patients on the importance of cybersecurity and provide them with resources to help protect their personal information. By taking these steps, telehealth organizations can better protect their IoT devices and ensure the safety and privacy of their patients [99].

11.5.3 AI-driven attacks

AI has become increasingly sophisticated, and its use in cyberattacks has grown in recent years, posing a significant threat to the telehealth industry [100]. AI-powered attacks can include advanced phishing attacks, deep fakes, and more targeted and automated attacks that bypass traditional security measures. These attacks are dangerous as they can mimic legitimate user behavior and bypass standard security measures. One potential solution to combat AI-powered attacks is using AI, employing ML algorithms to identify and prevent such attacks [101]. Also, telehealth organizations must implement adequate security protocols, such as two-factor authentication, access control, and encryption, to secure their networks and devices. Regular vulnerability assessments and penetration testing can also help identify potential vulnerabilities and reduce the risk of an AI-powered attack [102].

11.5.4 Eavesdropping attacks

Eavesdropping attacks are a type of cyberattack where a third party intercepts and monitors network communications, thereby gaining access to sensitive information. In telehealth, these attacks can expose confidential patient information, including medical records, financial leads, and personal identifiers [103]. Telehealth organizations can implement encryption technologies to ensure secure communication. Also, penetration testing and regular security audits can aid in identifying and addressing vulnerabilities in the telehealth system's infrastructure [104].

11.5.5 Password attacks

These attacks involve guessing or stealing passwords to gain unauthorized access to telehealth organizations' systems and data. Password attacks can take various forms, such as brute-force attacks, dictionary attacks, and phishing scams that trick users into revealing their passwords [105]. The effect of password attacks in telehealth can be severe, leading to data breaches, financial losses, and reputational damage. Attackers can use stolen passwords to access EHRs, alter patient data, and even issue fraudulent prescriptions. Strong password policies can enforce complex passwords, regular password changes, and password length requirements [106].

11.5.6 Cross-site scripting (XSS) attack

These attacks are cyberattacks where an attacker puts malicious code on a legitimate website [67,77]. This lets them take over user sessions, steal sensitive information, or spread malware. In the telehealth industry, XSS attacks can lead to the exposure of patient data, the manipulation of medical records, and even the compromise of medical devices [78]. Telehealth organizations should implement security measures such as input validation, output encoding, and content security policies to prevent XSS attacks. Input validation involves validating user input and rejecting malicious code, while output encoding involves converting user input into a format that cannot be executed as code [14]. The content security policy restricts the execution of any scripts that are not explicitly allowed by the website owner. Another solution is to use web application firewalls (WAFs) that monitor incoming web traffic and block any requests that contain malicious code. Additionally, organizations should regularly update their web applications and software to ensure they are protected against the latest vulnerabilities that could be exploited by XSS attacks [79,80].

11.5.7 Domain name system (DNS) tunneling

DNS tunneling is a technique cybercriminals use to bypass firewalls and security systems by encoding data within DNS queries and responses [94]. DNS tunneling can exfiltrate sensitive patient data or execute malicious code within a telehealth network. The effects of DNS tunneling attacks can be severe, as they allow attackers to establish unauthorized communication channels and evade detection [95,96]. One possible solution to prevent DNS tunneling is configuring DNS servers to block outbound traffic to suspicious domains or IP addresses, implementing DNS security extensions (DNSSEC) to validate DNS responses, and conducting regular network traffic monitoring and analysis [81]. Furthermore, regular employee training and awareness campaigns can aid in the prevention of social engineering attacks that take advantage of DNS tunneling vulnerabilities [82].

11.5.8 Structured query language (SQL) injection

In the telehealth industry, this can lead to unauthorized access, manipulation, or theft of sensitive patient data, such as medical history, insurance information, and personal identifiers. SQL injection attacks can cause significant damage to telehealth organizations, including financial losses, reputational damage, and legal liabilities. Telehealth organizations can implement several security measures to prevent SQL injection attacks. One solution is using parameterized queries that are less vulnerable to SQL injection attacks. Also, telehealth organizations can employ web application firewalls that can detect and block SQL injection attacks [83,98].

11.5.9 Distributed denial-of-service (DDoS) attack

DDoS is a category of cyberattack in which multiple sources flood a network or website with traffic, making it unable to handle real traffic and causing it to crash [25,84]. In the telehealth sector, DDoS attacks can disrupt medical services, preventing patients from receiving the care they need and causing financial losses for telehealth providers. They should also conduct regular risk assessments to identify potential vulnerabilities and implement appropriate mitigation strategies [39]. Moreover, telehealth organizations can engage with third-party vendors specializing in DDoS protection and mitigation to ensure the security of their networks and systems [40].

11.5.10 Phishing

Phishing is a cyberattack in which the attacker sends fake emails or messages to people, usually pretending to be a trustworthy organization, to get sensitive information like usernames, passwords, and financial information [41]. Phishing attacks in the telehealth industry can cause significant data breaches, compromise patient information, and harm the organization's reputation. There are many ways to stop phishing attacks, such as training employees, using anti-phishing software, and using multifactor authentication. Telehealth workers are taught how to spot and report suspicious emails and messages as part of their training. Anti-phishing software is made to find and stop phishing attacks by blocking access to suspicious websites and messages [42]. By implementing these measures, telehealth organizations can protect their systems and prevent phishing attacks from occurring.

11.6 Main imperatives for refining cybersecurity in healthcare

Many cyber threats to the telehealth industry can put patient data at risk and mess up medical services. Identify and rank critical assets. Telehealth organizations must identify and classify critical assets, such as patient data, medical devices, and critical infrastructure, to ensure they are well protected [43]. Develop and implement a cybersecurity framework: A cybersecurity framework helps organizations establish a structured approach to cybersecurity, including risk assessment, policies and procedures, and incident response plans [44]. Establish a strong security culture: A strong security culture involves training employees to recognize and report potential security threats, implementing security awareness programs, and regularly assessing and improving security practices. Implement robust access control: Access controls, such as multifactor authentication and privileged access management, help organizations limit access to sensitive data and systems and prevent unauthorized access [45].

Plans for responding to an incident: Make a complete plan for responding to an incident that includes clear roles and responsibilities, communication rules, and steps for getting services back up and running after an attack. Collaboration: Foster collaboration between telehealth organizations, government agencies, and cybersecurity experts to share information and best practices to improve overall cybersecurity in the industry [46].

11.6.1 Real-world telehealth data breaches

Telehealth data breaches are becoming a bigger problem in the modern world, and there have been a lot of real-life examples in the past few years. Unauthorized access, theft, or exposure of sensitive patient data, such as personal information and medical records, is involved in these breaches. The consequences of such violations can be severe, including financial losses, reputational damage, and even threats to patient safety [47,48].

Cybersecurity has become an increasingly important issue in the telehealth sector due to the vast amount of sensitive patient data stored in EHRs [49,51]. Telehealth providers must keep patient information private, accurate, and easy to access while ensuring their systems are safe from cyber threats. Unfortunately, despite different security measures that have been put in place, telehealth data breaches continue to happen [51]. This puts patient data at risk and could cost telehealth organizations money and hurt their reputation. Because of this, the telehealth industry needs to improve its cybersecurity measures to protect patient data.

With more people using technology and more health records being stored digitally, cyber threats to patient data have become a significant worry [52].

Telehealth records contain sensitive and valuable information, including personal identification details, medical history, and payment information, making them an attractive target for cybercriminals. Cybersecurity breaches in telehealth can have severe consequences, such as financial losses, reputational damage, and, most importantly, compromised patient care [53].

EHRs have many benefits, like better patient care, more efficient healthcare delivery, and easier access to patient information [54,55]. However, they also pose a significant cybersecurity risk. Telehealth data breaches have become more frequent in recent years, with cybercriminals targeting sensitive patient information such as names, addresses, social security numbers, medical history, and insurance details [56]. This has led to significant financial losses, reputational damage, and potential patient harm. As such, cybersecurity has become a crucial aspect of telehealth operations, and telehealth providers must take proactive steps to protect patient data from cyber threats [57–62]. Table 11.2 shows the actual medical data breaches with their reported details.

11.7 Telehealth infrastructure and data security threats

Telehealth systems are vulnerable to cyberattacks such as phishing, ransomware, and malware attacks, which can compromise patient data and disrupt critical infrastructure.

11.7.1 Cyberattacks

Addressing and mitigating cyberattacks in telehealth requires a comprehensive approach that includes regular security assessments, employee training, access control, data encryption, incident response planning, network segmentation, up-to-date technology, third-party vendor management, regulatory compliance, and continual monitoring [63–67]. Telehealth organizations must prioritize data security to protect patient data, infrastructure, and reputation. By implementing these measures, telehealth organizations can better prevent and respond to cyberattacks by lowering the risk of data breaches and other cyber threats [68].

11.7.2 Insider threats

Insider threats in telehealth can be lessened by putting in place strict access control policies, doing background checks and regular security checks on employees, giving all staff security training, and keeping an eye on system logs and network activities for signs of strange behavior [69]. Moreover, making patient data anonymous as much as possible can limit the amount of sensitive information that employees can see. Finally, telehealth organizations must maintain a culture of security awareness and encourage employees to report any suspicious behavior or potential security incidents [68]. By implementing these measures, telehealth organizations can reduce the risk of insider threats and protect patient data and privacy. Employees' or insiders' unauthorized access to sensitive patient data can lead to data breaches and compromise patient confidentiality.

Table 11.2 Telehealth data breaches

Date	Data breach	Impact (patients)	Compromised	Solution
September 2011	Tricare	5 million	Prescription information, lab tests, clinical notes, personal health data, phone numbers, addresses, names, social security numbers	Data encryption policies
April–June, 2014	Community Health Systems	4.5 million	Addresses, phone numbers, numbers, social security, birth dates, names	Teach employees to diagnose the threatening traits of malware injection attempts
July 2015	UCLA Health	4.5 million	Some medical data: identification number, health plan number, Medicaid number, social security numbers, dates of birth, names	Exhaustive investigation
August 2013	Advocate Health Care	4.03 million	Health insurance information, clinical information, demographic information, dates of birth, addresses, names	Physical security controls
July 2015	Medical Informatics Engineering	3.9 million	Birth statistics, names of children, medical conditions, doctor names, disability codes, diagnosis, lab results, social security numbers, dates of birth, email addresses	Monitor for sensitive data
July 2016	Newkirk Products	3.8 million	Invoice information, dates of birth, names of dependents, patient names, Medicaid ID number, and primary care provider information	Unceasingly scan servers for potential exploits.
August 2016	Banner Health	3.62 million	Information about the patient's health insurance, doctor appointments, social security number, birth date, address, and name	regular security rating risk and assessment monitoring
February 2022	Morley	521,046	Information about health insurance, treatment, medical diagnosis, client ID number, date of birth, social security number, addresses, and name	Data breach security controls

March, 2022	L'Assurance Maladie	510,000	Level of reimbursement, GP details, social security numbers, dates of birth, names	Data leak detection solution
February 2022	ARcare	345,000	Health insurance information, condition information, medical diagnosis information Financial account information, social security numbers; names	Third-party risk mitigation strategy
July 2022	One Touch Point	2.6 million	Patient medical records, diagnosis codes, health assessment test results, service descriptions and dates, Employee IDs, patient demographics	Sensitive patient data protection policies
May 2020	Trinity Health	3.3 million	Certain financial information, lab results, medical record numbers, vaccination addresses; telehealth provider; date and types of health care, full names	The consciousness of the ransomware attack sequence
March 2022	Shields Telehealth Group	2 million	Diagnosis Information, Patient IDs, medical record numbers, and full names Insurance numbers, Social Security numbers	A zero-trust approach
January 2022	Broward Health	1.3 million	Medical data, insurance information, driver's license numbers, birth dates, addresses, and names	Protect all privileged access supervision

11.7.3 Third-party breach

To mitigate the risk of a third-party breach in the telehealth industry, it is essential for telehealth organizations to meticulously screen and choose vendors and partners with a proven track record of data security. Contracts with third-party vendors must contain specific language detailing data security requirements and expectations [69,70]. Regular security assessments of third-party vendors by telehealth organizations should be conducted to ensure appropriate security measures are implemented.

Additionally, telehealth organizations must only share the required data for their services to limit the data shared with third-party vendors. They should contemplate using data encryption and other security measures when transmitting data [71]. Telehealth organizations must have a well-formulated plan to quickly respond to and investigate potential third-party breaches and notify patients who might be impacted [72]. By implementing these measures, telehealth organizations can significantly lower the risk of third-party violations, thereby preserving the security and privacy of patient data. Telehealth organizations often share patient data with third-party vendors or partners, who can become targets of cyberattacks or data misuse.

11.7.4 Physical security breach

Access control measures, like badge systems, biometric authentication, and security cameras, can stop physical security breaches in telehealth [73]. Only authorized personnel should have access to sensitive areas such as data centers and medication storage in telehealth organizations. Regular security assessments of physical infrastructure, including doors, locks, and windows, should be conducted to identify and address vulnerabilities [74]. Also, medical staff should receive training on physical security best practices and be encouraged to report any suspicious behavior or potential security incidents. Telehealth organizations can reduce the risk of physical security breaches by taking these measures and protecting patient data, infrastructure, and reputation.

11.7.5 Data theft

Telehealth organizations should also have policies and procedures for managing and monitoring user access to patient data, including regular reviews of user access logs and identifying unauthorized access attempts [93]. Furthermore, telehealth organizations should conduct regular security risk assessments and penetration testing to identify and address potential vulnerabilities in their systems [92]. Staff should receive regular training on data security best practices, including recognizing and reporting potential security incidents. Telehealth organizations should have an incident response plan to quickly respond to and investigate potential data theft incidents and notify affected patients if necessary [75,93].

11.7.6 Regulatory non-compliance

To mitigate the risk of regulatory non-compliance in healthcare, organizations must establish and maintain robust compliance programs that adhere to applicable laws, regulations, and industry standards [76]. This includes regular training for staff on compliance policies and procedures and appointing a designated compliance officer to oversee the program. Telehealth organizations must also do internal audits and assessments regularly to find any possible compliance gaps and take quick action to fix them [77]. Additionally, telehealth organizations should monitor regulatory changes and updates, adjust their compliance programs accordingly, and document all compliance-related activities.

11.7.7 Lack of encryption

Organizations must implement encryption measures for sensitive patient data in transit and at rest to mitigate the risk of data breaches caused by a lack of encryption in healthcare. This can be achieved using industry-standard encryption technologies and the following best practices for encryption key management [78]. Also, telehealth organizations should conduct regular vulnerability assessments and penetration testing to identify weaknesses in their encryption systems and promptly address them [14]. Staff should also receive training on encryption best practices, including how to encrypt properly and decrypt data. Telehealth organizations should have an incident response plan to respond to and investigate any potential encryption-related security incidents quickly and, if necessary, notify affected patients [79].

11.7.8 Outdated technology

Outdated technology in telehealth can be solved through various methods, such as upgrading existing systems, investing in new technologies, and implementing better training and education programs for telehealth professionals [80]. Upgrades can include software updates, hardware replacements, and improvements in system integration to enhance efficiency and accuracy. Investing in new technologies can involve adopting modern telehealth solutions such as EHRs, telemedicine, and AI-assisted diagnostics [95]. Telehealth professionals can be trained to use and integrate new technologies into their practices effectively. By combining these approaches, telehealth organizations can improve patient outcomes, reduce costs, and increase overall efficiency in care delivery [96].

11.7.9 Human error

Telehealth errors can be solved by implementing standardized procedures and protocols, increasing communication and teamwork, enhancing training and education programs, and utilizing technology to assist decision-making processes [81]. Standardized methods and protocols can help minimize errors and ensure consistency in patient care. Communication and teamwork can help reduce misunderstandings and increase collaboration among telehealth professionals [97]. Training and education programs can provide telehealth workers with the necessary skills and knowledge to perform their jobs effectively and efficiently [96]. Technologies such as decision support systems and automated alerts can assist in identifying potential errors and alerting telehealth workers to take appropriate

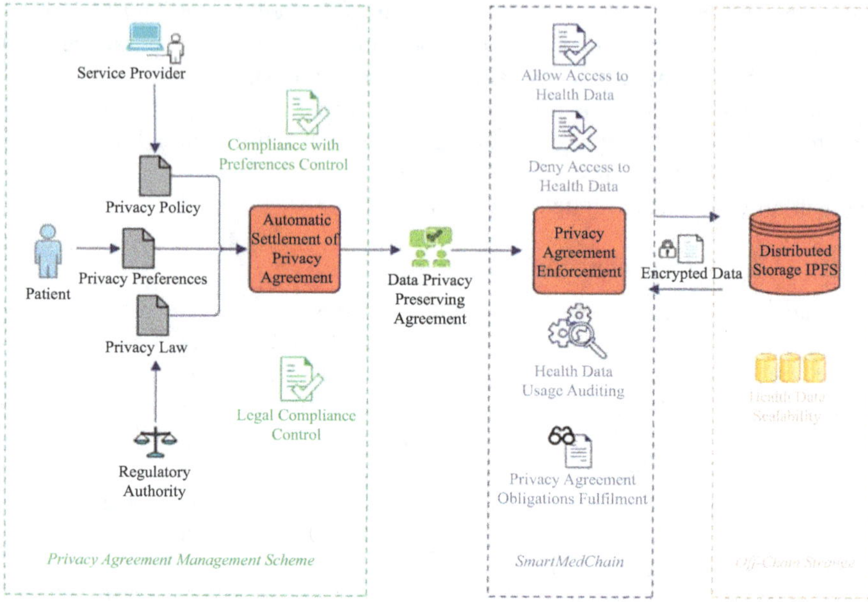

Figure 11.3 Proposed model summary

action. By combining these approaches, telehealth organizations can improve patient safety, reduce medical errors, and improve the quality of care provided [97].

11.7.10 Cloud security

Telehealth cloud security can be solved through various methods, such as implementing robust encryption protocols, utilizing multifactor authentication, conducting regular security assessments and audits, and maintaining strict access controls [81]. Robust encryption protocols can help protect sensitive data being transmitted or stored in the cloud. Multifactor authentication can provide an extra layer of security to prevent unauthorized access to cloud systems [82]. Regular security assessments and audits can help identify potential vulnerabilities and allow for timely remediation of any issues. Strict access controls can limit who has access to sensitive information and can help prevent data breaches [83,98]. We present a graphical framework inspired by Blockchain technology, and this approach demonstrates how privacy can be attained amidst patients' better quality of services, as in Figures 11.3 and 11.4.

11.8 The future of cybersecurity in telehealth

The telehealth industry increasingly relies on digital technology to manage sensitive patient data, including EHRs, insurance information, and personal details. As

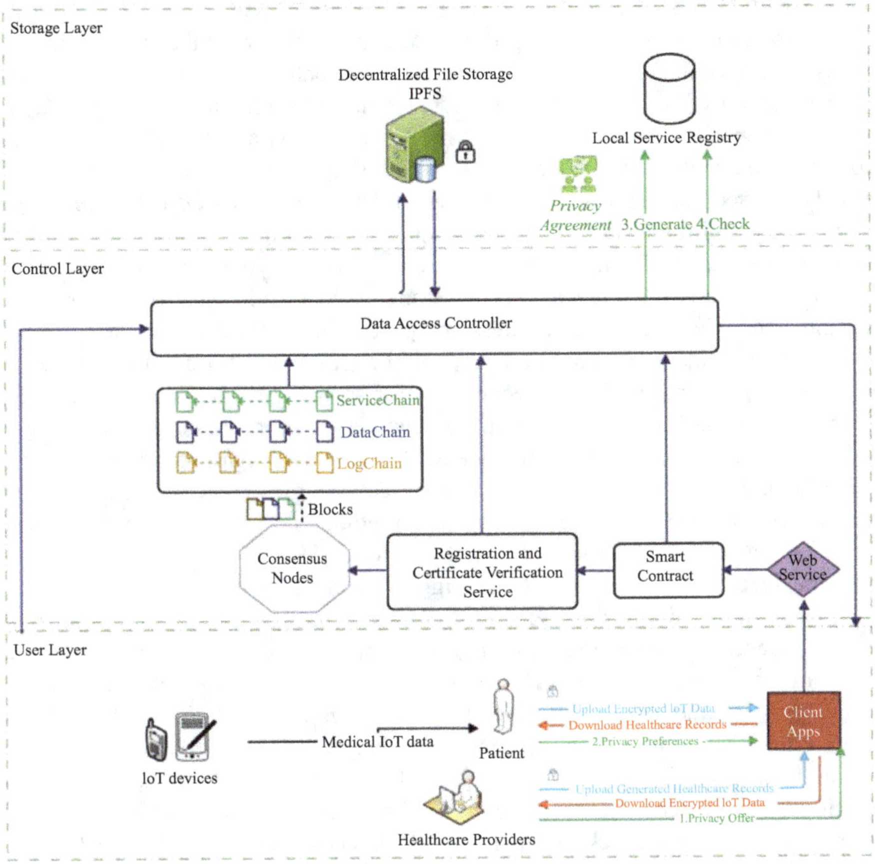

Figure 11.4 Proposed graphical secure privacy for telehealth system; it includes mainly three layers, namely, the user layer, control layer, and storage layer

such, cybersecurity has become a critical concern for telehealth providers, with data breaches and cybersecurity on the rise [98]. One research direction in cybersecurity in the current telehealth system is developing new tools and techniques to detect and prevent cyber threats [84,85]. This includes developing advanced firewalls and intrusion detection systems that can identify and respond to potential attacks in real time. Researchers are also exploring ML and AI to identify patterns and anomalies in network traffic that could indicate a possible attack.

Another research direction in cybersecurity in the current telehealth system is exploring the human factor in cybersecurity. For example, many data breaches occur due to human error, such as weak passwords, phishing scams, or employees failing to use social engineering tactics [86]. This includes developing new training materials, such as interactive simulations and games, to help employees better understand the risks and consequences of cyber threats [87]. Additionally, researchers are exploring behavioral analytics to identify potential insider threats, such as employees engaging in risky or suspicious behavior.

Developing effective methods for identifying and mitigating emerging cyber threats in telehealth systems. Investigating the role of AI and ML in detecting and responding to cybersecurity threats in telehealth systems [88]. Developing effective methods for securely storing and sharing patient data in cloud-based telehealth systems, developing new tools and techniques for securing mobile health applications and devices [89]. Studying the effectiveness of cybersecurity training and education programs for telehealth professionals and identifying the best practices for improving cybersecurity awareness and procedures. Investigating the impact of cybersecurity incidents on patient safety and developing risk mitigation strategies [90]. Developing new tools and techniques for securing medical devices and IoT systems in telehealth settings, developing new methods for assessing and managing third-party cybersecurity risks in telehealth systems, Investigating the effectiveness of Blockchain and other distributed ledger technologies for enhancing cybersecurity in telehealth systems Developing new methods for integrating cybersecurity and patient safety practices into telehealth systems [89].

Cybersecurity is now one of the biggest worries in the telehealth industry, which relies increasingly on digital technology to handle sensitive patient information. Telehealth providers, insurance companies, and patients have been the targets of data breaches and cyberattacks. The focus of research has been on coming up with and improving ways to protect against these threats [90]. In the current telehealth system, one direction for cybersecurity research is to make new tools and methods to find and stop cyber threats. Advanced firewalls, intrusion detection systems, security information, and event management systems are being made to find possible attacks in real-time [91]. These systems use algorithms for ML to look for patterns in network traffic that could be signs of an attack.

Another research direction in cybersecurity is exploring the human factor in cybersecurity. Studies have found that human error is a leading cause of data breaches, with employees being the weakest link in cybersecurity. Employee training and awareness programs are being developed as part of the research to help prevent these types of incidents. Interactive simulations, games, and behavioral analytics are designed to help employees better understand the risks and consequences of cyber threats [99].

Blockchain technology is being explored to enhance cybersecurity in healthcare. Blockchain technology provides a secure, decentralized platform for storing and sharing patient data. Researchers are exploring the use of Blockchain to improve data privacy, security, and interoperability in telehealth [100]. Blockchain can provide a secure and transparent way to share patient data between telehealth providers, reducing the risk of data breaches.

Telehealth providers are increasingly using cloud services to store and manage patient data. However, cloud services bring new security risks, such as data breaches, loss, and service interruptions [101,102]. The research focuses on finding new ways to make cloud services more secure. These include secure data encryption, access control, and identity management. These steps are meant to keep patient data safe while it is stored in the cloud [103]. Differential privacy is one algorithm that can help protect sensitive data while letting it be analyzed helpfully. In addition, these algorithms can stop patients from being reidentified in data sets.

Incident response and recovery are also important research areas in cybersecurity in healthcare. Despite our best efforts to prevent cyber threats, data breaches and cybersecurity breaches can still occur [104]. As a result, researchers are exploring new approaches to incident response and recovery, including developing new tools and techniques for detecting and responding to cyber threats and improving backup and recovery systems to help minimize the impact of cyber incidents [105]. These technologies can also enhance incident response and recovery by automating specific tasks and providing real-time analysis of cyber threats.

Standards and rules for cybersecurity in telehealth care are also being worked on as part of the research. Standards and regulations allow telehealth providers to meet the minimum cybersecurity requirements [106,107]. The development of standards and rules can help to ensure that patient data remains secure and that telehealth providers are held accountable for breaches and cybersecurity. As the use of digital technology continues to grow in telehealth, cybersecurity is an essential issue. Research is focused on developing and improving cybersecurity measures to protect against data breaches.

11.9 Lessons learned and future directions

The incorporation of AI and Blockchain technology can significantly enhance the security of telehealth systems. AI can be utilized to detect and respond to potential security threats in real time, allowing prompt action to be taken to mitigate the risk of data breaches or cyberattacks. This technology can also assist in identifying patterns and trends in data that may indicate a security threat, allowing for proactive measures to be taken to prevent a breach. Similarly, Blockchain technology can provide a tamper-proof and decentralized method of securing patient data. By using a distributed health system, patient data can be stored in a secure and immutable manner, reducing the risk of unauthorized access or modification. This can significantly improve patient privacy and confidentiality in telehealth systems, ensuring that sensitive information is only accessible to authorized individuals.

However, the implementation of AI and Blockchain technology in telehealth systems requires careful planning and consideration. Organizations must ensure that these technologies are appropriately integrated into their existing infrastructure and that their use complies with relevant regulatory frameworks. Additionally, staff members must be provided adequate training to ensure they understand how to effectively use these technologies.

The implementation of AI and Blockchain technology in telehealth systems requires a comprehensive and well-planned approach. Organizations must ensure that these technologies are appropriately integrated into their existing infrastructure, considering data security, network architecture, and data interoperability factors. Additionally, organizations must ensure that AI and Blockchain technology use complies with relevant regulatory frameworks, such as HIPAA and general data protection regulation, to avoid potential legal or ethical issues.

Moreover, organizations must provide adequate training to staff members to ensure that they understand how to effectively use these technologies. This includes training on properly handling patient data, identifying potential security threats, and using AI and Blockchain technology in day-to-day operations. Proper training can help ensure that staff members are able to effectively utilize these technologies, reducing the risk of errors or breaches.

Collaboration among industry stakeholders will be critical to the future success of AI and Blockchain technology in telehealth systems. As these technologies continue to evolve, it will be necessary for healthcare providers, technology vendors, and regulators to work together to develop common standards and best practices for cybersecurity. This collaboration can help ensure that telehealth systems are secure and that patient data is protected. Additionally, industry stakeholders must remain vigilant and continuously evaluate and improve the security of telehealth systems as new threats emerge, ensuring that patient data is always secure and protected.

The integration of AI and Blockchain technology in telehealth systems is expected to grow in the coming years. As healthcare organizations continue to embrace digital transformation and telehealth services, there is a growing need for robust and secure cybersecurity measures. AI and Blockchain technology are seen as critical solutions to these challenges, offering a range of benefits such as real-time threat detection, tamper-proof data storage, and decentralized data management.

AI algorithms may become even more sophisticated, allowing for more accurate threat detection and response. Similarly, Blockchain technology may evolve to incorporate additional features such as smart contracts and digital identities, further enhancing data security and privacy. As these technologies continue to evolve, it will be necessary for healthcare providers, technology vendors, and regulators to work together to develop common standards and best practices for cybersecurity. This collaboration can help ensure that telehealth systems are secure and that patient data is protected. Additionally, industry stakeholders must remain vigilant and continuously evaluate and improve the security of telehealth systems as new threats emerge, ensuring that patient data is always secure and protected.

The integration of Blockchain technology and AI in telehealth systems may also lead to increased patient empowerment and engagement. As patient data becomes more secure and easily accessible through telehealth systems, patients may be more willing to share their health information and become more engaged in their own care. Additionally, AI algorithms can help personalize care by analyzing patient data to identify individual health risks and needs. Blockchain technology can also enable patients to have more control over their health data, allowing them to grant or revoke access to their records as needed. As these technologies continue to evolve and become more widespread, patient empowerment and engagement may become critical drivers of the adoption of telehealth services. Ultimately, the integration of AI and Blockchain technology in telehealth systems has the potential to revolutionize the healthcare industry by improving patient outcomes, reducing costs, and enhancing the overall quality of care.

11.10 Conclusion

Cybersecurity concerns have grown as the telehealth industry has become more dependent on digital technology to manage patient data. Because of this cybersecurity, researchers are looking into different ways to protect against cyber threats and data breaches. Medical devices are one of the areas of focus for cybersecurity. Integrating medical devices with telehealth networks has rendered them vulnerable to cyber threats. Researchers are exploring novel ways to secure medical devices by implementing encryption, access control, and authentication measures. The goal is to protect the devices' integrity and prevent unauthorized access to sensitive patient data. In addition, telehealth organizations can reduce the risk of human error and data breaches by fostering a security culture. As evidenced by regulations, legal and regulatory compliance is critical to telehealth cybersecurity. In conclusion, cybersecurity is crucial to the telehealth industry, given its growing dependence on digital technology.

References

[1] J. Xu, K. Xue, S. Li, and H. Tian, "Healthchain: a blockchain-based privacy preserving scheme for large-scale health data," *IEEE Internet of Things Journal*, vol. 6, pp. 8770–8781, 2019, https://doi.org/10.1109/JIOT.2019.2923525.

[2] D. El Majdoubi, H. El Bakkali, and S. Sadki, "SmartMedChain: a blockchain-based privacy-preserving smart telehealth framework," *Journal of Telehealth Engineering*, 2021, https://doi.org/10.1155/2021/4145512.

[3] S. Silvestri, S. Islam, S. Papastergiou, C. Tzagkarakis, and M. Ciampi, "A machine learning approach for the NLP-based analysis of cyber threats and vulnerabilities of the telehealth ecosystem," *Sensors*, vol. 23, no. 2, pp. 651, 2023, https://doi.org/10.3390/s23020651.

[4] J. Lamba and E. Jain, "Advanced cyber security and internet of things for digital transformations of the Indian telehealth sector," *Research Anthology on Convergence of Blockchain, Internet of Things, and Security*, IGI Global, 2023, pp. 1037–1056, https://doi.org/10.4018/978-1-6684-7132-6.ch055.

[5] Y. Wu, L. Wu, and H. Cai, "Reinforced practical Byzantine fault tolerance consensus protocol for cyber physical systems," *Computer Communications*, vol. 203, pp. 238–247, https://doi.org/10.1016/j.comcom.2023.03.016.

[6] A. Awaludin, W. Sulistyadi, and A. F. Chandra, "Analysis of attacks and cybersecurity in the health sector during a pandemic COVID-19: scoping review," *Journal of Social Science*, vol. 4, no. 1, pp. 62–70, 2023, https://doi.org/10.46799/jss.v4i1.512.

[7] A. R. Javed, W. Ahmed, S. Pandya, P. K. Maddikunta, M. Alazab, and T. R. Gadekallu, "A survey of explainable artificial intelligence for smart cities," *Electronics*, vol. 12, no. 4, pp. 1020, 2023, https://doi.org/10.3390/electronics12041020.

[8] R. Montasari, "Internet of things and artificial intelligence in national security: applications and issues," In *Countering Cyberterrorism: The Confluence of Artificial Intelligence, Cyber Forensics and Digital Policing in US and UK National Cybersecurity*, 27–56, 2023. Cham: Springer International Publishing, https://doi.org/10.1007/978-3-031-21920-7_3.

[9] M. Mijwil, M. Aljanabi, and A. H. Ali, "ChatGPT: exploring the role of cybersecurity in the protection of medical information," *Mesopotamian Journal of Cybersecurity*, vol. 2023, pp. 18–21, 2023. https://doi.org/10.58496/MJCS/2023/004.

[10] G. Memmi, "Cyber attacks in healthcare: why they matter and how to defend against them," *British Journal of Telehealth Management*, vol. 29, no. 1, pp. 8–11, 2023, https://doi.org/10.12968/bjhc.2022.0134.

[11] M. Shukla, F. Ziya, S. Arun, and S. P. Singh, "Cyber security techniques management," *Holistic Approach to Quantum Cryptography in Cyber Security*, CRC Press, pp. 155–178, 2023, eBook ISBN9781003296034.

[12] A. U. Patel, C. L. Williams, S. N. Hart, *et al.*, "Cybersecurity and information assurance for the clinical laboratory," *The Journal of Applied Laboratory Medicine*, vol. 8, no. 1, pp. 145–161, 2023, https://doi.org/10.1093/jalm/jfac119.

[13] R. B. Claytor, M. D. Epstein, and G. Cox, "Cybersecurity: prevent, detect, respond," *Aesthetic Surgery Journal*, vol. 43, no. 3. Oxford University Press US, pp. 389–391, 2023, https://doi.org/10.1093/asj/sjac323.

[14] M. Paul, L. Maglaras, M. A. Ferrag, and I. AlMomani, "Digitization of telehealth sector: a study on privacy and security concerns," *ICT Express*, 2023. https://doi.org/10.1016/j.icte.2023.02.007.

[15] G. L. Tortorella, A. Prashar, J. Antony, F. S. Fogliatto, V. Gonzalez, and M. Godinho Filho, "Industry 4.0 adoption for healthcare supply chain performance during COVID-19 pandemic in Brazil and India: the mediating role of resilience abilities development," *Operations Management Research*, pp. 1–7, 2023 https://doi.org/10.1007/s12063-023-00366-z.

[16] P. Kanagala, "Effective cyber security system to secure optical data based on deep learning approach for telehealth application," *Optik*, vol. 272, pp. 170315, 2023. https://doi.org/10.1016/j.ijleo.2022.170315.

[17] M. D. Kalamkar and R. Prasad, "Impact of the COVID-19 pandemic on cyber security issues in the telehealth domain: a scoping review," *Cyber Security Threats and Challenges Facing Human Life*, pp. 24–41, 2023. https://doi.org/10.2196/29877.

[18] M. Parker, "Managing threats to health data and information: toward security," *Health Information Exchange*, Elsevier, 2023, pp. 149–196. https://doi.org/10.1016/B978-0-323-90802-3.00016-2.

[19] S. K. Shandilya, B. J. Choi, A. Kumar, and S. Upadhyay, "Modified firefly optimization algorithm-based IDS for nature-inspired cybersecurity," *Processes*, vol. 11, no. 3, pp. 715, 2023, https://doi.org/10.3390/pr11030715.

[20] S. Pahlevanynejad, S. R. Niakan Kalhori, M. R. Katigari, and R. H. Eshpala, "Personalized mobile health for elderly home care: a systematic review of benefits and challenges," *International Journal of Telemedicine and Applications*, 2023, https://doi.org/10.1155/2023/5390712.

[21] S. Khezr, M. Moniruzzaman, A. Yassine, and R. Benlamri, "Blockchain technology in healthcare: A comprehensive review and directions for future research," *Applied Sciences*, vol. 9, no. 9, pp. 1736, 2019, https://doi.org/10.3390/app9091736.

[22] W. Shafik and S. M., "Unmanned Aerial vehicles Analysis to Social Networks Performance," *The CSI Journal on Computer Science and Engineering*, vol. 18, no. 2, pp. 24–31, 2021.

[23] Z. F. Khan, and S. R. Alotaibi, "Applications of artificial intelligence and big data analytics in m-health: a healthcare system perspective," *Journal of Healthcare Engineering*, pp. 1–5, 2020, https://doi.org/10.1155/2020/8894694.

[24] Y. Tian, S. Wang, J. Xiong, R. Bi, Z. Zhou, and M. Z. A. Bhuiyan, "Robust and privacy-preserving decentralized deep federated learning training: focusing on digital telehealth applications," *IEEE/ACM Transactions on Computational Biology and Bioinformatics*, 2023. https://doi.org/10.1109/TCBB.2023.3243932.

[25] H. Miriam, D. Doreen, D. Dahiya, and C. R. Rene Robin, "Secured cyber security algorithm for telehealth system using blockchain technology," *Intelligent Automation & Soft Computing*, vol. 35, no. 2, 2023, http://dx.doi.org/10.32604/iasc.2023.028850.

[26] A Gerodimos, L. Maglaras, M. A. Ferrag, N. Ayres, and I. Kantzavelou, "IoT: communication protocols and security threats," *Internet of Things and Cyber-Physical Systems*, 2023, https://doi.org/10.1016/j.iotcps.2022.12.003

[27] J. Penfold, "The growing risk of cyber attacks in the NHS," *British Journal of Telehealth Management*, vol. 29, no. 1, pp. 5–7, 2023, https://doi.org/10.12968/bjhc.2022.0132.

[28] S. Gunasekaran, S. Shanmugam, D. P. Rajan, and P. Rontala, "Blockchain technology-enabled telehealth IoT to increase security and privacy using fog computing," *Machine Learning, Blockchain, and Cyber Security in Smart Environments*, Chapman and Hall/CRC, 2023, pp. 127–144, eBook ISBN9781003240310.

[29] W. Shafik, and S. M. Matinkhah, "Privacy issues in social Web of things," *5th International Conference on Web Research*, Tehran, Iran, pp. 208–214, 2019. IEEE, https://doi.org/10.1109/ICWR.2019.8765254.

[30] G. Neelamegam and P. Marikkannu, "Health data deduplication using window chunking-signature encryption in cloud," *Intelligent Automation & Soft Computing*, vol. 36, no. 1, 2023.

[31] R. Sathya Prabha, K. Kanagasabapathi, K. Sajeeth, and M. Aishwarya, "Health information sharing in cloud environment using modular encryption standard," *Recent Developments in Electronics and Communication Systems*, IOS Press, 2023, pp. 64–70, https://doi.org/10.3233/ATDE221238.

[32] H. H. Goldman, J. Porcino, G. Divita, *et al.*, "Informatics research on mental health functioning: decision support for the social security administration disability program," *Psychiatric Services*, vol. 74, no. 1, pp. 56–62, 2023, https://doi.org/10.1176/appi.ps.202200056.

[33] Y. Jun, A. Craig, W. Shafik, and L. Sharif, "Artificial intelligence application in cybersecurity and cyberdefense," *Wireless Communications and Mobile Computing*, 2021, https://doi.org/10.1176/appi.ps.202200056.

[34] S. Pahlevanynejad, S. R. Niakan Kalhori, M. R. Katigari, and R. H. Eshpala, "Personalized mobile health for elderly home care: a systematic review of benefits and challenges," *Journal of Telemedicine and Applications*, 2023, https://doi.org/10.1155/2023/5390712.

[35] P. Verma and D. S. Gupta, "A pairing-free data authentication and aggregation mechanism for Intelligent Telehealth System," *Computer Communications*, vol. 198, pp. 282–296, 2023, https://doi.org/10.1016/j.comcom.2022.12.009.

[36] R. Jiang, S. Han, Y. Yu, and W. Ding, "An access control model for medical big data based on clustering and risk," *Information Sciences*, vol. 621, pp. 691–707, 2023, https://doi.org/10.1016/j.ins.2022.11.102.

[37] W. Shafik, S. M. Matinkhah and M. Ghasemzadeh, "Theoretical understanding of deep learning in UAV biomedical engineering technologies analysis," *SN Computer Science*, vol. 1, no. 6, pp. 1–13, 2020, https://doi.org/10.1007/s42979-020-00323-8.

[38] F. Shokoor, W. Shafik, and S. M. Matinkhah, "Overview of 5G & beyond security," *EAI Endorsed Transactions on Internet of Things*, vol. 8, no. 30, 2022, http://dx.doi.org/10.4108/eetiot.v8i30.1624.

[39] L. Zhao, D. Zhu, W. Shafik, *et al.*, "Artificial intelligence analysis in cyber domain: a review," *International Journal of Distributed Sensor Networks*, vol. 18, no. 4, 2022, https://doi.org/10.1177/15501329221084882.

[40] J. Kaberuka and C. Johnson, "A case study in the application of STPA-sec and CHASSIS for socio-technical cyber security risk management in health care from developing nations," *Intelligent Sustainable Systems: Selected Papers of WorldS4*, vol. 1, Springer, pp. 383–390, 2023, https://doi.org/10.1007/978-981-19-7660-5_33.

[41] A. Renee Staton and M. Kielty, "A lurking threat: counselor practices to guard against cyber threats," *Journal of Mental Health Counseling*, vol. 45, no. 1, pp. 20–33, 2023, https://doi.org/10.17744/mehc.45.1.02.

[42] T. Manoj, K. Makkithaya, and V. G. Narendra, "A trusted IoT data sharing and secure oracle based access for agricultural production risk management," *Computers and Electronics in Agriculture*, vol. 204, pp. 107544, 2023, https://doi.org/10.1016/j.compag.2022.107544.

[43] A. Buzdugan and G. Căpăţână, "The trends in cybersecurity maturity models," *Education, Research and Business Technologies: Proceedings of 21st International Conference on Informatics in Economy*, pp. 217–228, 2023, https://doi.org/10.1007/978-981-19-6755-9_18.

[44] G. Zuccotti, and V. Calcaterra, "Telemedicine and E-Health: an innovative challenge in pediatric care," *International Journal of Environmental Research and Public Health*, vol. 20, no. 30, p. 2091, 2023. https://doi.org/10.3390/ijerph20032091.

[45] N. Omar, N. N. Nazirun, B. Vijayam B, A. A. Wahab, and H. A. Bahuri, "Diabetes subtypes classification for personalized health care: a review," *Artificial Intelligence Review*, vol. 56, no. 3, pp. 2697–2721, 2023, https://doi.org/10.1007/s10462-022-10202-8.

[46] H. Arimura, M. Soufi, H. Kamezawa, K. Ninomiya, and M. Yamada, Radiomics with artificial intelligence for precision medicine in radiation therapy. *Journal of Radiation Research*, vol. 60, pp. 150–157, 2019, https://doi.org/10.1093/jrr/rry077.

[47] U. Schmidt-Erfurth, A. Sadeghipour, B. S. Gerendas, S. M. Waldstein, and H. Bogunović, "Artificial intelligence in retina," *Progress in Retinal and Eye Research*, vol. 67, pp. 1–29, 2018, https://doi.org/10.1016/j.preteyeres.2018.07.004

[48] S. Kolluri, J. Lin, R. Liu, Y Zhang, and W. Zhang, "Machine learning and artificial intelligence in pharmaceutical research and development: a review," *The AAPS Journal*, vol. 24, p. 19, 2022, https://doi.org/10.1208/s12248-021-00644-3.

[49] S. Harrer, P. Shah, B. Antony, and J. Hu, "Artificial intelligence for clinical trial design," *Trends in Pharmacological Sciences*, vol. 40, pp. 577–591, 2019, https://doi.org/10.1016/j.tips.2019.05.005.

[50] X. Yang, Y. Wang, R. Byrne, G. Schneider, and S. Yang, "Concepts of artificial intelligence for computer-assisted drug discovery," *Chemical Reviews*, vol. 119, pp. 10520–10594, 2019, https://doi.org/10.1021/acs.chemrev.8b00728.

[51] A. Lusci, G. Pollastri, and P. Baldi, "Deep architectures and deep learning in chemoinformatics: the prediction of aqueous solubility for drug-like molecules," *Journal of Chemical Information and Modeling*, vol. 53, pp. 1563–1575, 2013, https://doi.org/10.1021/ci400187y.

[52] H. Y. Cheng, Y. C. Wu, M. H. Lin, *et al.*, "Applying machine learning models with an ensemble approach for accurate real-time influenza forecasting in Taiwan: development and validation study," *Journal of Medical Internet Research*, vol. 22, p. e15394, 2020, https://doi.org/10.2196/15394.

[53] M. Marini, N. Chokani, and R. S. Abhari, "COVID-19 epidemic in Switzerland: growth prediction and containment strategy using artificial intelligence and big data," *medRxiv*, 2020. https://doi.org/10.1101/2020.03.30.20047472.

[54] M. Akhtar, M. U. G. Kraemer, and L. M. A. Gardner, "Dynamic neural network model for predicting risk of Zika in real time," *BMC Medicine*, vol. 17, p. 171, 2019. https://doi.org/10.1186/s12916-019-1389-3.

[55] M.E. Celebi, C. Barata, A. Halpern, P. Tschandl, M. Combalia, and Y. Liu, "Guest Editorial Skin Image Analysis in the Age of Deep Learning," *IEEE Journal of Biomedical and Health Informatics*, vol. 27, no. 1, pp. 143–144, 2023.

[56] Y. Jin, C. Qin, Y. Huang, W. Zhao, and C. Liu, "Multi-domain modeling of atrial fibrillation detection with twin attentional convo-lutional long short-term memory neural networks," *Knowledge-Based Systems*, vol. 193, p. 105460, 2020, https://doi.org/10.1016/j.knosys.2019.105460.

[57] N. Shen, "AI regulation in health care: how Washington state can conquer the new territory of AI regulation," *Seattle Journal of Technology, Environmental & Innovation Law*, vol. 13, no. 1, 2023, https://digitalcommons.law.seattleu.edu/sjteil/vol13/iss1/5.

[58] H. Wang, D. Zhang, S. Ding, Z. Gao, J. Feng, and S. Wan, "Rib segmentation algorithm for X-ray image based on unpaired sample augmentation and multi-scale network," *Neural Computing and Applications*, pp. 1–15, 2021, https://doi.org/10.1007/s00521-021-06546-x.

[59] S. S. Ahmad, S. Khan, and M. A. Kamal, "What is blockchain technology and its significance in the current telehealth system? A brief insight," *Current Pharmaceutical Design*, vol. 25, no. 12, pp. 1402–1408, 2019, https://doi.org/10.2174/1381612825666190620150302.

[60] H. M. Hussien, S. M. Yasin, N. I. Udzir, M. I. Ninggal, and S. Salman, "Blockchain technology in the telehealth industry: trends and opportunities," *Journal of Industrial Information Integration*, vol. 22, pp. 100217, 2021, https://doi.org/10.1016/j.jii.2021.100217.

[61] P. Singh, and N. Singh, "Blockchain with IoT and AI: a review of agriculture and healthcare," *International Journal of Applied Evolutionary Computation*, vol. 11, no. 4, pp. 13–27, 2020, https://doi.org/10.4018/ijaec.2020100102.

[62] M. Y. Jabarulla, and H. N. Lee, "A blockchain and artificial intelligence-based, patient-centric telehealth system for combating the COVID-19 pandemic: opportunities and applications," In *Telehealth 2021*, vol. 9, no. 8, pp. 1019, 2021, https://doi.org/10.3390/healthcare9081019.

[63] P. Sharma, S. Namasudra, R. G. Crespo, J. Parra-Fuente, and M. C. Trivedi, "EHDHE: enhancing security of telehealth documents in IoT-enabled digital telehealth ecosystems using blockchain," *Information Sciences*, vol. 629, pp. 703–718, 2023, https://doi.org/10.1016/j.ins.2023.01.148.

[64] M. V. Baysal, Ö. Özcan-Top, and A. Betin-Can, "Blockchain technology applications in the health domain: a multivocal literature review," *The Journal of Supercomputing*, vol. 79, no. 3, pp. 3112–3156, 2023, https://doi.org/10.1007/s11227-022-04772-1.

[65] Z. Wenhua, F. Qamar, T. A. Abdali, R. Hassan, S. T. Jafri, and Q. N. Nguyen, "Blockchain technology: security issues, telehealth applications, challenges and future trends," *Electronics*, vol. 12, no. 3, pp. 546, 2023, https://doi.org/10.3390/electronics12030546.

[66] T. Nguyen, and T. Nguyen Gia, "Novel smart homecare IoT system with edge-AI and blockchain," In *Blockchain and Its Applications in Industry 4.0*, 293–317, 2023. Singapore: Springer Nature Singapore. https://doi.org/10.1007/978-981-19-8730-4_10.

[67] H. Sakly, M. Said, A. A. Al-Sayed, C. Loussaief, R. Sakly, and J. Seekins, "Blockchain technologies for internet of medical things (BIoMT) based telehealth systems: a new paradigm for COVID-19 pandemic. In *Trends of Artificial Intelligence and Big Data for E-Health*, pp. 139–165, 2023. Cham: Springer International Publishing, https://doi.org/10.1007/978-3-031-11199-0_8.

[68] A. Alabdulatif, M. Al Asqah, T. Moulahi, and S. Zidi, "Leveraging artificial intelligence in blockchain-based E-Health for safer decision making framework," *Applied Sciences*, vol. 13, no. 2, pp. 1035, 2023, https://doi.org/10.3390/app13021035.

[69] A. I. Taloba, A. Elhadad, A. Rayan, *et al.*, "A blockchain-based hybrid platform for multimedia data processing in IoT-Healthcare," *Alexandria Engineering Journal*, vol. 65, pp. 263–274, 2023,

[70] B. Rawat, A. S. Bist, D. Apriani, N. I. Permadi, and E. A. Nabila "AI based drones for security concerns in smart cities," *APTISI Transactions on Management (ATM)*, vol. 7, no. 2, pp. 125–130, 2023. https://doi.org/10.1080/10447318.2022.2041894.

[71] A. Goel, and S. Neduncheliyan, "An intelligent blockchain strategy for ecentralized telehealth framework," *Peer-to-Peer Networking and Applications*, 2023, https://doi.org/10.1007/s12083-022-01429-x.

[72] K. Pal, "Security implications of IoT applications with cryptography and blockchain technology in telehealth digital twin design," In *Digital Twins and Healthcare: Trends, Techniques, and Challenges*, pp. 229–252, 2023. IGI Global. https://doi.org/10.4018/978-1-6684-5925-6.ch015.

[73] W. Shafik and A. Tufail, "Energy optimization analysis on internet of things," In *Advanced Technology for Smart Environment and Energy*, 1–16, 2023. Cham: Springer International Publishing, https://doi.org/10.1007/978-3-031-25662-2_1.

[74] J. M. Roman-Belmonte, H. De la Corte-Rodriguez, and E. C. Rodriguez-Merchan, "Applications of blockchain technology in the COVID-19 era," In *Blockchain in Healthcare: From Disruption to Integration*, pp. 53–67, 2023. Cham: Springer International Publishing. https://doi.org/10.1007/978-3-031-14591-9_5.

[75] S. Raul, S. Das, C. Murty, and K. Devi, "A review on intelligent health care system using learning methods," *Recent Developments in Electronics and Communication Systems*, pp. 154–159, 2023. https://doi.org/10.3233/ATDE221251.

[76] A. Rejeb, K. Rejeb, H. Treiblmaier, *et al.*, "The Internet of Things (IoT) in healthcare: taking stock and moving forward," *Internet of Things*, vol. 100721, 2023, https://doi.org/10.1016/j.iot.2023.100721.

[77] M. Dionisio, S. J. de Souza Junior, F. Paula, and P. C. Pellanda, "The role of digital transformation in improving the efficacy of healthcare: a

systematic review," *Journal of High Technology Management Research*, vol. 34, no. 100442, 2023, http://dx.doi.org/10.1016/j.hitech.2022.100442.

[78] W. Shafik, M. Ghasemzadeh, and S. M. Matinkhah, "A fast machine learning for 5G beam selection for unmanned aerial vehicle applications," *Journal of Information Systems and Telecommunication*, vol. 4, no. 28, pp. 262, 2020, https://doi.org/10.7508/jist.2019.04.003.

[79] T. Shaik, X. Tao, N. Higgins, *et al.*, "Remote patient monitoring using artificial intelligence: current state, applications, and challenges," *Wiley Interdisciplinary Reviews: Data Mining and Knowledge Discovery*, pp. e1485, 2023, https://doi.org/10.1002/widm.1485.

[80] O. Ali, A. AlAhmad, and H. Kahtan, "A review of advanced technologies available to improve the telehealth performance during COVID-19 pandemic," *Procedia Computer Science*, vol. 217, pp. 205–216, 2023, https://doi.org/10.1016/j.procs.2022.12.216.

[81] L. B. Elvas, C. Serrão, and J. C. Ferreira, "Sharing health information using a blockchain," *Multidisciplinary Digital Publishing Institute*, vol. 11, no. 2, pp. 170, 2023, https://doi.org/10.3390/healthcare11020170.

[82] J. B. Awotunde, A. L. Imoize, O. B. Ayoade, M. K. Abiodun, D.T., Do, A. Silva, and S. N. Sur, "An enhanced hyper-parameter optimization of a convolutional neural network model for leukemia cancer diagnosis in a smart healthcare system," *Sensors*, vol. 22, no. 24, pp. 9689. https://doi.org/10.3390/s22249689.

[83] A. Belhadi, J. O. Holland, A. Yazidi, G. Srivastava, J. C. Lin, and Y. Djenouri, "BIoMT-ISeg: blockchain internet of medical things for intelligent segmentation," *Frontiers in Physiology*, vol. 13, no. 2744, 2023 https://doi.org/10.3389/fphys.2022.1097204.

[84] J. Liu, C. Jin, Y. Huang, K. Zhang, W. Li, and C. Cui, "Research on infectious disease surveillance and traceability system based on blockchain technology," In *Proceedings of the 4th International Conference on Economic Management and Model Engineering*, Nanjing, China, pp. 18–20, 2022, 2023. http://dx.doi.org/10.4108/eai.18-11-2022.2327112.

[85] P. Chinnasamy, A. Albakri, M. Khan, A. A. Raja, A. Kiran, and J. C. Babu, "Smart contract-enabled secure sharing of health data for a mobile cloud-based E-Health system," *Applied Sciences*, vol. 13, no. 6, pp. 3970, 2023, https://doi.org/10.3390/app13063970.

[86] W. Shafik, M. Matinkhah, and M. N. Sanda, "Network resource management drives machine learning: a survey and future research direction," *Journal of Communications Technology, Electronics and Computer Science*, pp. 1–5, 2020, http://dx.doi.org/10.22385/jctecs.v30i0.312.

[87] W. Shafik, "A Comprehensive cybersecurity framework for present and future global information technology organizations," In *Effective Cybersecurity Operations for Enterprise-Wide Systems*, pp. 56–79, 2023, IGI Global, http:doi.org/10.4018/978-1-6684-9018-1.ch002.

[88] S. P. Shankar, M. S. Supriya, D. Varadam, M. Kumar, H. Gupta, and R. Saha, "A comprehensive study on algorithms and applications of artificial intelligence in diagnosis and prognosis: AI for healthcare," In *Digital Twins*

and Healthcare: Trends, Techniques, and Challenges, pp. 35–54, 2023, IGI Global, https://doi.org/10.4018/978-1-6684-5925-6.ch003.

[89] Z. Yang, L. Jianjun, H. Faqiri, *et al.*, "Green internet of things and big data application in smart cities development," *Complexity*, pp. 1–5, 2021, https://doi.org/10.1155/2021/4922697.

[90] R. P. Puneeth, and G. Parthasarathy, "A survey on security and interoperability of electronic health records sharing using blockchain technology," *Acta Informatica Pragensia*, vol. 12, no. 1, 2023, https://doi.org/10.18267/j.aip.187.

[91] H. Meng, W. Shafik, S. M. Matinkhah, and Z. Ahmad, "A 5G beam selection machine learning algorithm for unmanned aerial vehicle applications," *Wireless Communications and Mobile Computing*, pp. 1–16, 2020, https://doi.org/10.1155/2020/1428968.

[92] P. K. Ghosh, A. Chakraborty, M. Hasan, K. Rashid, and A. H. Siddique, "Blockchain application in telehealth systems: a review," *Systems*, vol. 11, no. 1, pp. 38, 2023, https://doi.org/10.3390/systems11010038.

[93] B. Gupta, N. Sahay, K. Vinod, K. Sandhu, H. R. Basireddy, and R. K. Mudiganti, "Recent advances in system management, decision support systems, artificial intelligence and computing in anaesthesia," *Indian Journal of Anaesthesia*, vol. 67, no. 1, pp. 146–151, 2023, https://doi.org/10.4103/ija.ija_974_22.

[94] W. Wasswa. "Wearable Medical Electronics in Artificial Intelligence of Medical Things," In *Handbook of Security and Privacy of AI-Enabled Healthcare Systems and Internet of Medical Things*, pp. 21–40, 2023, http://doi.org/10.1201/9781003370321-2.

[95] W. Shafik, S. M Matinkhah, and F. Shokoor, "Recommendation system comparative analysis: internet of things aided networks," *EAI Endorsed Transactions on Internet of Things*, vol. 8, no. 29, 2022, http://dx.doi.org/10.4108/eetiot.v8i29.1108.

[96] W. Shafik, S. M. Matinkhah, F. Shokoor, and L. Sharif, "A reawakening of machine learning application in unmanned aerial vehicle: future research motivation," *EAI Endorsed Transactions on Internet of Things, vol.* 8, no. 29, 2022, http://dx.doi.org/10.4108/eetiot.v8i29.987.

[97] Z. Zhang, B. Tao, X. Li, and H. N. Dai, "An amalgamation of blockchain and connected health for combating COVID-19," In *Blockchain in Healthcare: From Disruption to Integration*, pp. 37–52, 2023. Cham: Springer International Publishing. https://doi.org/10.1007/978-3-031-14591-9_4.

[98] W. Shafik, S. M. Matinkhah, M. Asadi, Z., Ahmadi, and Z. Hadiyan, "A study on internet of things performance evaluation," *Journal of Communications Technology, Electronics and Computer Science*, pp. 1–19, 2020. http://dx.doi.org/10.22385/jctecs.v28i0.303.

[99] S. Olugbade, S. Ojo, A. L., Imoize, J., Isabona, and M. O. Alaba, "A review of artificial intelligence and machine learning for incident detectors in road transport systems," *Mathematical and Computational Applications*, vol. 27, no. 5, pp. 77, 2022, https://doi.org/10.3390/mca27050077.

[100] N. Shankar, M. K. Nallakaruppan, V. Ravindranath, M. Senthilkumar, and B. P. Bhagavath, "Smart IoMT framework for supporting UAV systems with AI," *Electronics*, vol. 12, no. 1, pp. 86, 2023, https://doi.org/10.3390/electronics12010086.

[101] S. N. Alaziz, B. Albayati, A. A. El-Bagoury, and W. Shafik, "Clustering of COVID-19 multi-time series-based K-means and PCA with forecasting," *International Journal of Data Warehousing and Mining (IJDWM)*, vol. 19, no. 3, 1–25, 2023, https://doi.org/10.4018/IJDWM.317374.

[102] D. Golinelli, E. Boetto, G. Carullo, A. G. Nuzzolese, A. G. Landini, and M. P. Fantini, "Adoption of digital technologies in health care during the COVID-19 pandemic: systematic review of early scientific literature," *Journal of Medical Internet Research*, vol. 22, no. 11, pp. e22280, 2020, https://doi.org/10.2196/22280.

[103] A. Kumar, V. Mani, V. Jain, H. Gupta, and V. G.Venkatesh, "Managing healthcare supply chain through artificial intelligence (AI): A study of critical success factors," *Computers & Industrial Engineering*, vol. 175, pp. 108815, 2023, https://doi.org/10.1016/j.cie.2022.108815.

[104] W. Shafik, S. M. Matinkhah, P. Etemadinejad, and M.N. Sanda, M. N., "Reinforcement learning rebirth, techniques, challenges, and resolutions," *JOIV: International Journal on Informatics Visualization*, vol. 4, no. 3, pp. 127–135. 2020, http://dx.doi.org/10.30630/joiv.4.3.376.

[105] E. R. D. Villarreal, J. García-Alonso, E. Moguel, and J. A. H. Alegría, "Blockchain for healthcare management systems: a survey on interoperability and security," *IEEE Access*, 11, 5629–5652,2023. https://doi.org/10.1109/ACCESS.2023.3236505.

[106] W. Shafik, "Cyber security perspectives in public spaces: drone case study," In *Handbook of Research on Cybersecurity Risk in Contemporary Business Systems*, pp. 79–97, 2023. IGI Global, http://doi.org/10.4018/978-1-6684-7207-1.ch004.

[107] O. C. Abikoye, E.T. Oladipupo, A.L. Imoize, J. B. Awotunde, C. C. Lee, and C. T. Li, "Securing critical user information over the internet of medical things platforms using a hybrid cryptography scheme," *Future Internet*, vol. 15, no. 3, pp. 99, 2023, https://doi.org/10.3390/fi15030099.

Chapter 12

Testing and validation of AI and blockchain-based models for application in telehealth systems

Lateef Adesola Akinyemi[1,2], *Comfort Oluwaseyi Folorunso*[3], *Oluwagbemiga Omotayo Shoewu*[1], *Stephen Obono Ekwe*[2,4], *Sunday Oladayo Oladejo*[5], *Quadri Ademola Mumuni*[1], *Oluwafemi Ipinnimo*[3], *Joseph Folorunsho Orimolade*[6] *and Abiodun Afis Ajasa*[1,7]

In the context of telehealth systems, this work addresses the capabilities of artificial intelligence (AI) and blockchain technology. Computer systems can behave intelligently thanks to AI, carrying out operations that would otherwise require human intellect. Blockchain is a decentralized digital ledger technology that securely logs network-wide transactional activity. The study aims to test and validate blockchain- and AI-based models for telehealth systems, spanning steps like data collection, training, blockchain validation, security assessment, legal compliance, in-app testing, and documentation. This chapter outlines the roles, difficulties, and blockchain-based methods in telehealth. It provides an up-to-date review and a helpful manual for researchers interested in conducting additional studies in this area. Despite the telehealth systems' infancy, the study outlines established

[1]Department of Electronic and Computer Engineering, Faculty of Engineering, Lagos State University, Epe Campus, Nigeria
[2]Department of Electrical Engineering, Faculty of Engineering and the Built Environment, University of Cape Town, South Africa
[3]Department of Systems Engineering, Faculty of Engineering, University of Lagos, Nigeria
[4]Department of Electrical, Electronic, and Computer Engineering, Cape Peninsula University of Technology (CPUT), South Africa
[5]School of Data Science and Computational Thinking, Stellenbosch University South Africa, South Africa
[6]School of Computing and Information Sciences, Caritas Institute of Higher Education (CIHE), Hong Kong
[7]School of Electrical Engineering, Faculty of Electrical Engineering, University of Technology Malaysia, Malaysia

standards for AI and blockchain models. There may be privacy and security problems with these models. Test scenarios scripted in PYTHON are used to gauge the model's performance and correctness. With this research, AI-inspired algorithms have been employed to predict chronic kidney diseases for their early detection and prevention. Classifiers such as Random Forest and eXtreme Gradient Boosting (XGBOOST) are utilized to carry out the forecast with the accuracy of such schemes ranging from 97.50% to 96.50%, respectively. The models' consistency and dependability are ensured through stress testing that involves high user loads, unpredictable data input, and network outages. By locating potential flaws and enhancing model performance, this technique increases resilience.

12.1 Introduction

Artificial intelligence (AI) is the ability of robots or computer systems to behave intelligently and carry out tasks that traditionally require human intelligence. This includes learning, problem-solving, decision-making, perception, and language understanding. Broadly speaking, there are two types of AI: strong or general AI and narrow or weak AI. Narrow AI, also referred to as weak AI, is restricted to carrying out the mission for which it was created. Voice assistants like Siri and Alexa, online shopping recommendation engines, and fraud detection tools used by financial institutions are all examples of narrow AI [1]. However, general AI, usually called strong AI, is a hypothetical AI system with the same level of cognition and intelligence as a human being. It would be able to comprehend, pick up knowledge, and carry out any intellectual work that humans can do. General AI, however, is still mostly a concept and has not yet been fully realized. Machine learning (ML), natural language processing (NLP), computer vision, robotics, and expert systems are just a few of the methods that can be used to create AI. With the use of these techniques, AI systems can evaluate data, spot patterns, make decisions, and adjust to new knowledge, enabling them to complete difficult jobs on their own or with little assistance from humans [1]. Numerous industries, including healthcare, banking, transportation, education, manufacturing, and entertainment, could benefit from AI. However, it brings up ethical, cultural, and privacy issues like biases in AI systems, potential job losses, and the effect of AI on human society. To ensure that AI is beneficial to humanity as a whole, careful evaluation of technological, ethical, legal, regulatory, and operational aspects must be made during the development and deployment of AI [2].

On the other hand, blockchain is a distributed and decentralized digital ledger technology used to securely and openly record transactions across a network of computers. It enables immutable and chronological data storage across a network of computers or 'nodes'. A chain of blocks is created by connecting each block in the blockchain using cryptographic methods. Each block in the blockchain comprises a collection of data, including transaction information, timestamps, and cryptographic signatures. The security of the blockchain is one of its fundamental characteristics. It is impossible to change or remove data after it has been stored in a block without the network's agreement, making it tamper-proof. This makes blockchain useful for applications like digital currencies (like Bitcoin), supply chain management, identity verification, and many more that demand trust, transparency, and security [3,4].

Blockchain relies on a consensus process in which network members agree on the legitimacy of transactions via a consensus algorithm. Peer-to-peer transactions are now possible, removing the need for intermediaries like banks or clearinghouses, boosting efficiency, and lowering costs. Blockchain technology offers decentralized, transparent, and secure solutions which have the potential to upend numerous sectors. Scalability, interoperability, and regulatory issues are difficulties it also faces. Despite these difficulties, blockchain technology is still developing and has the power to fundamentally alter the way that data are shared, saved, and verified in many facets of our daily lives [3–5]. With increased effectiveness, security, and patient outcomes, AI and blockchain technologies can revolutionize telehealth services. Some potential applications for AI and blockchain-based models in telehealth systems include automated triage and diagnosis recommendations. This is made possible by AI algorithms, which may examine patient information such as symptoms, medical history, and test results. This can aid telehealth systems in precisely and efficiently managing a huge volume of patients, enabling prompt and effective medical interventions. Another application area is remote patient monitoring using wearable devices like blood pressure cuffs, glucose meters, and heart rate monitors. AI may evaluate real-time data to look for patterns and trends that could point to patient health changes. Data quality and patient privacy can both be guaranteed by securely storing this information on a blockchain [6,7]. In addition, a patient's health data, including genetic data and treatment history, can be analysed by AI to produce individualized treatment plans. A blockchain can be used to store these plans, making it simple for healthcare providers to access and share them while yet protecting patient privacy. Medical records, prescriptions, and other documents connected to healthcare can be tracked and their legitimacy verified using blockchain's distributed ledger technology. AI algorithms can examine this data to identify and stop fraudulent behaviours. This includes forging prescriptions or filing duplicate claims, hence enhancing the security and integrity of telehealth systems as a whole [8]. Moreso, blockchain-based telehealth systems may be able to conduct payments, insurance claims, and consent management in a secure and automated manner. These transactions may be validated and verified using AI, reducing administrative work and increasing transparency.

Furthermore, AI can examine sizable datasets, such as posts on social media, meteorological information, and data on disease outbreaks. These data are used to forecast and stop the spread of diseases like pandemics or outbreaks. These forecasts can be kept on a blockchain, enabling decentralized access and teamwork between medical professionals and public health organizations [7]. AI and blockchain-based models can substantially impact telehealth systems by enhancing data security, privacy, and the precision of diagnosis and treatment recommendations. AI can analyse large amounts of data to produce insights and forecasts that can raise the standard of care. AI systems, for instance, can be trained on medical imagery to spot disease early warning signals or help with condition diagnosis. AI can also examine patient data to find trends and offer individualized therapies. By establishing an immutable ledger that records all transactions and modifications, blockchain technology can be utilized to improve the security and privacy of patient data. By doing so, one can guard against data breaches and guarantee that only authorized parties can access patient information. By allowing patients to authorize certain people or organizations to access their medical records, blockchain can also provide patients with more control over their data [7].

12.1.1 Contributions

In this book chapter regarding AI and blockchain-based models for telehealth systems, the following are the major contributions:

1. The thorough review presented herein gives up-to-date works on AI and blockchain-based models for telehealth systems, thereby serving as a hands-on for researchers who want to carry out further research in this field.
2. A few possible uses of AI and blockchain models for telehealth systems are detailed in this work.
3. Based on data from recent studies and trends, this book chapter presents some cultivated norms of the AI and blockchain model for telehealth systems, even though it is in the embryonic stage.
4. Challenges with security and confidentiality in the blockchain- and AI-based telehealth system models were identified.
5. The accuracy and performance of the models were assessed by subjecting them to various test scenarios using a Python environment.
6. To make sure the models function dependably and consistently under real-world circumstances, a case of chronic kidney disease is employed using some ML algorithms/classifiers to demonstrate the significance of AI/blockchain techniques in telehealth. This makes improving the models' resilience possible by identifying potential faults in them.

12.1.2 Chapter organization

Section 12.1 discusses the introductory section and contributions of the book chapter on AI and blockchain-based models for telehealth systems. Furthermore, Section 12.2 discusses the related work regarding AI and blockchain-based models for telehealth systems. A summary of the reviewed works is equally presented in a tabular form stating the strengths and weaknesses. The application of AI and blockchain-based models for telehealth systems is discussed in Section 12.3. Section 12.4 presents and discusses the outcomes of computational simulations. More importantly, lessons that have been learned and summarily discussed with AI and blockchain-based models for telehealth systems are presented in Section 12.5. Section 12.6 completes the book chapter by making conclusions regarding the AI and blockchain-based models for telehealth systems. The chapter organogram is shown in Figure 12.1.

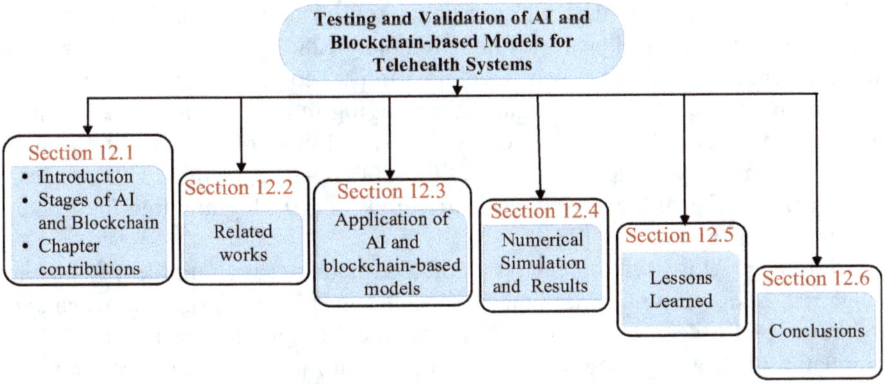

Figure 12.1 Organogram of the chapter

12.2 Overview of AI-based models and blockchain technology in telehealth

This literature review explores state-of-the-art research on AI-based models and blockchain technology in telehealth.

The application of telehealth in global health systems has been on the rise in recent years. With the emergence of AI and blockchain technologies, the potential for improving healthcare outcomes has become brighter than ever before [9–11]. There are several reasons why there is an increasing interest in AI-based models and blockchains in telehealth. Some of these include the provision of secured remote telehealth services in a decentralized, tamper-proof, transparent, traceable, reliable, and trustful manner, which is briefly highlighted in the works in [8,12–14]. Specifically, the application of blockchains to telehealth relies on six cardinal features of blockchains which are, namely [8,15,16]: (i) decentralization, (ii) immutability, (iii) transparency, (iv) open-source access, (v) auditability, and (vi) anonymity.

12.2.1 Related work

The authors in [17] posited that healthcare applications infrastructure and architectures could be categorized primarily into two, namely cloud- and blockchain-based solutions. Cloud-based solutions have been mainly used to address electronic health records (EHRs) and patient information challenges [18–21]. This is quite possible owing to the characteristically centralized model of cloud-based architectures. However, blockchains run on a decentralized model [8].

Moreover, AI has shown promise in several applications in telehealth. One of the significant applications is in decision support systems that can assist healthcare providers in diagnosing and treating patients [22–27]. For instance, Panigrahi *et al.* [26] developed a deep learning-based model that can predict the risk of hepatitis B among patients using their EHRs.

In telehealth, AI-based virtual assistants and chatbots are also used to assist patients in accessing healthcare services remotely [28–32]. A NLP-based chatbot with multilingual capabilities was developed in [28] to provide free health-related information and guidance to chronic patients living in rural communities in India. Similarly, in South Africa, technologies such as AI chatbots, robots, and mobile-based solutions were deployed to combat the COVID-19 epidemic [31]. Besides, a critical review of health chatbots was carried out in [29], highlighting their potential, limitations, and survey [33].

Moreover, AI is used to develop predictive models that could identify patients at high risk of developing certain medical conditions [11, 34–38]. Upadhyaya *et al.* [35] developed a deep learning-based model that can predict the risk of diabetic retinopathy (DR) and glaucoma. The deep-learning model incorporated DenseNet and Inception V3, based on a convolutional neural network (CNN), in the predictive models for DR and Glaucoma, respectively. Both models achieved an accuracy of over 90%.

The authors proposed a conceptual AI-based framework for telehealth [39] to address global health challenges such as the COVID-19 pandemic. The framework comprises six stages: an AI-based questionnaire unit; a telehealth unit; online monitoring unit; an emergency telehealth consultation unit; an AI-based lab unit; a training and monitoring unit; and a data bank. The proposed framework [39] did not consider patient data privacy and security that could be blockchain enhanced. Although leveraging AI-based models to telehealth opens greater possibilities in medical diagnosis, remote surgery, healthcare delivery, and treatment [40], the authors in [41,42] discussed at great length four fields of possibilities, i.e. information analysis cooperation, AI-based diagnosis, electronic healthcare information technology, and patient monitoring and control. The application of AI-based models in enhancing pharmacovigilance activities such as adverse drug effects detection and medication-related complications detection and prevention via electronic health and medical records were examined by Edrees *et al.* in [43].

A comprehensive overview of blockchain technology in healthcare, including potential applications in telehealth, was given in [44]. Khezr *et al.* in [44] also discussed in a great deal the open research areas and challenges of blockchains in healthcare. A blockchain-based telehealth system to facilitate remote consultations, medical testing, and drug administration during the COVID-19 pandemic was proposed in [8,45,46]. In [45,46], smart contracts were developed to ensure data integrity and generate secured and reliable alerts and notifications. The storage system ran on off-chain storage systems such as cloud storage or a decentralized storage system similar to the interplanetary file system (IPFS).

The works in [47–52] examined the potentials and challenges of blockchains for securing and trustful in telehealth. A secured digital medium that leverages 5G multi-access edge computing (MEC) with elliptical curve Qu-Vanstone (ECQV) authentication certificates in [47]. Besides, in [47], offloading storage was embedded in the design to account for the scalability of growing devices. A blockchain-based patient-centric framework for teleconsultation and telemonitoring services that exploit reliability, scalability, and security was proposed in [49].

The proposed framework in [49], HapiChain, was premised on three layers of interface layer for users' communications, a DApp layer for security and scalability, and a blockchain layer. Similarly, in [50,51], the authors put forward a blockchain-inspired foundation for secured EHR monitoring, storage, and maintenance. In this decentralized patient-centric framework [50], the patient has total control and ownership of her records. Additionally, the patient can monitor the transactions taking place with her records. A two-blockchain model was proposed in [51], with the first blockchain (i.e. private blockchain) designed for the EHR's maintenance, while the second blockchain (i.e. consortium blockchain) secures the EHR's indexes. Moreover, the EHRs are public-key encrypted to achieve secured access, data, search, and privacy tasks [51]. To predict, the authors proposed disease, a three-tier architecture in [52]. In [52], the first tier is the sensors layer, and it ensures patients' real-time monitoring using medical sensors. The second tier involves data storage using information entropy technology to enhance patients' privacy. The third tier relies on blockchain-based smart contracts. Smart contracts enable secure authorization and access control of EHR applications. The authors in [48] gave a detailed discussion of the opportunities and challenges of employing blockchains for secured medical systems. Besides, in [48], a thorough analysis of the literature was done regarding secured medical systems using blockchains.

In the literature, blockchains have been used as incentive mechanisms for information sharing by patients in telehealth systems. In [53], a blockchain-incentive mechanism for healthcare systems was proposed. The authors explored mathematical models based on game theory for two real-world scenarios. The blockchain models were to incentivize patients to exercise more and help recruit patients in a clinical trial of anticancer drugs. A blockchain-based crypto-economic token for information sharing among humans was explored in [54]. In the investigation in [54], the theory of self-determination was employed to determine the impact of blockchain-based tokens in human information sharing that could be extended to telehealth systems. Similarly, in [55], different incentive-based mechanisms and cost-pricing scenarios were investigated relative to blockchain-based data-sharing platforms. To cover the cost of data sharing, a cost compensation model was proposed to incentivize the participants. The model proposed in [55] could be applied to telehealth systems to encourage patients to share their data. In [56], a blockchain-based incentive mechanism, MedChain, was proposed to be integrated with proof of authority. In [56], the authors considered a patient's EHR as an asset belonging to the patient rather than a digital currency. The works in [53–56] considered a blockchain-based static incentive mechanism. However, in [57], a blockchain-based dynamic incentive mechanism to encourage data sharing was proposed. The dynamic incentive mechanism was premised on evolutionary game theory. The excitation parameters of the smart contract mechanism were dynamically controlled using the evolutionary game model.

Table 12.1 highlights the summary of selected literature regarding the use of AI and blockchain technological advances in telehealth systems by indicating the description; of technologies, weaknesses, and strengths of the models, frameworks, and implementations.

Table 12.1 Summary of literature review

Reference	Contributions/ description	Techniques/technologies	Weaknesses	Strengths
Ahmad *et al.* [8]	How blockchains can improve telehealth	Emphasis on blockchain technology	Did not address the actual implementation of blockchain in telehealth systems	Rigorous discussion on the benefits and challenges of adopting blockchain in telehealth systems
Younis *et al.* [12]	Development of a secured novel data-driven blockchain-based telehealth architecture	Proposed a blockchain-enabled data-driven access control and management system for smart healthcare applications (BeDaSH) architecture	Did not address the scalability issues and security challenges such as denial-of-service attacks peculiar to cloud-based systems	A secured platform that protects patients' rights, access, and data
Islam *et al.* [13]	Development of a blockchain-enabled decentralized,trustworthy framework for a secured telehealth system	The use of a blockchain framework enabled using an encryption key generator, a hash function system; and a health block data generator	Large size overhead of the data transactions owing to continuous monitoring and update of patient privacy and data security	Utilising parameters such as transaction data size, response time, transit delay, and efficiency, the suggested approach was assessed
Rajasekaran *et al.* [14]	Development of certificates and lightweight blockchain-based authentication scheme for patient-doctor data-sharing in a telehealth system	An elliptic curve cryptography and bilinear pairing running on blockchain technology	Scalability and data accessibility issues as the amount of stored data significantly increase	A secure and reliable authentication mechanism that avoids the re-authentication process by the patient in a multi-doctor communication instance. Designed to prevent several attacks

Antwi *et al.* [17]	Investigation of blockchain-enabled telehealth applications	Use of Hyperledger fabric and Hyperledger composer	Tests were carried out only in Fabric. Comparisons could have been done with other platforms.	Extensive evaluation of test case scenarios for telehealth applications
Panigrahi *et al.* [26]	Development of a clinical decision support system embedded with a machine learning model for prediction of the risk of hepatitis B among patients using their EHR	A hybrid of decision support systems and ML tools such as ANN. Use of ES-Builder web application tool	Did not address the challenges of security and data privacy peculiar to medical-based applications	The system is open-source and accessible
Ashwini *et al.* [28]	Development of an AI-based chatbot used in telehealth for rural healthcare	The use of a multilingual conversation-based NLP in a Dialogflow API environment	The training of the NLP model which is critical to model accuracy was not addressed. The scalability, security, and data privacy of the model were not discussed	The model can be deployed for low-resource languages in rural and semi-urban environments
Upadhyaya *et al.* [35]	An ML-based prediction model developed for diagnosing eye and ENT diseases such as diabetic retinopathy and glaucoma	Deep learning (i.e. DenseNet) and convolutional neural networks (i.e. Inception-V3)	The performance evaluation was limited to ML metrics such as accuracy, specificity, and sensitivity only. The telehealth and telemedicine testing metrics were not considered	Large training datasets with 61,458 retina photographs and 1500 glaucoma photographs
Yousaf *et al.* [39]	A conceptual telehealth framework for a global pandemic such as COVID-19 using telehealth systems	Use of AI-based chatbots and laboratories	Neither cloud-based nor blockchain-based. Did address patient data privacy and security that could be blockchain enhanced. Framework was not implemented	A quick guide for setting up telemedicine and telehealth during emergencies and pandemics

(Continues)

Table 12.1 (*Continued*)

Reference	Contributions/ description	Techniques/technologies	Weaknesses	Strengths
Hasan *et al.* [45], Ahmad *et al.* [46]	Blockchain-based decentralized smart-contracts solutions for telehealth and telemedicine	Interplanetary File System (IPFS) storage, cloud, permissioned Ethereum	The system was not fully deployed in a real Ethereum blockchain network	Fully decentralized with smart contracts made available privately and publicly
Hewa *et al.* [47]	Proposed a novel multi-access edge computing (MEC) and blockchain-based architecture with storage offloading capability for cloud scalability	Lightweight Elliptic Curve Qu-Vanstone certificates, IoT, MEC, and IPFS storage, cloud, smart contracts, Hyperledger Fabric blockchain platform	Did not address the security and privacy of the architecture. The smart contract implementation was not described	Introduction of a reward scheme to encourage patients and hospitals to share data via the blockchain to encourage
Kordestani *et al.* [49]	A blockchain-based patient-centric framework for telehealth that exploit reliability, scalability, and security was proposed	Smart contracts, IPFS, Ethereum blockchain	The framework's security was not tested against attacks to verify its performance and integrity	The use of probabilistic reasoning combines the Bayesian belief network with non-monotonic production rules to support the uncertainty in the data as well as the reasoning
Vora *et al.* [50]	Proposed a decentralized blockchain-based framework for EHR storage and maintenance	Five smart contracts, blockchain, cryptography	Scalability and latency issues arise as the number of users increases	Enable patients to have total control, ownership, and monitoring of their records

Shamshad *et al.* [51]	A two-blockchain model for a secured and private telemedicine system to improve diagnosis and treatment	Public encryption with keyword search (PEKS), proxy re-encryption technology (PRE), physically unclonable function (PUF) based protocols	Access control, availability, anonymity, and scalability of the model were not discussed	User authentication, privacy, and integrity of the telehealth system were fully addressed
Wang *et al.* [52]	A three-tier blockchain and machine learning-enabled architecture for disease prediction was proposed	Information entropy, blockchain-based smart contracts, transfer learning	An imbalanced and small sample size of the training dataset affects the practicability and scalability of the model	Blockchain-based backup of information summary to ensure the integrity of backtracking and anti-repudiation. The use of machine learning for disease prediction
Jung *et al.* [53]	A blockchain-incentive mechanism based on game theory to recruit participants in two real-world scenarios, i.e. physical exercise and a clinical trial of anticancer drugs programmes was proposed	Blockchain, game theory, convex optimization, token economy	The assumptions made are simplistic and may not apply to real-world scenarios and affect the practicability of the mechanisms	Application of game theory for incentive mechanism
Daraghmi *et al.* [56]	A blockchain-based incentive mechanism (MedChain), integrated with proof of authority was proposed	Smart contracts, encryption	Did not address user authentication, data privacy, and anonymity which are important in telehealth	A mechanism with strong access control and availability

12.2.2 Stages in the testing and validation of AI and blockchain-based models for telehealth systems

Blockchain and AI in telehealth systems can offer a complete answer for precise, secure, and individualized healthcare services. To ensure patient consent and address any biases in AI algorithms, as well as other ethical and regulatory considerations, it is crucial to consider the use of these technologies in healthcare. Assurance of these technologies' accuracy, dependability, security, testing, and validation of AI and blockchain-based models for telehealth systems is essential. The testing and validation procedures for blockchain- and AI-based models in telehealth systems include data gathering and preparation; training and evaluation of AI models; validation of blockchain-based models; security testing; regulation compliance; real-world testing; as well as reporting and documentation as depicted in Figure 12.2.

12.2.2.1 Data gathering and preparation

The first step is to gather and prepare the data that will be used to test and train the AI and blockchain-based models. This could consist of information from sensors, medical pictures, patient health records, and other pertinent data. To assure consistency and correctness, data preparation involves cleaning, converting, and normalising the data [58].

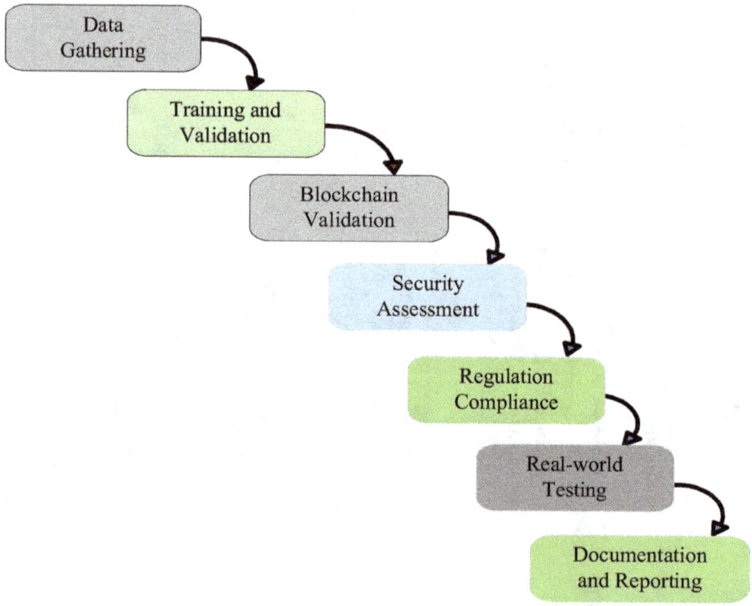

Figure 12.2 Stages in the testing and validation of AI and blockchain-based models for telehealth systems

12.2.2.2 Training and evaluation of AI models

After data gathering, the pre-processed data are used to train the AI models. To do this, ML algorithms must be used to discover patterns and relationships in the data. To obtain the necessary performance metrics, the models are adjusted and optimized. Following training, AI models are evaluated using a different set of data from the training set. This makes it easier to assess the model's effectiveness in accuracy, precision, recall, and F1 score. The generalizability and robustness of the model can be evaluated using a variety of testing methodologies, such as cross-validation [58].

12.2.2.3 Security assessment

This is essential since telehealth systems handle private patient information. Additional security concerns may apply to blockchain-based models, such as checking for flaws in encryption methods, consensus algorithms, and smart contracts. The protection of patient data is ensured by security testing. This assists in identifying and addressing potential security risks and weaknesses in AI and blockchain-based models. The integrity, validity, and transparency of the data stored in the blockchain are verified as part of the validation of blockchain-based models, including testing them. This involves confirming the immutability and consistency of the data, as well as validating the consensus processes and smart contracts [59].

12.2.2.4 Regulation compliance

Telehealth systems must adhere to several laws. Among these are the General Data Protection Regulation (GDPR), the Health Insurance Portability and Accountability Act (HIPAA), and others, and industry standards such as fast healthcare interoperability resources (FHIR). These laws, which cover data privacy, security, and consent requirements, should be complied with through testing and validating blockchain- and AI-based models [7].

12.2.2.5 Real-world testing

The AI and blockchain-based models may go through real-world testing in a controlled setting after initial testing and validation. This includes a pilot study with actual patients and healthcare professionals. Real-world testing identifies any problems that might occur during practical implementation. It also helps to evaluate how well the models function in realistic circumstances [6].

12.2.2.6 Reporting and documentation

To establish openness, repeatability, and accountability thoroughly, documenting the testing and validation methods, results, and findings is necessary. Write thorough summaries of the testing and validation findings that include any limits or suggestions for improvement [60].

AI and blockchain-based models have the potential to significantly improve telehealth systems. This can be achieved by facilitating secure and effective processing of patient data, individualized treatment plans, fraud detection, and public health predictive analytics. In telehealth systems, these technologies may help to enhance patient results, efficiency, and security. To secure patient privacy and data security, it is crucial to consider the ethical, legal, and regulatory ramifications of integrating AI and blockchain technology in telehealth.

The motivation of this chapter is as follows: First, telehealth systems with AI capabilities can automate repetitive operations like appointment booking, patient triage, and remote monitoring, which improves the effectiveness of healthcare delivery. Healthcare workers may quickly make educated decisions with the help of AI algorithms that can quickly evaluate enormous volumes of data and deliver real-time insights [61]. Second, AI algorithms can examine medical data, such as patient health records, symptoms, and medical imaging, to make precise diagnoses and treatment suggestions. Particularly in remote or underdeveloped locations where access to healthcare may be constrained, this can assist in decreasing errors and improve patient outcomes [62]. Third, the personal features of each patient, such as medical history, genetics, and lifestyle, can be considered by AI when creating individualized treatment regimens using patient data. This may make it possible to provide more specialized and targeted care, improving patient results and satisfaction. Blockchain can improve security and privacy in telehealth systems because of its decentralized and immutable nature. Patient data can be exchanged and maintained securely with the appropriate stakeholders to maintain data integrity, confidentiality, and consent management. This may increase patient and healthcare provider confidence and trust [63]. In addition, Blockchain can help with telehealth interoperability by offering a standardized platform for data transfer. This can facilitate the easy exchange of patient data among various healthcare professionals, resulting in coordinated care and a reduction in the need for extra tests or procedures. Also, blockchain can empower patients by allowing people to share their health data with healthcare professionals safely and giving them ownership over their data. Patients can use telehealth systems to contact healthcare practitioners remotely, which can be especially helpful in areas with limited access to healthcare services [8]. Lastly, telehealth systems powered by AI and blockchain can produce enormous volumes of data. These can be applied to research, innovation, and the creation of novel treatment procedures. It can develop medical technology and support evidence-based medicine. The benefits of applying AI and blockchain-based models to telehealth systems include their potential to boost productivity and improve diagnosis and treatment. It also delivers personalized care, improves telehealth security, and promotes interoperability and data exchange. It increases access to healthcare, and foster research and innovation, all of which could ultimately result in better patient care and outcomes [61].

However, to prevent data breaches, unauthorized access, and privacy violations, telehealth systems must have strong security mechanisms while collecting and transmitting sensitive patient data. Traditional telehealth systems might be exposed to cybersecurity dangers, resulting in data compromises and breaches. EHRs, remote monitoring tools, and other health IT systems are just a few examples of the numerous data sources and systems that telehealth applications frequently rely on. However, these systems could not be interoperable, which makes it challenging to efficiently communicate and interchange data, which might affect the precision and potency of AI models [64]. For telehealth technologies to be successfully adopted, patient, healthcare provider, and system trust must be established. Patients require confirmation that their data handling is secure and adheres to their right to privacy. To ensure the accuracy and dependability of AI algorithms, healthcare providers need to know how they are developed, tested, and updated. Concerns around data privacy, bias, transparency, accountability, and informed consent are raised by the use of AI in telehealth systems, from an ethical and legal standpoint. AI models could unintentionally reinforce bias, resulting in differences in healthcare outcomes. The liability and accountability for judgements made by AI models in telehealth settings may also have legal repercussions [65]. To deliver fast and accurate healthcare services, telehealth systems must manage massive volumes of data and process it in real-time. AI models must be scalable and performant to manage the rising demand for telehealth services, particularly during emergencies like pandemics. Regulations governing data protection, privacy, and medical standards are among those that apply to telehealth services. Incorporating AI and blockchain technologies into telehealth systems may complicate compliance and governance. Adhering to these rules might be complicated. It may be necessary to make large expenditures in technology infrastructure, data storage, and processing resources to implement and sustain blockchain-based and AI models in telehealth systems. Cost and resource limitations could be problematic, particularly for smaller healthcare organizations or those working in environments with few resources. These are some of the problems that will be addressed in the chapter.

12.3 The role of blockchain and artificial intelligence in telehealth: methods and challenges

Rapid technological advancements have resulted in significant changes to the healthcare landscape, paving the way for novel telehealth applications. These advancements are especially relevant in light of recent global problems, highlighting the significance of efficient, accessible, and secure healthcare delivery systems [8,66,67]. Blockchain and AI are two emerging technologies that have the potential to transform the healthcare industry. Both offer plausible solutions to significant problems in the telehealth and telemedicine fields [8]. This section examines the integration of blockchain technology, AI, and telehealth/medicine, focusing on the challenges and methods of these technologies in the healthcare industry.

12.3.1 Challenges of blockchain in telehealth systems

The decentralized, transparent, and secured characteristics nature of blockchain make it well-suited for usage in telehealth and telemedicine [8,67]. However, several challenges must be addressed before blockchain-based solutions may be successfully implemented and embraced [68]. This section investigates the most significant challenges encountered when integrating blockchain technology into telehealth and telemedicine systems.

12.3.1.1 Scalability and performance

When adopting blockchain technology for telehealth, scalability is a crucial concern [69] since these systems must be able to accommodate an increasing number of users and activities. Blockchain systems' transaction throughput, latency, and network capacity are currently constrained, particularly those that employ proof-of-work (PoW) consensus algorithms like Bitcoin and Ethereum [70]. It is crucial to develop flexible, high-performance blockchain systems to manage the increasing volume of telehealth and telemedicine transactions to ensure that healthcare services are delivered promptly and effectively. The scalability and effectiveness of blockchain networks may be increased in a number of ways. These include layer two techniques like the lightning network [71,72], off-chain transactions [73], and sharing [74]. But in the context of healthcare applications, these approaches frequently include trade-offs [75] in terms of security, decentralization, and complexity that must be carefully considered.

12.3.1.2 Security and privacy

In telehealth applications, protecting sensitive health information and patient privacy is of the uttermost importance. Blockchain technology may improve security and privacy because it allows storing data in a way that cannot be changed and is open to everyone. However, it presents new issues such as access control, data encryption, and anonymity that need to be solved to protect the privacy of private health information while maintaining the openness and reliability of blockchain [76]. Cryptographic methods like zero-knowledge proofs and homomorphic encryption have been suggested as ways to solve these problems by making it easier to process data on blockchain networks securely and privately [77]. Nonetheless, these methods often add more computational complexity and overhead, which could hurt the ability of blockchain systems to grow and work well [78]. More study is needed to ensure that cryptographic solutions for healthcare applications are safe and effective.

12.3.1.3 Interoperability

The successful implementation and incorporation of blockchain-based technology into existing healthcare systems necessitate addressing the interoperability issue. This entails the interchange and use of health information across different platforms, data formats, and standards [79]. It is been difficult to achieve interoperability in blockchain-based telehealth systems due to the diversity of data sources, such as EHRs, medical devices, and health information exchanges (HIEs), as well as the variability in data standards and protocols, such as HL7 (Health Level Seven International), FHIR, and DICOM (Digital Imaging and Communications in Medicine) [79]. In addressing this problem, researchers have proposed standardized data formats, ontologies, and application programming interfaces (APIs) for representing, sharing, and querying health information on blockchain networks [80]. In addition, developing cross-platform communication protocols and integration systems, such as Polkadot and Cosmos, can facilitate the exchange of data and value between blockchain networks [81]. Nonetheless, pervasive adoption of these standards and technologies requires collaboration and coordination among numerous stakeholders, including healthcare providers, technology vendors, and regulatory authorities.

12.3.1.4 Legal and regulatory compliance

Critical for the success of blockchain-based telehealth applications is compliance with healthcare regulations and data protection laws such as the Health Insurance Portability and Accountability Act (HIPAA) in the United States and the General Data Protection Regulation (GDPR) in the European Union [82]. These regulations have stringent data privacy, security, and permission standards that may clash with the immutability, transparency, and decentralization of blockchain [83]. Blockchain solutions must address these issues by implementing suitable data protection measures, such as access control, encryption, and anonymization, as well as by providing mechanisms for data correction and deletion by the GDPR [84]. Moreover, blockchain developers and healthcare providers must negotiate a dynamic regulatory landscape to guarantee their solutions conform to applicable local, state, national, and international norms.

12.3.1.5 Adoption and user experience

Though blockchain technology has the potential to advance telehealth systems, when developing for these sectors, it is critical to consider adoption and user experience. The successful use of blockchain technology is based on its capabilities and acceptability by healthcare professionals, patients, and other stakeholders. Many factors influence adoption, including usability, perceived value, and user experience quality. Although a blockchain system's user interface and user experience must be simple, intuitive, and user-friendly, some complexity is associated with the technology's use, such as managing cryptographic keys, which can be a barrier to adoption, especially for non-technically knowledgeable users [85]. As a result, measures for streamlining the user experience, such as task automation, guided learning, and reactive user assistance, should be used. The apparent adoption of blockchain-based technology has been largely motivated by its perceived benefit in enhancing healthcare services. As a result, it is vital to highlight the benefits and value addition of using blockchain to all stakeholders, such as better data security, patient ownership over data, and faster processes [11]. Infrastructure, system integration, maintenance, and training costs may deter healthcare practitioners, particularly small and medium clinics, from implementing blockchain technology. As a result, cost-benefit evaluations must be considered alongside the potential savings provided by the technology.

Although blockchain technology can change telehealth systems, certain challenges still need to be fixed before they can be successfully integrated and used. Figure 12.3 depicts a summary of these challenges. Future research and development should focus on coming up with innovative and practical solutions suitable for resolving the unique requirements of the telehealth and telemedicine industries.

12.3.2 Blockchain methods in telehealth systems

The application of blockchain-based technologies in the field of telehealth systems could provide some potential answers to problems that have been plaguing the healthcare sector. Here, we enumerate several methods that some works of literature have proposed.

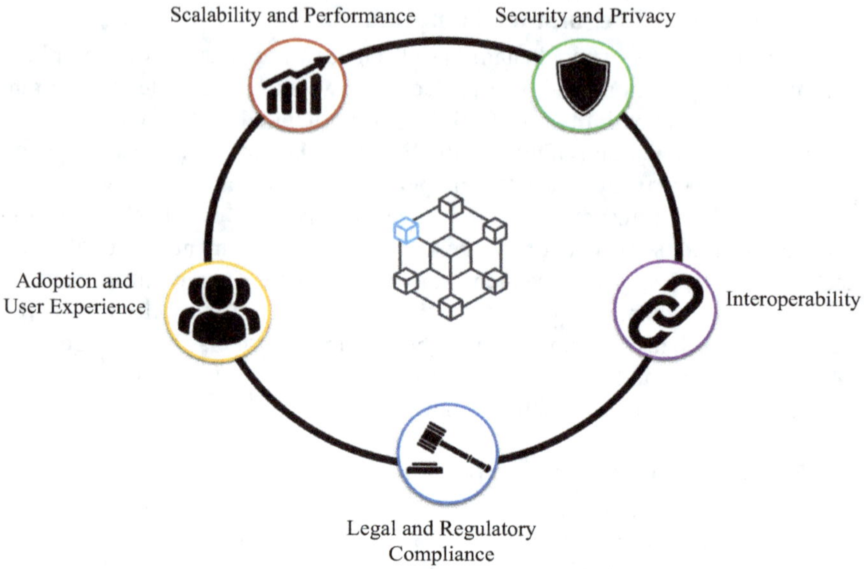

Figure 12.3 Challenges to blockchain-based integration in telehealth industries

12.3.2.1 Consensus algorithms

Consensus algorithms are critical to blockchain-based networks' continued operation, safety, and efficacy. These methods allow network users to agree on the legality and chronological sequence of transactions, hence eliminating inconsistencies and double-spending attacks [70,81]. PoW [86], proof-of-stake (PoS) [87], and practical byzantine fault tolerance (PBFT) [88] are common consensus methods used in blockchain systems. However, each consensus approach has its own set of trade-offs in terms of security, decentralization, energy consumption, and performance. PoW is computationally and energy-intensive, unlike PoS, which may lead to power consolidation among large-holding entities. In the context of telehealth and telemedicine, adopting consensus algorithms that optimize these trade-offs while meeting the special needs of healthcare applications, such as low latency, high throughput, and strong security guarantees [75], is crucial. Different consensus algorithms, such as proof-of-authority (PoA) [89] and delegated PoS (dPoS) [90], have recently been developed to improve the energy efficiency, performance, and security of healthcare applications. More research is required to assess whether or not these consensus algorithms are suitable for usage in real-world telehealth systems.

12.3.2.2 Smart contracts for healthcare services

Smart contracts, which are agreements that execute their terms and conditions, can be used to automate a range of operations in telehealth systems. They can, for example, be used to manage access to EHRs and the delivery of value-based care.

Smart contracts may boost efficiency, minimize paper waste, and lower the chance of fraudulent transactions by removing the need for human participation. Smart contracts are self-executing agreements that encode contractual terms and conditions directly into the blockchain, automating the execution of predetermined activities upon the fulfilment of specific circumstances [91]. Smart contracts may be used to automate procedures in telehealth systems such as patient consent management, accounting and payment, and treatment authorization [92]. Smart contracts, for example, might permit automated payments between patients and healthcare providers following the successful completion of telehealth sessions, lowering administrative expenses and assuring quick payment [93]. Furthermore, smart contracts may be used to enforce data access control measures, ensuring that sensitive health information is released only to authorized parties in compliance with data protection standards [91,92]. Nonetheless, the application of smart contracts in healthcare has obstacles, such as ensuring the privacy and security of sensitive data and resolving the legal and regulatory consequences of automated decision-making [92]. More research is needed to create privacy-preserving smart contract approaches and evaluate their legal and ethical implications in telehealth and telemedicine environments.

12.3.2.3 Decentralized identity management

Through the use of decentralized identity management technologies, individuals can create, manage, and distribute their digital identities independently of centralized institutions like governmental bodies or tech firms [94]. In telehealth systems, decentralized identity management can improve privacy, security, and data ownership over patients' health data by enabling patients to directly administer their credentials, permissions, and data access policies on the blockchain. Key components of decentralized identity management systems include decentralized identifiers (DIDs) and verified credentials, which allow for the safe and private transfer of identity data between users and service providers [94]. Patients, for instance, can use DIDs to establish their identity on telehealth platforms and control who has access to their medical records, while doctors and other medical professionals can utilize verified credentials to demonstrate their knowledge and training [95]. The widespread implementation of decentralized identity management in telehealth and telemedicine depends on the creation of standardized protocols and interoperable solutions that can be easily integrated into the preexisting infrastructure of the healthcare industry and its data standards [94]. Compliance with data protection regulations and the recognition of digital credentials across jurisdictions are just two examples of the legal and regulatory repercussions of decentralized identity management that need to be handled.

12.3.2.4 Data storage and sharing solutions

Telehealth systems applications may benefit from the transparent, secure, and tamper-proof storage and sharing of health data made possible by blockchain technology. Large amounts of health data, like medical photographs and genomic sequences, are generally impractical to store directly on the blockchain due to the network's constraints in scalability and throughput [96]. Hybrid data storage solutions combining the advantages of blockchain technology with those of off-chain storage systems such as distributed file systems, cloud storage services, and peer-to-peer networks have been proposed to address this issue [97]. While blockchain networks can be used to store metadata, access control policies, and cryptographic proofs of data integrity and provenance [98], they do not need to be utilized to store actual health data. One such distributed file system that has been proposed for use as off-chain storage in healthcare applications is the inter planetary file system (IPFS) [73]. Through content-addressable, distributed, and versioned file sharing, IPFS allows storing and retrieving data quickly and reliably. IPFS with blockchain integration provides scalable, performant, and cost-effective decentralized data storage options for telehealth and telemedicine systems [73,98].

12.3.2.5 Integration of blockchain technology with existing healthcare systems

EHRs, HIEs, and medical devices all need to be seamlessly integrated with blockchain technology for telehealth systems to reach their full potential [99]. To accomplish this, we need to create standardized data models, APIs, and middleware solutions to bridge existing healthcare systems and blockchain networks [100]. This will allow for the safe and seamless sharing of patient data across all participating platforms and parties. To make it easier to integrate telehealth systems solutions built on the distributed ledger technology with existing EHR systems and HIEs, the FHIR standard has been suggested as a framework for representing and transferring health data on blockchain networks [99]. In addition, blockchain-based device management and authentication systems can be used to safeguard remote patient monitoring and telehealth services by protecting data transmissions between medical devices and telehealth platforms.

The summary of the blockchain methods in telehealth systems is shown in Table 12.2.

12.3.3 Challenges of AI in telehealth systems

Incorporating AI into telehealth systems has the potential to revolutionize healthcare by facilitating better diagnosis, more individualized treatment plans, and enhanced patient outcomes. However, there are numerous challenges encountered when integrating AI into telehealth systems. These include data quality and bias issues, explainability and interpretability, AI ethics and fairness, AI deployment and maintenance, and legal and regulatory considerations.

12.3.3.1 Data quality and bias

AI models used in telehealth systems settings are only as good as the data on which they are trained. Inaccuracies, inconsistencies, or biases in the training data can lead to suboptimal or even detrimental consequences for AI algorithms when they discover correlations and base their forecasts or assessments on vast amounts of data [102]. The lacks of completeness, accuracy, timeliness, and/or representation in collected data are all indicators of poor data quality [103]. Concerns about data quality and bias can be mitigated using rigorous data collection, preprocessing, and validation methods, and ensuring

Table 12.2 Blockchain technology in telehealth systems

Method	Example	Description
Consensus Algorithms	*Proof-of-work (PoW)*	A consensus algorithm that requires nodes to solve difficult mathematical puzzles to certify transactions and generate new blocks [92,101]
	Proof-of stake (PoS)	A consensus algorithm selects a validator in distributed ledgers where the staked cryptocurrency is used as collateral [88]
	Practical byzantine fault tolerance (PBFT)	A method of multiple rounds of voting for attaining consensus, which can function in the presence of malicious or defective nodes [89]
	Proof-of-authority (PoA)	Energy efficiency, performance, and security are prioritized in a consensus process that chooses validators based on their reputation, identity, or competence [90]
	Delegated Proof-of-Stake (dPoS)	Stakeholders can distribute their voting authority across a small group of validators in this consensus process, which increases the efficiency and scalability of the system [91]
Smart contracts	*Healthcare services automation*	Smart contracts can be employed to automate various processes in telehealth systems, such as patient consent management, billing and reimbursement, and treatment authorization [92,93]
Decentralized identity management	*Decentralized identifiers (DIDs)*	Decentralized identifiers are unique, persistent, and globally resolvable identifiers that enable individuals to create, control, and share their digital identities without relying on centralized authorities [95,96]
	Verifiable credentials	Cryptographically secure, tamper-proof digital attestations that can be used to prove an individual's qualifications, licensure, or other attributes, enabling privacy-preserving identity verification in telehealth systems [97]
Data storage and sharing solutions	*Hybrid data storage solutions*	Combining the benefits of blockchain technology with off-chain storage systems, such as distributed file systems, cloud storage services, and peer-to-peer networks, to enable secure, transparent, and tamper-proof storage and sharing of health data while addressing the scalability and performance limitations of blockchain networks [100]

(Continues)

Table 12.2 (Continued)

Method	Example	Description
	Interplanetary file system (IPFS)	A distributed file system that enables efficient and resilient data storage and retrieval through content-addressable, distributed, and versioned file sharing, which can be integrated with blockchain technology to provide scalable, performant, and cost-effective data storage solutions for telehealth systems applications [73,98]
Integration with existing healthcare systems	*Fast healthcare interoperability resources (FHIR)*	A standardized data model and API for representing and exchanging health information on blockchain networks, enabling the integration of blockchain-based telehealth systems solutions with existing EHR systems and HIEs [102,103]
	Blockchain-based device management and authentication	Secure the communication and data exchange between medical devices and telehealth platforms by using blockchain-based device management and authentication solutions, enhancing the security and privacy of remote patient monitoring services [102]

the training data is diverse and representative [104]. To further uncover and reduce any biases and disparities in healthcare outcomes, multidisciplinary teams comprising physicians, data scientists, and ethicists should be involved in the creation of AI models.

12.3.3.2 Explainability and interpretability

The complexity and non-linearity of many AI models, especially deep learning models, make it difficult to understand and interpret their decision-making processes, leading to the common description of these models as 'black boxes' [105]. A major roadblock to the widespread use of AI in telehealth systems is the difficulty of explaining and interpreting the reasoning behind AI-driven judgements, which can make both healthcare providers and patients wary of using such technologies. Researchers have proposed several explainable AI (XAI) strategies to help explain the decisions made by AI models [106], such as feature importance analyses, surrogate models, and visualization tools. Guidelines and standards for evaluating and reporting AI model explainability and interpretability are also essential for ensuring the transparency, accountability, and trustworthiness of AI-driven healthcare choices [107].

12.3.3.3 AI ethics and fairness

Potential ethical concerns with AI-driven telehealth systems solutions include discriminatory decision-making, data breaches, and an imbalance of power among patients, doctors, and tech businesses. Adopting a value-sensitive design strategy that prioritizes human values such as autonomy, dignity, and equity throughout the development and deployment of AI systems [108] is crucial to ensuring that AI is utilized ethically and fairly in telehealth systems. Also, concepts like openness, accountability, justice, and respect for human rights should be incorporated into AI governance frameworks and ethical guidelines to direct AI's responsible development and use in telehealth and telemedicine [109]. So that AI-driven healthcare solutions are consistent with social values and ethical norms, clinicians, data scientists, ethicists, and policymakers need to work together [110].

12.3.3.4 AI deployment and maintenance

Due to the requirement for constant model updates, performance monitoring, and infrastructure management, deploying and sustaining AI models in telehealth systems contexts can be difficult. Regular retraining or fine-tuning of AI models may be necessary to accommodate shifts in medical understanding, clinical best practices, and patient demographics [111]. The continued provision of trustworthy suggestions or forecasts by AI models depends on their performance and is closely monitored. Robust AI deployment and maintenance procedures, such as routine model review, retraining, and validation, and monitoring tools to track model performance and identify potential real-time difficulties are necessary to overcome these obstacles [102]. Additionally, HIEs and EHRs must be integrated with scalable and secure infrastructure for AI model deployment in telehealth and telemedicine [103].

12.3.3.5 Legal and regulatory considerations

The application of AI in healthcare raises a tangle of legal and regulatory issues, particularly in the domains of telehealth systems. Many obstacles must be solved before AI methods may be employed in the medical industry. To preserve individual privacy and sensitive information, AI systems must adhere to rules such as HIPAA and GDPR [112]. Traditional liability models are largely focused on human actors, making assessing culpability in the context of AI-powered healthcare choices challenging. The incorporation of AI in telehealth systems, which introduces new legal and regulatory challenges, makes it challenging for legal experts, regulators, AI developers, healthcare providers, and ethicists to ensure AI's safe, ethical, and legal usage in healthcare. These demands are reconsidering existing legal frameworks and potentially building whole new ones tailored to the AI business. AI tools must adhere to the rules established by the Food and Drug Administration (FDA), the European Medicines Agency (EMA), and other comparable bodies throughout the world [113]. Cross-border healthcare service delivery via telehealth systems creates legal authority concerns. This area's legal and regulatory frameworks must be unified, which necessitates international collaboration.

12.3.4 AI methods in telehealth systems

The telehealth systems' use of AI has tremendous potential to alter the current status quo of healthcare delivery. Diagnostic accuracy, efficiency in managing patients, the effectiveness of treatment protocols, and individualization of medical care have greatly benefited from AI methodologies and models. ML algorithms,

NLP, computer vision and medical imaging, predictive analytics and risk assessment, and personalized health and treatment planning are all discussed in this section as examples of important AI methods currently being used and studied in the telehealth and telemedicine fields.

12.3.4.1 Machine learning algorithms

ML, a subfield of AI, makes use of statistical methods to train computers to learn from experience and make judgements or predictions based on that data. Supervised, unsupervised, and reinforcement learning are the three main types of ML algorithms [114]. ML models have found widespread application in telehealth systems for disease prediction, treatment prescription, and patient monitoring. Predicting patient outcomes and diagnosing diseases via supervised learning algorithms like decision trees, support vector machines, and neural networks based on a set of labelled training data [115]. For example, the medical professions of dermatology and radiology have greatly benefited from the accuracy with which images may be analysed using deep learning [116]. Clustering and dimensionality reduction methods are two examples of unsupervised learning algorithms that can be used on unlabelled data to reveal previously unseen patterns and associations. Segmenting patients, spotting outliers, and recognizing disease patterns are examples of these methods in telehealth [117]. Telehealth, in the form of individualized medical suggestions and robotic surgery, may benefit from reinforcement learning, in which an agent learns to make decisions by interacting with the environment to maximize some idea of cumulative reward [118].

12.3.4.2 Natural language processing

NLP facilitates communication between computers and humans via the use of natural language. It has demonstrated promising applications in numerous domains, including automated medical transcription services, sentiment analysis of patient feedback, and information extraction from EHRs [119]. Medical professionals can keep detailed records without sacrificing efficiency thanks to automated medical transcription systems that translate spoken words into text. Large amounts of unstructured feedback data, such as social media comments, online reviews, and patient surveys, can be processed and analysed with the help of sentiment analysis for patient feedback. Healthcare providers can learn about patient satisfaction, service quality, and areas for development by extracting and classifying the emotions conveyed in this data. It is possible to use NLP methods to glean useful data from EHRs, such as clinical notes, medical histories, and discharge summaries [119]. By sifting through mountains of health records, NLP can help with everything from clinical decision support and predictive modelling to community health management. Since NLP can automate mundane tasks, help extract useful information from unstructured data, and provide insights that drive improvements in patient care and healthcare service delivery, it holds great promise for boosting the efficacy and efficiency of telehealth and telemedicine services. Incorporating NLP into telehealth systems is likely to become more advanced as the discipline develops.

12.3.4.3 Computer vision and medical imaging

Computer vision, a multidisciplinary branch of AI, trains computers to recognize the visual world. It has been utilized to better analyse medical images, which has helped in the detection, diagnosis, and treatment planning of various diseases. Deep learning models, such as CNNs, have demonstrated outstanding performance in understanding medical pictures from many modalities, including X-rays, magnetic resonance imaging (MRI) scans, computed tomography (CT) scans, and ultrasound images [120]. These algorithms can automatically detect abnormalities in medical pictures, such as tumours in an MRI or pneumonia symptoms in a chest X-ray. AI-assisted diagnosis can lighten the load on radiologists and physicians by automating the preliminary screening process, offering second opinions, and highlighting areas of interest in medical pictures. Computer vision is a valuable tool for telehealth systems applications because it reduces the chance of human errors caused by fatigue or oversight. It can also be utilized for real-time image processing of video data in telehealth applications such as patient monitoring, gesture recognition, and health-related sign detection [121]. The automated segmentation of medical pictures can be used to distinguish between healthy and cancerous tissue in a scan, assisting in illness diagnosis and therapy planning. Incorporating computer vision methods into telehealth systems has the potential to greatly improve disease detection, diagnosis, and treatment. As AI and computer vision continue to develop, we may anticipate even greater use and efficacy in medical imaging and other areas of telehealth systems, leading to more precise diagnoses, better patient outcomes, and more effective healthcare delivery systems [122].

12.3.4.4 Predictive analytics and risk assessment

Predictive analytics uses data, statistical algorithms, and ML methodologies to predict future events based on previous data. It can predict patients' healthcare needs, readmission rates, prognoses, and other factors. ML algorithms may mine numerous forms of data for patterns and correlations that may indicate illness risks, such as EHRs, genetic data, and lifestyle data. Predictive models include factors such as the patient's medical history, the kind of underlying illness, treatment details, and socioeconomic determinants of health to forecast the probability of a patient being readmitted to a hospital after being discharged. AI models can predict disease development and patient survival [123]. The predictive capacity of these models is expected to expand as the quantity and diversity of health-related data grow, which will benefit the expansion of telehealth systems [124].

12.3.4.5 Personalized medicine and treatment planning

Personalized medicine considers the patient's genetic profile at every level of care, from prevention to diagnosis to therapy. The huge amounts and complexity of biological data, particularly in genomics, need the utilization of AI technological advancements for processing and interpretation. ML algorithms successfully assessed personalized treatment plans based on genetic data. Pharmacogenomics examines a patient's genetic data using ML algorithms to predict how they will react to a pharmaceutical and discover the most effective and safest treatment strategy [125]. Patients can be classified based on shared characteristics using ML techniques. Following these steps will help healthcare practitioners evaluate which treatment method is most beneficial for each patient subgroup [126]. Individuals at high risk of acquiring specific diseases based on their genetic profile, lifestyle, and other health characteristics may also be detected and provided individualized treatment regimens based on their health problems and projected responses to therapy using ML algorithms. The use of AI to analyse huge and complex health data sets is critical to reaching the goal of personalized care in telehealth systems. The impact of personalized medicine on telehealth systems is expected to grow as our understanding of the human genome and the capabilities of AI algorithms improve.

12.4 Models and numerical simulations

In this section, the numerical simulation and results obtained based on the availability of data as regards blockchain technology in healthcare systems are presented and discussed briefly. However, because of the paucity of resources and access to data to do more in-depth analysis, this book chapter will present preliminary results on account of the available data relating to the aforementioned and afore-discussed models and methods in Section 12.3.

12.4.1 Building of models

Here the stages involved in building the models are summarized for further illumination of the ideas of the application of AI to telehealth systems. There are two models employed in this study, namely random forest and XGBOOST.

A random forest classifier is essentially a group of decision tree classifiers, where each tree can vote for the prediction class that it thinks would be most accurate [127]. It uses ensemble learning, a technique that combines several classifiers to effectively predict outcomes in difficult situations. The acronym XGBOOST is a short form for the eXtreme Gradient Boosting framework. It takes a successful strategy for tree-based training and includes a capable linear model solver. It can perform various objective functions such as regression, classification, and ranking [128]. The implementation process involved is captured in Figure 12.4. The entire data were divided into k folds of equal size, of which onefold was used to test or validate the model, while other folds are used to train the model. The average performance will be determined once this process has been repeated k times, in this case, ten times.

12.4.2 Numerical results

This section discusses the numerical results obtained based on the datasets in [129] for health-related ailments specifically chronic diseases in the human body system to demonstrate the importance of AI/blockchain technology in proffering solutions to telehealth, telemedicine and other areas of human endeavours. A case study of the telehealth system is a prediction of chronic kidney disease using AI. The dataset

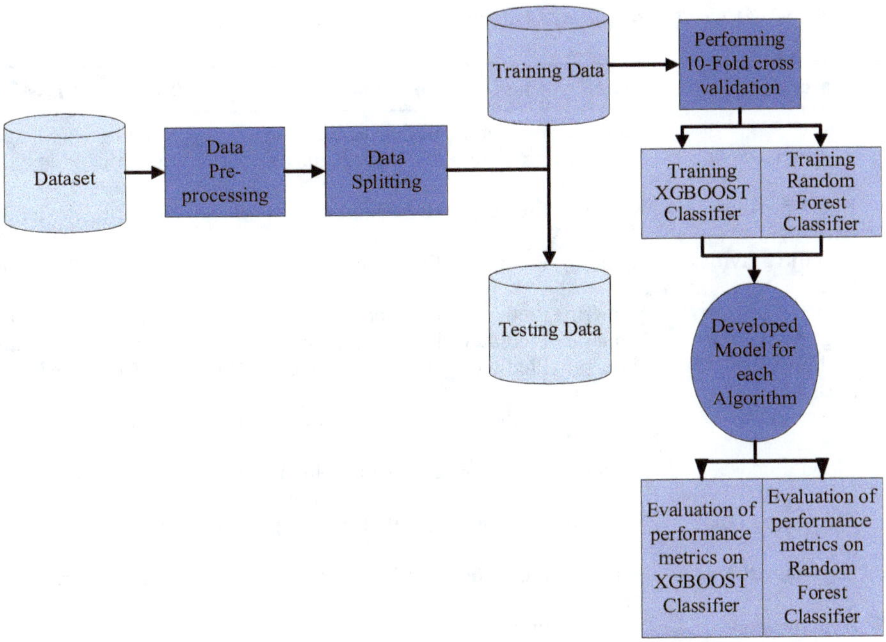

Figure 12.4 Implementation flowchart for model building

is obtained from UCI. The dataset consists of 400 records of patient data and 24 attributes. The dataset was obtained from Kaggle [129]. The attributes used are listed in Table 12.3.

The data were pre-processed and cleaned to get rid of unbalanced data, empty cells, and duplicate data within the dataset. The exploratory data analysis (EDA) was applied to the dataset to better understand the relationship among the various key attributes and the target variable in the dataset. Data visualization is done using violin plots, to interpret the relationship between these key attributes and the target variable (CKD status) as shown in Figure 12.5.

In this study, tenfold cross-validations (CVs) were employed to obtain the accuracy of each of the ML algorithms. CV was done to get rid of fluctuating accuracy. The original data were divided into tenfolds; accuracy was obtained for each fold, after which the mean of each fold was calculated to obtain the overall accuracy of each ML algorithm. The accuracy of each algorithm is given in Table 12.4. Furthermore, the confusion matrix for XGBOOST and random forest is depicted in Figures 12.6 and 12.7, respectively. The bar charts and ROC for XGBOOST and random forest are shown in Figures 12.8–12.11, correspondingly.

12.4.3 Discussion of numerical results

Based on the classifiers employed in this study, it is observed that the random forest classifier with a numerical value of 97.50% performs better in comparison to that of

Table 12.3 Attributes of the dataset employed in this research

No	Feature	Type	Class	No	Type	Type	Class
1.	Age	Numeric	Predictor	14	Anaemia	Nominal	Predictor
2	Red blood cells (RBC)	Numeric	Predictor	15	Blood glucose	Numeric	Predictor
3	Blood pressure (BP)	Numeric	Predictor	16	Blood urea	Numeric	Predictor
4	Specific gravity (SG)	Numeric	Predictor	17	Serum creatinine	Numeric	Predictor
5	Albumin	Numeric	Predictor	18	Sodium	Numeric	Predictor
6	Sugar	Numeric	Predictor	19	Potassium	Numeric	Predictor
7	Red blood cells (RBC)	Nominal	Predictor	20	Haemoglobin (HM)	Numeric	Predictor
8	Pus cell (PC)	Nominal	Predictor	21	Packed cell volume (PCV)	Numeric	Predictor
9	Blood glucose random (BGR)	Numeric	Predictor	22	White blood cell count (WBCC)	Numeric	Predictor
10	Blood urea (BU)	Numeric	Predictor	23	Red blood cell count (RBCC)	Numeric	Predictor
11	Serum creatinine	Numeric	Predictor	24	Diabetes mellitus (DM)	Nominal	Predictor
12	Hypertension	Nominal	Predictor	25	Appetite	Nominal	Predictor
13	Coronary artery disease (CAD)	Nominal	Predictor	26	Ckd_Status	Nominal	Target

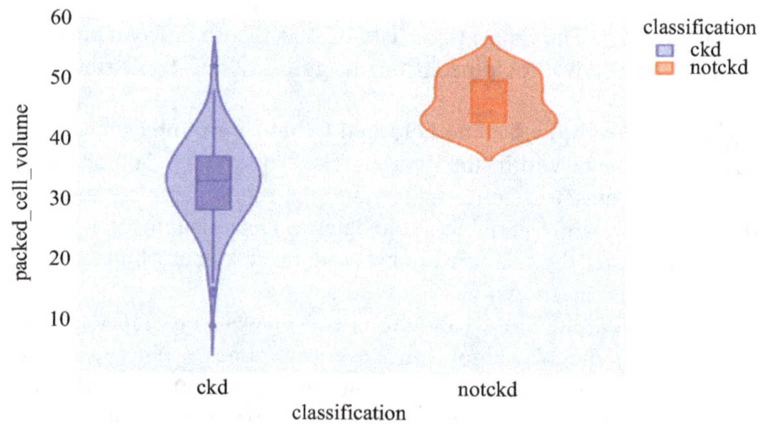

Figure 12.5 Violin plot showing the relationship between ckd_status and pcv

Table 12.4 Accuracy of ML algorithm using tenfold CV

ML algorithms	Accuracy (%)
XGBOOST	96.50
Random forest	97.50

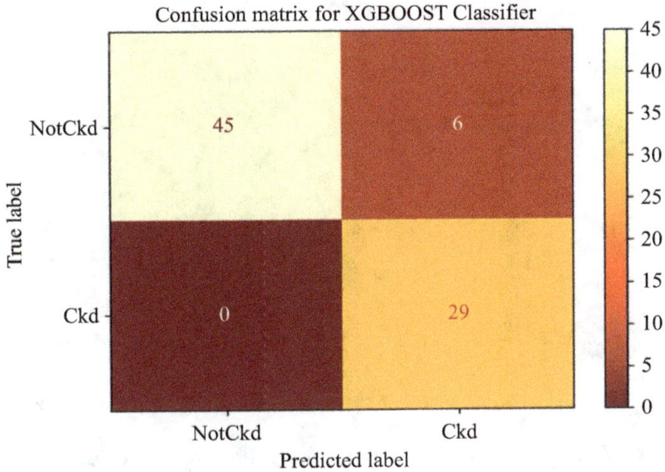

Figure 12.6 Confusion matrix for XGBOOST classifier

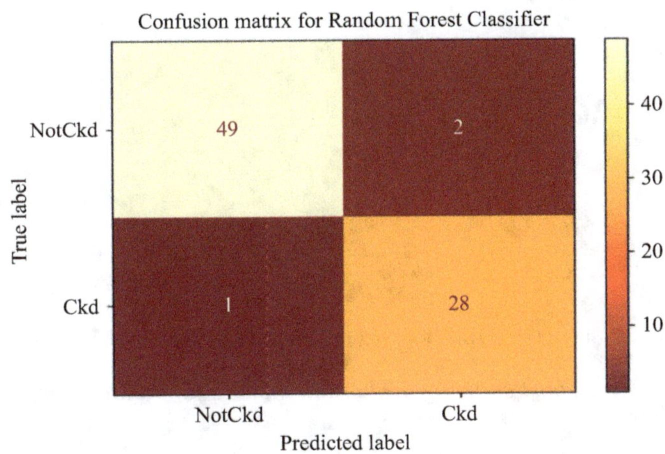

Figure 12.7 Confusion matrix for random forest classifier.

XGBOOST with 96.50% in the prediction of chronic kidney diseases as tabulated in Table 12.4. Furthermore, in terms of the confusion matrix in Figures 12.6 and 12.7, it is equally noticed that the random forest outperforms the other. Additionally, in Figures 12.8 and 12.9, where various metrics such as sensitivity, F-measure, accuracy, and precision were utilized to gauge the effectiveness of each classifier for the prediction of chronic kidney disease, it was observed that at some point, the sensitivity recorded for XGBOOST was better than that of random forest. Noticeably, in Figures 12.10 and 12.11 regarding the ROC curve, the random forest algorithm converges faster than the XGBOOST in the prediction of chronic kidney

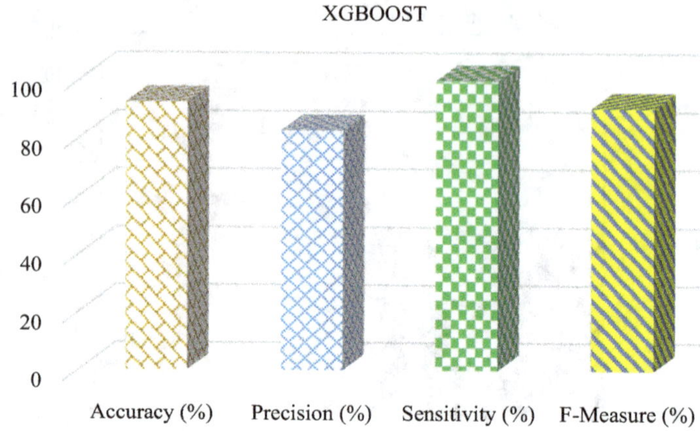

Figure 12.8 Bar chart showing evaluation metrics for XG BOOST classifier

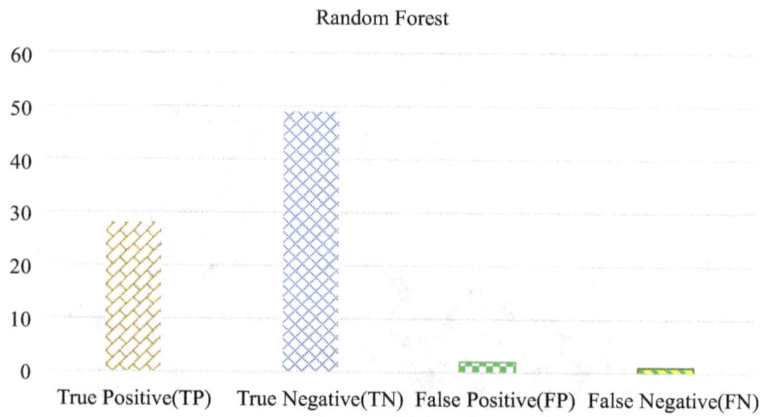

Figure 12.9 Bar chart showing evaluation metrics for random forest classifier

diseases. It should be noted that other schemes or classifiers and metaheuristic algorithms can be employed to forecast health-related ailments/diseases soon based on the availability of data on such diseases in the areas of telehealth systems using AI-inspired schemes or blockchain-based technology.

12.5 Lessons learned

Blockchain technology is now widely used in financial sectors, healthcare systems, and systems technology. Additionally, during the COVID-19 epidemic, AI and blockchain played a crucial role. More importantly, though, they have helped telehealth systems become more popular around the world. Centralization is a significant hurdle in current telehealth systems that raise the risk of a single point of

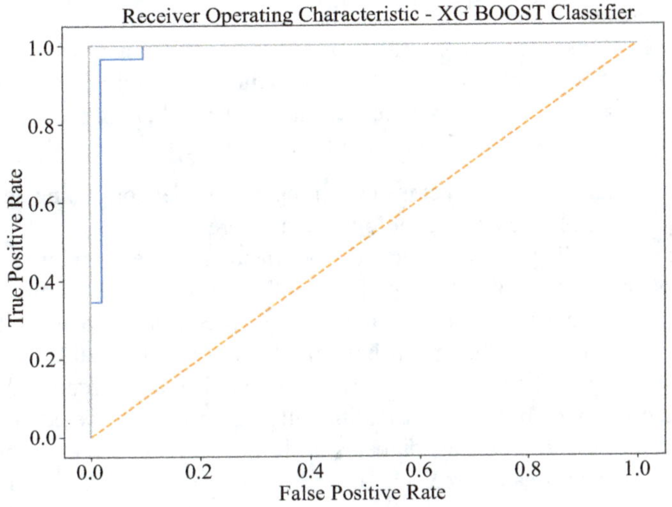

Figure 12.10 *ROC curve for XGBOOST classifier*

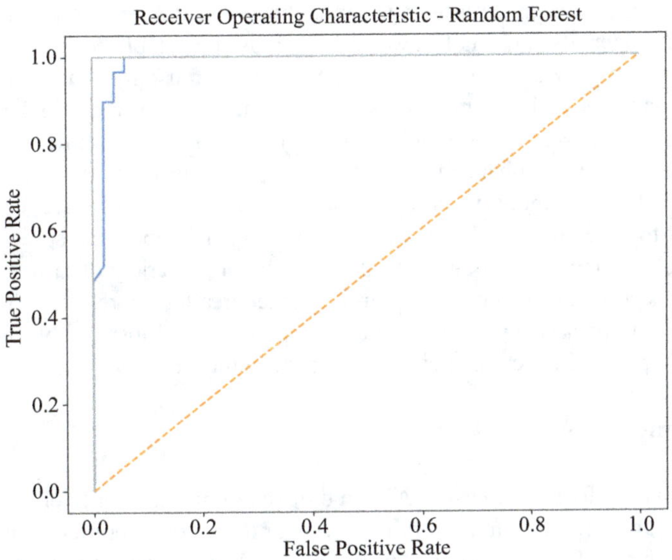

Figure 12.11 *ROC curve for random forest classifier*

failure. A variety of both internal and external data breaches also pose a danger to the dependability and accessibility of modern telehealth systems. The lessons or takeaways from the usage of the blockchain, AI, and ML in telehealth systems are thus as follows. By fixing the primary issues with the telehealth systems currently in use concerning dependability, traceability, indestructibility, accountability, background data, inspection, credibility, and safety, solutions based on blockchain technology might significantly improve them. Due to several issues, existing telehealth systems cannot completely take advantage of blockchain technology. In this section, various lessons learned are highlighted as follows:

- Given how quickly the subject is developing, the model combining deep learning techniques and blockchain technology needs more in-depth study. Deep learning may be used to diagnose myopia and other inside disorders, and when combined with blockchain technology, the patient's information is accurate and secure. It is crucial to conduct an extensive study earlier presenting a plan of the recommended design to collaborate in both fields, and this may also be one of our future research goals. An overview of the potential future is provided by the fact that these kinds of models will additionally be capable of detecting long-term conditions, including cancer, diabetes, arthritis, and some serious heart conditions, with much greater precision and retain the security of the data.
- The security and privacy of blockchain technology enabled by AI still have a lot of room for advancement. Future studies could focus on implementing the most recent hash algorithms and employing a stricter validation system. For this study subject, it is impractical to establish the benefits and drawbacks of using dual-factor verification and multi-stage authentication for every node on the decentralized ledger. It would not be wise to employ the established consensus protocols, such as PoW and PoS, given they have been in use for roughly the previous 10–11 years and have numerous flaws. The AI-powered blockchain could implement new consensus protocols like evidence-of-elapsed-time and delegation of PoS, which will enhance the effectiveness and privacy of the entire system.
- Compared to an intransigent computing technique, collaborative computing is thought to speed up calculating a block's hashing. The operating speed of a driven by AI blockchain might be increased by combining a variety of different methods, and connecting it with current systems is another area for future research. Enhancing security and preserving privacy are also important if AI-inspired blockchain solutions are planned for commercial deployment in the healthcare sector.

12.6 Conclusion

This book chapter focuses on using AI and blockchain models for telehealth systems. This chapter also provides an in-depth analysis of recent developments on the testing and validation of AI and blockchain-inspired model on telehealth systems. Using AI and blockchain for telehealth holds great potential for transforming healthcare delivery. From the chapter, the various benefits of using AI and blockchain in telehealth were identified, which include increased diagnostic precision, effective remote monitoring, greater data security and privacy, increased trust and transparency, compliance with regulations and scalability, amongst others. Telehealth can transform healthcare delivery by utilising these technologies, expanding access to high-quality care, and enhancing patient outcomes. However, for successful acceptance and fulfilment of the full potential of AI and blockchain technology in telehealth systems, cautious deployment, ongoing review, and addressing ethical considerations are essential. Crucially, modern AI algorithms have been employed to predict chronic kidney disorders proactively, enabling early detection and prevention of these conditions easier. Advanced classifiers, such as Random Forest and eXtreme Gradient Boosting (XGBOOST), are used to achieve this. These strong models have outstanding prediction rates ranging from 97.50% to 95.50%, and they are exceptionally accurate, depicting a promising result in this area. These findings aid in assessing the models' readiness and suitability for additional processing and deployment in telehealth settings. In addition, the early detection of chronic kidney disease and a prevention case study using some ML classifiers show promising results in this area. For future scope or directions, it is recommended that transformative telehealth service improvements be made possible through further research and development in areas like enhanced real-time monitoring, better interoperability, stringency on regulatory compliance, improved privacy and security measures, system optimization, and user experience improvement.

References

[1] E. Brynjolfsson, "The turing trap: the promise & peril of human-like artificial intelligence," *Augmented Education in the Global Age*, Routledge, pp. 103–116, 2023.

[2] P. Rajpurkar, E. Chen, O. Banerjee, and E. J. Topol, "AI in health and medicine," *Nat. Med.*, vol. 28, no. 1, pp. 31–38., 2022.

[3] A. Hayes, "Blockchain Facts: What is it, how it works, and how it can be used," *Investopedia*, 2023. [Online]. Available: https://www.investopedia.com/terms/b/blockchain.asp. [Accessed: 24-Apr-2023].

[4] A. S. Rajasekaran, M. Azees, and F. Al-Turjman, "A comprehensive survey on blockchain technology," *Sustain. Energy Technol. Assess.*, vol. 52, p. 102039, 2022.

[5] L. K. Ramasamy, F. K. KP, A. L. Imoize, J. O. Ogbebor, S. Kadry, and S. Rho, "Blockchain-based wireless sensor networks for malicious node detection: a survey," *IEEE Access*, vol. 9, pp. 128765–128785, 2021.

[6] W. Y. Ng, T. E. Tan, P. V. Movva, *et al.*, "Blockchain applications in health care for COVID-19 and beyond: a systematic review," *Lancet Digit. Heal.*, vol. 3, no. 12, pp. e819–e829., 2021.

[7] M. Y. Jabarulla and H.-N. Lee, "A blockchain and artificial intelligence-based, patient-centric healthcare system for combating the COVID-19 pandemic: opportunities and applications," *Heal. MDPI*, vol. 9, no. 8, p. 1019, 2021.

[8] R. W. Ahmad, K. Salah, R. Jayaraman, I. Yaqoob, S. Ellahham, and M. Omar, "The role of blockchain technology in telehealth and telemedicine," *Int. J. Med. Inform.*, vol. 148, p. 104399, 2021, doi: 10.1016/j.ijmedinf.2021.104399.

[9] C. Drago, A. Gatto, and M. Ruggeri, "Telemedicine as technoinnovation to tackle COVID-19: A bibliometric analysis," *Technovation*, p. 102417, 2021.

[10] J. Yi, H. Zhang, J. Mao, Y. Chen, H. Zhong, and Y. Wang, "Review on the COVID-19 pandemic prevention and control system based on AI," *Eng. Appl. Artif. Intell.*, p. 105184, 2022.

[11] J. P. Li, H. Liu, D. S. Ting, *et al.*, "Digital technology, tele-medicine and artificial intelligence in ophthalmology: a global perspective," *Prog. Retin. Eye Res.*, vol. 82, p. 100900, 2021.

[12] M. Younis, W. Lalouani, N. Lasla, L. Emokpae, and M. Abdallah, "Blockchain-enabled and data-driven smart healthcare solution for secure and privacy-preserving data access," *IEEE Syst. J.*, vol. 16, no. 3, pp. 3746–3757, 2022.

[13] M. S. Islam, M. A. B. Ameedeen, M. A. Rahman, H. Ajra, and Z.B. Ismail, "Healthcare-chain: blockchain-enabled decentralized trustworthy system in healthcare management Industry 4.0 with cyber safeguard," *Computers*, vol. 12, no. 2, p. 46, 2023.

[14] A. S. Rajasekaran, A. Maria, M. Rajagopal, and J. Lorincz, "Blockchain enabled anonymous privacy-preserving authentication scheme for internet of health things," *Sensors*, vol. 23, no. 1, p. 240, 2022.

[15] T. Gadekallu, T. Reddy Huynh-The, W. Wang, *et al.*, "Blockchain for the metaverse: a review," *Future Generation Computer Systems*. vol. 143. pp. 401–419, 2023.

[16] S. Yaqoob, M. M. Khan, R. Talib, *et al.*, "Use of blockchain in healthcare: a systematic literature review," *Int. J. Adv. Comput. Sci. Appl.*, vol. 10, no. 5, 2019.

[17] M. Antwi, A. Adnane, F. Ahmad, R. Hussain, M. H. ur Rehman, and C. A. Kerrache, "The case of HyperLedger Fabric as a blockchain solution for healthcare applications," *Blockchain Res. Appl.*, vol. 2, no. 1, p. 100012, 2021.

[18] E. Markakis, Y. Nikoloudakis, E. Pallis, and M. Manso, "Security assessment as a service cross-layered system for the adoption of digital, personalised and trusted healthcare," *IEEE 5th World Forum Internet Things (WF-IoT)*, Limerick, Irel., pp. 91–94, 2019, doi: 10.1109/WF-IoT.2019.8767249.

[19] V. Koufi, F. Malamateniou, and G. Vassilacopoulos, "Ubiquitous access to cloud emergency medical services," *Proc. 10th IEEE Int. Conf. Inf. Technol. Appl. Biomed. Corfu*, Greece, pp. 1–4, 2010, doi: 10.1109/ITAB.2010.5687702.

[20] C. Chakraborty and A. Kishor, "Real-time cloud-based patient-centric monitoring using computational health systems," *IEEE Trans. Comput. Soc. Syst.*, vol. 9, no. 6, pp. 1613–1623, 2022, doi: 10.1109/TCSS.2022.3170375.

[21] V. K. Quy, N. V. Hau, D. V. Anh, and L.A. Ngoc, "Smart healthcare IoT applications based on fog computing: architecture, applications and challenges," *Complex Intell. Syst.*, vol. 8, no. 5, pp. 3805–3815, 2022.

[22] S. Tutun, M. E. Johnson, A. Ahmed, *et al.*, "An AI-based decision support system for predicting mental health disorders," *Inf. Syst. Front.*, vol. 25, no. 3, pp. 1261–76, 2023.

[23] M. Knop, S. Weber, M. Mueller, and B. Niehaves, "Human factors and technological characteristics influencing the interaction of medical professionals with artificial intelligence–enabled clinical decision support systems: literature review," *JMIR Hum. Factors*, vol. 9, no. 1, p. e28639, 2022.

[24] S. van Baalen, M. Boon, and P. Verhoef, "From clinical decision support to clinical reasoning support systems," *J. Eval. Clin. Pract.*, vol. 27, no. 3, pp. 520–528, 2021.

[25] M. A. Al-Antari, "Artificial intelligence for medical diagnostics—existing and future AI technology," *Diagnostics*, vol. 13, no. 4, p. 688, 2023.

[26] N. Panigrahi, I. Ayus, and O.P. Jena, "An expert system-based clinical decision support system for Hepatitis-B prediction & diagnosis," *Mach. Learn. Healthc. Appl.*, pp. 57–75, 2021.

[27] M. Braun, P. Hummel, S. Beck, and P. Dabrock, "Primer on an ethics of AI-based decision support systems in the clinic," *J. Med. Ethics*, vol. 47, no. 12, pp. e3–e3, 2021.

[28] A. Ashwini, N. R. Rajalakshmi, P. V. Paul, and L. Jayakumar, "Dynamic NLP enabled chatbot for rural health care in India," *Second Int. Conf. Comput. Sci. Eng. Appl. (ICCSEA)*, Gunupur, India, pp. 1–6, 2022, doi: 10.1109/ICCSEA54677.2022.9936389.

[29] M. Almalki and F. Azeez, "Health chatbots for fighting COVID-19: a scoping review," *Acta Inform. Medica*, vol. 28, no. 4, pp. 1–6, 2022.

[30] A. Khamis, J. Meng, J. Wang, *et al.*, "Robotics and intelligent systems against a pandemic.," *Acta Polytech. Hungarica*, vol. 18, no. 5, pp. 13–35, 2021.

[31] E. Mbunge, J. Batani, G. Gaobotse, and B. Muchemwa, "Virtual healthcare services and digital health technologies deployed during coronavirus disease 2019 (COVID-19) pandemic in South Africa: A systematic review," *Glob. Heal. J.*, vol. 6, no. 2, pp. 102–113, 2022.

[32] D. Golinelli, E. Boetto, G. Carullo, A. G. Nuzzolese, M. P. Landini, and M. P. Fantini, "Adoption of digital technologies in health care during the COVID-19 pandemic: systematic review of early scientific literature," *J. Med. Internet Res.*, vol. 22, no. 11, p. e22280, 2020.

[33] A. L. Imoize, P. A. Gbadega, H. I. Obakhena, D. O. Irabor, K. V. N. Kavitha, and C. Chakraborty, "Artificial Intelligence-enabled Internet of Medical Things for COVID-19 pandemic data management," *Explain. Artif. Intell. Med. Decis. Support Syst.*, pp. 357–380, 2023.

[34] V. Subbhuraam and D. Panigrahi, "Telemedicine," *Predict. Anal. Heal. Transform. Futur. Med. IOP Publ.*, vol. 1, 2021.

[35] P. Upadhyaya, S. K. Upadhyay, A. Shrestha, *et al.*, "Use of telemedicine and artificial intelligence in Eye and ENT: a boon for developing countries.," *4th IEEE Int. Conf. Artif. Intell. Speech Technol.*, pp. 1–6, 2022.

[36] S. Tiribelli, A. Monnot, S. F. Shah, A. Arora, P. J. Toong, and S. Kong, "Ethics principles for artificial intelligence–based telemedicine for public health," *Am. J. Public Health*, vol. 113, no. 5, pp. 577–584, 2023.

[37] D. M. El-Sherif, M. Abouzid, M. T. Elzarif, A. A. Ahmed, A. Albakri, and M.M. Alshehri, "Telehealth and artificial intelligence insights into healthcare during the COVID-19 pandemic," *Heal. MDPI*, vol. 10, no. 2, p. 385, 2022.

[38] I. Oke, "The pursuit of generalizability and equity through artificial intelligence-based risk prediction models," *JAMA Ophthalmol.*, vol. 140, no. 8, pp. 798–799, 2022.

[39] W. Yousaf, A. I. Umar, S. H. Shirazi, *et al.*, "Telehealth for COVID-19: a conceptual framework.," *J. Healthc. Eng.*, vol. 2023, 8pp, 2023. Article ID 3679829. https://doi.org/10.1155/2023/3679829

[40] S. Ranasinghe, G. Gamage, H. Moraliyage, *et al.*, "An artificial intelligence framework for the detection of emotion transitions in telehealth services," *15th Int. Conf. Hum. Syst. Interact.*, pp. 1–5, 2022, doi: 10.1109/HSI55341.2022.9869503.

[41] A. Kadu and M. Singh, "Comparative analysis of e-Health care telemedicine system based on internet of medical things and artificial intelligence," 2nd Int. Conf. Smart Electron. Commun. (ICOSEC), Trichy, India, pp. 1768–1775, 2021, doi: 10.1109/ICOSEC51865.2021.9591941.

[42] A. Amjad, P. Kordel, and G. Fernandes, "A review on innovation in healthcare sector (telehealth) through artificial intelligence," *Sustainability*, vol. 15, no. 8, p. 6655, 2023.

[43] H. Edrees, W. Song, A. Syrowatka, A. Simona, M. G. Amato, and D.W. Bates, "Intelligent telehealth in pharmacovigilance: a future perspective," *Drug Saf.*, vol. 45, no. 5, pp. 449–458, 2022.

[44] S. Khezr, M. Moniruzzaman, A. Yassine, and R. Benlamri, "Blockchain technology in healthcare: a comprehensive review and directions for future research," *Appl. Sci.*, vol. 9, no. 9, p. 1736, 2019.

[45] H. R. Hasan, K. Salah, R. Jayaraman, I. Yaqoob, M. Omar, and S. Ellahham, "Blockchain-enabled telehealth services using smart contracts," *IEEE Access*, vol. 9, pp. 151944–151959, 2021.

[46] R. W. Ahmad, K. Salah, R. Jayaraman, I. Yaqoob, S. Ellahham, and M. Omar, "Blockchain and COVID-19 pandemic: applications and challenges," *Cluster Comput.*, pp. 1–26, 2023.

[47] T. Hewa, A. Braeken, M. Ylianttila, and M. Liyanage, "Multi-access edge computing and blockchain-based secure telehealth system connected with 5G and IoT," *IEEE Glob. Commun. Conf. (GLOBECOM)*. Taipei, Taiwan, pp. 1–6, 2020, doi: 10.1109/GLOBECOM42002.2020.9348125.

[48] Q. Liu, Y. Liu, M. Luo, D. He, H. Wang, and K. -K. R. Choo, "The security of blockchain-based medical systems: research challenges and opportunities," *IEEE Syst. J.*, vol. 16, no. 4, pp. 5741–5752, 2022, doi: 10.1109/JSYST.2022.3155156.

[49] H. Kordestani, K. Barkaoui, and W. Zahran, "HapiChain: a blockchain-based framework for patient-centric telemedicine," *IEEE 8th Int. Conf.*

Serious Games Appl. Heal. (SeGAH), Vancouver, BC, Canada, pp. 1–6, 2020, doi: 10.1109/SeGAH49190.2020.9201726.

[50] J. Vora, A. Nayyar, S. Tanwar, *et al.*, "BHEEM: A blockchain-based framework for securing electronic health records," *IEEE Globecom Work. (GC Wkshps)*, pp. 1–6, 2018.

[51] S. Shamshad, K. Mahmood, S. Kumari, and C.M. Chen, "A secure blockchain-based e-health records storage and sharing scheme," *J. Inf. Secur. Appl.*, vol. 55, p. 102590, 2020.

[52] W. Wang, H. Zhang, H. Wu, G. Li, and K. Gai, "Blockchain-based secure medical data management and disease prediction," *Proc. Fourth ACM Int. Symp. Blockchain Secur. Crit. Infrastruct*, pp. 71–82, 2022.

[53] S. Y. Jung, T. Kim, H. J. Hwang, and K. Hong, "Mechanism design of health care blockchain system token economy: development study based on simulated real-world scenarios," *J. Med. Internet Res.*, vol. 23, no. 9, p. e26802, 2021.

[54] M. C. Ballandies, "To incentivize or not: impact of blockchain-based cryptoeconomic tokens on human information sharing behavior," *IEEE Access*, vol. 10, pp. 74111–74130, 2022, doi: 10.1109/ACCESS.2022.3189774.

[55] V. Jaiman, L. Pernice, and V. Urovi, "User incentives for blockchain-based data sharing platforms," *PLoS One*, vol. 17, no. 4, p. e0266624, 2022.

[56] E.-Y. Daraghmi, Y.-A. Daraghmi, and S. -M. Yuan, "MedChain: a design of blockchain-based system for medical records access and permissions management," *IEEE Access*, vol. 7, pp. 164595–164613, 2019, doi: 10.1109/ACCESS.2019.2952942.

[57] S. Xuan, L. Zheng, I. Chung, *et al.*, "An incentive mechanism for data sharing based on blockchain with smart contracts," *Comput. Electr. Eng.*, vol. 83, p. 106587, 2020.

[58] S. Hannah, A. J. Deepa, V. S. Chooralil, *et al.*, "Blockchain-based deep learning to process IoT data acquisition in cognitive data," *Biomed Res. Int.*, 2022.

[59] M. Imran, U. Zaman, J. Imtiaz, M. Fayaz, and J. Gwak, "Comprehensive survey of IoT, machine learning, and blockchain for health care applications: a topical assessment for pandemic preparedness, challenges, and solutions," *Electronics*, vol. 10, no. 20, p. 2501, 2021.

[60] Y. Zhang, F. Xiong, Y. Xie, X. Fan, and H. Gu, "The impact of artificial intelligence and blockchain on the accounting profession," *IEEE Access*, vol. 8, pp. 110461–110477, 2020.

[61] S. K. Rana, S. K. Rana, K. Nisar, *et al.*, "Blockchain technology and artificial intelligence based decentralized access control model to enable secure interoperability for healthcare," *Sustainability*, vol. 14, no. 15, p. 9471, 2022.

[62] J. Almalki, W. Al Shehri, R. Mehmood, *et al.*, "Enabling blockchain with IoMT devices for healthcare," *Information*, vol. 13, no. 10, p. 448, 2022.

[63] S. B. Junaid, A. A. Imam, A. O. Balogun, *et al.*, "Recent advancements in emerging technologies for healthcare management systems: a survey," *Heal. MDPI*, vol. 10, no. 10, p. 1940, 2022.

[64] Q. Mamun, "Blockchain technology in the future of healthcare," *Smart Heal.*, vol. 23, p. 100223, 2022.

[65] E. Nehme, R. El Sibai, J. B. Abdo, A. R. Taylor, and J. Demerjian, "Converged AI, IoT, and blockchain technologies: a conceptual ethics framework," *AI Ethics*, pp. 1–15, 2022.

[66] R. Ftouni, B. AlJardali, M. Hamdanieh, L. Ftouni, and N. Salem, "Challenges of telemedicine during the COVID-19 pandemic: a systematic review," *BMC Med. Inform. Decis. Mak.*, vol. 22, no. 1, 2022, doi: 10.1186/s12911-022-01952-0.

[67] H. Bitar and S. Alismail, "The role of eHealth, telehealth, and telemedicine for chronic disease patients during COVID-19 pandemic: a rapid systematic review," *Digit. Heal.*, vol. 7, p. 205520762110093, 2021, doi: 10.1177/20552076211009396.

[68] T. McGhin, K.-K. R. Choo, C. Z. Liu, and D. He, "Blockchain in healthcare applications: research challenges and opportunities," *J. Netw. Comput. Appl.*, vol. 135, pp. 62–75, 2019.

[69] S. Ramzan, A. Aqdus, V. Ravi, D. Koundal, R. Amin, and M. A. Al Ghamdi, "Healthcare applications using blockchain technology: motivations and challenges," *IEEE Trans. Eng. Manage.*, pp. 1–17, 2022.

[70] D. K. Sharma, S. Pant, M. Sharma, and S. Brahmachari, "Cryptocurrency mechanisms for blockchains: models, characteristics, challenges, and applications," *Handb. Res. Blockchain Technol.*, pp. 323–348, 2020, doi: 10.1016/b978-0-12-819816-2.00013-7.

[71] C. Sguanci, R. Spatafora, and A. M. Vergani, "Layer 2 Blockchain Scaling: a Survey," arXiv.org, 2021.

[72] I. A. Seres, L. Gulyás, D. A. Nagy, and P. Burcsi, "Topological analysis of Bitcoin's lightning network," *Math. Res. Blockchain Econ.*, pp. 1–12, 2020, doi: doi:10.1007/978-3-030-37110-4_1.

[73] J. Jayabalan and N. Jeyanthi, "Scalable blockchain model using off-chain IPFS storage for healthcare data security and privacy," *J. Parallel Distrib. Comput.*, vol. 164, pp. 152–167, 2022, doi: 10.1016/j.jpdc.2022.03.009.

[74] F. Hashim, K. Shuaib, and N. Zaki, "Sharding for scalable blockchain networks," *SN Comput. Sci.*, vol. 4, no. 1, 2022, doi: 10.1007/s42979-022-01435-z.

[75] N. Kannengießer, S. Lins, T. Dehling, and A. Sunyaev, "Trade-offs between distributed ledger technology characteristics," *ACM Comput. Surv.*, vol. 53, no. 2, pp. 1–37, 2020, doi: 10.1145/3379463.

[76] S. Singh, S. K. Sharma, P. Mehrotra, P. Bhatt, and M. Kaurav, "Blockchain technology for efficient data management in healthcare system: opportunity, challenges and future perspectives," *Mater. Today Proc.*, vol. 62, pp. 5042–5046, 2022, doi: 10.1016/j.matpr.2022.04.998.

[77] J. Jedlicka and E. S. Grant, "Data privacy through zero-knowledge proofs," in *Fourth International Conference on Emerging Research in Electronics, Computer Science and Technology (ICERECT)*, 2022, doi: 10.1109/icerect56837.2022.10060661.

[78] R. Antwi, J. D. Gadze, E. T. Tchao, *et al.*, "A survey on network optimization techniques for blockchain systems," *Algorithms*, vol. 15, no. 6, p. 193, 2022, doi: 10.3390/a15060193.

[79] E. G. Spanakis, S. Sfakianakis, S. Bonomi, C. Ciccotelli, S. Magalini, and V. Sakkalis, "Emerging and established trends to support secure health information exchange," *Front. Digit. Heal.*, vol. 3, 2021, doi: 10.3389/fdgth.2021.636082.

[80] A. Telenti and X. Jiang, "Treating medical data as a durable asset," *Nat. Genet.*, vol. 52, no. 10, pp. 1005–1010, 2020, doi: 10.1038/s41588-020-0698-y.

[81] Y. Pang, "A new consensus protocol for blockchain interoperability architecture," *IEEE Access*, vol. 8, pp. 153719–153730, 2020, doi: 10.1109/access.2020.3017549.

[82] J. M. Roman-Belmonte, H. D. la Corte-Rodriguez, and E. C. Rodriguez-Merchan, "How blockchain technology can change medicine," *Postgrad. Med.*, vol. 130, no. 4, pp. 420–427, 2018, doi: 10.1080/00325481.2018.1472996.

[83] S. Seebacher and R. Schüritz, "Blockchain technology as an enabler of service systems: a structured literature review," in *Lecture Notes in Business Information Processing*, 2017, pp. 12–23, doi: 10.1007/978-3-319-56925-3_2.

[84] C. Wirth and M. Kolain, "Privacy by blockchain design: a blockchain-enabled GDPR-compliant approach for handling personal data," in *Proceedings of 1st ERCIM Blockchain Workshop 2018. European Society for Socially Embedded Technologies (EUSSET)*, 2018.

[85] E. Ducas and A. Wilner, "The security and financial implications of blockchain technologies: regulating emerging technologies in Canada," *Int. J. Canada's J. Glob. Policy Anal.*, vol. 72, no. 4, pp. 538–562, 2017, doi: 10.1177/0020702017741909.

[86] A. Gervais, G. O. Karame, K. Wüst, V. Glykantzis, H. Ritzdorf, and S. Capkun, "On the security and performance of proof of work blockchains," in *Proceedings of the 2016 ACM SIGSAC Conference on Computer and Communications Security*, 2016, doi: 10.1145/2976749.2978341.

[87] F. Saleh, "Blockchain without waste: proof-of-stake," *Rev. Financ. Stud.*, vol. 34, no. 3, pp. 1156–1190, 2020, doi: 10.1093/rfs/hhaa075.

[88] X. Hao, L. Yu, L. Zhiqiang, L. Zhen, and G. Dawu, "Dynamic practical byzantine fault tolerance," in IEEE Conference on Communications and Network Security (CNS), 2018, doi: 10.1109/cns.2018.8433150.

[89] Y. Fernando and R. Saravannan, "Blockchain technology: energy efficiency and ethical compliance," *J. Gov. Integr.*, vol. 4, no. 2, pp. 88–95, 2021, doi: 10.15282/jgi.4.2.2021.5872.

[90] Q. Hu, B. Yan, Y. Han, and J. Yu, "An improved delegated proof of stake consensus algorithm," *Procedia Comput. Sci.*, vol. 187, pp. 341–346, 2021, doi: 10.1016/j.procs.2021.04.109.

[91] S. Nzuva, "Smart contracts implementation, applications, benefits, and limitations," *J. Inf. Eng. Appl.*, 2019, doi: 10.7176/jiea/9-5-07.

[92] L. W. Cong and Z. He, "Blockchain disruption and smart contracts," *Rev. Financ. Stud.*, vol. 32, no. 5, pp. 1754–1797, 2019, doi: 10.1093/rfs/hhz007.

[93] N. Z. Bawany, T. Qamar, H. Tariq, and S. Adnan, "Integrating healthcare services using blockchain-based telehealth framework," *IEEE Access*, vol. 10, pp. 36505–36517, 2022, doi: 10.1109/access.2022.3161944.

[94] L. Stockburger, G. Kokosioulis, A. Mukkamala, R. R. Mukkamala, and M. Avital, "Blockchain-enabled decentralized identity management: the case of self-sovereign identity in public transportation," *Blockchain Res. Appl.*, vol. 2, no. 2, p. 100014, 2021, doi: 10.1016/j.bcra.2021.100014.

[95] I. T. Javed, F. Alharbi, B. Bellaj, T. Margaria, N. Crespi, and K. N. Qureshi, "Health-ID: a blockchain-based decentralized identity management for remote healthcare," *Healthcare*, vol. 9, no. 6, p. 712, 2021, doi: 10.3390/healthcare9060712.

[96] B. A. Dedeturk, A. Soran, and B. Bakir-Gungor, "Blockchain for genomics and healthcare: a literature review, current status, classification and open issues," *Peer J*, vol. 9, p. e12130, 2021, doi: 10.7717/peerj.12130.

[97] M. A. Acquah, N. Chen, J.-S. Pan, H.-M. Yang, and B. Yan, "Securing fingerprint template using blockchain and distributed storage system," *Symmetry (Basel)*., vol. 12, no. 6, p. 951, 2020, doi: 10.3390/sym12060951.

[98] J. Eberhardt, "Scalable and privacy-preserving off-chain computations," *Scalable and Privacy-Preserving Off-Chain Computations*, 2021, MSc Thesis, Electrical Engineering and Computer Science of the Technical University, Berlin. Retrieved from https://api-depositonce.tu-berlin.de/server/api/core/bitstreams/2b81beb7-5b0f-4048-a56f-104317a82675/content

[99] K. Wilson and L. Khansa, "Migrating to electronic health record systems: a comparative study between the United States and the United Kingdom," *Health Policy (New. York)*., vol. 122, no. 11, pp. 1232–1239, 2018, doi: 10.1016/j.healthpol.2018.08.013.

[100] A. Jnr. Bokolo, "Exploring interoperability of distributed ledger and decentralized technology adoption in virtual enterprises," *Inf. Syst. E-bus. Manag.*, vol. 20, no. 4, pp. 685–718, 2022, doi: 10.1007/s10257-022-00561-8.

[101] M. Ball, A. Rosen, M. Sabin, and P. N. Vasudevan, "Proofs of work from worstcase assumptions," In *Advances in Cryptology–CRYPTO 2018: 38th Annual International Cryptology Conference*, Santa Barbara, CA, USA, August 19–23, 2018, Proceedings, Part I 38 2018, pp. 789–819. Springer International Publishing.

[102] Q. D. Buchlak, N. Esmaili, J. C. Leveque, *et al.*, "Machine learning applications to clinical decision support in neurosurgery: an artificial intelligence augmented systematic review," *Neurosurg. Rev.*, vol. 43, pp. 1235–1253, 2020.

[103] A. Rajkomar, E. Oren, K. Chen, *et al.*, "Scalable and accurate deep learning with electronic health records," *NPJ Digit. Med.*, vol. 1, no. 1, p. 18, 2018.

[104] M. A. Gianfrancesco, S. Tamang, J. Yazdany, and G. Schmajuk, "Potential biases in machine learning algorithms using electronic health record data,"

JAMA Intern. Med., vol. 178, no. 11, p. 1544, 2018, doi: 10.1001/jamainternmed.2018.3763.

[105] D. Castelvecchi, "Can we open the black box of AI?," *Nature*, vol. 538, no. 7623, pp. 20–23, 2016, doi: 10.1038/538020a.

[106] A. B. Arrieta, N. Díaz-Rodríguez, J. Del Ser, *et al.*, "Explainable artificial intelligence (XAI): concepts, taxonomies, opportunities and challenges toward responsible AI," *Inf. Fusion*, vol. 58, pp. 82–115, 2020, doi: 10.1016/j.inffus.2019.12.012.

[107] R. Guidotti, A. Monreale, S. Ruggieri, F. Turini, F. Giannotti, and D. Pedreschi, "A survey of methods for explaining black box models," *ACM Comput. Surv.*, vol. 51, no. 5, pp. 1–42, 2018, doi: 10.1145/3236009.

[108] C. Burr and D. Leslie, "Ethical assurance: a practical approach to the responsible design, development, and deployment of data-driven technologies," *AI Ethics*, vol. 3, no. 1, pp. 73–98, 2022, doi: 10.1007/s43681-022-00178-0.

[109] J. Matthews, "Patterns and anti-patterns, principles and pitfalls: accountability and transparency in AI," *AI Mag.*, vol. 41, no. 1, pp. 82–89, 2020, doi: 10.1609/aimag.v41i1.5204.

[110] R. Wehrens, M. Stevens, J. Kostenzer, A. M. Weggelaar, and A. de Bont, "Ethics as discursive work: the role of ethical framing in the promissory future of data-driven healthcare technologies," *Sci. Technol. Hum. Values*, p. 016224392110536, 2021, doi: 10.1177/01622439211053661.

[111] R. Poojary, R. Raina, and A. Kumar Mondal, "Effect of data-augmentation on fine-tuned CNN model performance," *IAES Int. J. Artif. Intell.*, vol. 10, no. 1, p. 84, 2021, doi: 10.11591/ijai.v10.i1.pp84-92.

[112] T. Ke and K. Sudhir, "Privacy rights and data security: GDPR and personal data driven markets," *SSRN Electron. J.*, 2020, doi: 10.2139/ssrn.3643979.

[113] Y. S. Liu, Y. Liang, Q. Shao, and K. Rascati, "PNS199 a review of policies regarding patient-reported outcomes (pro) from the Food and Drug Administration (FDA) and European Medicines Agency (EMA)," *Value Heal.*, vol. 23, p. S320, 2020, doi: 10.1016/j.jval.2020.04.1192.

[114] S. Russell and P. Norvig, "A modern, agent-oriented approach to introductory artificial intelligence," *ACM SIGART Bull.*, vol. 6, no. 2, pp. 24–26, 1995, doi: 10.1145/201977.201989.

[115] A. L. Beam and I. S. Kohane, "Big Data and Machine Learning in Health Care," *JAMA*, vol. 319, no. 13, p. 1317, 2018, doi: 10.1001/jama.2017.18391.

[116] K. Fujimoto, K. Hayashi, R. Katayama, *et al.*, "Deep learning-based image deconstruction method with maintained saliency," *Neural Networks*, vol. 155, pp. 224–241, 2022, doi: 10.1016/j.neunet.2022.08.015.

[117] J. Yang, Y. Shi, and Z. Qi, "Learning deep feature correspondence for unsupervised anomaly detection and segmentation," *Pattern Recognit.*, vol. 132, p. 108874, 2022, doi: 10.1016/j.patcog.2022.108874.

[118] L. Yu, Z. Xu, T. Zhang, X. Guan, and D. Yue, "Energy-efficient personalized thermal comfort control in office buildings based on multi-agent deep reinforcement learning," *Build. Environ.*, vol. 223, p. 109458, 2022, doi: 10.1016/j.buildenv.2022.109458.

[119] A. Kormilitzin, N. Vaci, Q. Liu, and A. Nevado-Holgado, "Med7: A transferable clinical natural language processing model for electronic health records," *Artif. Intell. Med.*, vol. 118, p. 102086, 2021, doi: 10.1016/j.artmed.2021.102086.

[120] G. Zhu, H. Chen, B. Jiang, F. Chen, Y. Xie, and M. Wintermark, "Application of Deep Learning to Ischemic and Hemorrhagic Stroke Computed Tomography and Magnetic Resonance Imaging," *Semin. Ultrasound, CT MRI*, vol. 43, no. 2, pp. 147–152, 2022, doi: 10.1053/j.sult.2022.02.004.

[121] S. Rajput and S. Ramesh, "Real time image based gesture recognition model for dynamic applications using transfer learning," *SSRN Electron. J.*, 2023, doi: 10.2139/ssrn.4268582.

[122] M. McGuigan and J. Christmas, "Automating RTI: automatic light direction detection and correcting non-uniform lighting for more accurate surface normals," *Comput. Vis. Image Underst.*, vol. 192, p. 102880, 2020, doi: 10.1016/j.cviu.2019.102880.

[123] K. Cameron and D. Singh, "When to account for the patient? The effect of clinical treatment of social determinants of health on patient health outcomes," *SSRN Electron. J.*, 2021, doi: 10.2139/ssrn.3778987.

[124] A. Miracolo, M. Mills, and P. Kanavos, "POSB29 can predictive tools and analytics foresee health outcomes or identify patient subgroups with higher risk of progression in the management of inflammatory bowel disease? A systematic literature review," *Value Heal.*, vol. 25, no. 1, p. S30, 2022, doi: 10.1016/j.jval.2021.11.139.

[125] G. Ciliberto, R. Giuliani, M. Zambon, and C. Nicholl, "Genomes over a lifetime (GOAL): an innovative approach to personalized patient empowerment through early diagnosis and treatment for cancer patients and rare disease," *Popul. Med.*, vol. 5, 2023, doi: 10.18332/popmed/165769.

[126] E. Bose and K. Radhakrishnan, "Using unsupervised machine learning to identify subgroups among home health patients with heart failure using telehealth," *CIN Comput. Informatics, Nurs.*, vol. 36, no. 5, pp. 242–248, 2018, doi: 10.1097/cin.0000000000000423.

[127] E. R. Sruthi, "Understand Random Forest Algorithms With Examples," *Analytics Vidhya*, 2023. [Online]. Available: https://www.analyticsvidhya.com/blog/2021/06/understanding-random-forest/. [Accessed: 28-Apr-2023].

[128] GuestBlog, "Introduction to XGBoost Algorithm in Machine Learning," *ANALYTICS VIDHYA*, 2023. [Online]. Available: https://www.analyticsvidhya.com/blog/2018/09/an-end-to-end-guide-to-understand-the-math-behind-xgboost/. [Accessed: 28-Apr-2023].

[129] M. Iqbal, "Chronic KIdney Disease dataset," *kaggle*, 2017. [Online]. Available: https://www.kaggle.com/datasets/mansoordaku/ckdisease. [Accessed: 24-Apr-2023].

Chapter 13

Mitigating cyber threats in healthcare systems: the role of artificial intelligence and machine learning

Daniel Dauda Wisdom[1], Olufunke Rebecca Vincent[2], Kingsley T. Igulu[3], Michael O. Arowolo[4], Eneh Agozie Hyacinth[5], Arinze Uchechukwu Christian[5] and Garba Alpha Baba[6]

As we move further into the digital era, the importance of cybersecurity becomes increasingly apparent, especially in the healthcare industry, where sensitive patient data is stored and transmitted through various technological systems. The advancement of technology makes safeguarding healthcare systems from cyber threats more critical than ever. Cybercriminals target patient information, financial data, and medical records, resulting in severe consequences like reputational damage, loss of trust, financial losses, legal consequences, and potential harm to patients. Despite attempts to regulate healthcare cybersecurity, the rising number of cyberattacks remains an important challenge. To tackle this issue, the adoption of artificial intelligence (AI) and machine learning (ML) has shown promise. AI can detect and prevent real-time cyberattacks, providing an additional layer of security. ML algorithms can predict and thwart future attacks by analyzing cybercriminal behaviors and patterns. Additionally, secure communication channels are vital for healthcare systems to protect sensitive data. Encrypted communication methods, such as secure messaging systems and virtual private networks, significantly enhance healthcare system security. This book chapter provides an overview of the importance of cybersecurity in healthcare, exploring various cyber threats faced by healthcare systems, including malware attacks, ransomware attacks, and social engineering attacks. It also examines the impact of these threats on healthcare, such

[1]Department of Computer Science, Chrisland University, Nigeria
[2]Department of Computer Science, Federal University of Agriculture, Nigeria
[3]Department of Computer Science, Ignatius Ajuru University, Nigeria
[4]Bond Life Sciences Centre, University of Missouri, USA
[5]Department of Computer Science, University of Nigeria, Nigeria
[6]Department of Computer Science, Kaduna State College of Education, Nigeria

as patient privacy breaches, financial losses, and reputational damage. Furthermore, the chapter delves into the regulatory and legal requirements that healthcare organizations must adhere to in order to safeguard patient privacy and security. It outlines various cybersecurity measures that healthcare organizations can adopt, such as risk assessments, staff training, network segmentation, access controls, and incident response plans. Lastly, the chapter discusses emerging technologies like blockchain and AI, demonstrating their potential to enhance cybersecurity in healthcare systems.

13.1 Introduction

In recent years, the healthcare industry has undergone a remarkable transformation with the integration of advanced technologies into its systems and processes. As we embrace the benefits of the digital age, healthcare organizations have reaped substantial advantages, ranging from streamlined patient care to improved operational efficiency [1]. However, this rapid digitalization has also introduced new challenges, particularly in the realm of cybersecurity. The healthcare sector holds a vast amount of sensitive and private information, making it an attractive target for cybercriminals. Patient records, financial data, and critical medical information are stored and transmitted through interconnected technological systems, making them susceptible to cyber threats and attacks. The consequences of successful cyberattacks can be devastating, resulting in reputational damage, loss of trust among patients, financial losses, and, most alarmingly, endangering patients' well-being [2]. To combat this ever-evolving landscape of cyber threats, the integration of cutting-edge technologies has become imperative. artificial intelligence (AI) and machine learning (ML) have emerged as potent tools in the arsenal of cybersecurity professionals. Their ability to analyze vast amounts of data in real time, detect anomalies, and proactively respond to potential threats has revolutionized the way healthcare systems approach cybersecurity. Mitigating cyber threats in healthcare systems is an increasingly critical task in today's digital age. As healthcare organizations embrace technological advancements to improve patient care and optimize processes, they must also confront the escalating risks posed by cybercriminals [3]. The sensitive and private nature of patient data, coupled with the interconnectivity of healthcare networks, makes the industry an attractive target for malicious actors seeking financial gain or strategic advantage. Traditional cybersecurity measures alone are no longer sufficient to combat the sophistication and persistence of cyber threats. Cyberattacks in the healthcare sector can have dire consequences, ranging from the compromise of patient privacy and financial data to the disruption of critical medical services and even potential harm to patients. AI and ML have emerged as game-changers in the realm of cybersecurity. Their ability to analyze vast volumes of data, identify patterns, and detect anomalies in real time presents a transformative opportunity to strengthen the defense of healthcare systems against cyber threats. One of the key advantages of AI in healthcare cybersecurity is its capacity to augment human capabilities significantly.

AI-driven security solutions can continuously monitor network activity, detect unusual behaviors, and rapidly respond to threats at a speed and scale beyond human capacity. This proactive approach can thwart cyberattacks before they cause substantial damage, minimizing the risk to patient safety and organizational reputation. ML complements AI by enabling systems to learn from past cyber incidents and adapt to new attack methodologies [4]. By constantly updating its knowledge base, ML algorithms improve their ability to identify and prevent emerging threats, reducing false positives and enhancing overall system efficiency.

Moreover, AI and ML can play a vital role in safeguarding patient privacy. Advanced encryption algorithms and privacy-preserving techniques ensure that sensitive patient data remains secure even as it is processed for essential healthcare research and analysis. As healthcare organizations adopt AI and ML technologies, there are challenges that must be addressed. These include the integration of new systems into existing infrastructure, ensuring regulatory compliance, and addressing the shortage of skilled cybersecurity professionals with expertise in AI and ML [5].

Collaboration between healthcare organizations, researchers, and technology providers is essential to foster innovation and share knowledge in the field of healthcare cybersecurity. By pooling resources and expertise, the industry can build robust cybersecurity solutions and stay ahead of evolving threats.

In addition, the role of AI and ML in mitigating cyber threats in healthcare systems cannot be overstated. These transformative technologies offer unparalleled opportunities to fortify the cybersecurity defenses of healthcare organizations, protect patient data, and ensure the continuity of quality healthcare services. Embracing AI and ML in healthcare cybersecurity is not only a necessity but a strategic imperative to safeguard patient trust, privacy, and safety in an increasingly interconnected world [6].

This book chapter delves into the crucial role of AI and ML in mitigating cyber threats in healthcare systems. It explored the challenges faced by the healthcare industry in safeguarding sensitive data and maintaining the trust of patients and stakeholders. The book chapter provides an in-depth analysis of how AI and ML technologies can be leveraged to strengthen cybersecurity measures, detect and prevent cyberattacks, and ensure the privacy and integrity of patient information.

13.2 Related work

The study [1] put forth a proposal to critically analyze the available literature regarding the utilization of AI applications in the construction sector. The main objective was to scrutinize the application of AI techniques, identify both the potential opportunities and challenges in implementing AI in construction, and offer insights into the significant AI applications that are pertinent to the construction industry's unique challenges.

The research aimed to achieve the following goals: (a) uncover the various AI applications within the construction industry, encompassing activities like

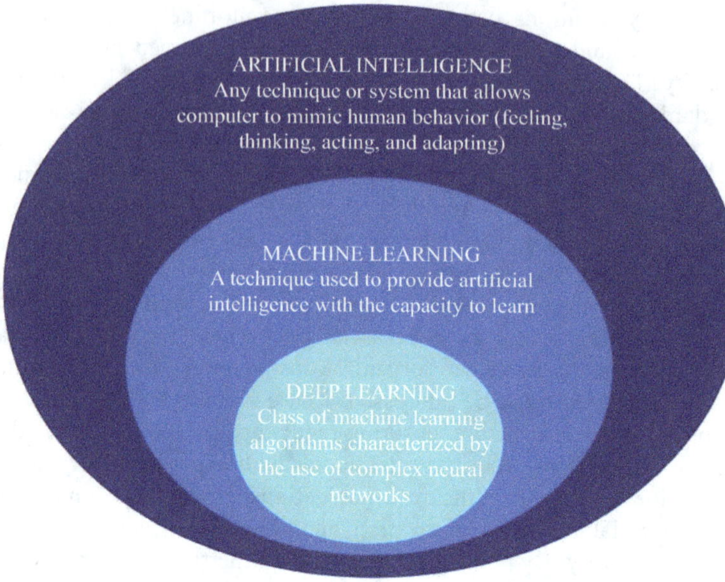

Figure 13.1 The basic concept of artificial intelligence

monitoring tasks, managing risks, optimizing resources, and minimizing waste; (b) recognize the potential opportunities and challenges that come with employing AI in the construction domain; (c) investigate the extent of AI integration within the construction sector; (d) conduct an exhaustive review of relevant research publications spanning the last six decades across diverse areas of construction applications; (e) categorize AI subfields within construction research based on their developmental stages – emerging, ripe, or mature technologies; (f) develop a "hype cycle" model to forecast the timeline for the maturation of each AI subfield; (g) identify additional prospects and unresolved research topics in the realm of AI research for construction; and (h) offer recommendations to address the challenges that hinder the adoption of AI in the construction industry (Figure 13.1).

The study embraced a qualitative approach by analyzing trends in publications regarding AI and its subfields within the construction sector. Researchers conducted searches in robust databases such as SCOPUS, Science Direct, IEEE, and ACM over a span of six decades (1960–2020) to ensure credibility and reduce bias. The study's primary focus was to qualitatively review literature and trends related to the implementation of AI applications in the construction industry. The study's findings unveiled the application of diverse AI technologies in construction research. However, while recent advancements in these technologies have shown significant improvement, the integration of advanced and potent AI technology has been comparatively gradual. Notably, the adoption of deep learning, with its potential for enhanced prediction accuracy compared to conventional ML methods, has been limited. The study also categorized AI subfields within construction research based on their stages of development and introduced a “hype cycle” to project the anticipated timeline for the maturation of each subfield.

Furthermore, the study identified additional prospects and unresolved research topics within AI research for construction. It emphasized the relevance of combining AI with emerging trends like building information modeling, Internet of things (IoT), quantum computing, augmented reality, cybersecurity, and blockchain. The study concluded by offering recommendations to address the challenges that impede the adoption of AI in the industry. Future research endeavors include conducting more comprehensive studies to explore the precise applications of AI technologies in construction, comprehending the obstacles to adoption, and formulating strategies for successful implementation. Additionally, research could delve into harnessing the potential of AI in conjunction with emerging technologies to further enhance construction processes and address industry-specific challenges.

The paper [2] aims to utilize techniques involving AI and the IoT-driven methodologies to analyze and optimize e-government services. This utilization of AI and IoT is anticipated to enhance the efficiency and effectiveness of e-government services, all while minimizing the vulnerability to cyberattacks. The research objectives encompass the following: (a) creating a reference model that is not reliant on technical platforms or organizational structures, to facilitate the deployment of e-government services; (b) investigating and improving e-government services through the application of AI-driven IoT techniques; (c) identifying the factors that influence the acceptance and integration of e-government services; (d) confronting challenges linked to the utilization of IoT and AI for intelligent governance within the public sector; (e) proposing a comprehensive framework that amalgamates both IoT and AI elements for intelligent governance; and (f) exploring potential avenues of future research concerning the implementation of IoT and AI systems. The study involves an extensive literature review intended to explore the challenges tied to employing IoT and AI for intelligent governance in the public sector.

Although the paper doesn’t specify the utilization of any particular algorithm or computational model, it does propose the implementation of AI-driven IoT techniques to enhance e-government services. However, the exact algorithms or methodologies that will be utilized remain unspecified. The paper proposed employment of AI-driven IoT techniques to augment e-government services, but it fails to provide any empirical findings or data to substantiate these claims. Consequently, they lack concrete empirical results, data, and specific insights into the research methodology employed. The effectiveness of the AI-driven IoT techniques in elevating e-government services is not discussed. The forthcoming work entails the execution of domain-specific studies pertaining to the implementation of IoT and AI systems. This extends beyond mere adoption studies to delve into the practical implementation and assessment of these systems, particularly focusing on the specific challenges that hinder the effective integration of IoT and AI systems. However, the paper refrains from providing further elaboration on potential directions for future research or other unexplored facets that could be considered in future investigations.

The study [3] introduced an innovative approach to counteract poisoning attacks on ML models. This was accomplished by integrating data provenance into a filtering algorithm. The objective was to identify and eliminate harmful data points inserted into the training set by adversaries, which aimed to manipulate the model's predictions. The research pursued the following goals: (a) create a methodology that leverages contextual information regarding the source and transformation of data points (referred to as data provenance) to discern and eliminate toxic data in ML training sets; (b) empower online and regularly retrained ML applications to effectively process data sources even within potentially hostile environments; (c) introduce two variations of the methodology, tailored for partially trusted datasets and fully untrusted datasets, respectively; and (d) assess the proposed methodology against existing approaches for poison data detection, showcasing an enhancement in the detection rate.

The methodology harnessed tamper-free provenance frameworks to incorporate data provenance as an integral component of the filtering algorithm. The research presented two adaptations of the provenance defense strategy, designed to address both partially trusted and fully untrusted datasets. An empirical evaluation was undertaken to compare the effectiveness of the proposed strategy with baseline methods for detecting poison data. The research primarily centers on the methodology's application of data provenance for the identification and removal of harmful data within ML training sets. Empirical results highlighted that the proposed provenance-based defense strategy outperformed the baseline methods, making it possible to deploy online and regularly retrained ML models in adversarial environments, where reliable provenance data could be sourced. Nevertheless, the text does not furnish specific quantitative outcomes or metrics. Moreover, the intricate algorithmic specifics and particular attributes utilized in the data provenance-based filtering algorithm are not exhaustively expounded upon.

The paper introduces numerous intriguing avenues for future exploration. This encompasses investigating scenarios where multiple data sources may collaborate to contaminate the ML model, examining various calibration techniques to discern the impact of diverse provenance features on model precision, and undertaking an exhaustive evaluation of the fully untrusted model. Regrettably, the text does not delve into precise strategies or trajectories for pursuing these prospective research directions.

The study [4] put forth a conceptual framework designed to foster the creation of secure applications within the realm of the Internet of medical things (IoMT). This framework's primary aim is to offer a strategic guide for constructing secure IoMT applications, taking into account the advancements made in the domain of AI. Furthermore, the framework seeks to address and mitigate vulnerabilities and cyberattacks existing within distinct layers of a specified IoMT. To achieve this, the framework integrates pertinent machine and deep learning methods. The research's objectives encompass the following: (a) formulating an all-encompassing framework that effectively tackles the security challenges entailed by IoMT from its early developmental phases; (b) furnishing a roadmap comprising strategic methodologies for cultivating secure IoMT applications; (c) ensuring the inclusion of security design principles and security attributes throughout the entire developmental trajectory; (d) defining security practices through an initiative-based approach, enabling meticulous assessment of compliance and completion at any developmental stage; (e) identifying cybersecurity threats linked with each layer of the IoMT architecture and proposing AI-based methods to counteract these threats; and (f) establishing three pivotal documents encompassing security goal mapping, elaboration of precise activities for each initiative, and evaluating adherence to security objectives at any juncture.

The paper undertook a comprehensive literature review and analysis of prevailing security frameworks and practices that pertain to IoMT applications. The study's primary focus revolves around crafting a comprehensive framework to ensure the security of IoMT applications, rather than presenting a specific algorithmic solution. Notably, empirical evidence or case studies to substantiate the practical efficacy of the proposed framework are absent from the study. Additionally, the paper does not furnish specific particulars regarding the integration of AI-driven mitigating methods into the framework. Future prospects for the research include potential extensions such as the development of an automated tool for streamlining framework processes, enhancing accessibility and monitoring during the assessment process. Another potential avenue for future research involves the integration of the proposed framework with existing frameworks beyond the security domain, used for different purposes in the development of IoMT technologies. However, the paper does not expound upon the granular details or guidelines for pursuing these prospective research directions.

The article [5] introduced a proposition concerning a survey and analysis directed toward the identification of prospective security threats originating from malicious applications of AI technologies. The study also endeavored to put forth methods aimed at predicting, preventing, and mitigating these threats. The research objectives encompassed the following aspects: identification of plausible security threats emerging from the malevolent utilization of AI technologies; devising strategies to anticipate, forestall, and alleviate these threats; examination of the long-term equilibrium existing between attackers and defenders within the domain of AI security; and deliberation on potential interventions that could be implemented by professionals in the AI development community and other institutions. The paper adopts a survey-based methodology as a means to recognize possible security threats associated with the malicious use of AI technologies. It scrutinizes the landscape of AI security threats while concurrently exploring potential interventions to counteract these challenges. This methodology constitutes a combination of literature review, evaluation of existing AI security practices, and an exploration of potential policy interventions' implications. The study's central focus is on discussing strategic frameworks and policy considerations rather than offering a particular algorithmic solution. The paper provides insights into plausible AI security threats and suggests strategies to tackle them. However, it does not conclusively resolve the issue of the long-term balance between attackers and defenders within the AI security sphere. Nevertheless, it emphasizes the vital importance of preemptive measures to counter malicious AI applications. The paper does not incorporate empirical data or experimental outcomes to substantiate its proposed interventions. Moreover, it abstains from furnishing a distinct algorithmic remedy to address AI security threats. Instead, the primary emphasis remains on policy recommendations and strategic approaches, rather than delving into the implementation of tangible technical solutions. The paper advocates for a collaborative effort between the AI development community, policymakers, and legal institutions to effectively counteract AI security threats. It underscores the necessity for continuous cooperation and discourse aimed at shaping public policies and regulations concerning the safety and security of AI applications. Prospective directions for further research encompass an in-depth exploration of the enduring equilibrium between attackers and defenders in the realm of AI security, as well as the development of concrete technical remedies to mitigate specific AI security risks. Additionally, evaluating the effectiveness of plausible policy interventions and analyzing the implications of different governance levels concerning various types of risks are noteworthy avenues for future investigation.

The chapter [6] proposed the application of explainable AI (XAI) as a solution to address the lack of transparency and interpretability in traditional AI technologies, particularly deep learning, when applied to cybersecurity in smart city-based solutions. The main objective of the research was to conduct a comprehensive study of ML applications in cybersecurity in the context of smart cities. The study aimed to emphasize the need for explainability in AI systems to understand their decision-making processes and biases, and how it impacts the security and trustworthiness of data-driven automated applications. The chapter utilized a secondary data analysis approach to conduct the study. It gathered existing research and literature on ML applications in cybersecurity and XAI to present an overall analysis of the prospect of XAI in smart city applications. The paper discussed the need to transition from black-box to white-box AI systems, emphasizing interpretability, transparency, and understandability of AI-based technologies. The chapter presented insights into the significance of XAI in addressing cybersecurity challenges in smart cities. It discussed the potential benefits of XAI platforms in enhancing the credibility of AI-based cybersecurity components, ensuring security, privacy, and trustworthiness in smart city deployments. However, the chapter lacks specific details on the implementation of XAI algorithms or tools. It does not provide empirical results from experiments or case studies to demonstrate the effectiveness of XAI in improving cybersecurity in smart cities. The chapter suggested future challenges and opportunities in the domain of XAI. However, it did not explicitly outline specific areas for further research. Future work could involve conducting empirical studies to evaluate the effectiveness of various XAI techniques in enhancing cybersecurity in real-world smart city applications and exploring new approaches to address interpretability challenges in AI systems.

The research study [7] explores the role of AI in enhancing healthcare security. It focuses on five key areas: anomaly detection, predictive analytics, access control, threat intelligence, and incident response. The main objective is to investigate how AI can contribute to improving healthcare security by detecting and preventing security breaches, predicting future attacks, managing user access, staying updated with the latest security threats, and providing real-time incident response. The study presents a literature review or exploratory study, discussing the potential applications of AI in healthcare security based on existing knowledge and previous studies. The paper discusses AI's potential applications in different areas such as anomaly detection, predictive analytics, access control, threat intelligence, and incident response. The passage does not present empirical results or findings as it is more of a theoretical exploration and analysis of the potential benefits of AI in healthcare security. The paper lacks specific details about the research design, data collection, and empirical analysis, making it difficult to determine any concrete results or outcomes from the study. The paper highlights challenges and issues related to AI adoption in healthcare security, including the need for standardized data, addressing data privacy and security concerns, building trust in AI-generated diagnoses, overcoming integration difficulties, mitigating biases in AI algorithms, and addressing legal and ethical implications. These challenges could potentially guide future research in the field of AI and healthcare security.

The paper [8] proposed the use of XAI for intrusion detection and mitigation in intelligent connected vehicles (ICVs). It aims to enhance the security of ICVs by providing transparency and interpretability to AI models used in intrusion detection systems. The research studies review the application of XAI in ICV intrusion detection systems, explore the capabilities and use cases of existing XAI frameworks, and identify outstanding research problems related to XAI's applicability in ICV security. The ultimate goal was to improve the network efficiency and security of ICVs. The paper used a review methodology to assess the application of XAI in ICV intrusion detection. It involved a comprehensive background study of existing XAI frameworks, their capabilities, and real-world use cases. The paper also analyzed the current state of XAI's applicability to ICV security and identified research challenges. The paper did not propose a specific algorithm. Instead, it focused on the application of XAI in ICV intrusion detection and discussed the capabilities of existing XAI frameworks. The study found that XAI is a promising research direction for improving the security of ICVs. While still in its infancy in the context of ICVs, XAI offers the potential to enhance transparency, reliability, and interpretability in AI-based intrusion detection systems. It was also observed that XAI's increased transparency would foster its acceptability in the automobile industry. The paper did not present a specific implementation of an XAI model for ICV intrusion detection. It focused on the review of existing XAI frameworks and their potential applications in ICVs without providing empirical results or practical demonstrations. The paper identified several research issues for further exploration, such as ensuring reliability, addressing computational complexity, and incorporating user-friendly XAI modules in ICV security systems. Additionally, the issue of bias introduced by rule-based XAI needs to be addressed to gain acceptance in critical industries like the automobile industry. Future work could involve developing and evaluating specific XAI models for ICV intrusion detection and mitigation, considering the identified research challenges.

The researchers [9] proposed an IoT architecture called "BlockIoTIntelligence" that combines blockchain and AI to support effective big data analysis in the context of the industrial IoT. The architecture aims to overcome challenges related to centralized architecture, security, privacy, resource constraints, and lack of sufficient training data for big data analysis using AI. The main goal of the research was to design and develop an IoT architecture that leverages the benefits of both blockchain and AI to enable efficient big data analysis. The architecture's objectives were to achieve scalability, accuracy, security, and privacy in real-time data analysis for IoT applications. The research involved a combination of literature review, conceptual design, and architectural development. The researchers analyzed existing IoT architectures, AI models, and blockchain frameworks to identify challenges and opportunities for convergence. The proposed architecture was evaluated through simulations or experiments to assess its performance in terms of accuracy, centralization, security, and latency. The paper design and development of an IoT architecture that integrates blockchain and AI. The proposed BlockIoTIntelligence architecture outperformed existing IoT architectures and addressed the challenges related to centralized control and AI data analysis. The research suggests future directions for the convergence of blockchain and AI in IoT applications, including cloud intelligence, fog intelligence, edge intelligence, and device intelligence. The authors identify several research challenges, such as scalability enhancement, interoperability, resource management, standardization, data integrity, heterogeneity, costs, energy efficiency, and traffic monitoring. Possible solutions to these challenges may be explored in future research endeavors.

The authors [10] proposed a decentralized, patient-centric healthcare framework based on the integration of blockchain and AI technologies to combat the challenges posed by the COVID-19 pandemic. The main objectives of the research were to explore how blockchain and AI can be utilized to improve the digital healthcare workflow during the COVID-19 pandemic, provide decentralized healthcare data sharing, protect users' privacy, empower patients with their data, and optimize clinical workflows. The paper is conceptual and focuses on proposing a decentralized, patient-centric healthcare system based on the integration of blockchain and AI technologies. It provides an overview of digital healthcare services and problems during the COVID-19 pandemic and explores potential applications of blockchain and AI in public healthcare strategies for tackling COVID-19. The paper does not explicitly mention any specific algorithm. Instead, it discusses the integration of blockchain and AI technologies to create a patient-centric healthcare system for handling COVID-19. The paper primarily discusses a conceptual framework for the proposed patient-centric healthcare system based on blockchain and AI integration. It highlights the potential benefits, such as improved interoperability, enhanced privacy, and better medical research and treatment through predictive diagnosis and analysis. The paper lacks detailed empirical results or specific implementations of the proposed framework. It mainly presents a conceptual approach rather than a practical implementation. The paper does not explicitly outline future research directions. However, potential future work could involve the development and implementation of the proposed patient-centric healthcare system, addressing technical challenges and evaluating its effectiveness in real-world scenarios.

The paper [11] proposed an IoT-enabled AI smart home architecture to support stable and confidential applications in intelligent cities, with a focus on analyzing security risks, problems, and solutions using the LR (logistic regression) algorithm. The objectives of the research were to develop a modern architecture for IoT-enabled AI smart home applications, analyze security risks in cloud computing, and propose solutions using the LR algorithm to enhance data security.

The paper involves a literature review, analysis of security risks in cloud computing, and application of the LR algorithm to address these risks. The paper proposed the use of the LR algorithm as a solution to address security risks in cloud computing and enhance data security in IoT-enabled AI smart home applications. The paper does not provide specific details about the results obtained from the research. The abstract lacks specific details about the results and findings of the research. It does not mention the scope and scale of the study, the data used, the actual implementation of the proposed architecture, and any empirical results or evaluations. The future work includes practical implementation and evaluation of the proposed architecture, as well as further exploration of AI technologies to address security challenges in IoT-based networks.

The paper [12] proposed a review of how ML techniques are used in cyber-security to enhance the process of malware detection and mitigate cybersecurity threats. The primary objective of the research was to assess the effectiveness of ML techniques in cybersecurity, specifically in making the process of malware detection more actionable, scalable, and effective than traditional approaches. The study also aimed to discuss existing cybersecurity threats and how ML techniques have been applied to mitigate them. The study is a review of ML techniques implemented on cybersecurity data and the effectiveness of these techniques in addressing cybersecurity threats. it discusses several ML and statistical methods such as deep learning, support vector machines, and Bayesian classification that have proven effective in mitigating cyberattacks. The future work discussed in the paper includes a feasibility analysis of ML for real-time traffic monitoring, particularly dealing with diverse Internet packets and encryption challenges. The research also aims to explore homomorphic encryption, a technique to handle encrypted data, and investigate threats related to quantum computing and its impact on public key encryption. However, the paper does not elaborate further on these future research directions.

The research article [13] proposed to demonstrate the various areas where AI plays a crucial role in managing the risk of cyberattacks within the field of Computer Science and Engineering (CSE) and cyber risk management. The objectives of the research were to highlight the significance of AI and ML in reducing the risk of cybercrimes, especially in the context of cyber risk management within the CSE and management fields. The article aimed to discuss the increasing number of malwares and cyberattacks in the business world and emphasize the importance of cybersecurity management. The methodology used in the research involved a literature review on the selected topic, focusing on the role of AI in cyber-security and spotting malware. It also utilized various journal articles, secondary sources, and primary survey questionnaires based on responses from 50 employees working in the IT industry. The paper does not mention any specific ML algorithms proposed in the research. The paper lacks specific details about the actual findings and results of the study. It does not provide any empirical data or quantitative results from the primary survey questionnaires conducted with IT industry employees. The paper does not explicitly mention future work or areas of further research. However, it can be assumed that future work may involve further exploration of AI's potential in cybersecurity and risk management, as well as conducting more extensive studies with a larger sample size to gather more comprehensive data on the topic. Additionally, future research may focus on evaluating the effectiveness of AI-based security systems in enhancing security measures in various industries, from technology to healthcare.

The research article [14] proposed the use of AI and the IoT to enhance e-government services and improve the efficiency and effectiveness of government service delivery. The objectives of the research were to identify the challenges faced by governments in providing e-government services, promote the use of AI and IoT to overcome these challenges, and develop a reference model that comprehends the framework and guidelines to deploy e-government services and improve their usability for citizens. Future work involve further exploration of AI and IoT applications in e-government services and addressing potential threats related to data privacy and security. Additionally, developing and implementing the proposed reference model to assess its effectiveness in enhancing e-government services, respectively.

The research [15] proposed the use of AI and ML to enhance healthcare systems' response to COVID-19. The integration of these techniques into healthcare systems is suggested to better utilize resources, provide personalized patient management plans, inform policy, and expedite clinical trials. The objectives were to address five important challenges in responding to COVID-19 and demonstrate how recent developments in AI and ML can help in each of these challenges. The research aimed to show how the integration of AI and ML techniques into healthcare systems can save lives and propose specific methods for swift and efficient implementation. The mainly discusses the use of AI and ML techniques to address challenges in healthcare systems' response to COVID-19.

The paper, however, lacks specific details about the methodology and results of the research. It does not provide empirical data or findings from any studies conducted. Future work involve developing and implementing safe and trustworthy ML methodologies to assist decision-making processes in healthcare systems' response to COVID-19.

The research [16] proposed an enhanced cyberattack detection process for Internet of Health Things (IoHT) devices using a deep neural network (DNN)-based system. The research aimed to develop a resilient cyberattack detection system for IoHT devices to mitigate security risks and prevent cyberattacks. The focus was on multiclass classification to detect specific types of attacks (ARP Spoofing, DoS attacks, Nmap attacks, and Smurf attacks) in the healthcare domain using the ECU-IoHT dataset. The methodology involved building a DNN-based cyberattack detection system using AI on the ECU-IoHT dataset. The system utilized a DNN approach for anomaly detection and multiclass classification to identify different types of cyberattacks. The proposed algorithm was a DNN that utilized AI for cyberattack detection in the IoHT environment. The proposed DNN-based cyberattack detection system achieved an average higher performance accuracy of 99.85%, an average area under the receiver operator characteristic curve (AUC-ROC) of 0.99, and a false positive rate of 0.01. The experimental results demonstrated that the proposed system outperformed existing methods in terms of detection rate, precision, recall, and F1 score.

The paper does not provide specific details about the size and characteristics of the ECU-IoHT dataset used for training and evaluation. Additionally, it lacks information about the DNN architecture and hyperparameters used in the proposed system. The future work suggested testing the proposed DNN-based system in a real-time IoHT environment and expanding its scalability to detect other types of attacks in IoHT devices. Further research may focus on improving the efficiency and adaptability of the system to evolving cyber threats in the healthcare domain.

The research [17] proposed to provide a review of cybersecurity considerations for radiology departments involved with AI projects. The objectives of the research were to introduce cybersecurity concepts as they relate to medical imaging and AI, provide background information on general and healthcare-specific cybersecurity challenges, discuss approaches to enhancing security through detection and prevention techniques, and suggest potential risk mitigation strategies for radiology AI projects. The paper is a review, which involves a comprehensive literature review and analysis of existing research and cybersecurity concepts. Future work involve conducting in-depth studies or empirical research to validate the suggested risk mitigation strategies and to explore further improvements in cybersecurity for radiology AI projects, respectively.

The researchers [18] proposed a novel federated deep learning scheme called "DeepFed" for detecting and mitigating cyber threats against industrial cyber-physical systems (CPSs).

The main objectives of the research were to develop a comprehensive intrusion detection model for industrial CPSs using deep learning techniques, create a federated learning framework to enable multiple industrial CPSs to collectively build the intrusion detection model in a privacy-preserving manner, and demonstrate the effectiveness of the proposed DeepFed scheme in detecting various types of cyber threats compared to state-of-the-art schemes. The researchers used a combination of deep learning techniques, specifically a convolutional neural network (CNN) and a gated recurrent unit (GRU), to design an intrusion detection model for industrial CPSs. They then developed a federated learning framework that allowed multiple industrial CPSs to collaboratively build the model in a privacy-preserving way. They also employed a Paillier cryptosystem-based secure communication protocol to protect the security and privacy of model parameters during the training process. The main algorithm proposed in the research is the "DeepFed" federated deep learning scheme, which involves a CNN–GRU-based intrusion detection model and a federated learning framework with a Paillier-based secure communication protocol. The experiments on a real industrial CPS dataset demonstrated that the DeepFed scheme was highly effective in detecting various types of cyber threats to industrial CPSs. It outperformed state-of-the-art schemes in terms of intrusion detection accuracy. The paper does not provide specific details about the real-world industrial CPS dataset used in the experiments or elaborate on the specific types of cyber threats that were detected and mitigated by the proposed DeepFed scheme. The researchers suggest that future research should focus on addressing cybersecurity issues by federating data resources from different-domain industrial CPSs. This means extending the proposed federated intrusion detection model to work with CPSs from diverse industries and domains, which could present new challenges and opportunities for enhancing cybersecurity in industrial systems.

The research [19] proposed exploring the potential of AI and ML to combat COVID-19 and identified existing opportunities for low- and middle-income countries (LMIC) through a scoping review. The objectives were to identify the potential applications of AI and ML in addressing the COVID-19 pandemic, especially in LMIC, and to highlight the benefits of using AI-driven tools to optimize healthcare research and improve health outcomes. The researchers conducted a literature search through the PubMed database using specific keywords related to COVID-19, AI, ML, and LMIC. They screened 43 articles for eligibility and included 13 articles in the final review. The review followed the guidelines for PRISMA extension for scoping reviews (PRISMA-ScR). The research identified and synthesized results under four themes: the need for AI during the pandemic, the utility of AI in COVID-19 screening and diagnosis, the use of AI in patient monitoring and drug development, and the opportunities for LMIC to benefit from AI beyond COVID-19. The study highlighted the potential benefits of AI in speeding up identification, screening, and diagnosis of COVID-19 cases and in predictive and preventive healthcare. However, the paper does not provide detailed quantitative results or data on the specific AI models used, their performance metrics, or the exact impact on healthcare systems in LMIC. The paper suggests that further research is needed to explore additional utilities of AI-based tools in healthcare and to continue investigating how AI can ease the burden on healthcare systems, especially in LMIC, respectively.

The article [20] proposed a combined software-defined networking (SDN) and reinforcement learning (RL) approach for modeling, detecting, and mitigating cyber threats against industrial healthcare systems, particularly focusing on the IEC 60 870-5-104 protocol widely adopted in the healthcare sector. The research aimed to investigate and assess the severity of IEC 60 870-5-104 cyberattacks, introduce an intrusion detection and prevention system (IDPS) using ML and SDN to automatically detect and mitigate cyberattacks, and evaluate the efficiency of the proposed IDPS in terms of intrusion detection accuracy and automated mitigation performance. The research utilized a quantitative threat model based on attack–defense trees and Common Vulnerability Scoring System v3.1 to evaluate the severity of IEC 60 870-5-104 cyberattacks. It introduced an IDPS that combines ML and SDN technologies. ML was used to detect cyberattacks using TCP/IP network flow statistics and IEC 60 870-5-104 payload flow statistics. Automated mitigation was formulated as a multi-armed bandit problem and solved using the Thomson sampling method and SDN. The proposed algorithm used a CART (classification and regression trees) classifier for intrusion detection, based on TCP/IP network flow statistics and IEC 60 870-5-104 payload flow statistics. For automated mitigation, the algorithm utilized a RL method called Thomson sampling and SDN to address the multi-armed bandit problem. The evaluation analysis showed that the proposed IDPS achieved high efficiency in terms of intrusion detection accuracy and automated mitigation performance. The detection accuracy and F1 score of the IDPS were reported as 0.831 and 0.8258, respectively, while the mitigation accuracy reached 0.923. The research does not explicitly mention the specific datasets used for training and evaluating the proposed IDPS, nor does it elaborate on the computational resources or hardware configurations used for the experiments. The future work of this research is focused on enhancing the proposed IDPS to detect multistep cyberattacks related to IEC 60 870-5-104 and other industrial and IoMT protocols utilized in the healthcare sector, such as Modbus, MQTT, and EtherCAT. The adoption of ML-based association rules techniques is mentioned as a part of this future plan as well.

The handbook [21] proposed to address the security issues and privacy concerns in AI-enabled healthcare systems and the Internet of medical things (AIoMT). It aimed to offer new insights, solutions, and practical AI-based approaches to handle security challenges in the healthcare ecosystem. The objectives of the research were to do the following: examine real-world scenarios related to the deployment, application, management, and benefits of AIoMT in healthcare systems; assess the existing security designs and propose solutions to enhance traditional security architecture; develop efficient intrusion detection algorithms and attack prevention techniques; offer cryptographic and non-cryptographic solutions to enhance security; and address critical security and privacy issues that impact all stakeholders in the healthcare ecosystem. They proposed a handbook, which involve a compilation of expert contributions, literature reviews, case studies, and practical applications, respectively. The provided excerpt does not mention a specific proposed algorithm. Instead, it indicates that the handbook offers new designs of efficient intrusion detection algorithms, attack prevention techniques, and both cryptographic and non-cryptographic solutions. The provided excerpt outlines the topics covered in the handbook but does not mention any empirical findings or data analysis. The book does not explicitly mention future work. However, a section that discusses future work might be included in the book chapters.

The chapter [22] proposed an insightful privacy-aware energy-efficient architecture using AI of medical things (AIoMT) for COVID-19 pandemic data handling. The goal was to secure sensitive medical records of patients and other stakeholders in the healthcare domain and to address the limitations related to power usage and security risks associated with data transmission over open wireless channels. The objectives of the research were to the following: introduce the concept of AIoMT in healthcare data management for addressing the heterogeneity and complexity of the collected data; develop an architecture to enable the autonomous operation of sensors and devices for providing a favorable and secure environment for healthcare personnel and patients; present methods for improving

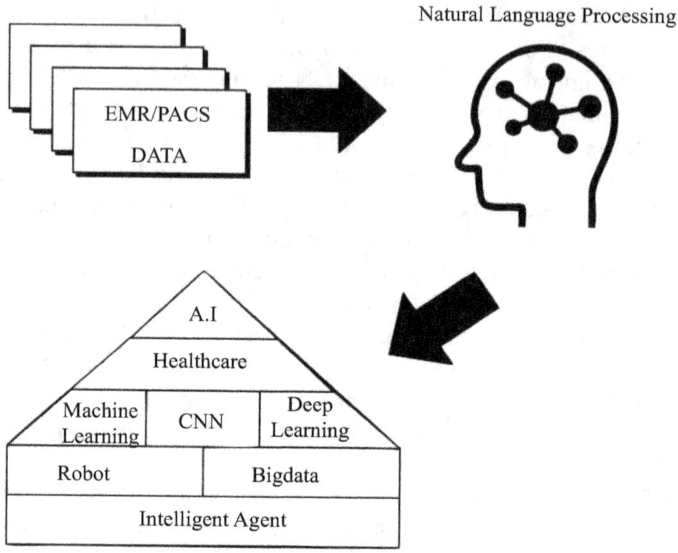

Figure 13.2 Schematic diagram of healthcare artificial intelligence

energy efficiency and minimizing communication cost in handling COVID-19-related medical data; and enhance healthcare information security by proposing privacy-aware measures. The chapter seems to be more theoretical in nature, discussing the concept of AIoMT and its potential applications in healthcare data management. The methodology involved a literature review, analysis of existing AIoMT technologies, and theoretical discussions thereafter. The chapter primarily focuses on the conceptual framework of AIoMT and does not go into technical details about any particular algorithm or model. The chapter discusses the proposed architecture and its potential benefits in enhancing healthcare data security and efficiency. The chapter lacks specific details about the architecture itself. It doesn't describe the technical aspects of the proposed privacy-aware energy-efficient architecture using AIoMT. Additionally, there are no data or evidence presented to support the claims made in the text. The paper briefly mentions the chapter's highlight of open research issues and possible lines of future research in AIoMT. However, it does not provide specific details about what these future research directions might be (Figure 13.2).

13.3 Understanding cyber threats in healthcare systems

This chapter explored the various types of cyber threats faced by healthcare systems, including malware attacks, ransomware incidents, social engineering exploits, and insider threats. It emphasizes the consequences of successful cyber-attacks on healthcare organizations and their impact on patient care and data security.

Understanding cyber threats in healthcare systems is of paramount importance in today's digital landscape. The healthcare industry has become a prime target for cybercriminals due to the wealth of sensitive patient information it holds and the critical nature of its services. As healthcare organizations increasingly rely on interconnected technologies and store patient data electronically, the attack surface for cyber threats has expanded, necessitating a deeper comprehension of the risks involved [7].

13.3.1 Several types of cyber threats pose significant challenges to healthcare systems

1. **Ransomware attacks:** Ransomware is a prevalent and disruptive threat in the healthcare sector. Cybercriminals use malicious software to encrypt critical data and demand ransom payments in exchange for decryption keys. Hospitals and healthcare providers can face dire consequences when their systems are locked down, leading to temporary disruptions in patient care and operational paralysis [8].
2. **Data breaches and patient privacy:** The compromise of patient data through data breaches can have severe consequences for both patients and healthcare organizations. Personal health information is highly valuable on the black market, and its exposure can result in identity theft, medical fraud, and reputational damage to the affected institutions.
3. **Phishing and social engineering:** Cyberattackers often use social engineering techniques like phishing emails to trick healthcare staff into revealing sensitive information or granting unauthorized access to systems. These tactics prey on human vulnerabilities, making employees the weakest link in the cybersecurity chain [9].
4. **Insider threats:** Insider threats occur when current or former employees, contractors, or partners misuse their access to systems and data for malicious purposes. These threats can be particularly challenging to detect and prevent due to the familiarity of the insider with the organization's infrastructure and security protocols.
5. **IoT vulnerabilities:** As healthcare systems integrate IoT devices and wearables, they introduce potential vulnerabilities. Poorly secured IoT devices can serve as entry points for cyberattackers to infiltrate larger healthcare networks.

Understanding these threats is crucial because the consequences of cyberattacks on healthcare systems can be far-reaching as follows [10,23,24].

13.3.2 Consequences of cyberattacks on healthcare

1. Impact on patient safety: A successful cyberattack on healthcare systems can disrupt medical services, leading to delays in patient care and potential harm to patients in critical conditions.
2. Financial losses: The financial repercussions of cyber incidents can be substantial. Organizations may face significant costs for remediation, recovery, and potential legal penalties.

3. Reputational damage: A cybersecurity breach can tarnish the reputation of healthcare organizations, eroding patient trust and damaging relationships with partners and stakeholders.
4. Regulatory non-compliance: The healthcare industry is subject to strict data protection regulations, such as the Health Insurance Portability and Accountability Act (HIPAA) in the United States [7]. A cybersecurity breach can result in regulatory fines and legal actions for non-compliance. To effectively address cyber threats in healthcare systems, organizations must adopt a comprehensive and proactive approach to cybersecurity:
   i. Robust cybersecurity infrastructure: Invest in advanced cybersecurity technologies and tools to protect against known and emerging threats.
   ii. Employee training and awareness: Educate healthcare staff about cyber threats, phishing prevention, and the importance of strong password management.
   iii. Data encryption and access controls: Implement strong encryption protocols and access controls to safeguard patient data.
   iv. Incident response planning: Develop and regularly test incident response plans to ensure a swift and effective response to cyber incidents.
   v. Regular security audits and assessments: Conduct periodic security audits and risk assessments to identify and address vulnerabilities proactively.

Finally, understanding cyber threats in healthcare systems is essential for healthcare organizations to safeguard patient data, maintain operational continuity, and protect patient safety. A proactive and multilayered cybersecurity strategy, combined with a culture of security awareness, is crucial in defending against the evolving landscape of cyber threats in the healthcare sector.

13.4 The role of artificial intelligence in healthcare cybersecurity

This book chapter delves into the capabilities of AI in detecting and responding to cyber threats in real time. It discusses the different AI-powered security solutions available, such as behavior-based anomaly detection, threat intelligence analysis, and predictive analytics. The chapter showcases real-world case studies of AI applications in healthcare cybersecurity [7,25].

AI is revolutionizing the field of cybersecurity in healthcare, offering innovative solutions to combat the increasing complexity and frequency of cyber threats. With the rapid digitization of healthcare systems and the exponential growth of sensitive patient data, the need for robust cybersecurity measures has become paramount. AI's ability to process vast amounts of data, analyze patterns, and make real-time decisions has positioned it as a game-changer in healthcare cybersecurity. This discussion explores the role of AI in various aspects of healthcare cybersecurity and its potential to transform the industry's defense against cyber threats [7,26].

1. **Real-time threat detection and response**: AI-powered cybersecurity solutions excel at detecting anomalies and identifying malicious activities in real time. Traditional rule-based systems often struggle to keep pace with rapidly evolving cyber threats, whereas AI's ML capabilities enable it to learn from new patterns and adapt its response accordingly. By continuously monitoring network traffic and behavior, AI-driven systems can swiftly respond to emerging threats and prevent potential cyberattacks before they cause significant damage[9,27].
2. **Advanced malware detection:** Malware attacks, including ransomware and trojans, are a significant concern for healthcare organizations. AI algorithms can analyze the behavior and characteristics of malware to identify and block them effectively. This dynamic approach enhances malware detection rates and reduces false positives, allowing healthcare systems to focus on genuine threats.
3. **User and entity behavior analytics (UEBA):** AI can analyze user and entity behavior within a healthcare system to identify deviations from normal patterns. UEBA tools can detect insider threats, suspicious activities by employees, and potential data breaches. By flagging unusual behaviors, AI helps healthcare organizations respond proactively to potential security incidents.
4. **Threat intelligence analysis:** AI can leverage threat intelligence data from various sources to enrich its knowledge base. By assimilating information on known threats, cyber trends, and attacker techniques, AI systems can enhance their ability to detect and counter emerging threats effectively.
5. **Predictive security analytics:** AI-driven predictive analytics assesses historical data to forecast potential cyber threats. By analyzing patterns and trends, AI can identify vulnerabilities in healthcare systems, predict potential attack vectors, and advise proactive security measures to mitigate risks [10,28].
6. **Automated incident response:** AI can streamline incident response by automating repetitive and time-consuming tasks. It can prioritize incidents based on severity, trigger responses to mitigate attacks, and facilitate forensic investigations, thereby reducing response times and minimizing the impact of cyber incidents.
7. **Cybersecurity awareness training:** AI can play a crucial role in cybersecurity awareness training for healthcare staff. It can simulate phishing attacks and tailor training modules to address individual vulnerabilities, thereby improving the organization's human firewall.
8. **Protecting medical devices and IoT:** As the use of medical devices and IoT in healthcare increases, so does the attack surface for cyber threats. AI can be deployed to monitor and secure these devices, ensuring their integrity and protecting them from potential exploitation.
9. **Privacy-preserving techniques:** AI can be applied to perform analytics on sensitive patient data while preserving privacy. Techniques like federated learning and differential privacy enable data analysis without compromising

individual patient records, facilitating secure collaboration and research within the healthcare community [23,29].

10. **Scalability and efficiency:** AI-driven cybersecurity solutions can scale effortlessly to handle large and complex healthcare systems, providing consistent protection across the entire network.

Despite its many advantages, AI in healthcare cybersecurity also presents some challenges which are, namely, as follows:

1. Data quality and bias: The accuracy and effectiveness of AI models rely on the quality and diversity of data they are trained on. Biased or incomplete data may lead to skewed predictions and reduced performance.
2. Adversarial attacks: AI systems themselves can be vulnerable to adversarial attacks, where malicious actors attempt to trick the AI model or manipulate its decisions.
3. Human oversight: While AI can automate many cybersecurity tasks, human oversight and intervention remain essential to ensure the accuracy and ethical use of AI in healthcare cybersecurity [20].
4. Regulatory compliance: Healthcare organizations must navigate regulatory frameworks and ensure that AI-driven cybersecurity solutions adhere to data protection and privacy laws.

Finally, the role of AI in healthcare cybersecurity is transformative. By augmenting human capabilities and offering advanced threat detection and response mechanisms, AI empowers healthcare organizations to safeguard sensitive patient data and maintain the integrity of critical medical services. As AI continues to evolve, its potential to revolutionize healthcare cybersecurity and protect patient well-being grows, making it an indispensable tool in the fight against cyber threats in the healthcare sector. To fully harness AI's benefits, healthcare organizations must embrace AI-driven solutions, invest in training and skill development, and ensure ongoing collaboration between human cybersecurity experts and AI systems for a comprehensive and robust defense against cyber threats [19,30] (Figure 13.3).

13.4.1 Empowering cybersecurity with machine learning algorithms

This chapter focuses on the role of ML algorithms in healthcare cybersecurity. It highlights how ML algorithms can identify patterns in cybercriminal behavior, predict future attacks, and continuously adapt security measures based on emerging threats. The chapter also explores the challenges and limitations of ML in cybersecurity [17].

Empowering cybersecurity with ML algorithms has become a game-changing approach in combating the ever-evolving landscape of cyber threats. ML brings a new dimension to cybersecurity by allowing systems to learn from data, adapt to changing environments, and make data-driven decisions autonomously. This discussion explores how ML algorithms empower cybersecurity and revolutionize the way organizations defend against cyber threats [3,31].

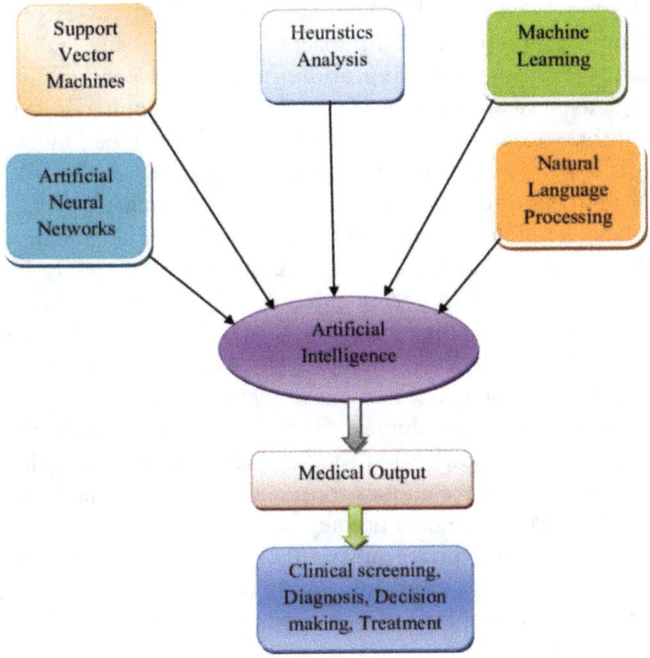

Figure 13.3 Process charts of artificial intelligence in the medicals

1. **Threat detection and anomaly detection:** ML algorithms excel at detecting patterns and anomalies in large datasets. In cybersecurity, ML can analyze network traffic, user behavior, and system logs to identify abnormal activities indicative of potential cyberattacks. By learning from historical data, ML can distinguish between normal and suspicious behavior, significantly reducing false positives and improving threat detection accuracy [1,32].
2. **Behavioral analysis:** ML enables behavioral analysis of users and entities within a system. By continuously monitoring and profiling user actions, ML algorithms can identify deviations from normal behavior, helping detect insider threats and unauthorized access attempts.
3. **Dynamic malware detection:** Traditional signature-based antivirus solutions are limited in detecting new and unknown malware. ML-based antivirus solutions can learn from malware characteristics and behavior to identify previously unseen malware and adapt their defenses accordingly [11].
4. **Predictive analytics:** ML algorithms can analyze historical cybersecurity data to predict potential future threats and vulnerabilities. By identifying patterns and trends in cyber incidents, organizations can proactively address security weaknesses and implement preventive measures.
5. **Automated response and incident management:** ML-driven automation can expedite incident response processes. ML algorithms can automatically

trigger responses, such as blocking suspicious IP addresses or quarantining infected devices, mitigating the impact of cyberattacks in real time.

6. **Continuous learning and adaptation:** ML models continually update their knowledge as new data becomes available. This continuous learning allows ML algorithms to evolve and stay up-to-date with emerging cyber threats, ensuring a dynamic and adaptive cybersecurity defense.
7. **Security analysis and forensics:** ML algorithms can analyze vast amounts of security data, helping security analysts quickly identify root causes of security incidents and perform forensic investigations more efficiently [11,33].
8. **User authentication and access control:** ML algorithms can enhance user authentication mechanisms by analyzing user behavior and context to assess the risk associated with login attempts. This helps in preventing unauthorized access and strengthening access control measures.
9. **Privacy-preserving technologies:** ML techniques like federated learning and homomorphic encryption enable secure analysis of sensitive data while preserving privacy. These techniques are particularly beneficial in healthcare and finance industries, where data privacy is paramount.
10. **Scaling cybersecurity operations:** ML allows organizations to scale their cybersecurity operations efficiently. With ML automation, security teams can handle large volumes of data and incidents without compromising the quality of their responses.

Despite its numerous advantages, ML in cybersecurity also presents challenges, namely:

1. **Data quality and bias:** The quality and diversity of data used to train ML models can significantly impact their effectiveness. Biased or incomplete data can lead to biased predictions and may not accurately represent all real-world scenarios [12].
2. **Adversarial attacks:** ML models can be vulnerable to adversarial attacks, where cyberattackers manipulate input data to mislead the model's decision-making process.
3. **Interpretability:** Some ML models, such as DNNs, can be challenging to interpret, making it difficult to understand how they arrive at their decisions.
4. **Model overfitting:** ML models trained on limited or noisy data can lead to overfitting, where the model performs well on the training data but fails to generalize to new, unseen data.

Finally, empowering cybersecurity with ML algorithms represents a significant advancement in defending against cyber threats. ML's ability to learn from data, identify patterns, and adapt to new challenges makes it an invaluable tool for security teams. As ML continues to evolve, organizations must invest in skilled personnel, interpretability, and robust data collection to harness its full potential. By leveraging ML's capabilities, organizations can stay ahead of cyber threats, strengthen their cybersecurity posture, and safeguard critical data and systems from malicious actors [13].

13.4.2 Enhancing privacy and data protection in healthcare

Data privacy is of utmost importance in the healthcare sector. Chapter 5 examines how AI and ML technologies can be utilized to enhance privacy and protect sensitive patient data. It explores privacy-preserving techniques, data anonymization, and secures communication methods.

Enhancing privacy and data protection in healthcare is of paramount importance as the industry relies heavily on sensitive patient information to deliver quality care and improve medical outcomes. With the digitization of healthcare records and the increasing use of technology in medical practices, ensuring the confidentiality and security of patient data has become a complex and multifaceted challenge. This discussion explores various strategies and technologies aimed at enhancing privacy and data protection in healthcare [14].

1. **Data encryption:** Encryption is a fundamental technique for protecting patient data. By converting sensitive information into an unreadable format, even if unauthorized access occurs, the data remains incomprehensible. Healthcare organizations must adopt strong encryption methods for data at rest, in transit, and during processing.
2. **Access controls and authentication:** Implementing robust access controls and authentication mechanisms is crucial to limit data access to authorized personnel only. Multifactor authentication, role-based access, and fine-grained access controls help prevent unauthorized individuals from accessing patient records.
3. **Privacy-preserving technologies:** Techniques like differential privacy and federated learning allow healthcare organizations to analyze aggregated patient data without exposing individual-level details. These privacy-preserving technologies enable secure data sharing for research and analytics without compromising patient privacy [15].
4. **Secure data storage:** Healthcare organizations must prioritize secure data storage practices. Storing data in encrypted databases and utilizing secure cloud storage solutions with strong security measures can mitigate the risk of data breaches.
5. **Data minimization and retention policies:** Adopting data minimization principles means collecting and retaining only the minimum amount of patient data necessary for medical purposes. Establishing clear data retention policies helps ensure that patient information is not stored longer than necessary, reducing exposure to potential data breaches.
6. **Data access logs and auditing:** Monitoring and logging data access activities are essential for identifying suspicious behavior and tracking potential security incidents. Regular audits of data access logs help identify and address any anomalous activities promptly.
7. **Secure communication channels:** Securing communication channels is vital to protect patient data during transmission. Implementing encrypted communication methods, such as virtual private networks (VPNs) and secure messaging systems, ensures that sensitive data remains protected [16].

8. **Employee training and awareness:** Employees play a significant role in safeguarding patient data. Comprehensive cybersecurity training programs can raise awareness about data protection best practices and the importance of adhering to privacy policies.
9. **Vendor and third-party security:** Healthcare organizations often collaborate with vendors and third-party service providers. Ensuring that these partners adhere to stringent security and privacy standards is critical to prevent potential data breaches through external channels.
10. **Compliance with data protection regulations:** Healthcare organizations must comply with data protection regulations such as the HIPAA in the United States, the General Data Protection Regulation (GDPR) in the European Union, and other relevant local regulations. Adhering to these regulations demonstrates a commitment to protecting patient privacy and data security.
11. **Incident response planning:** Developing a comprehensive incident response plan helps healthcare organizations respond swiftly and effectively in case of a data breach or cybersecurity incident. Timely containment and mitigation of security breaches are critical to minimizing the impact on patients and the organization's reputation.

In addition, enhancing privacy and data protection in healthcare requires a multifaceted approach that combines technological solutions, organizational policies, and employee awareness. Healthcare organizations must prioritize data security, employ the latest encryption and privacy-preserving technologies, and adhere to relevant data protection regulations. By continuously improving cybersecurity practices and staying vigilant against emerging threats, healthcare providers can maintain patient trust and protect the integrity of sensitive medical information [17].

13.4.3 Implementing solutions to mitigating cyber threats in healthcare

Implementing effective measures to counteract cyber threats in healthcare holds significant importance due to the sensitive nature of patient data and the critical status of medical infrastructure. Healthcare institutions are increasingly falling victim to cyberattacks, underscoring the necessity of adopting robust strategies to safeguard patient information, uphold patient safety, and preserve the reliability of healthcare systems [34,35] to be precise, a comprehensive approaches are given as follows:

1. **Cyber threat landscape in healthcare:** The healthcare sector has become a prime target for cyber threats due to the immense value of patient data and the critical nature of medical services. Cyberattacks such as ransomware, data breaches, and malware infections can compromise patient privacy, disrupt medical operations, and even impact patient care. The increasing interconnectedness of medical devices and systems amplifies the potential risks. Thus, implementing effective solutions to mitigate these threats is imperative [36,37].

2. **Strategies for mitigation:** Mitigating cyber threats in healthcare requires a multifaceted approach involving proactive measures and advanced technologies. One crucial strategy is conducting comprehensive risk assessments to identify vulnerabilities and potential entry points for cyberattacks. This assessment forms the basis for developing a robust risk management plan that prioritizes and addresses these vulnerabilities. Additionally, employee training and awareness campaigns are vital to educate healthcare staff about cybersecurity best practices and the importance of safeguarding patient data. Staff plays a pivotal role in preventing threats like phishing attacks [38].

   Another key aspect is network security, involving the implementation of advanced firewalls, intrusion detection systems, and encryption protocols to secure data transmission and prevent unauthorized access. Regular patch management is essential to address known vulnerabilities and prevent exploitation. Access control and identity management mechanisms, including two-factor authentication, ensure that only authorized personnel can access sensitive patient information. An incident response plan is crucial to handle cyber incidents effectively, including identifying, containing, mitigating, and recovering from attacks. Data encryption both at rest and in transit ensures that even if breached, the data remains unreadable and unusable to attackers [39,40].
3. **Utilizing emerging technologies:** Emerging technologies offer promising solutions to bolster healthcare cybersecurity. Blockchain technology can enhance data security and privacy by providing a tamperproof and transparent record of transactions, preventing unauthorized changes to patient records. AI and ML can analyze vast datasets to detect abnormal patterns and potential security breaches. They can automate threat detection and response, improving real-time defense capabilities. With the rise of IoT medical devices, ensuring their security is essential. Proper authentication, encryption, and regular updates are necessary to safeguard patient data and maintain the integrity of healthcare systems [41,42].
4. **Compliance, collaboration, and future direction:** Healthcare organizations must adhere to regulations like the HIPAA to ensure patient data protection and guide cybersecurity measures. Collaboration and information sharing among healthcare institutions, cybersecurity experts, and governmental agencies are crucial to staying ahead of evolving threats. Sharing threat intelligence and best practices enhances collective defense efforts and strengthens the overall cybersecurity posture. As the cyber threat landscape continues to evolve, healthcare organizations must remain vigilant, continually improve their strategies, and adapt to new challenges to effectively mitigate cyber threats and safeguard patient data and healthcare systems' integrity [41,43].

   i. **Blockchain technology:** By providing an immutable and transparent record of transactions, blockchain enhances the security and privacy of patient data. Unauthorized changes to patient records can be thwarted [42].
   ii. **Utilizing AI and ML:** Large datasets can be analyzed by AI and ML to detect abnormal patterns and potential security breaches. Automation of threat detection and response is also possible.

iii. **IoT security considerations:** In light of the proliferation of IoT medical devices, ensuring their security is crucial. Rigorous authentication, encryption, and consistent updates are pivotal [41].

i. **Risk evaluation and management:** Thorough assessments of vulnerabilities and potential points of entry for cyber threats are essential. Developing a plan to manage these risks prioritizes and addresses vulnerabilities.
ii. **Training and sensitization of personnel:** Equipping healthcare staff with knowledge of cybersecurity best practices is crucial to fend off prevalent threats like phishing attacks. Employees play a pivotal role in protecting patient data [44].
iii. **Enhanced network security:** Implementation of robust network security measures, including firewalls, intrusion detection systems, and encryption, is vital to secure data transmission and prevent unauthorized access.
iv. **System patching and maintenance:** Ensuring regular updates and patches for software, operating systems, and medical devices is essential to address known vulnerabilities and thwart exploitation [45].
v. **Access control and identity management:** The deployment of stringent access controls guarantees that only authorized personnel can access sensitive patient data. Augmenting security through two-factor authentication is advisable.
vi. **Incident response planning:** The creation of a comprehensive plan for addressing cyber incidents is imperative. It encompasses the identification, containment, mitigation, and recovery stages of cyberattacks.
vii. **Encryption of data:** Safeguarding patient data, both during transmission and when at rest, through encryption is paramount. In the event of a breach, encrypted data remains indecipherable and unusable to attackers [40].
viii. **Management of vendor risks:** Ensuring that third-party vendors and suppliers adhere to established cybersecurity standards is essential, as their vulnerabilities can serve as potential entry points for attackers.

Harnessing emerging technologies which are, namely, as follows:

1. **The significance of collaboration and information sharing:** Establishing collaborative ties with cybersecurity experts, governmental agencies, and fellow healthcare institutions to exchange threat intelligence and best practices enhances overall defense capabilities.

Finally, the multifaceted challenge of combating cyber threats in healthcare necessitates a comprehensive approach encompassing technology, procedural enhancements, and collaborative endeavors. Ongoing vigilance, adaptation to evolving threats, and continual enhancement of cybersecurity strategies are indispensable in safeguarding patient data and the reliability of healthcare systems [42,43].

13.4.4 Implementing AI and ML solutions in healthcare organizations

This practical chapter focuses on the implementation of AI and ML solutions in healthcare organizations. It addresses the challenges and considerations healthcare providers may face in integrating these technologies into their existing systems and processes. Best practices and success stories from leading healthcare institutions are presented.

Implementing AI and ML solutions in healthcare organizations presents a transformative opportunity to enhance patient care, streamline operations, and optimize healthcare outcomes. The integration of AI and ML technologies enables healthcare providers to leverage data-driven insights, improve decision-making, and address some of the industry's most pressing challenges. This discussion explores the key considerations and benefits of implementing AI and ML solutions in healthcare organizations [18].

1. **Clinical decision support:** AI and ML can assist healthcare professionals in making more informed and accurate clinical decisions. By analyzing vast amounts of patient data, including medical history, lab results, and imaging studies, AI-driven clinical decision support systems can provide personalized treatment recommendations and flag potential issues, leading to improved patient outcomes.
2. **Disease diagnosis and detection:** AI and ML algorithms can aid in early disease diagnosis and detection. Image recognition technologies, for example, can analyze medical images, such as X-rays and MRIs, to identify abnormalities and assist radiologists in detecting diseases like cancer at an early stage.
3. **Predictive analytics for patient care:** AI and ML can predict patient outcomes and potential health risks based on historical patient data. This predictive analytics capability enables healthcare providers to intervene proactively and deliver targeted interventions to high-risk patients, thereby preventing complications and reducing hospital readmissions [5].
4. **Personalized medicine and treatment plans:** AI and ML can analyze individual patient data, including genetic information, lifestyle factors, and treatment history, to create personalized medicine and treatment plans tailored to each patient's specific needs and characteristics.
5. **Healthcare operations and resource management:** AI and ML can optimize healthcare operations by analyzing patient flow, resource allocation, and staffing needs. Predictive models can help healthcare organizations manage resources efficiently, leading to improved patient access and reduced wait times.
6. **Drug discovery and development:** AI and ML technologies can accelerate drug discovery and development processes by analyzing vast datasets, predicting potential drug interactions, and identifying potential drug candidates more efficiently than traditional methods.
7. **Remote patient monitoring:** AI and ML can facilitate remote patient monitoring by analyzing data from wearable devices and IoT sensors. Continuous monitoring of patient vitals and health parameters enables early detection of health issues and timely interventions [7].
8. **Natural language processing (NLP) for electronic health records (EHRs):** NLP technology can convert unstructured clinical data in EHRs into

structured and actionable information, enabling healthcare providers to extract valuable insights from patient records and improve data accessibility.

9. **Reduced administrative burden:** AI-driven automation can streamline administrative tasks, such as appointment scheduling, billing, and claims processing, reducing the administrative burden on healthcare staff, and allowing them to focus more on patient care.
10. **Enhanced patient engagement and experience:** AI-powered chatbots and virtual assistants can engage with patients, providing timely responses to inquiries, appointment reminders, and post-treatment follow-ups, thus enhancing patient experience and satisfaction.

However, there are some challenges and considerations in implementing AI and ML solutions in healthcare organizations [4,5]:

1. Data quality and privacy: The success of AI and ML models depends on the quality and quantity of data. Ensuring data accuracy, reliability, and privacy is essential to achieve meaningful and trustworthy results.
2. Regulatory compliance: Healthcare organizations must comply with data protection regulations, such as HIPAA, and ensure that AI and ML solutions adhere to ethical and legal guidelines.
3. Interoperability: Integrating AI and ML solutions with existing healthcare systems and EHRs can be complex, requiring compatibility and interoperability between different platforms [19].
4. Data bias and fairness: ML algorithms can inherit biases present in the data used for training. It is essential to address these biases to ensure fairness and equity in healthcare decision-making.
5. Training and expertise: Healthcare organizations need skilled data scientists, AI engineers, and clinicians who understand both healthcare domain knowledge and AI/ML techniques to develop and deploy effective solutions.

Moreso, implementing AI and ML solutions in healthcare organizations holds immense potential to revolutionize patient care, enhance operational efficiency, and advance medical research. By leveraging AI and ML technologies responsibly and ethically, healthcare providers can improve patient outcomes, reduce costs, and pave the way for a more data-driven and patient-centric healthcare ecosystem. It is crucial for healthcare organizations to approach AI and ML implementation with a well-defined strategy, robust data governance, and a commitment to patient privacy and regulatory compliance to fully realize the transformative benefits of these technologies [20].

13.4.5 Building a cybersecurity culture in healthcare organizations

The success of any cybersecurity initiative depends on fostering a culture of security awareness and responsibility. Chapter 7 discusses the importance of promoting a cybersecurity-conscious culture within healthcare organizations. It outlines strategies for training employees, conducting simulated cyber drills, and creating a sense of shared responsibility for cybersecurity.

Building a cybersecurity culture in healthcare organizations is crucial to establish a proactive and resilient defense against the increasing cyber threats faced by the industry. A cybersecurity culture fosters a collective awareness, responsibility, and commitment to safeguarding sensitive patient data and critical medical systems. This section explores the key elements and strategies to cultivate a cybersecurity culture in healthcare organizations [7,30].

1. **Leadership commitment:** A cybersecurity culture starts at the top. Leadership must demonstrate a strong commitment to cybersecurity by prioritizing it in the organization's mission and goals. Executives should actively participate in cybersecurity initiatives, allocate resources, and champion security best practices.
2. **Education and training:** Regular cybersecurity training and education for all employees are essential. Training programs should cover topics such as identifying phishing attempts, handling sensitive data, and recognizing potential cyber threats. Employees should be aware of their role in protecting patient information and the consequences of security breaches.
3. **Clear policies and procedures:** Establishing clear and comprehensive cybersecurity policies and procedures is critical. Employees should know the organization's expectations regarding data protection, password management, device usage, and incident reporting [4].
4. **Continuous awareness campaigns:** Conduct ongoing awareness campaigns to keep cybersecurity top-of-mind for employees. Utilize newsletters, posters, email reminders, and other communication channels to share cybersecurity tips, recent threats, and success stories.
5. **Leading by example:** Leaders and IT personnel should lead by example, practicing strong security habits and demonstrating the importance of cybersecurity in their daily work. This sets a positive tone and encourages others to follow suit.
6. **Encouraging reporting and accountability:** Encourage a culture of reporting potential security incidents without fear of repercussions. Employees should feel empowered to report suspicious activities or security concerns promptly. Promptly addressing reported incidents and providing feedback fosters a sense of accountability [2].
7. **Involving all departments:** Cybersecurity is not solely the responsibility of the IT department. Engage all departments, including clinical staff, administrative staff, and management, in cybersecurity efforts. Each department plays a role in safeguarding patient data and protecting the organization from cyber threats.
8. **Third-party risk management:** Extend cybersecurity culture to third-party vendors and partners. Establish stringent security requirements for vendors, conduct regular audits, and ensure that they adhere to the same cybersecurity standards as the organization.
9. **Incident response planning and drills**: Develop a robust incident response plan and conduct regular drills to prepare employees for handling

cybersecurity incidents effectively. This ensures a coordinated and swift response to potential breaches [3].

10. **Continuous improvement and adaptation:** Cybersecurity threats are continuously evolving. Promote a culture of continuous improvement, where the organization adapts to new threats, implements new security measures, and learns from past incidents to strengthen its security posture.
11. **Rewarding positive security behaviors:** Recognize and reward employees who actively contribute to the cybersecurity culture. Positive reinforcement reinforces good security practices and motivates employees to remain vigilant.

In addition, building a cybersecurity culture in healthcare organizations requires a multifaceted approach that involves leadership commitment, employee education, clear policies, and a collective responsibility for data protection. By creating a cybersecurity-aware environment and fostering a sense of ownership among employees, healthcare organizations can establish a robust defense against cyber threats and better protect patient data and critical healthcare systems. The cybersecurity culture must be ingrained in the organization's values, and it should continuously evolve to address new challenges and stay ahead of emerging threats [5,23].

13.4.6 The future of AI and ML in healthcare cybersecurity

The final chapter looks ahead to the future of AI and ML technologies in healthcare cybersecurity. It explores emerging trends, potential advancements, and the continuous evolution of cyber threats. The chapter discusses the need for ongoing research, collaboration, and adaptation to ensure robust cybersecurity measures in the ever-changing digital landscape of healthcare.

The chapter emphasizes the pivotal role of AI and ML in mitigating cyber threats and reinforces the importance of a proactive approach to cybersecurity in healthcare systems. The chapter concludes by underlining the collective responsibility of healthcare organizations, researchers, and policymakers in safeguarding patient data and securing the future of healthcare cybersecurity [15].

The future of AI and ML in healthcare cybersecurity holds great promise as these technologies continue to advance and evolve. The integration of AI and ML in cybersecurity is expected to reshape the landscape of healthcare data protection, threat detection, and incident response. This discussion explores some key aspects that illustrate the exciting prospects and potential challenges for AI and ML in healthcare cybersecurity namely.

1. **Enhanced threat detection and prevention:** AI and ML algorithms will become even more adept at identifying and mitigating cyber threats in real time. As cybercriminals develop more sophisticated attack methods, AI-driven cybersecurity solutions will continuously learn and adapt to detect new patterns and anomalies, providing healthcare organizations with a proactive defense against evolving threats [41].

2. **Behavioral biometrics and continuous authentication:** AI and ML will facilitate the adoption of behavioral biometrics for continuous authentication. Analyzing user behavior, such as typing patterns or mouse movements, can establish a unique profile for each user, making it easier to identify potential unauthorized access attempts [16].
3. **Zero-trust architecture:** AI and ML will play a significant role in implementing a zero-trust architecture, where every user and device is treated as potentially untrusted. AI-driven security measures will continuously assess the risk associated with each user and transaction, allowing access only to authorized users with the necessary permissions.
4. **Improved privacy-preserving techniques:** AI and ML will continue to advance privacy-preserving techniques, ensuring that patient data remains protected while being used for analysis and research. Techniques like federated learning and homomorphic encryption will enable secure collaboration and data sharing across healthcare organizations without compromising individual privacy [17].
5. **Automated incident response and threat hunting:** AI and ML will increasingly automate incident response processes, enabling rapid identification, containment, and mitigation of cybersecurity incidents. Threat hunting will also benefit from AI-driven analytics, allowing cybersecurity experts to proactively search for threats and vulnerabilities.
6. **Cybersecurity autonomous response (CAR):** The future may see the emergence of cybersecurity autonomous response systems that can autonomously detect and respond to cyber threats, potentially neutralizing threats before human intervention is required.
7. **Interoperability and integration:** AI and ML solutions will become more interoperable and seamlessly integrated into existing healthcare systems and workflows. This integration will enhance efficiency and enable seamless data sharing and analysis across various healthcare platforms.
8. **Ethical AI and bias mitigation:** As AI and ML play increasingly critical roles in healthcare decision-making, addressing ethical concerns and mitigating biases will be of paramount importance. Healthcare organizations must ensure that AI algorithms are fair, transparent, and free from any unintended discrimination.
9. **Addressing adversarial attacks:** AI and ML models will need to be strengthened against adversarial attacks, where malicious actors attempt to manipulate the models' decision-making process. Robustness against such attacks will be crucial to maintaining the integrity of cybersecurity defenses [18].
10. **Advanced threat intelligence and threat hunting:** AI and ML will enable the processing of vast amounts of threat intelligence data, improving threat hunting capabilities and enabling more proactive cybersecurity strategies.

Challenges:

1. Data quality and integration: The success of AI and ML in healthcare cybersecurity relies heavily on high-quality, integrated, and standardized data.

Healthcare organizations must address data silos and ensure data accuracy and reliability.

2. Regulatory compliance: Healthcare organizations must navigate complex regulatory environments and ensure that AI and ML solutions comply with data protection and privacy regulations [1,2].
3. Skilled workforce: The shortage of skilled cybersecurity professionals with expertise in AI and ML poses a challenge. Healthcare organizations must invest in training and developing cybersecurity experts who understand the complexities of these technologies.
4. Explainability and transparency: AI and ML models can be complex and difficult to interpret. Ensuring the explainability and transparency of AI-driven cybersecurity decisions will be crucial to building trust in these technologies.

In addition, the future of AI and ML in healthcare cybersecurity is promising, with the potential to revolutionize threat detection, incident response, and data protection. Healthcare organizations that embrace these technologies responsibly and invest in the necessary infrastructure, talent, and ethical considerations stand to gain a significant advantage in defending against the ever-evolving cyber threats in the healthcare sector. By leveraging the power of AI and ML, healthcare organizations can safeguard patient data, enhance patient care, and fortify their cybersecurity defenses for a safer and more resilient healthcare ecosystem [3].

13.4.6.1 Implications for the future of healthcare cybersecurity

The future of healthcare cybersecurity is likely to be shaped by several key implications, driven by technological advancements, evolving threats, and regulatory changes. Here are some important implications to consider:

1. Growing importance of AI and ML: AI and ML will play an increasingly significant role in healthcare cybersecurity. These technologies can continuously analyze vast amounts of data to detect anomalies, identify potential cyber threats, and respond in real time to prevent attacks [26]. AI-driven cybersecurity solutions can provide proactive protection and adapt to emerging threats more effectively than traditional approaches.
2. Integration of IoT devices and wearables: The IoT devices and wearables are becoming more prevalent in the healthcare industry. While they offer numerous benefits, their widespread use also increases the attack surface for cybercriminals. Securing these devices will be critical to prevent unauthorized access to sensitive patient data and protect the integrity of medical devices [13].
3. Challenges in securing telehealth services: The rise of telehealth services, especially during global events like the COVID-19 pandemic, has improved healthcare accessibility. However, it has also exposed new vulnerabilities in the healthcare system. Securing telehealth platforms and ensuring secure

communication between healthcare providers and patients will be vital to safeguard patient information.

4. Emergence of cybersecurity regulations: As the importance of healthcare data security becomes more evident, governments and regulatory bodies are likely to introduce stricter cybersecurity regulations for the healthcare sector. Healthcare organizations will need to stay compliant with these regulations and invest in robust security measures to protect patient data adequately [25].
5. Cybersecurity workforce shortage: The demand for skilled cybersecurity professionals will continue to outpace supply, leading to a workforce shortage in the healthcare industry and beyond. Healthcare organizations may need to explore partnerships with cybersecurity firms or invest in training existing staff to bridge this gap effectively.
6. Ransomware and extortion threats: Ransomware attacks, where cybercriminals encrypt data and demand a ransom for its release, have been on the rise in recent years. Healthcare institutions are particularly vulnerable to such attacks due to the sensitive nature of patient data. As a result, investing in robust backup solutions and implementing security best practices will become crucial to mitigate these threats.
7. Interconnected ecosystems and third-party risks: The interconnected nature of healthcare ecosystems, involving multiple providers, insurance companies, and vendors, can introduce security vulnerabilities. Cybercriminals may target third-party partners to gain access to larger healthcare networks. Healthcare organizations will need to perform due diligence on third-party vendors and establish clear security standards in contracts [4,26].
8. Importance of user education and training: Human error is a significant factor in cybersecurity breaches. Educating and training healthcare staff about cybersecurity best practices, identifying phishing attempts, and recognizing social engineering tactics will be essential to reinforce the human firewall and reduce the risk of successful attacks.
9. Zero-trust architecture: The adoption of zero-trust architecture will likely increase in healthcare to ensure a strong security posture. This model requires constant verification of users and devices, regardless of their location, before granting access to sensitive data or systems.
10. Ethical considerations in data usage: As healthcare organizations collect and analyze vast amounts of patient data for various purposes, ethical considerations regarding data privacy and consent will become more pronounced. Ensuring transparent data usage and obtaining patient consent for data sharing and analytics will be critical for maintaining trust with patients [16].

In conclusion, the future of healthcare cybersecurity will require a multifaceted approach that combines advanced technologies, regulatory compliance, and a proactive cybersecurity mindset. Healthcare organizations must remain vigilant in adapting to emerging threats while also prioritizing patient privacy and data protection.

13.4.6.2 Call to action for healthcare organizations and researchers

Call to action for healthcare organizations:

1. Invest in cybersecurity infrastructure: Healthcare organizations must prioritize cybersecurity by investing in robust and up-to-date cybersecurity infrastructure. This includes adopting advanced security technologies, employing AI-driven threat detection systems, and implementing encryption protocols to protect patient data [4].
2. Establish a cybersecurity culture: Foster a cybersecurity-conscious culture within the organization. This involves providing regular cybersecurity training to all staff members, raising awareness about the latest threats, and promoting a sense of responsibility among employees to safeguard patient data.
3. Collaborate and share information: Healthcare organizations should collaborate with each other and share information about cyber threats and incidents. By pooling knowledge and resources, the industry can better prepare and respond to emerging cybersecurity challenges.
4. Third-party risk management: Implement a robust third-party risk management program. Healthcare organizations often rely on various vendors and partners, making it crucial to assess their security practices and ensure they meet cybersecurity standards [6].
5. Regular security audits and assessments: Conduct regular security audits and risk assessments to identify vulnerabilities and areas for improvement. Regular evaluations help healthcare organizations stay proactive in addressing potential security gaps.
6. Incident response planning: Develop comprehensive incident response plans to effectively handle cybersecurity breaches. This includes defining roles and responsibilities, establishing communication protocols, and practicing simulated cyber incident drills.
7. Compliance with regulations: Stay updated with cybersecurity regulations and comply with relevant data protection laws. Adhering to industry standards and legal requirements helps build trust with patients and regulatory authorities [8].
8. Continuous monitoring and threat hunting: Implement continuous monitoring and threat hunting practices to detect and respond to cyber threats in real time. This proactive approach enables early detection and minimizes the impact of potential breaches.
9. Data minimization and encryption: Minimize the collection and retention of unnecessary patient data to reduce the potential impact of a breach. Additionally, employ strong encryption techniques to protect data both at rest and in transit.
10. Transparent communication with patients: Be transparent with patients about data security measures and any potential security incidents. Open communication builds trust and allows patients to take necessary precautions to protect their information.

13.4.6.3 Call to action for researchers

1. Research on emerging threats: Researchers should focus on studying and understanding emerging cyber threats specific to the healthcare industry. This includes analyzing new attack vectors, threat actors' behavior, and potential vulnerabilities unique to healthcare systems.
2. Develop advanced security solutions: Create innovative cybersecurity solutions tailored to the healthcare sector. This may involve developing AI-powered threat detection algorithms, secure communication protocols, or advanced authentication methods [9].
3. Privacy-preserving technologies: Researchers can explore and develop privacy-preserving technologies that allow data analysis without compromising patient privacy. Techniques such as homomorphic encryption and differential privacy can be valuable in healthcare data analytics.
4. Collaboration with healthcare organizations: Collaborate with healthcare organizations to gain insights into real-world challenges and to validate the effectiveness of proposed cybersecurity solutions. Such partnerships can bridge the gap between academia and practical implementation [10].
5. Ethical considerations: Consider the ethical implications of cybersecurity research in healthcare, particularly when dealing with patient data and vulnerabilities. Ensure research adheres to ethical guidelines and prioritizes patient privacy and consent.
6. Standardization and best practices: Contribute to the development of cybersecurity standards and best practices for the healthcare industry. Standardization promotes consistency and ensures that organizations can adopt proven methodologies.
7. Education and awareness: Researchers can contribute to raising awareness about cybersecurity issues in healthcare through publications, conferences, and public engagements. By disseminating knowledge, they can help healthcare professionals and the public better understand and address cybersecurity risks.
8. Focus on usability: Develop cybersecurity solutions that are user-friendly and easy to implement. Usability is crucial in encouraging [20] widespread adoption and ensuring that healthcare organizations can effectively integrate these solutions into their existing systems.
9. Responsible disclosure: Researchers who discover vulnerabilities or weaknesses in healthcare systems should follow responsible disclosure practices. This involves notifying the affected organization and providing adequate time to address the issue before making it public.
10. Long-term impact assessment: Research efforts should assess the long-term impact of cybersecurity measures and technologies in healthcare. Understanding how these solutions evolve over time can help improve their effectiveness and address potential challenges. By collectively taking action, healthcare organizations and researchers can strengthen cybersecurity in the healthcare sector, protect patient data, and ensure the continuity of quality healthcare services in an increasingly digital world.

13.5 Conclusion

As we enter the digital age, the significance of cybersecurity becomes increasingly evident, particularly in the healthcare sector, where sensitive patient data is stored and transmitted through various technological systems. With advancing technology, safeguarding healthcare systems from cyber threats has become more critical than ever before. Cybercriminals target patient information, financial data, and medical records, leading to severe consequences like reputational damage, loss of trust, financial loss, legal repercussions, and even potential harm to patients. Despite efforts to regulate cybersecurity in healthcare, the increasing number of cyberattacks remains a challenge. To address this, implementing AI and ML has shown promise. AI can detect and prevent cyberattacks in real time, providing an additional layer of security. ML algorithms can predict and prevent future attacks by analyzing cybercriminal behaviors and patterns. Secure communication channels are also crucial for healthcare systems to protect sensitive data. Encrypted communication methods, such as secure messaging systems and VPNs, significantly enhance the security of healthcare systems. This book chapter presents an overview of the importance of cybersecurity in healthcare, exploring various cyber threats faced by healthcare systems, including malware attacks, ransomware attacks, and social engineering attacks. It delves into the impact of cyber threats on healthcare, such as patient privacy breaches, financial losses, and reputational damage. Additionally, the chapter discusses the regulatory and legal requirements that healthcare organizations must follow to safeguard patient privacy and security. Furthermore, the chapter outlines cybersecurity measures that healthcare organizations can adopt, such as risk assessments, staff training, network segmentation, access controls, and incident response plans. Finally, emerging technologies like blockchain and AI were discussed, illustrating their potential to enhance cybersecurity in healthcare systems.

References

[1] Abioye, S. O., Oyedele, L. O., Akanbi, L., *et al.* (2021). Artificial intelligence in the construction industry: A review of present status, opportunities and future challenges. *Big Data, Enterprise and Artificial Intelligence Laboratory (Big-DEAL), Bristol Business School*, University of the West of England, Bristol, United Kingdom; DOI: 10.1016/j.jobe.2021.103299.

[2] Al-Besher, A., and Kumar, K. (2022). Use of artificial intelligence to enhance e-government services. *College of Computing and Informatics, Saudi Electronic University, Riyadh, 11673*, Saudi Arabia. DOI: 10.1016/j.measen.2022.100484

[3] Baracaldo, N., Chen, B., Ludwig, H., and Safavi, J. A. (2017). Mitigating poisoning attacks on machine learning models: A data provenance based approach. *Session: Defense against Poisoning. AISec'17*, November 3, 2017, Dallas, TX.

[4] Alsammari, B. M. (2023). A framework for developing secure Internet of Medical Things: A comprehensive roadmap from an artificial intelligence perspective. *Journal of Theoretical and Applied Information Technology*, 101(4).

[5] Brundage, M., Avin, S., Clark, J., *et al.* (2018). *The Malicious Use of Artificial Intelligence: Forecasting, Prevention, and Mitigation*. February, 2018.

[6] Kabir, M. H., Hasan, K. F., Hasan, M. K., and Ansari, K. (2021). Explainable artificial intelligence for smart city application: A secure and trusted platform. Springer Nature. 2021.

[7] Telo, J. (2017). AI for enhanced healthcare security: An investigation of anomaly detection, predictive analytics, access control, threat intelligence, and incident response. *Journal of Advanced Analytics in Healthcare Management*. 2017.

[8] Nwakanma, C. I., Ahakonye, L. A. C., Njoku, J. N., *et al.* (2023). Explainable artificial intelligence (XAI) for intrusion detection and mitigation in intelligent connected vehicles: a review. *Applied Sciences*, 13(3), 1252. https://www.mdpi.com/, https://doi.org/10.3390/app13031252.

[9] Singh, S. K., Rathore, S., and Park, J. H. (2019). BlockIoTIntelligence: A Blockchain-enabled Intelligent IoT Architecture with Artificial Intelligence. *Department of Computer Science and Engineering, Seoul National University of Science and Technology (SeoulTech)*, Seoul Korea. Elsevier, 2019.

[10] Jabarulla, M. Y., and Lee, H.-N. (2021). A blockchain and artificial intelligence-based, patient-centric healthcare system for combating the COVID-19 pandemic: opportunities and applications. *Healthcare*, 9, 1019. https://doi.org/10.3390/healthcare9081019

[11] Kavitha, S., Bora, A., Naved, M., Raj, K. B., and Nadh Singh, B. R. (2021). An internet of things for data security in cloud using artificial intelligence. *International Journal of Grid and Distributed Computing*, 14(1), 1257–1275.

[12] Ahsan, M., Nygard, K. E., Gomes, R., Chowdhury, M. M., Rifat, N., and Connolly, J. F. (2022). Cybersecurity Threats and Their Mitigation Approaches Using Machine Learning—A Review. JCP, Volume(Issue), Page numbers. Retrieved from https://www.mdpi.com/journal/jcp.

[13] Jakka, G., Yathiraju, N., and Ansari, M. F. (2022). Artificial intelligence in terms of spotting malware and delivering cyber risk management. *Journal of Positive School Psychology*, 6(3), 6156–6165. Retrieved from http://journalppw.com.

[14] Al-Besher, A., and Kumar, K. (2022). Use of artificial intelligence to enhance e-government services. *Measurement & Sensors*, 24(Suppl. C), 100484. Retrieved from file:///C:/journal/measurement-sensors/vol/24/suppl/C.

[15] van der Schaar, M., Alaa, A. M., Floto, A., *et al.* (2021). How artificial intelligence and machine learning can help healthcare systems respond to

COVID-19. *Machine Learning*, 110(1), 1–14. https://doi.org/10.1007/s10994-020-05928-x.

[16] Vijayakumar, K. P., Pradeep, K., Balasundaram, A., and Prusty, M. R. (2023). Enhanced Cyber Attack Detection Process for Internet of Health Things (IoHT) Devices Using Deep Neural Network. School of Computer Science and Engineering, *Vellore Institute of Technology, Chennai 600127, India*. Retrieved from https://www.mdpi.com/.

[17] Kelly, B. S., Quinn, C., Belton, N., Lawlor, A., Killeen, R. P., and Burrell, J. (2023). Cybersecurity considerations for radiology departments involved with artificial intelligence. *European Radiology*. https://doi.org/10.1007/s00330-023-09860-1.

[18] Li, B., Wu, Y., Song, J., Lu, R., Li, T., and Zhao, L. (2021). DeepFed: federated deep learning for intrusion detection in industrial cyber–physical systems. *IEEE Transactions on Industrial Informatics*, 17(8), 5658–5667. DOI: 10.1109/TII.2021.3060480.

[19] Naseem, M., Akhund, R., Arshad, H., and Ibrahim, M. T. (2020). Exploring the potential of artificial intelligence and machine learning to combat COVID-19 and existing opportunities for LMIC: a scoping review. *Journal of Primary Care & Community Health*, 11, 1–11. DOI: 10.1177/2150132720963634. https://journals.sagepub.com/home/jpc.

[20] Radoglou-Grammatikis, P., Rompolos, K., Sarigiannidis, P., *et al.* (2022). Modeling, detecting, and mitigating threats against industrial healthcare systems: a combined software defined networking and reinforcement learning approach. *IEEE Transactions on Industrial Informatics*, 18(3), 2022.

[21] Imoize, A. L., Balas, V. E., Solanki, V. K., Lee, C. C., and Obaidat, M. S. (Eds.). (2023). *Handbook of Security and Privacy of AI-Enabled Healthcare Systems and Internet of Medical Things* (1st ed.). Boca Raton: CRC Press. https://doi.org/10.1201/9781003370321

[22] Imoize, A. L., Gbadega, P. A., Obakhena, H. I., Irabor, D. O., Kavitha, K. V. N., and Chakraborty, C. (2022). Artificial Intelligence-enabled Internet of Medical Things for COVID-19 pandemic data management. In *Explainable Artificial Intelligence in Medical Decision Support Systems* (pp. 357–380). (Vol. 50). Web of Science. https://covidwho-2323747., doi: 10.1049/PBHE050E_ch13.

[23] Wisdom, D. D., Tambuwal, A. Y., Chun, P. B., Adamu, H. K., and Ajayi, E. A. (2018). Enhanced model for computer viruses counter measures. 1st International Conference on Education and Development (ITED), Baze University, Abuja, Nigeria 2018.

[24] Gudu, E. B., Wisdom, D. D., Gudu, G. J., Ahmad, M. A., Isaac, S., and Akinyemi, A. E. (2020). Data science for Covid-19 (Mathematical Recipe for Curbing CoronaVirus (Covid-19) Transmission Dynamics), *Elsevier* (pp. 527–545). (Vol. 2021). https://doi.org/10.1016%2FB978-0-12-824536-1.00013-7.

[25] Wisdom, D. D., Obiniyi, A. A., Igulu, K. T., *et al.* Industrial IoT security threats and counter measures, *Springer Nature*, 2023.

[26] Gudu, E. B., Wisdom, D. D., Ahmed, M. A., Akinyemi, A. E., Isaac, S., and Dazi, A. J. (2020). Mathematical model for the spread and control of ebola virus by quarantine techniques, *Anals Journal of Computer Science Series*, 19(1), 2021.

[27] Imoize, A. L., Irabor, D. O., Peter, G., and Chakraborty, C. (2022). Blockchain technology for secure COVID-19 pandemic data handling. In *Smart Health Technologies for the COVID-19 Pandemic: Internet of medical things perspectives* (pp. 141–179). DOI: 10.1049/PBHE042E_ch6. University of Lagos, University of KwaZulu-Natal, Birla Institute of Technology, Mesra.

[28] Wisdom, D. D., Vincent, O. R., Igulu, K., *et al.* (2023). Cybersecurity in the Industry 4.0 and 5.0. Taylor and Francis group, 2023.

[29] Gudu, E. B., Wisdom, D. D., Hyacinth, E. A., *et al.* (2023). Transmission dynamics of COVID-19 virus disease. *Artificial Intelligence in Biomedical and Modern Healthcare Informatics*, Elsevier, August, 2023.

[30] Wisdom, D. D., Ajayi, E. A., Arinze, U. C., Idris, H., Bello, U. M., and Aladesote, O. I. An optimized TWIN battery resource management scheme in wireless networks, lecture notes in networks, Vol. 217. *Proceedings of Sixth International Congress on Information and Communication Technology, Springer Nature*, 2021. 978-981-16- 2101-7,511607.

[31] Wisdom, D. D., Tambuwal, A. Y., Mohammed, A., Audu, A., Soroyewun, M. B., and Isaac, S. A delay aware power saving scheme (DAPSS-BT) based on load on traffic in IEEE 802.16e WiMAX Networks, *Institute of Electrical and Electronic Engineers Conference IEEE, Ahmadu Bello University Zaria, Kaduna State, Nigeria, 2019*.

[32] Isaac, S., Wisdom, D. D., Ahmed, M. A., and Arinze, U. C. Battery-life management with an efficient sleep-mode power saving scheme (BM-ESPSS) in IEEE 802.16e Networks, *International Journal of Mechatronics, Electrical and Computer Technology (JMEC)*, 7(2), 2020.

[33] Wisdom, D. D., Saidu, I., Tambuwal, A. Y., Ahmad, M. A., Isaac, S., and Farouk, N. An efficient sleep- window-based power saving scheme (ESPSS) in IEEE 802.16e Networks, *15th International Conference on Electronics Computer and Computation ICECCO* 2019.

[34] Imoize, L., Hemanth, J., Do, D.-T., and Sur, S. N. (Eds.). (2022). *Explainable Artificial Intelligence in Medical Decision Support Systems*. Institution of Engineering and Technology. https://doi.org/10.1049/PBHE050E.

[35] Ramasamy, L. K., Khan K. P., F., Imoize, A. L., Ogbebor, J. O., Kadry, S., and Rho, S. (2021). Blockchain-based wireless sensor networks for malicious node detection: a survey. *IEEE Access*, 9, 128765–128785. https://doi.org/10.1109/ACCESS.2021.3111923.

[36] Awotunde, J. B., Imoize A. L., Ayoade O. B., *et al.* (2022). An enhanced hyper-parameter optimization of a convolutional neural network model for leukemia cancer diagnosis in a smart healthcare system. *Sensors*, 22(24), 9689. https://doi.org/10.3390/s22249689.

[37] Sei, Y., Ohsuga, A., and Imoize, A. L. (2022). Statistical test with differential privacy for medical decision support systems. In L. Imoize, J. Hemanth, D.-T. Do, and S. N. Sur (Eds.), *Explainable Artificial Intelligence in Medical Decision Support Systems* (pp. 401–433). Institution of Engineering and Technology. https://doi.org/10.1049/PBHE050E_ch15.

[38] Rufai, A. T., Dukor, K. F., Ageh, O. M., and Imoize, A. L. (2022). XAI robot-assisted surgeries in future medical decision support systems. In L. Imoize, J. Hemanth, D.-T. Do, and S. N. Sur (Eds.), *Explainable Artificial Intelligence in Medical Decision Support Systems* (pp. 167–195). Institution of Engineering and Technology. https://doi.org/10.1049/PBHE050E_ch6

[39] Wisdom, D. D., Isaac, S., Ahmed, M. A., Farouk, N., Magami, S., and Elijah, Y. (2020). An improved battery-life power saving scheme (IBPSS) in IEEE 802.16e Networks. *International Journal of Information Processing and Communication (IJIPC)*, 8(2).

[40] Ayoade, O. B., Oladele T. O., Imoize A. L., *et al.* (2022). Explainable artificial intelligence (XAI) in medical decision systems (MDSSs): healthcare systems perspective. In L. Imoize, J. Hemanth, D.-T. Do, and S. N. Sur (Eds.), *Explainable Artificial Intelligence in Medical Decision Support Systems* (pp. 1–43). Institution of Engineering and Technology. https://doi.org/10.1049/PBHE050E_ch1

[41] Kumar, R. L., Wang, Y., Poongodi, T., and Imoize, A. L. (2021). *Internet of Things, Artificial Intelligence and Blockchain Technology*. Cham: Springer International Publishing. https://doi.org/10.1007/978-3-030-74150-1.

[42] Abikoye, O. C., Oladipupo, E. T., Imoize, A. L., Awotunde, J. B., Lee, C.-C., and Li, C.-T. (2023). Securing critical user information over the internet of medical things platforms using a hybrid cryptography scheme. *Future Internet*, 15(3), 99. https://doi.org/10.3390/fi15030099.

[43] Wisdom, D. D., Farouk, N., Ahmed, M. A., Isaac, S., Idris, H., and Hassan, J. B. (2020). An enhanced power saving scheme (EPSS) in IEEE 802.16e Networks. *International Journal of Information Processing and Communication (IJIPC)*, 8(2).

[44] Oyebiyi, O. G., Abayomi-Alli, A., Arogundade, O. 'T., Qazi, A., Imoize, A. L., and Awotunde, J. B. (2023). A systematic literature review on human ear biometrics: approaches, algorithms, and trend in the last decade. *Information*, 14(3), 192. https://doi.org/10.3390/info14030192.

[45] Kavitha, K. V. N., Sharmila A., Imoize A. L., *et al.* (2022). On the use of wavelet domain and machine learning for the analysis of epileptic seizure detection from EEG signals. *Journal of Healthcare Engineering*, 2022, 1–16. https://doi.org/10.1155/2022/8928021

Chapter 14

Government regulatory policies on telehealth data protection using artificial intelligence and blockchain technology

Abubakar Aliyu[1], *Emeka Ogbuju*[1,2], *Taiwo Kolajo*[1], *Ihinkalu Olalekan*[1] *and Francisca Oladipo*[3]

Patients, healthcare providers, and healthcare systems can benefit from telehealth, a fast-growing field of medicine. Although telehealth services are becoming increasingly popular, patient data security and privacy issues present significant difficulties. Blockchain and artificial intelligence (AI) technology development opens up new possibilities for improving telehealth data privacy and addressing these issues. This chapter investigates how blockchain and AI technology could be used to strengthen regulatory frameworks for telehealth data protection. By utilizing AI algorithms, security vulnerabilities in telehealth systems can be identified and mitigated. For example, abnormal data access patterns or potential phishing attempts can be detected. AI can detect and respond to threats in real-time by continuously monitoring telehealth platforms, which lowers the chance of data breaches and illegal access, and using blockchain technology to establish secure, decentralized data storage and sharing, and telehealth providers can ensure patient confidentiality while improving the efficiency and accessibility of healthcare services. The chapter also reviews current telehealth regulatory frameworks that can foster innovation and ensure patient safety in the rapidly changing telehealth landscape.

14.1 Introduction

The integration of blockchain and artificial intelligence (AI) technology has significantly advanced telehealth, a fast-developing area of healthcare. These developments could fundamentally alter how healthcare data is protected, assuring

[1]Department of Computer Science, Faculty of Science, Federal University Lokoja, Nigeria
[2]Department of Computer Science, School of Computing, Miva Open University, Nigeria
[3]Department of Computer Science, Faculty of Computing and Applied Science, Thomas Adewumi University, Nigeria

confidentiality, safety, and adherence to legal requirements [1]. This chapter analyses how blockchain and AI can be used to augment existing regulations governing the safeguarding of telehealth data. The delivery of healthcare services remotely while enabling patients and healthcare practitioners to communicate through digital communication channels is referred to as telehealth, which includes telemedicine and telehealthcare. Protecting patient data has become a top priority as telemedicine usage increases. Global regulatory authorities have set guidelines to control the protection of telehealth data because they understand how important it is to do so [2]. Regulations are essential for maintaining telehealth data's integrity, confidentiality, and privacy. Although they differ depending on the country, these policies often cover data protection, patient consent, security requirements, data retention, and breach reporting. Compliance with these principles is crucial to promote trust, uphold patient privacy, and reduce the risks linked with the digital transmission of sensitive healthcare information [3]. AI technology offers powerful tools for enhancing telehealth data protection. Data encryption, anonymization, and de-identification can be facilitated by AI algorithms, protecting patient privacy. Additionally, telehealth system security measures are strengthened by AI-powered anomaly detection, which can spot potential security breaches or unauthorized access attempts [4]. Blockchain offers a solid platform for increasing telemedicine data privacy since it is a decentralized, immutable ledger. Telehealth systems can provide secure data storage, traceability, and transparency. Blockchain's decentralized structure reduces the dangers associated with centralized data repositories, while its cryptographic algorithms guarantee data integrity. By facilitating consent management, data access control, and compliance enforcement, smart contracts on the blockchain can strengthen regulatory rules [5]. The application of blockchain and AI in telehealth systems has enormous promise. AI may examine enormous amounts of telehealth data to find patterns, spot anomalies, and improve data security protocols [6]. In turn, blockchain offers a transparent and safe framework for managing, storing, and exchanging the data. The symbiotic relationship between AI and blockchain strengthens regulatory frameworks by promoting strong data security frameworks, safeguarding patient privacy, and enhancing general healthcare outcomes [7].

14.1.1 Key contributions of the chapter

The following are the chapter's main contributions:

1. The convergence of telemedicine, AI, blockchain technology, and regulatory policies are explored in this chapter's thorough analysis of the body of previous research on the subject.
2. The chapter emphasizes the difficulties and dangers related to telehealth data protection. It explores the risks associated with applying AI and blockchain technologies, including cybersecurity dangers, privacy issues, and ethical issues.
3. The chapter explores the standards and regulatory frameworks currently in place that are pertinent to protecting telehealth data. It examines the legal environment in numerous nations, including the United States, the European

Union, Singapore, and China. This gives readers an understanding of how various legal systems approach the regulatory issues around AI and blockchain in telehealth.

4. The chapter addresses how blockchain and AI might help reduce the risks associated with data protection. It looks at how AI algorithms are used for data encryption, access management, and cybersecurity threat detection. Additionally, it looks into the usage of smart contracts for data sharing and consent control and other possible uses for blockchain technology.
5. The chapter offers a list of recommendations for telehealth data protection policy development based on the findings and observations. These suggestions cover topics like thorough rules, openness and explainability of AI systems, bolstering data protection standards, encouraging moral AI use, interoperability standards, encouraging cooperation, and ongoing regulation monitoring.

14.1.2 Chapter organization

Section 14.2 of this chapter thoroughly investigates telehealth data security and privacy. It starts with a thorough examination of the relevant literature, looking at previously published studies and academic papers. Section 14.3 describes the methodology used throughout the chapter. Section 14.4 covered data protection in detail, along with the difficulties and dangers that may arise and how crucial it is to maintain security and privacy. Section 14.5 highlights the significance of AI integration in telehealth systems and how it might be used to strengthen telehealth data protection procedures. Section 14.6 discusses how blockchain technology can be used for safeguarding patient data, data transmission, and data storage. Section 14.7 discusses the regulatory policies for telehealth data protection. Section 14.8 of this chapter examines the legal and regulatory frameworks governing the protection of telehealth data, highlighting commonalities and distinctions between various nations. Section 14.9 outlines the major lessons learned. Section 14.10 concludes the chapter and suggests further research actions. Section 14.11 finishes the chapter with actionable suggestions for enhancing telehealth data protection, considering policy concerns, technology improvements, and best practices for healthcare providers and stakeholders in the telehealth ecosystem. These suggestions are based on the findings and analyses.

14.2 Related work

In recent years, telehealth, the use of technology to provide healthcare remotely, has become increasingly popular. It provides several advantages, including increased patient convenience, cheaper healthcare, and easier access to services. But the growing popularity of telehealth also prompts concerns about how to safeguard private patient information.

1. Privacy and security risks in telehealth
   Sensitive medical data and patient identifiers are among the types of personal health information that are transmitted, stored, and processed as part of

telehealth. The potential of unwanted access, data breaches, and privacy violations rises due to this data's digitization and distant exchange [8].

2. Regulatory requirements
   Health Insurance Portability and Accountability Act (HIPAA) in the United States and the General Data Protection Regulation (GDPR) in the European Union (EU) are two examples of the strict regulations that apply to healthcare data. To guarantee patient data security, privacy, and confidentiality, telehealth providers must abide by these rules [9].

Maintaining patient trust, protecting privacy rights, and minimizing potential consequences related to data breaches and unauthorized access depend on adequate data protection in telehealth. The following points help explain the importance of telehealth data protection.

1. Patient confidentiality
   The communication of private medical data between patients and healthcare professionals is essential to telehealth. Maintaining patient confidentiality is essential to upholding ethical standards, preserving the doctor-patient relationship, and encouraging people to seek care remotely [10].
2. Data integrity and accuracy
   Making informed clinical decisions requires access to reliable and accurate health data. In order to avoid unauthorized changes, data tampering, or falsification that can result in inaccurate diagnoses or treatments, it is essential to ensure data integrity in telehealth [11].
3. Trust and adoption
   For telehealth services to be used and successful, patient trust is essential. Patients are given trust by effective data protection measures, such as strict security rules and privacy safeguards, and are more likely to accept telehealth as a dependable method of receiving treatment [12].
4. Legal and ethical obligations
   Healthcare organizations are required by law and morality to secure patient information. Inadequate data protection procedures may have legal ramifications, harm one's reputation, and undermine public trust [13].

Using AI and blockchain technology to protect telehealth data, different jurisdictions may have distinct regulatory policies. However, several broad concepts and guidelines are frequently used to ensure data security in telehealth systems using AI and blockchain. These guidelines are outlined and briefly described in Table 14.1.

In order to promote trust, safeguard patient rights, and guarantee the seamless delivery of telehealth services, regulatory laws for telehealth data protection are essential. The integration of AI and blockchain technology presents unprecedented opportunities to strengthen these regulations by boosting security, privacy, transparency, and accountability. By embracing these cutting-edge technologies, healthcare organizations can create a solid framework that safeguards patient information, meets legal requirements, and encourages the wider use of telehealth services, ultimately leading to better patient outcomes globally.

Table 14.1 Guidelines used to ensure data security in telehealth systems using AI and blockchain technology

Reference	Guideline	Description
[14]	*General regulations for data protection*	There are laws governing data protection in several nations, such as the California Consumer Privacy Act (CCPA) in the United States or the General Data Protection Regulation (GDPR) of the European Union. These laws establish standards for the gathering, storing, and handling of personal data, including health data. These rules must be followed while managing patient data by telehealth systems.
[6]	*Informed consent*	Before any data is gathered, retained, or shared about patients, their informed consent must be obtained. According to telehealth systems, patients should be properly informed about the goal, scope, and potential hazards associated with the use of AI and blockchain in data processing. Patients should have the freedom to revoke their agreement at any moment, and the consenting procedure should be open and clear.
[15]	*De-identification and anonymization*	Telehealth systems can use AI and blockchain technologies to anonymize or de-identify patient data to protect privacy. Anonymization involves removing identifying information from the data, while de-identification involves replacing identifying information with pseudonyms. These techniques help minimize the risk of re-identification and ensure patient confidentiality.
[16]	*Data reduction and purpose restriction*	Telehealth systems should collect and retain only the necessary data for the intended purpose. Implementing data minimization and purpose limitation principles helps reduce the risk of unauthorized access or use of sensitive patient information.
[17]	*Security Protocols*	To protect telemedicine data, strong security measures are necessary. To protect data transmission, storage, and access, encryption should be used. Access restrictions, authentication procedures, and audit trails should be put in place to guarantee that only authorized users can access the data. To discover and remedy any gaps, it is advised to conduct regular security audits and vulnerability assessments.
[18]	*Recognizing healthcare regulations*	Telehealth systems must also abide by national and international healthcare laws, such as the Personal Data Protection Act (PDPA) in Singapore and the Health Insurance Portability and Accountability Act (HIPAA) in the United States. Additional standards for handling patient data are outlined in these regulations, including security precautions, breach reporting procedures, and patient rights.

(Continues)

Table 14.1 (Continued)

Reference	Guideline	Description
[19]	*Ownership and control of data*	Telehealth systems should specify data ownership and control procedures in detail. Patients should be able to view, alter, and remove their personal health information as permitted by laws. The system should also outline the terms under which, with whom, and how data is exchanged.
[20]	*Governance and accountability in transparency*	Blockchain and AI enabled telehealth systems should set up open governance processes to ensure responsibility for data management and processing. To deal with any breaches or unauthorized access to patient data, clear protocols and processes should be in place. System providers should be responsible for ensuring regulatory compliance and openness regarding their data protection procedures.
[21]	*Data retention and disposal*	Systems for telehealth should provide explicit guidelines for data retention and deletion. Only the amount of time required by applicable rules should be used to maintain patient data. Data should be securely removed once it is no longer required to reduce the danger of illegal access or use.
[22]	*Ethical-related considerations*	Blockchain and AI utilized in telehealth should abide by moral standards. Fairness, accountability, and openness in AI systems should be prioritized to prevent biases or discrimination. Blockchain technology implementations should consider the energy and environmental costs of mining and validating transactions.
[23]	*International data transfers*	Compliance with international data transfer laws should be enforced if telehealth systems entail the transfer of data across international boundaries. To ensure the privacy and security of the transferred data, adequate protections should be put in place, such as data transfer agreements or procedures like Standard Contractual Clauses or Privacy Shield (where applicable).
[24]	*Monitoring and auditing on a continuous basis*	To find and address any potential vulnerabilities, breaches, or non-compliance with data protection rules, telehealth systems should be regularly monitored and audited. This enables prompt rectification of any discovered flaws and assures continuing adherence to privacy and security requirements.

An investigation of this issue provides an in-depth examination of security and privacy risks in telehealth systems. In addition to discussing the application of AI and blockchain technology for telehealth data protection, the research analyses the regulatory obstacles and the role of policies in addressing these issues [25]. In another perspective, a report by [26], the current state of privacy and security in telehealth. It addresses the legal frameworks and laws in place to safeguard telehealth data and the potential contribution of cutting-edge technology like blockchain and AI. Another initiative aims to leverage blockchain technology to improve access control and privacy in electronic health records. It talks about the possibilities of blockchain-based frameworks for telehealth data protection and guaranteeing regulatory compliance. These studies offer insightful information on the laws, problems, and technological advancements relating to safeguarding telehealth data employing blockchain and AI technologies [5].

A research work [27] examines how telemedicine, AI, and privacy connect. It investigates the privacy-preserving strategies and legislative barriers for AI-driven telehealth systems, emphasizing the significance of regulations for safeguarding patient data. Islam *et al.* [28] concentrate on the usage of blockchain technology in healthcare. The study examines how blockchain technology might protect telehealth data, including regulatory compliance and secure data exchange. Fernández-Alemán *et al.* [29] compare the various regulatory strategies used for telemedicine services. The study looks at the regulatory frameworks in place across the world and considers the consequences for telehealth data protection, including the use of blockchain and AI. The research work by [30] emphasizes eHealth systems' data privacy and security. The work examines the legal considerations, difficulties, and potential remedies for telehealth data protection, including the application of AI and blockchain technologies.

Zhang *et al.* [31] evaluate how blockchain technology is being used in electronic health records (EHRs). It talks about the possible advantages, difficulties, and legal ramifications of implementing blockchain for safe EHR management in telehealth networks. This chapter explores a number of legislative policies, privacy, security, and technological solutions connected to protecting telehealth data using blockchain and AI technology. Khan *et al.* [32] discuss the issues and methods for telehealth systems' AI-powered privacy protection. It examines the regulatory issues and emphasizes the necessity of strong regulations governing the use of AI to protect patient privacy. ElHassan *et al.* [33] examine how well-regulated telemedicine platforms for remote diagnostics are. It analyses the difficulties with compliance and looks at how regulatory rules, including the use of AI and blockchain technology, might ensure data safety. Yao *et al.* [34] propose a blockchain-based platform for privacy-aware telehealthcare apps. The work examines the legal requirements for safeguarding patient privacy and data security, putting special emphasis on how blockchain technology may improve telehealth data security.

According to [35], explores utilizing blockchain to share medical data in telemedicine applications securely. It looks at the difficulties with regulations and the possibility of blockchain technology to secure patient privacy and data in telehealth services. The research offers more details on the legal considerations, difficulties, and technological solutions pertaining to the protection of telehealth data using blockchain and AI technologies. In another research work by [36], the work investigates the telemedicine system integration of AI with blockchain technology during COVID-19. The potential of AI technology to improve telehealth data protection and privacy in accordance with regulatory standards is examined, along with the regulatory challenges that already exist [37], the work highlights blockchain technology's application in healthcare. It talks about the prospective uses of blockchain in telehealth data protection, including safe data sharing, patient consent management, and adherence to privacy laws. It also analyses the regulatory ramifications of these uses. Khan *et al.* [38] focus on telehealth's usage of AI. It looks at the legal issues and analyses how AI could improve telehealth systems' data security, privacy, and protection.

A policy-based approach was established by Edmunds *et al.*, [39] to integrate telehealth's clinical, operational, and legal components. Live video conferencing, remote monitoring, help with safe electronic transfer of X-rays, CT scans, and digital images, together with regulatory agencies, quality standards, privacy protection, and payment models, are a few of the significant topics covered. However, these frameworks provide very little functionality and neglect to address significant issues like privacy, security, and trust in all ICT-based systems. In order to address these issues, Yaqoob *et al.* [40] focus on integrating blockchain with healthcare systems. The authors discuss a blockchain-based payment platform, clinical trials, patient data, health insurance, and drug traceability.

MyPCR, the first-ever comprehensive personal care record platform powered by blockchain, was presented by Guardtime and its business partners. MyPCR is a blockchain-based governance system for health data. They assert that up to 30 million NHS patients have smartphone access to the platform. The platform offers irrefutable evidence of the provenance and integrity of health data in line with the GDPR data rights management [41]. The developers interpreted it as a "bulletin board" for health services. A decentralized platform called Medicalchain [42] allows for the safe, quick, and transparent sharing and use of medical data. A marketplace for health data is offered with a doctor-to-patient telemedicine service on the platform. A patient can consult a doctor remotely via the telemedicine programme while maintaining control over their data. Through the use of telecommunications technologies, in order to facilitate direct communication between a patient and professionals, HealPoint.io [43] provides telehealth services. With any internet-enabled device, this platform enables patients to simultaneously visit a number of experts to get a second opinion on their diagnosis. Blockchain-based AI algorithms estimate the likelihood of a diagnosis and link the patient with appropriate medical professionals in the selected nation. Even though these platforms support virtual consultations, only MedX can guarantee the credibility of the doctors there.

14.3 Methodology

In this chapter, a combination of a literature review and a policy analysis was employed as the study methodology, as clearly depicted in Figure 14.1. We thoroughly analyse the body of research on blockchain, regulatory issues, AI, and telemedicine. Find pertinent research findings, scholarly writings, business reports, and policy documents that touch on the junction of these issues. We examine the present legislative frameworks and policies pertaining to telehealth data protection,

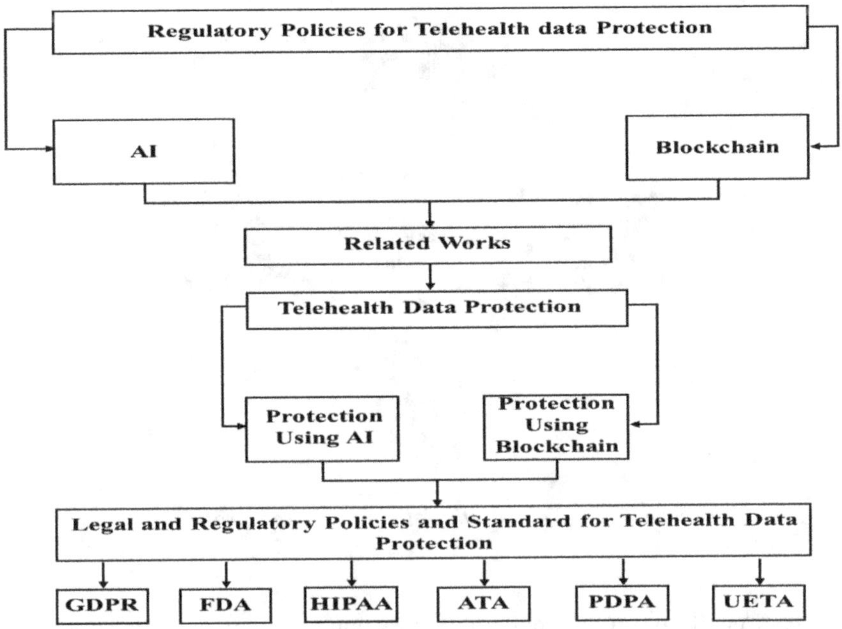

Figure 14.1 Study methodology flow

AI, and blockchain technology to thoroughly understand the state of knowledge in this sector. We also analyse the literature's findings, methodologies, and significant insights. We conduct a comparative analysis of the regulatory frameworks and policies across different countries and compare how different jurisdictions address telehealth data protection, AI, and blockchain in their legal and regulatory frameworks in order to identify the specific policies, laws, and guidelines that govern data protection, privacy, security, and ethical considerations in telehealth. Based on the literature study and policy analysis, we create a set of recommendations for regulatory policies in telehealth data protection using blockchain and AI. By using this methodology, the chapter can present a comprehensive review of the current legal landscape, pinpoint areas for improvement, and make helpful recommendations for improving telehealth data protection in the context of AI and blockchain.

14.4 Telehealth data protection

The processes and policies implemented to guarantee patient data confidentiality, security, and integrity in telehealth services are referred to as telehealth data protection, as depicted in Figure 14.2. Given the sensitivity of healthcare information, safeguarding patient data is crucial for upholding patient confidence, adhering to legal requirements, and reducing the likelihood of data breaches and unauthorized access.

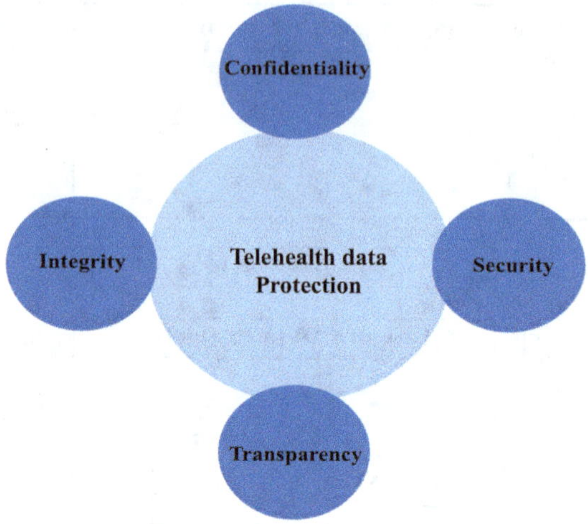

Figure 14.2 Telehealth policies for data protection

It is crucial to protect patient data when using telehealth services for numerous reasons. First and foremost, it ensures that patients' privacy, confidentiality, and trust in the healthcare system are protected [44]. During telehealth contacts, patients must feel confident that their private health information will be handled safely and kept private. This trust is essential for preserving the doctor–patient relationship and promoting distant care for patients. Second, protecting patient data is crucial for telehealth services to adhere to legal specifications such as the United States HIPAA [59]. HIPAA establishes requirements for security and privacy in the healthcare industry and regulates the protection of patient health information. These rules must be followed by telehealth providers in order to guarantee the privacy, accuracy, and accessibility of patient data. Safeguarding patient information in telehealth services reduces the dangers of data breaches and illegal access. The possible vulnerabilities that bad actors could exploit are increased by the digitalization and remote transfer of patient information [45]. It is crucial to implement strong security measures to protect patient data from misuse and unauthorized disclosure. Furthermore, preserving the security and authenticity of patient data is essential for providing top-notch care. Correct health information is crucial for clinical decision-making in telehealth [20]. To guarantee that healthcare practitioners have access to accurate and trustworthy information during telehealth consultations, it is crucial to safeguard patient data from tampering or unauthorized adjustments [46]. Protecting patient data in telehealth services is essential for upholding patient confidence, adhering to legal obligations, reducing the risk of data breaches, and guaranteeing the accuracy and integrity of medical records [20]. Some key challenges and risks associated with data protection in telehealth are outlined and described in Table 14.2.

Table 14.2 Challenges and risks associated with data protection in telehealth

References	Challenge	Description
[47]	*Data breaches*	Data breaches can leave telehealth systems open to illegal access, disclosure, or theft of patient data. These hacks may be the result of telehealth platform's security flaws or the interception of data in transit.
[21]	*Cybersecurity threats*	Cybersecurity threats to telehealth services include ransomware, phishing, malware, and distributed denial-of-service (DDoS) attacks. These dangers could jeopardize patient privacy and confidence by jeopardizing patient data's availability, confidentiality, and integrity.
[20]	*Authentication and authorization are inadequate*	Unauthorized access to patient data may result from insufficient authentication and authorization mechanisms. Telehealth systems may be more vulnerable to unauthorized usage or data breaches if their passwords are weak if they do not use multi-factor authentication.
[48]	*Compliance with the law and regulations*	Telehealth providers face difficulties adhering to data privacy laws, including GDPR and HIPAA. Careful installation and ongoing compliance are required to satisfy the criteria for patient consent, data storage, and privacy rights in a telehealth scenario.
[49]	*Data interoperability*	The sharing of patient data between various platforms and systems in telehealth might hamper data interoperability and standardization. Systems and data format inconsistencies increase the risk of data loss or corruption, making it more difficult to securely share data.
[46]	*Human errors and training*	In telehealth contexts, human errors, such as unintentional patient data exposure or incorrect handling, might happen. These dangers may be exacerbated by healthcare personnel who have insufficient training or awareness of data protection procedures.
[50]	*Telehealth device security*	Devices used for telehealth, like smartphones, tablets, and wearable technology, must be secure. These gadgets might be more prone to theft, loss, or unauthorized access, which might expose patient data.

14.5 Protection of telehealth data using AI

AI significantly improves telehealth data protection in several ways. The identification of unexpected patterns or behaviours in patient data that can point to security breaches or illegal access is one important use of AI-powered anomaly detection. AI systems can identify and notify healthcare professionals of potential hazards or suspicious activity by analysing enormous volumes of data and learning from trends, enabling proactive interventions to reduce risks [51]. Intelligent data encryption and access control systems are also made possible by AI. Patient data is protected from illegal disclosure or modification with the aid of cutting-edge encryption techniques and AI-driven access control systems. AI algorithms can improve encryption methods, maintaining strong data security while enabling authorized individuals to access the data as needed [52]. Furthermore, automated monitoring and analysis of telehealth interactions is made possible by AI-powered natural language processing (NLP) approaches. Real-time text or speech data analysis by NLP algorithms can assist spot any potential lapses in patient confidentiality or the improper disclosure of sensitive information. This proactive monitoring improves data protection by assuring compliance with privacy laws and upholding patient confidence [53]. AI-based machine learning models also aid in the development of predictive analytics for risk assessment and preventive security measures. By examining historical data, AI algorithms can find patterns and trends linked to data breaches or security flaws. This makes it possible for healthcare institutions to put in place focused security measures, spend resources efficiently, and reduce any possible dangers to patient data [21].

According to Rajkomar *et al.* [54], AI technology can also help anonymize and de-identify patient data, protecting privacy while enabling secondary analysis for research and population health management objectives. By automatically removing or encrypting personally identifiable information, AI algorithms can lower the risk of re-identification while maintaining the data's usefulness. AI plays a significant role in telehealth data protection by providing anomaly detection, intelligent encryption, access control, real-time monitoring, risk assessment, and anonymization approaches. In telehealth contexts, these AI-driven methods improve patient data's security, privacy, and integrity.

14.5.1 Role of AI in identifying and mitigating cybersecurity threats

AI plays a significant part in recognizing and mitigating cybersecurity threats by utilizing cutting-edge algorithms and machine learning approaches. AI makes it possible to actively identify threats, act quickly, and continuously monitor systems and networks to improve their security posture. In order to find trends and abnormalities that might point to cybersecurity risks, AI-powered threat detection systems examine a tremendous quantity of data, including network traffic, system logs, and user activity. These systems use machine learning techniques to recognize well-known attack patterns by learning from past data. AI algorithms may swiftly identify deviations from expected patterns by continually studying network traffic and system activity, enabling the early detection of cyberthreats [50]. AI makes it possible for cybersecurity operations to be automated, which cuts down on the time and effort needed to respond to threats. AI systems can independently analyse and classify security alerts, prioritize incidents according to their seriousness, and offer instantaneous incident response advice. As a result, security teams can work more efficiently and react to threats more quickly [53].

According to [49], AI also makes creating predictive analytics models for evaluating cybersecurity risk easier. AI systems can forecast possible weaknesses, attack methods, or new dangers by examining past data and seeing trends. Organizations are able to devote resources to regions that are most likely to be attacked and take proactive security measures thanks to these predictive capabilities. AI-driven threat detection technologies collect and examine vast amounts of data from a variety of sources, such as social media, dark web surveillance, and security feeds. This improves an organization's ability to recognize and respond to new hazards by keeping them current on the most recent cybersecurity threats and trends [50]. By enabling proactive threat detection, automation of security procedures, predictive analytics, and extensive threat intelligence analysis, AI plays a crucial role in identifying and mitigating cybersecurity threats.

14.5.2 Use of AI-powered tools for real-time monitoring and detection of data breaches

AI-powered technologies are being used more and more to monitor and detect data breaches in real-time, allowing enterprises to quickly recognize and address security concerns. These technologies examine network traffic, system logs, and user behaviour using cutting-edge algorithms and machine learning approaches, improving the effectiveness and efficiency of data breach detection.

The use of anomaly detection algorithms is a significant use of AI in the detection of data breaches. AI algorithms can provide a baseline of typical network and system behaviour by learning patterns from past data. Any departures from this norm may be detected as potential anomalies, signalling a possible security incident or data breach [55]. Tools with AI capabilities can also identify suspicious behaviour and potential signs of data breaches by using behaviour-based analytics. AI algorithms can spot unusual or unauthorized acts that may point to a data breach by tracking user behaviour, such as access patterns, file transfers, or data requests. Instantaneous identification and action are made possible through real-time monitoring and analysis. AI systems can continuously learn from new threat vectors and develop attack strategies thanks to machine learning algorithms. These algorithms are able to examine massive amounts of data and spot trends or signs of data breaches that were previously undetected. The AI models' performance in identifying and categorizing data breach instances can be improved as they learn from new data [52]. Natural language processing (NLP) techniques are also used by AI-powered technologies to evaluate textual data, such as system logs, incident reports, or user conversations, in order to find signs of data breaches. The use of NLP algorithms by AI technologies can help security teams prioritize and analyse potential events by identifying keywords or linguistic patterns that could indicate the presence of a data breach [51]. Anomaly detection, behaviour-based analytics, machine learning, and NLP approaches are used by AI-powered systems for real-time monitoring and detection of data breaches to quickly identify and respond to security problems, enhancing the overall cybersecurity posture of businesses [56].

14.5.3 AI algorithms for data encryption and access control in telehealth systems

In telehealth systems, AI algorithms make data encryption and access control procedures possible. These algorithms use cutting-edge methods for encryption, authentication, and authorization to improve the security and privacy of patient data. AI algorithms facilitate the development of reliable encryption techniques to safeguard sensitive patient data. Machine learning techniques can be employed to optimize cryptographic algorithms and key management protocols to increase the effectiveness and efficiency of data encryption. AI algorithms can strengthen encryption techniques to fend off prospective assaults and maintain patient data security by analysing data trends and spotting flaws [55]. In telehealth systems, AI algorithms also support the access control measures that make sure that only authorized users can access patient data. AI systems can recognize legitimate access requests and potentially unwanted access attempts by using machine learning techniques to learn from past access patterns and user behaviour. By doing so, data breaches and illegal data disclosures are reduced [57].

The development of adaptive access control models, which dynamically modify access credentials in response to shifting contextual elements, is made possible by AI algorithms. AI algorithms, for instance, can choose the right amount of access for certain scenarios by looking at elements like user location, access time, and device attributes. This solution to adaptive access control aids in preserving data security while taking into account telehealth systems' dynamic nature [58]. AI algorithms can help with multi-factor authentication procedures by examining a variety of user behaviours and data points to verify the legitimacy of access requests. AI algorithms can improve the precision and dependability of access control methods by merging numerous authentication factors, such as biometrics, device information, and behaviour patterns [53]. By optimizing encryption techniques, enabling adaptive access control, and boosting multi-factor authentication procedures, AI algorithms significantly contribute to data encryption and access control in telehealth systems.

14.6 Protection of telehealth data with blockchain technology

The recommended technique for improving data privacy in telehealth systems is blockchain technology. Blockchain offers a number of advantages in preserving the integrity, confidentiality, and privacy of patient data due to its decentralized and tamper-resistant nature. The immutability and transparency of blockchain technology are two of its main benefits for telehealth data protection. The immutability of transactions and data entries on the blockchain prevents their modification or tampering without the agreement of network users. This function protects the confidentiality of patient information and renders it impervious to unauthorized changes [59]. Blockchain uses cryptographic methods to further improve data security. The confidentiality of patient data recorded on the blockchain is guaranteed by encryption and association with a special code or hash. Cryptographic keys can be used to enable access to patient data, allowing for the secure and regulated sharing of sensitive information [60]. Blockchain also makes it possible for telehealth systems to share data safely and audibly. Data sharing and access can be made easier through smart contracts, self-executing contracts with established rules inscribed on the blockchain. These agreements ensure that only authorized parties can access and distribute patient data by enforcing access control policies and enabling fine-grained permission management [61]. By giving patients access to their own data, blockchain can enhance the privacy of patient data. Patients can retain ownership and control over their private health information by using self-sovereign identity models and decentralized identity management systems, and they can give or revoke access as necessary [62].

Blockchain technology can also improve the data in telehealth systems' traceability and auditability. An auditable trail of data exchanges is made possible by the timestamped and connected nature of every transaction recorded on the blockchain. This function makes it possible to track the source of data, ensuring responsibility and openness in the processing of patient data [63]. With immutability, cryptographic security, secure data exchange, patient data control, and traceability, this technology gives telehealth systems strong data protection features.

14.6.1 The use of blockchain for secure and decentralized storage of telehealth data

Blockchain technology offers a safe and decentralized method of telehealth data storage, addressing issues with data accessibility, privacy, and integrity. Blockchain offers a novel way to store and manage private patient data as shown in Figure 14.3, by using its immutability, anonymity, auditability, transparency, and decentralized consensus features. These feature guaranty data protection and privacy in telehealth systems. Blockchain decentralized structure ensures that telehealth data is dispersed over a network of nodes rather than stored in a single central location. A copy of the complete blockchain, with a history of all transactions and data entries, is kept on file by each node. Because of this decentralization, there is no longer a single point of failure, which lowers the possibility of data loss or unwanted access [64]. Data integrity is also guaranteed by blockchain technology's immutability feature. Without the agreement of the network's users, data that has been stored on the blockchain cannot be changed or tampered with. A chain of blocks that is computationally secure and impermeable is formed by each new data entry being cryptographically linked to the one before it [65]. Blockchain offers improved security and privacy for the storing of telemedicine data. On the blockchain, patient data can be encrypted and stored to maintain privacy and guard against illegal access. Cryptographic keys can be used to restrict access to the data, enabling only legitimate people or organizations to access and view the data [60].

Data accountability is facilitated by the transparency and auditability of blockchain system. On the blockchain, each transaction and data entry is transparently and tamper-proofly timestamped and recorded. This improves confidence

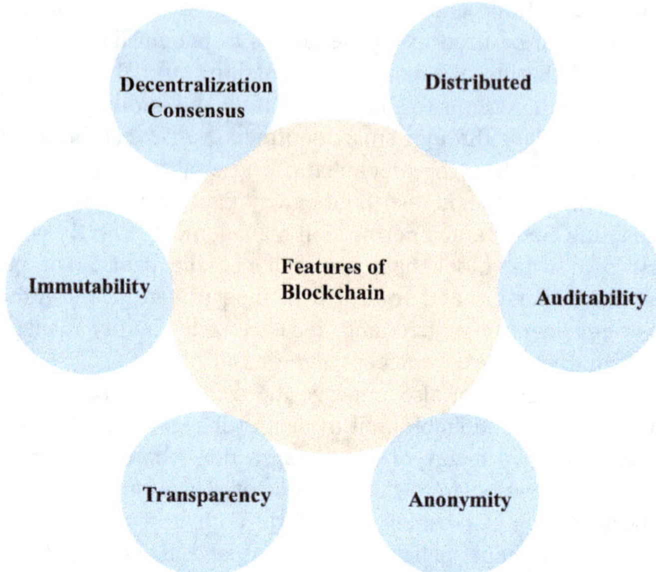

Figure 14.3 Features of blockchain that guaranty data protection and privacy in telehealth systems

and accountability by enabling healthcare providers, patients, and regulatory agencies to follow and confirm the history of data flows [64]. Smart contracts, which are self-executing contracts with established rules encoded on the blockchain, are made possible by blockchain technology. In order to ensure that data is safely saved and available depending on present conditions or permissions, smart contracts can automate the data storage and access processes. As a result, data storage and retrieval operations become more effective and rely less on manual intervention [60]. Blockchain offers benefits, including decentralized design, data integrity, privacy, security, transparency, and automation, through smart contracts when used for the secure and decentralized storage of telehealth data [24].

14.6.2 Blockchain-based smart contracts for data sharing and consent management

Smart contracts built on the blockchain in telehealth systems offer a secure, automated way to handle consent and data sharing. By serving as self-executing contracts with specified rules and conditions that are inscribed on the blockchain, smart contracts enable trusted and open communication between parties participating in data sharing. Smart contracts enforce predetermined rules and permissions to make data sharing easier. Smart contracts can be used to create access controls and the circumstances for data sharing when a patient's data is kept on the blockchain. According to Liang *et al.* [66], a smart contract could, for instance, stipulate that only approved healthcare practitioners are allowed to access data for a given reason and duration. By managing consent, smart contracts give patients authority over their own data. By digitally signing the smart contract, patients can express their clear authorization to share specified data with approved parties. Giving patients complete control over the scope and length of data sharing guarantees that patient data is shared in an open and accountable manner [67]. Through immutability and transparency, blockchain technology improves the security and dependability of data exchange and consent management. The agreed-upon guidelines for data sharing are preserved after a smart contract is deployed on the blockchain since they cannot be changed or interfered with after that point. All stakeholders can check and follow the execution of the smart contract thanks to the transparency of blockchain technology, which increases responsibility and confidence. Additionally, smart contracts based on blockchain can ease administrative constraints and facilitate automated operations. Self-executing smart contracts can automate data sharing and consent management, decreasing the need for manual intervention and middlemen, speeding the data sharing process, and lowering the likelihood of mistakes or disagreements [68]. For data sharing and consent management in telehealth systems, blockchain-based smart contracts offer advantages like automated access control enforcement, patient-centric consent management, increased security and trust through immutability and transparency, and streamlined procedures.

14.7 Regulatory policies for telehealth data protection

Regarding the privacy of patient data, telehealth services, which use technology to deliver healthcare remotely, create significant concerns. In the context of cutting-edge technology like blockchain and AI, protecting the security, privacy, and integrity of telehealth data requires regulations. Regulatory standards that address the moral use and responsible handling of patient data are necessary for AI-based telehealth technology. As an illustration, the GDPR of the European Union establishes stringent guidelines for the processing and protection of personal data, including data pertaining to healthcare. The GDPR highlights the values of transparency, purpose limitation, and minimal data collection, and it mandates that enterprises acquire explicit consent before processing data [9].

Regulatory policies may particularly address the usage of AI algorithms in telehealth in addition to GDPR. For instance, the United States Food and Drug Administration (FDA) has published recommendations for creating and verifying AI algorithms used in healthcare, highlighting the necessity for openness, comprehensibility, and continuous algorithm performance monitoring [69]. Blockchain technology requires legislative standards for telehealth data protection since it has the ability to improve data security and privacy. Although the legislative environment may differ between jurisdictions, general principles like data protection, consent management, and security still apply. For instance, the United States' HIPAA stipulates rules for the protection of patient health information, including clauses for electronic health records and data security [70]. The regulatory laws may address certain blockchain-related issues, including data integrity, access restrictions, and transparency. Businesses using blockchain in telehealth may have to abide by current laws while making sure that the technology does not threaten patient security and privacy. Regulatory policies should balance promoting innovation and protecting patient data to boost the adoption and application of blockchain and AI in telehealth. The development of trust among patients, healthcare professionals, and other stakeholders involved in telehealth services should be supported by these regulations, which should set forth clear criteria for the responsible use of AI algorithms and the secure implementation of blockchain technology.

14.7.1 Regulations and standards for telehealth data protection

Several sets of laws and standards that protect patient information and guarantee privacy and security apply to telehealth data protection. These regulations and standards provide guidelines and obligations for healthcare providers, technology vendors, and other stakeholders in telehealth services. The HIPAA, which establishes guidelines for the security of patient health information (PHI), is one of the most well-known laws in the United States. PHI handling, storing, and transfer are subject to the Privacy Rule and Security Rule under HIPAA [70]. The Security Rule specifies safeguards to secure the confidentiality, integrity, and availability of electronic PHI (ePHI), whereas the Privacy Rule regulates the use and disclosure of PHI [71]. Data privacy for telehealth services is significantly influenced by laws other than HIPAA, like the General Data Privacy Regulation (GDPR) in the EU. According to the [72], the GDPR establishes stringent guidelines for the processing, archiving, and transfer of personal data, including data pertaining to healthcare. The law sanctions fines for non-compliance and strongly emphasizes individual rights, permission, and data minimization [9].

International standards like ISO/IEC 27799 and ISO/IEC 27001 offer direction for the implementation of particular controls for healthcare organizations and information security management systems, respectively [73]. These guidelines include a range of data protection topics, including risk management, access controls, encryption, and incident response. Regulatory organizations and business associations might provide standards and suggestions for telehealth data protection. For instance, the American Telemedicine Association (ATA) offers recommendations on privacy and security issues for telehealth services [72]. The safety of patient data in telehealth services depends on compliance with these laws and standards, and vendors of technology and healthcare organizations alike must abide by them to ensure sensitive data's privacy and security [73].

14.7.2 Need for comprehensive and up-to-date policies to address emerging challenges

In order to protect patient data, the quickly changing telehealth environment brings new dangers and problems that call for thorough and current rules. Regulatory frameworks must change as technology develops and new data protection threats materialize to meet these changing issues. For instance, worries regarding data privacy, algorithm transparency, and bias reduction have been raised by the rising usage of AI algorithms and machine learning in telehealth. To ensure the moral and responsible use of AI in telehealth, comprehensive protocols are required, including rules for data anonymization, the explicability of algorithms, and continual monitoring to find and correct any biases [57]. Similar problems and legal implications arise when blockchain technology is incorporated into telemedicine. To ensure the secure and privacy-preserving usage of blockchain in telehealth systems, policies should cover topics including data integrity, encryption techniques, and access controls [20]. Strong cybersecurity standards are also required given the interconnection of telehealth systems and the rising reliance on linked devices and networks. Platforms for telehealth must be secured against unwanted access, data breaches, and online dangers. To reduce potential hazards, policies should include risk management, incident response strategies, and ongoing security measure monitoring [20]. Regulating authorities must continually examine and revise current regulations in order to successfully meet these new problems. As a result, regulatory frameworks are kept current with emerging threats and technological improvements. Additionally, cooperation among stakeholders is necessary to create complete regulations that strike a balance between innovation and data security, including healthcare providers, technology suppliers, lawmakers, and privacy activists [57].

Comprehensive and current policies are required to handle the new issues in telehealth data privacy. Regulatory frameworks can offer a strong foundation for guaranteeing patient data privacy, security, and integrity in telehealth systems by proactively addressing challenges connected to AI, blockchain, cybersecurity, and other developing technologies.

14.8 Legal and regulatory frameworks

The use, development, and deployment of particular technologies or activities inside a given jurisdiction are governed by a number of laws, regulations, and policies collectively referred to as the legal and regulatory framework. It offers a well-organized framework outlining the rights, duties, and commitments of people, groups, and governing entities. Using AI and blockchain technology to protect telehealth data, different jurisdictions may have distinct regulatory policies. However, some broad ideas and guidelines that are frequently used to guarantee data privacy in telehealth systems utilizing blockchain and AI are as are outlined and described in Table 14.3.

The legal and regulatory frameworks around AI and blockchain technology differ from one country to another, so it's necessary to be aware of this fact. To find out the precise legal and regulatory requirements in a particular jurisdiction, it's advisable to consult official government sources and legal experts.

14.8.1 Legal and regulatory frameworks in some selected countries

This section briefly discusses the legal and regulatory frameworks in some countries.

Table 14.3 Guidelines used to guarantee data privacy in telehealth systems utilizing blockchain and AI

Reference	Guideline	Description
[13]	*General Data Protection Regulation (GDPR)*	The European Union (EU) has a comprehensive data protection law known as the GDPR that addresses the handling and safeguarding of personal data. It creates standards, legal protections, and responsibilities for businesses using AI and blockchain technology to handle personal data.
[74]	*Health Insurance Portability and Accountability Act (HIPAA)*	Protected health information (PHI) privacy and security are governed by HIPAA, a United States federal law. It establishes guidelines for how healthcare providers, health plans, and other organizations – including telehealth services – use and disclose PHI.
[75]	*Personal Data Protection Act (PDPA)*	Singapore's PDPA data protection law regulates the gathering, use, and disclosure of personal data. It outlines data protection obligations and is applicable to AI and blockchain systems processing personal data in Singapore.
[9]	*Digital Economy Act 2017*	The United Kingdom's Digital Economy Act covers a variety of topics linked to the digital economy, including measures for cybersecurity, electronic communications, and data protection. It offers a regulatory framework for the application of blockchain and artificial intelligence (AI) in several industries
[76]	*Law on Personal Data (Russia)*	The Personal Data Law governs the processing and protection of personal data in Russia. It outlines rules for data protection and is applicable to AI and blockchain systems processing personal data.
[13]	*Emerging AI-specific regulations*	Several nations are thinking about or putting AI-specific laws into place. For instance, in an effort to control the creation, implementation, and utilization of AI systems within the EU, the European Commission proposed the Artificial Intelligence Act.

1. United States
   No explicit federal law in the United States fully regulates blockchain and AI. But different laws and rules cover particular topics. The Federal Trade Commission Act (FTC Act), which applies to AI, forbids unfair or misleading acts, including those connected to AI applications [77]. State laws governing blockchain technology have been passed in several states, including the Uniform Electronic Transactions Act (UETA) and the Uniform

Regulation of Virtual-Currency Businesses Act from the Uniform Law Commission [78].

2. European Union

   The EU has made tremendous advancements in data protection and AI regulation. Principles and standards for the processing of personal data, including AI systems, are established by the GDPR [12]. The Artificial Intelligence Act, which the European Commission has also suggested, proposes to control the deployment and usage of AI systems by concentrating on high-risk AI applications [13].
3. Singapore

   The Personal Data Protection Act (PDPA) in Singapore governs the gathering, use, and disclosure of personal information, including information processed by blockchain and AI systems [26]. Additionally, rules are provided by the Monetary Authority of Singapore (MAS) for applying blockchain technology in the financial sector, covering concerns such as technological risk management and client safety [79].
4. Russia

   Blockchain technology and AI are governed by several laws and rules in Russia. The Law on Personal Data governs the handling and protection of personal data, including information handled by blockchain and AI systems [76]. The Law on Digital Financial Assets also establishes rules for digital assets and provides a legal framework for using blockchain technology in financial transactions [80].
5. China

   China has put in place a number of laws and attempts to control blockchain and AI. The People's Republic of China's Cybersecurity Law for AI addresses issues with cybersecurity and the protection of private data [81]. A legal foundation for the development and regulation of blockchain technology in China is provided by the Law on the Promotion of the Development of the Blockchain Industry, which strongly emphasizes the protection of rights and interests as well as the avoidance of fraud and unlawful activity. The strategic development objectives for AI are described in China's National New Generation AI Development Plan, which addresses topics such as technical research, industry applications, talent cultivation, and ethical considerations [82].

14.9 Lessons learned

The chapter illuminated regulatory laws for telehealth data protection employing AI and blockchain technology. Several major conclusions may be drawn from the techniques used to investigate telehealth data protection, AI and blockchain technology, regulatory policies, and legal frameworks.

1. Data privacy in telehealth is clearly a difficult and complex issue. Telehealth technologies pose new problems and hazards that must be properly handled to protect patient data privacy, security, and integrity.

2. It is critical to put in place strong and comprehensive data protection safeguards. This involves using secure data transfer protocols, putting in place strong authentication and identity verification systems, and implementing encryption and access control mechanisms to safeguard sensitive data.
3. Regulatory policies are critical to the safeguarding of telehealth data. Existing legislation, including HIPAA in the United States and the GDPR in the European Union, must be followed to protect patient privacy and uphold legal and ethical standards. Furthermore, specific legislative frameworks adapted to the unique challenges of telehealth are required to address developing difficulties and give clear data protection standards.
4. Emerging technologies such as AI and blockchain hold great promise for improving telehealth data security. AI can help spot abnormalities and potential breaches, but blockchain can provide immutable and transparent records that ensure data integrity and traceability.

Finally, the lesson learned from this chapter is that data protection in telehealth necessitates a multifaceted approach. It entails putting in place strong technical safeguards, adhering to regulatory laws, and using emerging technology to manage risks and preserve patient data effectively. We can provide the confidence, privacy, and security required for the effective integration and expansion of telehealth services by prioritizing data protection in telehealth.

14.10 Recommendations

Stakeholder cooperation is essential to creating regulatory frameworks. In order to balance innovation and data protection, healthcare providers, technology suppliers, policymakers, and privacy activists should collaborate regarding laws governing the use of AI and blockchain technology to protect telehealth data; this chapter makes the following recommendations:

1. Develop comprehensive and harmonized regulations
   Governments and regulatory organizations should work together to create thorough, unified rules that are specially suited to telehealth data protection. The privacy, security, and integrity of patient data should be guaranteed by these regulations, which should also address the particular difficulties presented by blockchain and AI technology.
2. Enhance transparency and explainability
   AI algorithms utilized in telehealth should be transparent and comprehensible to foster confidence between patients and healthcare professionals. The development and use of AI systems that can clearly explain their decision-making processes should be encouraged by regulatory rules.
3. Strengthen data protection standards
   Strong data protection standards, like encryption, access controls, and safe storage techniques, should be emphasized by regulatory frameworks. To

ensure compliance and uniformity, these standards should be in line with recognized data protection legislation like GDPR, HIPAA, or PDPA.

4. Promote ethical use of AI
   Ethical principles for the application of AI in telehealth should be incorporated into regulatory policies. By addressing issues like algorithmic bias, data privacy, and informed permission, these principles should promote the appropriate and moral use of AI technologies.
5. Establish interoperability standards
   Regulatory policies should support creating and implementing interoperability standards to enable easy data exchange and interoperability between various telehealth systems. These guidelines should guarantee that healthcare professionals may exchange patient data securely and effectively while respecting patient privacy and security.
6. Encourage research and development
   Governments and funding organizations ought to promote blockchain and AI research and development for telehealth data security. This entails providing financing for research initiatives, encouraging collaboration between academia and industry, and encouraging innovation in the industry.
7. Foster collaboration and information sharing
   Regulatory agencies, healthcare providers, technology vendors, and other stakeholders should cooperate and share information to stay informed about new dangers, best practices, and technical breakthroughs. This partnership can promote a proactive strategy for tackling the problems associated with telehealth data privacy and assist build a shared awareness of those challenges.
8. Continuously monitor and update regulations
   Regulatory regulations should be continually reviewed, examined, and updated to maintain their relevance and efficacy, given the nature of technology's rapid evolution and the hazards associated with data protection. To help identify opportunities for improvement and adaptation, close communication with pertinent parties and continuing regulatory landscape assessment are recommended.

These recommendations are meant to encourage the safe and responsible application of blockchain and AI in telehealth while protecting patient information and upholding public confidence. By putting these suggestions into practice, we can create strong regulatory frameworks that encourage innovation, safeguard privacy, and guarantee the long-term survival of telehealth services. The suggestions made here are generic in nature and ought to be further customized and improved in light of certain regulatory environments and stakeholder considerations. Future work, as shown in Figure 14.4, should focus on the advancement of technical solutions, the exploration of the possibilities of emerging technologies, the refinement of regulatory frameworks, and the implementation of frequent assessments to ensure the continuous improvement of data protection in telehealth.

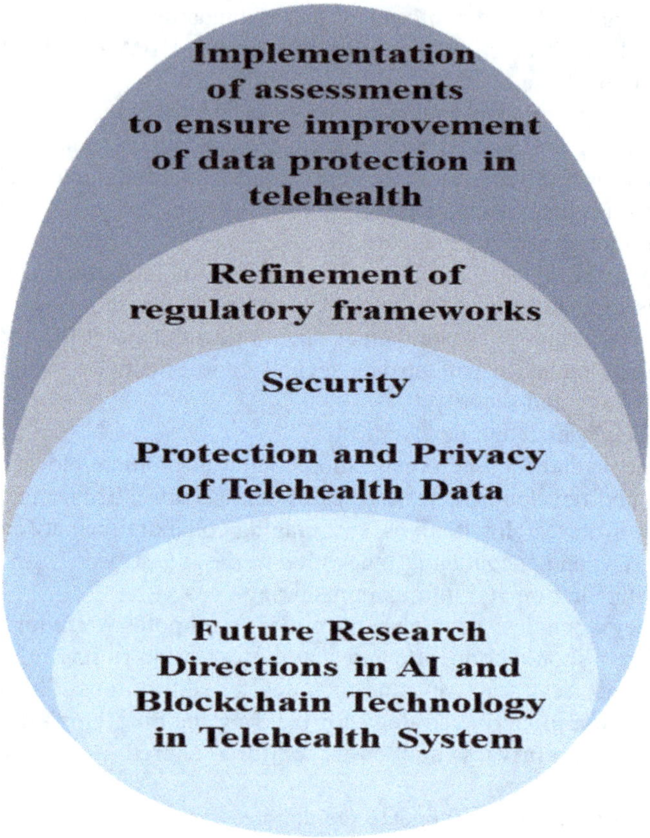

Figure 14.4 Future research directions

14.11 Conclusion

The regulatory frameworks for telehealth data protection employing AI and blockchain technologies have been covered in this chapter. The use of telehealth, fuelled by developments in blockchain and AI, can potentially transform the way that healthcare is provided completely. However, it also creates distinct challenges and concerns in terms of data security, privacy, and protection. It is crucial to safeguard patient information when using telehealth services. Maintaining trust and adhering to healthcare standards depend on the secrecy, integrity, and availability of sensitive patient information. The fusion of blockchain and AI technologies offers ground-breaking approaches to these problems as well as improved healthcare data security. AI is essential for telehealth system cybersecurity threat detection and mitigation. AI-powered technologies make real-time monitoring and breach detection possible, improving overall security posture. Data encryption and access control, which ensure that only authorized individuals may access and process critical medical information, are also made possible by AI algorithms. Blockchain technology offers a decentralized and secure method of storing telehealth data. Blockchain provides transparency, immutability, and auditability through its distributed ledger technology and cryptographic methods, lowering the possibility of data tampering and unauthorized access. Smart contracts built on blockchain technology allow for efficient and reliable data exchange and consent management, giving patients control over their data and enabling access to healthcare providers as needed. However, implementing AI and blockchain in telehealth necessitates thorough regulatory frameworks that keep up with emerging dangers and technical breakthroughs. Governments and regulatory agencies must create and revise legislation that handles the particular difficulties posed by AI and blockchain in safeguarding telehealth data. These rules should strongly emphasize data security, privacy protections, openness, and moral considerations. Our knowledge of telehealth data protection will continue to grow as a result of ongoing study, development, and information sharing, which will also encourage regulatory policies to be constantly improved. We can harness the transformational potential of telehealth while protecting patient data by adopting AI and blockchain technology and putting in place strict regulatory measures. The protection of telehealth data is essential for the future of healthcare delivery because it is not only morally and legally required.

References

[1] S. D. Patil and D. Toshniwal, "Secure blockchain framework for sharing electronic health records using attribute-based encryption," *J. Ambient Intell. Humaniz. Comput.,* vol. 11, no. 3, pp. 1451–1465, 2020.

[2] U. Yilmaz and S. A. Adams, "Telehealth privacy and security: Current landscape and future directions," *J. Am. Med. Inform. Assoc.*, vol. 27, no. 6, pp. 1066–1074, 2020.

[3] M. Görög and F. Sušilović-Đurević, "Regulatory approaches for telemedicine services: A comparative analysis," *Health Policy Technol.*, vol. 10, no. 1, pp. 76–85, 2021.

[4] H. Wu, N-K. Chan, C.J.P. Zhang, and W.-K. Ming. The role of the sharing economy and artificial intelligence in health care: Opportunities and challenges. *J. Med. Internet Res.,* vol. 21, pp. e13469, 2019.

[5] A. I. Newaz, A. K. Sikder, M. A. Rahman, and A. S. Uluagac, "A survey on security and privacy issues in modern healthcare systems: Attacks and defenses," *ACM Trans. Comput. Healthc.*, vol. 2, no. 3, pp. 1–44, 2021.

[6] L. F. Nakayama, L. Zago Ribeiro, F. Novaes, *et al.*, "Artificial intelligence for telemedicine diabetic retinopathy screening: A review," *Ann. Med.*, vol. 55, no. 2, p. 2258149, 2023.

[7] R. Dwivedi, D. Mehrotra, and S. Chandra, "Potential of Internet of Medical Things (IoMT) applications in building a smart healthcare system: A systematic review," *J. Oral Biol. Craniofac. Res.*, vol. 12, no. 2, pp. 302–318, 2022.

[8] A. N. Gohar, S. A. Abdelmawgoud, and M. S. Farhan, "A patient-centric healthcare framework reference architecture for better semantic interoperability based on blockchain, cloud, and IoT," *IEEE Access*, vol. 10, pp. 92137–92157, 2022.

[9] European Commission, "General Data Protection Regulation (GDPR)," [Online]. Available: https://ec.europa.eu/commission/priorities/justice-and-fundamental-rights/data-protection/2018-reform-eu-data-protection-rules_en.

[10] U.S. Department of Health & Human Services, "Health information privacy," [Online]. Available: https://www.hhs.gov/hipaa/index.html.

[11] European Commission, "General Data Protection Regulation (GDPR)," [Online]. Available: https://ec.europa.eu/commission/priorities/justice-and-fundamental-rights/data-protection/2020-reform-eu-data-protection-rules_en.

[12] European Commission, "General Data Protection Regulation (GDPR)," [Online]. Available: https://ec.europa.eu/commission/priorities/justice-and-fundamental-rights/data-protection/2019-reform-eu-data-protection-rules_en.

[13] European Commission, "Proposal for a Regulation on a European approach for Artificial Intelligence," [Online]. Available: https://ec.europa.eu/info/law/better-regulation/have-your-say/initiatives/12544-European-approach-to-artificial-intelligence, 2021.

[14] S. Agarwal and A. Lyles, "Regulatory compliance of telemedicine platforms for remote diagnosis," *Int. J. Healthcare Inf. Syst. Informatics.*, vol. 15, no. 2, pp. 1–15, 2020.

[15] M. A. Khan, N. Xiong, and J. Ma, "AI-powered privacy protection in telehealthcare systems: Challenges, approaches, and future directions," *IEEE. Trans. Serv. Comput.*, 2021, Early Access.

[16] D. M. El-Sherif, M. Abouzid, M. T. Elzarif, A. A. Ahmed, A. Albakri, and M. M. Alshehri, "Telehealth and Artificial Intelligence insights into healthcare during the COVID-19 pandemic," *Healthcare*, vol. 10, no. 2, p. 385, 2022.

[17] C. C. Agbo, Q. H. Mahmoud, and J. M. Eklund, "Blockchain technology in healthcare: A systematic review," *Healthcare.*, vol. 7, no. 2, pp. 56, 2019.

[18] United States Department of Health & Human Services. (n.d.), "HIPAA for Professionals," [Online]. Available: https://www.hhs.gov/hipaa/for-professionals/index.html

[19] Personal Data Protection Commission Singapore. (n.d.), "Key Concepts," [Online]. Available: https://www.pdpc.gov.sg/legislation-and-guidelines/overview/key-concepts

[20] M. Huang, M. Elad, Y. Y. Zeevi, and Y. Birk, "Security and privacy in telemedicine and e-health," *IEEE Trans. Inf. Forensics Security.*, vol. 15, pp. 2354–2369, 2020.

[21] J. Choi, J. S. Park, and J. Hong, "Privacy and security in telemedicine: An overview," *J. Med. Syst.*, vol. 42, no. 12, pp. 256, 2018.

[22] S. Lee, H. Kim, and S. G. Lee, "Blockchain-based secure data exchange for telehealth systems," *Sensors.*, vol. 20, no. 23, pp. 6718, 2020.

[23] U. Yilmaz and S. A. Adams, "Telehealth privacy and security: Current landscape and future directions," *J. Am. Med. Inform. Assoc.*, vol. 27, no. 6, pp. 981–984, 2020.

[24] G. G. Dagher, J. Mohler, M. Milojkovic, and P. B. Marella, "Ancile: Privacy-preserving framework for access control and interoperability of electronic health records using blockchain technology," *Sustainable. Cities. Soc.*, vol. 39, pp. 283–297, 2018.

[25] A. Ali, E. Ahmed, J. Siddiqi, and S. Lee, "Data security and privacy in cloud-based eHealth: A systematic literature review," *IEEE Access.*, vol. 8, pp. 111457–111477, 2020.

[26] Personal Data Protection Commission Singapore. (n.d.), "Personal Data Protection Act (PDPA)," [Online]. Available: https://www.pdpc.gov.sg/legislation-and-guidelines/legislation.

[27] A. B. Smith, C. D. Johnson, and E. F. Brown, "Telehealth in the age of artificial intelligence: Current regulations and challenges," *J. Telemed. Telecare.*, vol. 27, no. 7, pp. 393–402, 2021.

[28] R. Karim, H. Chiroma, M. Uddin, A. Gital, and T. Herawan, "Toward context-aware access control for IoT healthcare," *IEEE Access.*, vol. 6, pp. 33783–33793, 2018.

[29] J. L. Fernández-Alemán, I. C. Señor, P. Á. O. Lozoya, and A. Toval, "Security and privacy in electronic health records: A systematic literature review." *J. Biomed. Inf.*, 103458, 2020.

[30] M. Ali, F. Naeem, M. Tariq, and G. Kaddoum, "Federated learning for privacy preservation in smart healthcare systems: A comprehensive survey," *IEEE J. Biomed. Health Inform.*, vol. 27, no. 2, pp. 778–789, 2022.

[31] A. Haddad, M. H. Habaebi, M. R. Islam, N. F. Hasbullah, and S. A. Zabidi, "Systematic review on ai-blockchain based e-healthcare records management systems," *IEEE Access*, vol. 10, pp. 94583–94615, 2022.

[32] A. Shaban-Nejad, M. Michalowski, and D. L. Buckeridge, "Health intelligence: How artificial intelligence transforms population and personalized health," *NPJ Digit. Med.*, vol. 1, no. 1, p. 53, 2018.

[33] M. Magdy, K. M. Hosny, N. I. Ghali, and S. Ghoniemy, "Security of medical images for telemedicine: a systematic review," *Multimedia Tools Appl.*, vol. 81, no. 18, pp. 25101–25145, 2022.

[34] I. V. Pustokhina, D. A. Pustokhin, and K. Shankar, "Blockchain-based secure data sharing scheme using image steganography and encryption techniques for telemedicine applications," in *Wearable Telemedicine Technology for the Healthcare Industry*. New York: Academic Press, 2022, pp. 97–108.

[35] Anushree Tandon, Amandeep Dhir, A.K.M. Najmul Islam, Matti Mäntymäki, Blockchain in healthcare: A systematic literature review, synthesizing framework and future research agenda, Computers in Industry, vol. 122, 2020, 103290, ISSN 0166-3615, https://doi.org/10.1016/j.compind.2020.103290.

[36] T.P. Mashamba-Thompson, and E.D. Crayton, Blockchain and artificial intelligence technology.

[37] N. Z. Bawany, T. Qamar, H. Tariq, and S. Adnan, "Integrating healthcare services using blockchain-based telehealth framework," *IEEE Access*, vol. 10, pp. 36505–36517, 2022.

[38] F. Pesapane, C. Volonté, M. Codari, and F. Sardanelli, "Artificial intelligence as a medical device in radiology: Ethical and regulatory issues in Europe and the United States," *Insights Imaging.,* vol. 9, pp. 745–753, 2018.

[39] FDA, "Digital Health Policies and Public Health Solutions for COVID-19." FDA, Silver Spring, MD, USA, 2020.

[40] V. Shah, R. Keniya, A. Shridharani, M. Punjabi, J. Shah, and N. Mehendale, "Diagnosis of COVID-19 using CT scan images and deep learning techniques," *Emerg. Radiol.*, vol. 28, pp. 497–505, 2021.

[41] C. R. Simpson, C. Robertson, S. Kerr, *et al.*, "External validation of the QCovid risk prediction algorithm for risk of COVID-19 hospitalization and mortality in adults: National validation cohort study in Scotland," *Thorax*, vol. 77, no. 5, pp. 497–504, 2022.

[42] A. Gillissen, T. Kochanek, M. Zupanic, and J. Ehlers, "Medical students' perceptions towards digitization and artificial intelligence: A mixed-methods study," *Healthcare*, vol. 10, no. 4, p. 723, 2022.

[43] J. Hermansson, and T. Kahan, "Systematic review of validity assessments of Framingham risk score results in health economic modelling of lipid-modifying therapies in Europe," *Pharmacoeconomics.*, vol. 36, pp. 205–213, 2018.

[44] H. Ko, J. Ahn, S. Kim, J. Kim, and H. Hwang, "Security and privacy in blockchain-based telemedicine," *J. Med. Syst.,* vol. 44, no. 4, pp. 77, 2020.

[45] R. H. Hylock, X. Zeng, and Y. Moon, "Telemedicine privacy and security considerations in the age of COVID-19," *J. Am. Med. Inform. Assoc.*, vol. 27, no. 7, pp. 1142–1146, 2020.

[46] P. Kierkegaard, A. Kaushal, J. R. Vest, and N. Menachemi, "Challenges to the privacy and security of patient data," *J. Am. Med. Inform. Assoc.*, vol. 26, no. 8–9, pp. 840–844, 2019.

[47] A. Bansal, A. Singh, and R. Girdhar, "Securing telemedicine data during the COVID-19 pandemic," *Health Technol.*, vol. 11, no. 2, pp. 357–364, 2021.

[48] H. Kasiviswanathan, N. Ramakrishnan, N. Shah, and A. Verma, "Telemedicine in the age of artificial intelligence," *EAI Endorsed Trans. Scalable Inf. Syst.*, vol. 18, no. 15, pp. e5, 2018.

[49] K. K. R. Choo, C. Liu, Y. Wang, and X. Yang, "Cybersecurity analytics and artificial intelligence: An overview," *IEEE Access.*, vol. 7, pp. 105247–105257, 2019.

[50] M. Mehdi, M. Elhoseny, N. Agarwal, and A. Rajput, "Artificial intelligence and cybersecurity: A comprehensive survey," *J. Cybersecurity Privacy.*, vol. 3, no. 2, pp. 103–143, 2020.

[51] M. Althobaiti, J. H. Weber-Jahnke, and J. Weber-Jahnke, "A survey of natural language processing techniques in cybersecurity," *J. Cybersecurity Privacy.*, vol. 3, no. 2, pp. 61–88, 2020.

[52] J. L. Viegas, J. T. Souza, L. R. Lima, and L. H. Gomes, "Artificial intelligence techniques for detection and prevention of data breaches: A systematic literature review," *J. Inf. Secur. Appl.*, vol. 46, pp. 68–83, 2019.

[53] A. N. Mahmood, K. K. R. Choo, H. Abbas, and A. Gani, "AI-based secure authentication framework for healthcare systems," *IEEE Access.*, vol. 8, pp. 182119–182132, 2020.

[54] A. Rajkomar, J. Dean, and I. Kohane, "Machine learning in medicine," *New Engl. J. Med.*, vol. 380, no. 14, pp. 1347–1358, 2018.

[55] X. Yang, Q. Li, Y. Wu, Y. Zhu, and R. Xie, "An improved efficient certificateless encryption scheme based on machine learning," *IEEE Access.*, vol. 8, pp. 11122–11130, 2020.

[56] J. Jiang, J. Lai, J. Liu, and N. Xiong, "A survey on secure access control in fog computing," *IEEE Access.*, vol. 7, pp. 152052–152068, 2019.

[57] M. Chui, J. Manyika, and M. Miremadi, "How artificial intelligence can deliver real value to companies," McKinsey Global Institute, [Online]. Available: https://www.mckinsey.com/business-functions/mckinsey-digital/our-insights/how-artificial-intelligence-can-deliver-real-value-to-companies.

[58] S. Angraal, H. M. Krumholz, and W. L. Schulz, "Blockchain technology: Applications in health care," *Circulation: Cardiovasc. Qual. Outcomes.*, vol. 14, no. 4, pp. e007707, 2021.

[59] X. Yue, H. Wang, D. Jin, M. Li, and W. Jiang, "Healthcare data gateways: Found healthcare intelligence on blockchain with novel privacy risk control," *J. Med. Syst.*, vol. 42, no. 8, pp. 1–9, 2018.

[60] R. Chen, R. Lu, H. Zhu, X. Zhang, and Y. Xiang, "Blockchain-based fine-grained access control for electronic health records," *IEEE Trans. Ind. Informatics.*, vol. 16, no. 8, pp. 5464–5473, 2020.

[61] P. Zhang, D. C. Schmidt, J. White, G. Lenz, and S. T. Rosenbloom, "FHIRChain: Applying blockchain to securely and scalably share clinical data," *Comput. Struct. Biotechnol. J.*, vol. 18, pp. 1987–1996, 2020.

[62] Á. Rocha, G. André, and A. Zaslavsky, "Blockchain-based privacy-preserving access control for electronic health records," *IEEE Trans. Serv. Comput.*, vol. 12, no. 4, pp. 577–589, 2019.

[63] H. Wu, Z. Xu, J. Li, M. Zhang, X. Huang, and L. Zhao, "A traceable blockchain-based system for secure sharing of personal health records," *IEEE Trans. Ind. Informatics*, vol. 17, no. 1, pp. 571–582, 2021.

[64] L. Hammell, L. Hoffman-Goetz, and L. Lévesque, "Use of blockchain technology to maintain privacy and security of personal health information

in the era of digital health," *J. Med. Internet Res.*, vol. 21, no. 10, pp. e14394, 2019.

[65] X. Li, X. Huang, X. Luo, J. Xu, and Z. Zhang, "Blockchain-based data sharing and patient consent management in healthcare systems," *J. Med. Syst.*, vol. 43, no. 10, pp. 306, 2019.

[66] A. Al Omar, R. Ramadan, and A. Abuarqoub, "Privacy-aware blockchain-based framework for telehealthcare applications," *Comput. Mater. Continua.*, vol. 60, no. 2, pp. 529–546, 2019.

[67] X. Chen, M. Goyal, and C. Kamhoua, "A survey on security and privacy issues in telehealth systems," *IEEE Access.*, vol. 7, pp. 131014–131038, 2019.

[68] S. M. S. Islam, D. Kwak, M. H. Kabir, M. A. Hossain, and K. S. Kwak, "Blockchain in healthcare: A systematic literature review, synthesizing framework, and future research agenda," *Int. J. Med. Inform.*, vol. 144, pp. 1–17, 2020.

[69] U.S. Food and Drug Administration, "Artificial Intelligence/Machine Learning (AI/ML)-Based Software as a Medical Device (SaMD)," [Online]. Available: https://www.fda.gov/medical-devices/software-medical-device-samd/artificial-intelligencemachine-learning-ai-ml-based-software-medical-device-samd.

[70] U.S. Department of Health & Human Services, "Health information privacy," [Online]. Available: https://www.hhs.gov/hipaa/index.html.

[71] Federal Trade Commission, "Federal Trade Commission Act," [Online]. Available: https://www.ftc.gov/about-ftc/what-we-do/enforcement-authority.

[72] American Telemedicine Association, "Practice guidelines for video-based online mental health services," [Online]. Available: https://www.americantelemed.org/.

[73] H. Saeed, H. Malik, U. Bashir, *et al.*, "Blockchain technology in healthcare: A systematic review," *PLoS One*, vol. 17, no. 4, p. e0266462, 2022.

[74] United States Department of Health & Human Services. (n.d.), "Health Insurance Portability and Accountability Act (HIPAA)," HIPAA for Professionals. Retrieved from https://www.hhs.gov/hipaa/for-professionals/index.html

[75] Personal Data Protection Commission Singapore. (n.d.), "Personal Data Protection Act (PDPA)," Key Concepts. Retrieved from https://www.pdpc.gov.sg/legislation-and-guidelines/overview/key-concepts

[76] Federal Law No. 152-FZ, "On Personal Data," [Online]. Available: http://www.consultant.ru/document/cons_doc_LAW_34683/ 2019.

[77] Y. Wang, L. Kung, and T. A. Byrd, "Big data analytics: Understanding its capabilities and potential benefits for healthcare organizations," *Technol. Forecast. Soc. Change.*, vol. 126, pp. 3–13, 2018.

[78] U.S. Department of Health & Human Services, "Summary of the HIPAA Security Rule," [Online]. Available: https://www.hhs.gov/hipaa/for-professionals/security/laws-regulations/index.html.

[79] Federal Trade Commission. (n.d.). Federal Trade Commission Act. Retrieved from https://www.ftc.gov/about-ftc/what-we-do/enforcement-authority
[80] Federal Law No. 259-FZ, "On Digital Financial Assets," [Online]. Available: http://www.consultant.ru/document/cons_doc_LAW_349955/, 2020
[81] National People's Congress, "Cybersecurity Law of the People's Republic of China," [Online]. Available: http://www.npc.gov.cn/englishnpc/Law/2018-11/07/content_2065111.htm.
[82] The State Council of the People's Republic of China, "Law on the Promotion of the Development of the Blockchain Industry," [Online]. Available: http://www.gov.cn/zhengce/content/2019-01/10/content_5359357.htm.

Chapter 15

Legal frameworks for artificial intelligence and blockchain technology in telehealth systems

Abdulwaheed Musa[1,2,3], *Abdulhakeem Abdulfatai*[1], *Daniel Oluyemi*[1], *Segun Jacob*[1] *and Agbotiname Lucky Imoize*[4]

In recent years, the rapid advancements in artificial intelligence (AI) and blockchain technology have brought numerous possibilities and transformative applications in the field of telehealth systems. However, the integration of these technologies also raises important legal considerations and regulatory challenges. This chapter investigates and addresses the legal frameworks surrounding the utilization of AI and blockchain in telehealth systems. Key aspects, such as data privacy, security, liability, consent, and intellectual property rights, are examined in the context of these emerging technologies. By analyzing existing regulations and proposing potential solutions, this study aims to contribute to the development of comprehensive legal frameworks that promote the responsible and ethical implementation of AI and blockchain in telehealth systems.

15.1 Introduction

Today, telehealth systems encompass a broad range of applications, such as teleconsultations, remote monitoring, telesurgery, and telepsychiatry, leveraging advancements in artificial intelligence (AI), machine learning (ML), and Internet of Things (IoT) technologies. These technologies enhance the accuracy of diagnoses, personalize treatment plans, and streamline healthcare workflows [1]. Telehealth systems have become an integral part of modern healthcare, providing cost-effective, efficient, and patient-centered care. As the demand for accessible and efficient healthcare services continues to rise, integrating innovative technologies becomes crucial to enhance the capabilities of telehealth systems [2]. AI and blockchain

[1]Department of Electrical and Computer Engineering, Kwara State University, Nigeria
[2]Centre for Artificial Intelligence and Machine Learning Systems, Kwara State University, Nigeria
[3]Institute for Intelligent Systems, University of Johannesburg, South Africa
[4]Department of Electrical and Electronics Engineering, Faculty of Engineering, University of Lagos, Nigeria

technology have gained significant attention for their potential to revolutionize the field. When applied to telehealth systems, AI can enable remote patient monitoring, assist in accurate diagnosis, provide treatment recommendations, and support personalized care plans [3]. In parallel, blockchain technology, originally developed for cryptocurrencies, has found relevance in healthcare, offering a decentralized and secure ledger to ensure data immutability, traceability, and privacy [4].

Figure 15.1 shows the different ways AI and blockchain technology can be used in telehealth systems. These technologies have the potential to enable more access to care by enhancing the effectiveness and accuracy of telehealth services, which will enhance patient health outcomes. AI can analyze patient data to identify potential health problems, provide personalized treatment recommendations, as well as automate tasks such as appointment schedules and prescriptions, while blockchain can securely store patient data, track medical devices and medications, as well as enhance payments in telehealth services.

The integration of AI and blockchain technology into telehealth brings forth a range of legal and regulatory challenges that must be carefully addressed. One significant concern revolves around data privacy and security [5]. Telehealth platforms that utilize AI algorithms rely on vast amounts of patient data for accurate diagnoses and personalized treatment recommendations. Compliance with data protection laws, such as the General Data Protection Regulation (GDPR) in the European Union [6] or the Health Insurance Portability and Accountability Act (HIPAA) in the United States [7], becomes crucial. Additionally, the use of blockchain technology introduces questions regarding data ownership, consent, and the right to be forgotten, given its decentralized and immutable nature. Balancing the need for data accessibility and innovation with strict privacy safeguards poses a key challenge for regulators and healthcare providers.

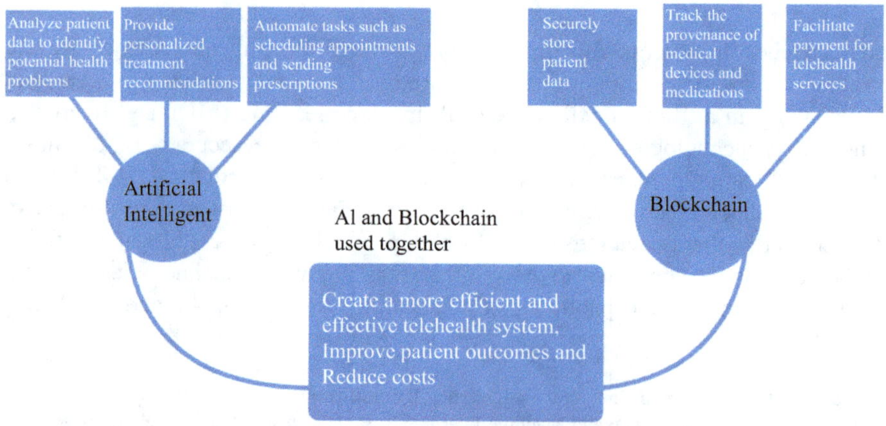

Figure 15.1 Artificial intelligence and blockchain technology use in telehealth system

Against this background, this study investigates and addresses the legal frameworks surrounding the utilization of AI and blockchain technology in telehealth systems. The goal is to ensure ethical use, protect rights and interests, establish accountability, foster innovation, and maintain public trust and confidence in these transformative technologies. The study serves as a guidepost for responsible and beneficial deployment, striking a balance between the potential benefits and the associated risks and challenges.

15.1.1 Key contributions of the chapter

The following are the significant contributions of this chapter:

1. Reviews of AI and blockchain technology in telehealth systems were conducted.
2. The chapter presents the history and evolution of telehealth systems.
3. The chapter outlines key promising AI and blockchain technology–based security frameworks to support telehealth systems.
4. The legal frameworks for AI and blockchain technology in telehealth systems have been investigated and addressed.
5. The chapter also provides far-reaching recommendations on how to improve the legal frameworks for AI and blockchain technology in telehealth systems.

15.1.2 Chapter organization

The remaining sections of this chapter are structured as follows: Section 15.2 provides a historical overview of telehealth systems, including their deployment and the transformation of healthcare delivery. Section 15.3 discusses the application of AI and blockchain technology in telehealth systems. Section 15.4 reviews security frameworks for telehealth systems, and Section 15.5 investigates the legal frameworks for AI and blockchain technology. While the lessons learned and future directions are highlighted and discussed in Section 15.6, the chapter is concluded with recommendations in Section 15.7.

15.2 History of telehealth systems

Human civilization has always included efforts to communicate outside of the hearing range, such as smoke signals, drums, and pigeon carriers. They were also employed to obtain medical care. Even then, there was a gap between the upper and lower classes regarding access to high-quality healthcare, with access to the best care being restricted to kings and other aristocrats. The elderly and infirm frequently sent messengers or used messages to send home a diagnosis and treatment options, as well as information on symptoms. The development of telecommunication, as we know it today, came after the 19th-century discovery of electricity. The concepts underlying telehealth started to take shape as technology advanced and wired connectivity became more prevalent. Telegraphs were employed to send soldiers' mortality lists and medical supplies during the American Civil War. Access to the public also started to arise since the telephone was simpler to use than the telegraph. In 1876, the invention of telemedicine by Alexander Graham Bell led to the first recorded case. After spilling acid on his pants, he sought assistance from his assistant, Mr. Watson [8]. The Lancet published a story in 1879 about a doctor who successfully diagnosed a child over the phone in the middle of the night and then talked about the possibility of remote patient care to reduce the need for unneeded house visits [9].

A Dutch scientist who used the telephone to transmit and monitor heart sounds and rhythms helped develop the idea of telemedicine in 1905. Nearly as soon as it began, bicycle-powered radios were used to call for medical assistance from Australia's flying doctors. When two-way television and audio signals were employed for communication in the 1920s, the word "telemedicine" first received official acceptance. In the 1940s, radiography was transmitted among cities located 20 miles apart using telephone circuits in Pennsylvania. In the late 1950s and early 1960s, telemedicine was first used to send complicated medical data, videos, and photographs. The University of Nebraska broadcast neurological tests using interactive television (IATV) in 1959, which is largely regarded as the first instance of a real-time video telemedicine consultation. The next step was remote counseling and telepsychiatry.

The need for telemedicine was made abundantly evident when the National Aeronautics and Space Administration (NASA) started making plans to send astronauts into space. Telemedicine features were incorporated into the earliest spacecraft and spacesuits for monitoring purposes. As part of the Space Technology Applied to Rural Papago Advanced Health Care (STARPAHC) project, NASA, Lockheed Corporation, and the U.S. Indian Health Service collaborated in the 1960s to bring telemedicine to an American Indian reservation using telecommunications systems similar to those found in space stations. To realize the great potential of this discovery, many projects were sponsored throughout North America and Canada. The transfer of medical data, including X-rays, electrocardiograms (ECGs), stethoscope heart and chest sounds, and fluoroscopy images, and images followed. These early projects' primary driving forces were as follows: providing rural communities with access to healthcare and emergencies in medicine.

In the 1980s, telemedicine was first fully embraced by the field of radiology. The enterprise-level digitalization of medical pictures, which was a natural advancement from Picture Archiving and Communication System (PACS), was accomplished here. PACSs were created as a means of storing X-ray images in a digital format while saving money and space. This gave users of computer monitors located throughout the radiology department and in the wards immediate access to both recent and old images. The next stage was to provide remote access, which was done first for the hospital's radiologists so they could submit reports from their homes. They can now report from anywhere in the world.

In 1975, the Indian city of Gwalior built one of the first telecardiology systems for sending electrocardiograms over the Internet. With the use of this technology, electrocardiogram data could be wirelessly transmitted from an intensive care unit (ICU) van that was traveling or a patient's home to the central station in the hospital's ICU. The background noise in transmission was reduced thanks to frequency modulation. The monitoring of pacemaker patients in remote locations also utilized this technique. Arrhythmia was accurately deciphered by the ICU's central control unit. Even though it was widely used by the turn of the century, telehealth was not affected until much later since the early systems needed more bandwidth than was initially available. Specialties relying on the interpretation of audio or visuals, either still or moving, were some of the first to profit (video). Speech therapy, patient discussions, and heart sounds are some examples of the former, while dermatology, cardiology (electrocardiograms, echo, and angiograms), ophthalmology, and pathology are examples of the latter. A third category was whether care could be provided through video conferencing (psychiatry). Tele-stethoscopes and tele-electrocardiograms are two examples of specialist tools that have been developed to facilitate the transfer. There are also dedicated microscopes for telepathology that allow for real-time zooming and remote control of the slide viewer's movement.

India has long been a pioneer in telecare among underdeveloped nations. The need was highlighted by the fact that between 60 and 70 percent of the population lived in rural areas and that even the few doctors who had been officially placed would rarely be on call. The Indian Space Research Organization (ISRO) and a specialized school for telemedicine that was developed in the city of Lucknow led the initiative. During the Kumbh event in 2001, this center offered consultations to pilgrims assembled in Allahabad to bathe in the Ganges [10]. It became incredibly well known and well liked after offering high-altitude trekkers in the Himalayas emergency remote support following an avalanche. Since nearly the beginning, CPCs and medical seminars have been held, drawing participants from all around the nation. There are telemedicine connections to numerous hospitals in African nations as well as clinics in far-off places like Ladakh and the Andaman Islands. The ISRO gave neighboring nations like Nepal and Bhutan the chance to use Indian satellites for their initiatives. China has also assisted Iran, Argentina, and Mongolia.

Early telemedicine deployments almost always required significant organizational and personnel changes as well as specific staffing. The majority of the large projects were for the military or the government. They were unsustainable because they were cumbersome and costly. For a particular use, such as telepsychiatry, specialized gear and software had been developed. There was a constant need for maintenance, which was not available nearby. The inability of different software to communicate with one another sparked efforts toward standardization. Due to the quick advancements and changes in technology, even the few ideas that made it through the earliest stages quickly became obsolete. The primary determining factor for projects was the connectivity option, which initially consisted of phone lines (dial-up Internet), general packet radio service, or satellite.

ISDN was a less unpredictable and more affordable alternative to satellite, but it only held influence for a short period before being replaced by broadband Internet and, more recently, mobile technologies like 3G, 4G, and 5G. Other developments include memory and storage (databases, object-store for large files like images and videos), as well as accessibility—through backup servers that can dynamically increase capacity in response to demand load, normalization (MP4, PNG, etc.), protection (encryption, password protection, access levels, etc.), application development with open-source software, frameworks, and modern programming languages (Java, JavaScript, DotNet, etc.) (Apache), techniques for digitizing data; the cloud and virtual servers like Amazon Web Services (AWS); (digital cameras, scanners, etc.).

The 1990s marked a turning point for telehealth systems with the rapid expansion of the Internet and the development of videoconferencing technologies [11]. This enabled real-time audiovisual communication between healthcare providers and patients, facilitating remote consultations and diagnosis. Additionally, advancements in medical imaging technology allowed for the transmission of high-quality images, facilitating remote radiology and pathology consultations.

In the early 2000s, telehealth systems gained further momentum with the proliferation of broadband Internet and the widespread availability of affordable digital devices. This led to the development of remote patient monitoring systems, which allowed healthcare providers to remotely track patients' vital signs, chronic conditions, and medication adherence [12]. Moreover, telehealth systems started to integrate electronic health records, facilitating seamless information exchange and continuity of care [13].

The COVID-19 pandemic, which emerged in 2019, acted as a catalyst for the widespread adoption of telehealth systems. To minimize in-person contact and curb the spread of the virus, healthcare providers rapidly scaled up their telehealth capabilities. Virtual visits became the norm, allowing patients to receive medical advice, prescriptions, and follow-up care from the safety and convenience of their homes. This shift highlighted the potential of telehealth systems to improve healthcare accessibility, especially for underserved populations and remote areas.

Today, telehealth systems encompass a wide range of applications, including teleconsultations, remote monitoring, telesurgery, and telepsychiatry [14]. They leverage advancements in AI, ML, and IoT technologies to enhance diagnosis accuracy, personalize treatment plans, and streamline healthcare workflows [15]. Telehealth systems have become an integral part of the modern healthcare ecosystem, delivering cost-effective, efficient, and patient-centered care.

Public health has been significantly impacted by smartphones. Over 325,000 health applications are available today, some of which serve as daily activity trackers, communicate health data, and remind patients to take their medications. The collection of health data can be improved with the use of features like Global Positioning System and cameras. It is possible to use a clip-on lens, software, hardware, and attachments to turn a mobile device into an e-stethoscope, slit lamp, or microscope. A special device created can be equipped with an ultrasound probe, a pulse oximeter, and a monitor, allowing information to be seamlessly obtained and transmitted. Internet-based electronic medical record vendors give patients and medical professionals access to medical data. Additionally, patient portals have emerged, enabling patients to access their lab results, request prescription refills, or communicate securely with their doctor. Parents can work thanks to baby monitors. Portable monitors identify cardiac arrhythmias and falls and inform the clinician about them. By being able to deliver blood samples, medications, and medical support to a remote site, drones are enabling emergency care.

Today, it is common practice for an ambulance to transport a patient from a trauma site straight to the operating room, with a surgeon waiting nearby. The general public is choosing telecare over a doctor visit [16]. Search engines, social media, and occasionally email, WhatsApp, Skype, or even desktop sharing are used to accomplish this instead of specialist software. Many of the former raise privacy issues and are typically disliked by academics and professionals. It is a little dismal how things are in emerging nations. Even though the developed and developing worlds have nearly equal access to the newest software and hardware—the absence of this parity invites software piracy—poor connectivity is still a problem. Even in areas with information and communication technology (ICT) infrastructure, more fundamental health issues like water and sanitation—and occasionally even food—take precedence, which telehealth will never be able to address.

An overview of the key development of telehealth systems is provided in Table 15.1. The history of telehealth systems is a testament to the transformative power of technology in healthcare. From the early telephonic experiments to the current era of advanced digital platforms, telehealth has evolved to overcome geographical barriers, improve access to care, and enhance patient outcomes. The integration of AI and ML algorithms for data analysis, diagnosis support, and personalized treatment plans from around 2010, as well as the advancements in telecommunication infrastructure, high-speed Internet, and improved video conferencing software, have all combined to enhance the expansion of telehealth services globally.

Table 15.1 Development of telehealth

Reference	Period	Key developments
[17]	Early 20th century	Use of telegraphy to transmit radiographic images for diagnostic purposes.
[18]	1960s–1970s	Development of telephonic transmission of medical data, such as electrocardiograms.
[19]	1980s–1990s	Introduction of teleconferencing and video communication technologies in telehealth.
[20]	2000s	Integration of electronic health records (EHRs) into telehealth systems for seamless information sharing.
[21]	Mid-2000s	Adoption of telehealth for remote patient monitoring, including vital signs and chronic condition management.
[22]	The late 2000s	The emergence of mobile health (mHealth) applications, leveraging smartphones and wearables for health tracking and remote consultations.
[23,24]	2010s	Integration of artificial intelligence (AI) and machine learning (ML) algorithms for data analysis, diagnosis support, and personalized treatment plans.
[25]	Present day	Advancements in telecommunication infrastructure, high-speed Internet, and improved video conferencing software. Expansion of telehealth services globally.

15.3 Artificial intelligence and blockchain technology for telehealth systems

As the demand for accessible and efficient healthcare services continues to grow, the integration of innovative technologies becomes imperative to enhance the capabilities of telehealth systems. In this context, AI and blockchain technology have garnered significant attention for their potential to revolutionize the field. When applied to telehealth systems, AI can enable remote patient monitoring, assist in accurate diagnosis, provide treatment recommendations, and even support personalized care plans [1,26]. In parallel, blockchain technology, originally developed as the underlying technology for cryptocurrencies [27], has evolved beyond its financial origins and found relevance in healthcare. Blockchain offers a decentralized and secure ledger, ensuring the immutability, traceability, and privacy of healthcare data [28]. By leveraging blockchain technology in telehealth systems, sensitive patient information can be securely stored and shared, enabling interoperability, consent management, and efficient supply chain management for pharmaceuticals. In this section, we delve into the applications, challenges, and opportunities surrounding the integration of AI and blockchain in telehealth systems. We examine the role of AI in remote patient monitoring, diagnosis, and personalized care, as well as the potential benefits of blockchain in data security, interoperability, and supply chain management.

15.3.1 Artificial intelligence in telehealth systems

The telehealth system is one area where AI's impact has been particularly significant. AI has the potential to enhance telehealth systems by improving diagnosis accuracy, enabling remote monitoring, personalizing care, and enhancing the overall patient experience. One of the primary applications of AI in telehealth systems is improving diagnosis accuracy [29]. AI algorithms can analyze vast amounts of patient data, including medical records, lab results, and imaging studies, to identify patterns and detect abnormalities that may be missed by human clinicians. This can lead to more accurate and timely diagnoses, enabling earlier interventions and improved patient outcomes. AI-powered diagnostic systems have shown promising results in various medical specialties, including radiology, pathology, and dermatology [30].

Another key area where AI can be utilized in telehealth is remote patient monitoring. With the help of wearable devices and sensors, AI algorithms can continuously monitor patients' vital signs, such as heart rate, blood pressure, and glucose levels [31]. These algorithms can detect deviations from normal values and alert healthcare providers in real time, enabling timely interventions and proactive care. Remote monitoring systems powered by AI can be particularly beneficial for patients with chronic conditions who require regular monitoring and for those who are geographically distant from healthcare facilities [32].

Personalizing care is another advantage of AI in telehealth systems. AI algorithms can analyze patient data, including medical history, genetic information, lifestyle factors, and treatment responses, to develop personalized treatment plans [33]. This can help healthcare providers make more informed decisions about the most appropriate interventions for individual patients. By considering a patient's unique characteristics, AI-powered telehealth systems can optimize treatment outcomes and minimize the risk of adverse effects. Furthermore, AI can support shared decision-making by providing patients with evidence-based information and recommendations tailored to their specific circumstances [34].

AI also plays a crucial role in improving the overall patient experience in telehealth. Natural language processing algorithms enable AI chatbots and virtual assistants to engage in interactive conversations with patients, addressing their queries and concerns [35]. These AI-powered systems can provide basic healthcare information, schedule appointments, remind patients about medication schedules, and offer emotional support. They can also assist in triaging patients, directing them to the most appropriate level of care based on their symptoms and urgency. By automating routine tasks and providing round-the-clock support, AI enhances accessibility and convenience for patients, leading to increased patient satisfaction.

In Figure 15.2, some key AI algorithms, namely: convolutional neural networks (CNNs), support vector machines (SVMs), random forests, and naive Bayes, that are used in the healthcare system are highlighted. CNN is designed to learn complex patterns and features within images, enabling them to detect abnormalities, identify specific conditions, and aid in diagnostic decision-making. SVM is a powerful algorithm that finds an optimal hyperplane to separate different classes of

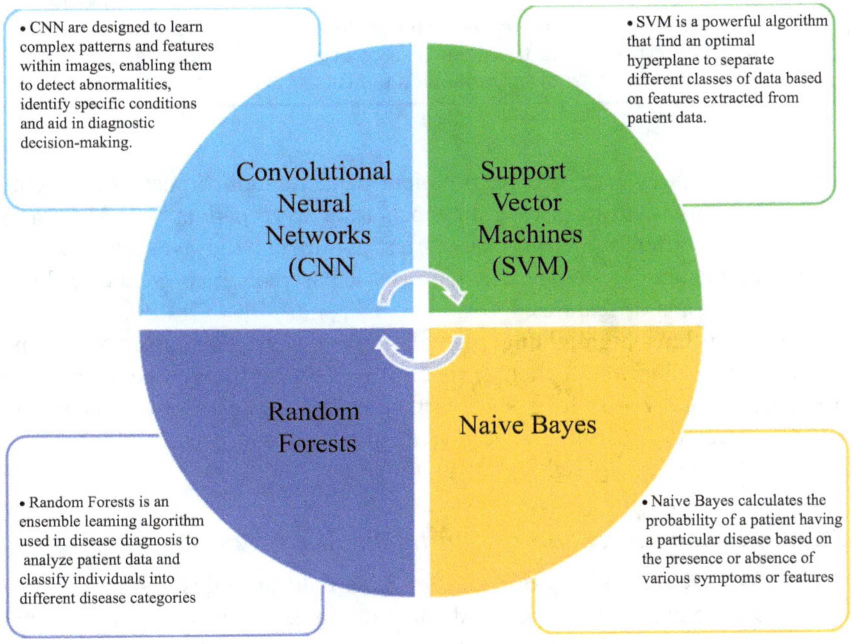

Figure 15.2 Some artificial intelligence algorithms in healthcare

Table 15.2 Artificial intelligence algorithms for healthcare

Reference	Algorithm	Methodology	Use
[36]	Decision trees	The tree-based model makes decisions based on conditions	Diagnosing diseases, predicting outcomes, and risk assessment
[37]	Artificial neural networks (ANNs)	Interconnected layers of artificial neurons	Disease prediction, medical imaging analysis, genomics
[38]	Recurrent neural networks (RNNs)	Designed to analyze sequential data with memory	Time series analysis, patient monitoring, clinical notes
[39]	Long short-term memory (LSTM)	Type of RNN with memory units to retain information	Predicting patient outcomes, anomaly detection
[40]	Generative adversarial networks (GAN)	Comprises generator and discriminator models	Synthetic data generation, medical image synthesis
[41]	Reinforcement learning (RL)	Learning from trial and error through rewards and penalties	Optimizing treatment plans, personalized medicine
[42]	*k*-Nearest neighbors (*k*-NN)	Classifies data points based on similarity to neighbors	Disease diagnosis, patient stratification, data clustering
[43]	Hidden Markov models (HMM)	A probabilistic model with hidden states and observed outputs	Speech recognition, gesture analysis, disease modeling
[44]	Gaussian mixture models (GMM)	Represents probability distributions as a combination of Gaussian components	Clustering patient populations, anomaly detection

data based on features extracted from patient data. Random forests are ensemble learning algorithms used in disease diagnosis to analyze patient data and classify individuals into different disease categories, while naive Bayes calculates the probability of a patient having a particular disease based on the presence or absence of various symptoms or features.

Other algorithms highlighting methodology and applications are shown in Table 15.2. The algorithms include decision trees, artificial neural networks, recurrent neural networks, long short-term memory, generative adversarial networks, reinforcement learning, *k*-nearest neighbors (*k*-NN), and hidden Markov models. The table also highlights their methodology and uses.

15.3.2 Blockchain technology in telehealth systems

Traditional healthcare systems often suffer from data breaches and unauthorized access due to centralized storage and vulnerabilities in existing infrastructure. Blockchain, on the other hand, employs a distributed ledger that records transactions across multiple nodes, ensuring that data is replicated and secured in a decentralized manner [10]. This decentralized architecture makes it extremely difficult for malicious actors to tamper with or compromise patient data. Each transaction recorded on the blockchain is cryptographically secured and linked to previous transactions, creating an immutable audit trail that can be audited and verified by authorized participants [45]. This transparency and immutability contribute to a higher level of trust in the telehealth system.

Interoperability is another challenge in healthcare that can be addressed by blockchain technology. In telehealth systems, where patients may seek care from different providers or across multiple platforms, it is essential to have seamless data exchange and interoperability standards. Blockchain enables the creation of a unified and standardized platform where patient data can be securely shared and accessed by authorized parties [46]. By utilizing smart contracts, which are self-executing agreements with predefined rules and conditions, blockchain can facilitate automated and secure data sharing between different healthcare organizations. This interoperability can significantly improve care coordination and enable healthcare providers to make more informed decisions based on comprehensive patient information [47].

Patient privacy is a crucial aspect of telehealth systems, and blockchain technology can help protect sensitive patient data. Blockchain networks allow patients to have greater control over their health information by granting them ownership and consent rights [48]. Patients can determine who can access their data and under what conditions, empowering them to make informed decisions about sharing their health information. Additionally, blockchain can enable secure and auditable consent management, where patient consent transactions are recorded on the blockchain, ensuring transparency and accountability in data-sharing practices. This patient-centric approach to data privacy can foster trust between patients and healthcare providers and encourage greater participation in telehealth services.

Blockchain technology can also facilitate the secure integration of IoT devices into telehealth systems [48]. IoT devices such as wearables and remote monitoring sensors generate vast amounts of patient data [49]. By connecting these devices to a blockchain network, the data can be securely transmitted, stored, and analyzed [47]. This integration ensures data integrity and authenticity, as each data transaction is recorded on the blockchain, making it highly resistant to tampering or manipulation [46]. Furthermore, blockchain can enable the creation of smart contracts that automate data processing and incentivize data contributors, fostering a decentralized ecosystem of health data sharing and analysis [50].

These are just a few examples of how blockchain technology is being utilized in the healthcare industry. Table 15.3 is an overview of key elements and features of blockchain technology in telehealth systems. The inherent qualities of blockchain technology, such as transparency, immutability, audibility, and user and data anonymity, are highlighted in the table. Decentralization is a feature that makes it possible for multiple locations to be used to store, access, and manage electronic health records. Similarly, anonymity features do not only make the identities of participants in telemedicine to be anonymous, but they also make data and transactions to be protected.

Table 15.3 Key elements and features of blockchain technology in telehealth

Reference	Key elements	Features
[51]	Decentralization	Multiple locations are used to store, access, and manage electronic health records. Several entities govern the network. The network is governed by consensus protocols.
[52]	Immutability	Patients' PHR and EHR cannot be modified. Consensus mechanisms and asymmetric key encryption assure the immutability of medical records.
[47,52]	Transparency	Because of the transparency, remote patient-centered data control is made easier and information users can discuss and ask about any questionable activity.
[53]	Open-source access	Before making an appointment for remote consulting, patients can view a doctor's profile. Accessibility for all users (public data)
[54]	Auditability	Drug administration authorities can track a drug's lineage. To ensure regulatory compliance procedures, the medical records are protected.
[47]	Anonymity	The identities of participants in telemedicine are anonymous. Data and transactions are protected

Table 15.4 Comparison of traditional, centralized, and blockchain-supported telehealth systems [47]

	Traditional healthcare	Centralized telemedicine	Blockchain-supported telehealth
Cost	High	Low	Low
Patient waiting time	Very high	Low	Low
Fault tolerance	NO	NO	NO
Requirement for in-person visit	YES	NO	YES
Data provenance	NO	NO	YES
Health record manipulation	YES	YES	NO
Documentation system	YES	YES	NO
Administration	Centralized	Centralized	Decentralized
Audit trials	NO	NO	YES
Data privacy and security	Hard	Hard	Easy
Transparency	NO	NO	YES
Reliability and integrity	Low	Low	High

Table 15.4 shows a comparison of traditional healthcare, centralized telemedicine, and blockchain-supported telehealth systems. The table highlights the distinctive qualities and advantages of using blockchain technology to digitize healthcare and telemedicine services. Important factors, such as cost, patient

waiting time, fault tolerance, requirement for in-person visit, health record manipulation, documentation system, administration, audit trials, data privacy and security, reliability and integrity, as well as transparency, have been considered for the comparison.

15.3.3 Convergence of artificial intelligence and blockchain in telehealth systems

AI, with its ability to analyze vast amounts of healthcare data, can significantly benefit from the integration with blockchain [1]. Blockchain technology provides a secure and decentralized platform for storing and sharing sensitive patient data, ensuring data integrity and privacy. By leveraging blockchain's immutable ledger, AI algorithms can access a comprehensive dataset while maintaining patient confidentiality [15]. This allows AI models to learn from a diverse range of patient information without exposing personal identifiers. The integration of AI and blockchain thus enables the development of more robust and accurate predictive models, leading to better diagnostic accuracy, treatment recommendations, and patient care.

The integration of AI and blockchain also addresses the issue of data interoperability in telehealth systems [46]. Currently, healthcare data is often siloed across different organizations and systems, making it challenging to access and share comprehensive patient information. Blockchain provides a decentralized framework that enables secure data exchange and interoperability between various healthcare providers, systems, and AI applications. Patient data stored on the blockchain can be accessed by authorized AI algorithms, facilitating seamless integration and collaboration across different healthcare entities. This interoperability enhances care coordination, reduces duplicate testing, and ensures healthcare providers have access to complete patient histories, leading to more informed decision-making and personalized care.

The integration of AI and blockchain in telehealth systems also enhances patient privacy and control over personal health information. Blockchain's decentralized architecture and cryptographic techniques provide patients with greater ownership and control of their data. Patients can grant and revoke access to their health information, monitor how their data is being used, and have greater transparency into data-sharing practices. AI algorithms operating on the blockchain can access patient data only with the patient's explicit consent and within the defined parameters set by the patient. This patient-centric approach ensures that individuals have autonomy over their health information, fostering trust and engagement in telehealth services.

15.3.4 Challenges and considerations

It is crucial to foster a multidisciplinary approach that combines expertise in AI, blockchain, healthcare, ethics, and regulation to develop robust solutions that maximize the benefits while mitigating potential risks [55]. By carefully addressing challenges, such as computational complexity, scalability, regulatory compliance, interoperability, and data quality, the integration of AI and blockchain in telehealth systems can pave the way for more efficient, secure, and patient-centric healthcare delivery.

1. **Computational complexity and scalability**: AI algorithms, particularly deep learning models, often require significant computational power and resources. Running these resource-intensive algorithms on a blockchain network can present challenges due to the inherent limitations of blockchain, such as consensus mechanisms and transaction processing speed. Scaling AI computations on a blockchain while maintaining efficiency and responsiveness is a complex task that requires innovative solutions, such as off-chain processing and layer-two protocols [56].
2. **Regulatory compliance**: Integrating AI and blockchain in telehealth systems necessitates compliance with existing healthcare regulations, data privacy laws, and security standards. Healthcare data is subject to stringent regulations, such as the Health Insurance Portability and Accountability Act (HIPAA) in the United States and the General Data Protection Regulation (GDPR) in the European Union. Blockchain's decentralized nature and immutability may pose challenges in meeting certain compliance requirements, such as the "right to be forgotten." Developing regulatory frameworks that address the unique aspects of AI and blockchain in healthcare is essential to ensure legal compliance while fostering innovation.
3. **Interoperability**: Achieving seamless data exchange and interoperability across different blockchain networks, healthcare systems, and AI applications is a significant challenge. Different organizations and systems may employ varying blockchain platforms, data structures, and standards, making it difficult to achieve uniform data representation and sharing protocols. Establishing interoperability standards and protocols that enable seamless integration and data exchange between different entities and systems is crucial to unlock the full potential of AI and blockchain in telehealth.
4. **Data quality and integrity**: AI algorithms heavily rely on high-quality and reliable data for training and validation. While blockchain provides immutability and transparency, it does not guarantee the accuracy and integrity of the data entered into the system. Data sources feeding into the blockchain need to be carefully vetted, and mechanisms should be in place to detect and address inaccuracies, errors, or malicious entries. Ensuring data quality and integrity is essential to maintain the trustworthiness and effectiveness of AI models operating on the blockchain.
5. **User experience and adoption**: The successful integration of AI and blockchain in telehealth systems depends on user acceptance and adoption. User interfaces and experiences should be designed to be intuitive, user-friendly, and seamlessly integrated into existing healthcare workflows. Educating and training healthcare professionals on the benefits and functionalities of AI and blockchain technologies is crucial to ensure their successful adoption and utilization.

6. **Ethical considerations**: AI algorithms operating on blockchain may introduce ethical considerations, such as bias, fairness, transparency, and accountability. Bias in training data can perpetuate existing healthcare disparities, and it is important to address these biases during algorithm development. Transparent AI models that provide explanations for their decisions can help build trust and facilitate ethical decision-making. Additionally, ensuring accountability and responsibility for the actions and decisions made by AI algorithms operating on the blockchain is essential.

Addressing these challenges requires collaboration among healthcare stakeholders, policymakers, technologists, and regulatory bodies.

15.3.5 Case studies

Several noteworthy case studies demonstrate the application and benefits of integrating AI and blockchain technology in telehealth systems. These case studies showcase how these technologies can improve diagnosis accuracy, enhance data security, streamline healthcare processes, and empower patients. Here are a few examples:

1. Shivom
   Shivom is a blockchain-based genomics platform that utilizes AI to provide personalized healthcare solutions. It allows users to securely store their genetic data on the blockchain and control access to it. With AI algorithms, Shivom analyzes genetic information to generate insights related to disease risk, drug response, and personalized treatment options. This integration of AI and blockchain enables secure and personalized genomics analysis, enhancing healthcare decision-making and patient outcomes.
2. Medicalchain
   Medicalchain is a blockchain platform that enables patients to have control over their health records and securely share them with healthcare providers. By integrating AI, Medicalchain facilitates automated data analysis and decision support. AI algorithms can process patient data stored on the blockchain to identify patterns, detect abnormalities, and provide clinical recommendations. This integration enhances data security, interoperability, and enables personalized care based on comprehensive patient records.
3. Coral Health
   Coral Health is a blockchain-based platform that focuses on improving healthcare data exchange and interoperability. By combining blockchain and AI, Coral Health enables the secure sharing of patient health information across healthcare providers. AI algorithms integrated into the platform can analyze patient data from multiple sources, identify insights, and generate predictive models to assist in early diagnosis, disease management, and treatment planning. This integration fosters collaboration and care coordination among healthcare providers, leading to better patient outcomes.
4. Doc.ai
   Doc.ai is an AI-powered healthcare platform that utilizes blockchain for data security and patient consent management. The platform allows users to

securely store and share their health data, while AI algorithms provide personalized health insights and recommendations. By integrating blockchain, Doc.ai ensures patient privacy, transparency, and control over data sharing. The AI capabilities enhance patient engagement, enabling individuals to make informed decisions about their health and wellness.

5. Nebula Genomics
   Nebula Genomics is a blockchain-powered genomics platform that leverages AI to provide insights into genetic data. The platform allows users to securely store their genomic information on the blockchain and control access to it. AI algorithms analyze the data to identify genetic predispositions, provide ancestry information, and support research initiatives. The integration of AI and blockchain ensures data security and privacy and empowers individuals to contribute to scientific advancements while maintaining control over their genomic data [56,57].

These case studies demonstrate the potential of integrating AI and blockchain in telehealth systems. By combining the power of AI for data analysis, decision support, and personalized care with blockchain for data security, privacy, and interoperability, these platforms are driving innovation and transforming the healthcare landscape.

15.4 Security frameworks for telehealth systems

Ensuring the security and privacy of patient data is of paramount importance in telehealth systems, where healthcare services are delivered remotely through digital technologies. Robust security frameworks are crucial to protect sensitive information, maintaining the trust of patients, and complying with regulatory requirements [58]. The following outline key considerations for security frameworks in telehealth systems.

First, implementing strong access controls and authentication mechanisms is essential to restrict unauthorized access to patient data. Multi-factor authentication, strong passwords, and secure user authentication protocols help verify the identity of healthcare providers and patients accessing telehealth platforms. Role-based access control ensures that individuals only have access to the information necessary for their roles, reducing the risk of unauthorized data exposure.

Encryption is another vital aspect of telehealth security frameworks. Data encryption should be employed to protect data both in transit and at rest. Robust encryption algorithms and protocols safeguard patient information from interception or unauthorized disclosure. Encryption ensures that even if data is compromised, it remains unreadable and unusable to unauthorized individuals, providing an additional layer of protection.

Figure 15.3 shows the different security frameworks, including physical security, information security, operational security, and risk management, which can be used to protect telehealth systems. Measures to protect the physical infrastructure of telehealth systems, such as data centers, servers, and networks, have

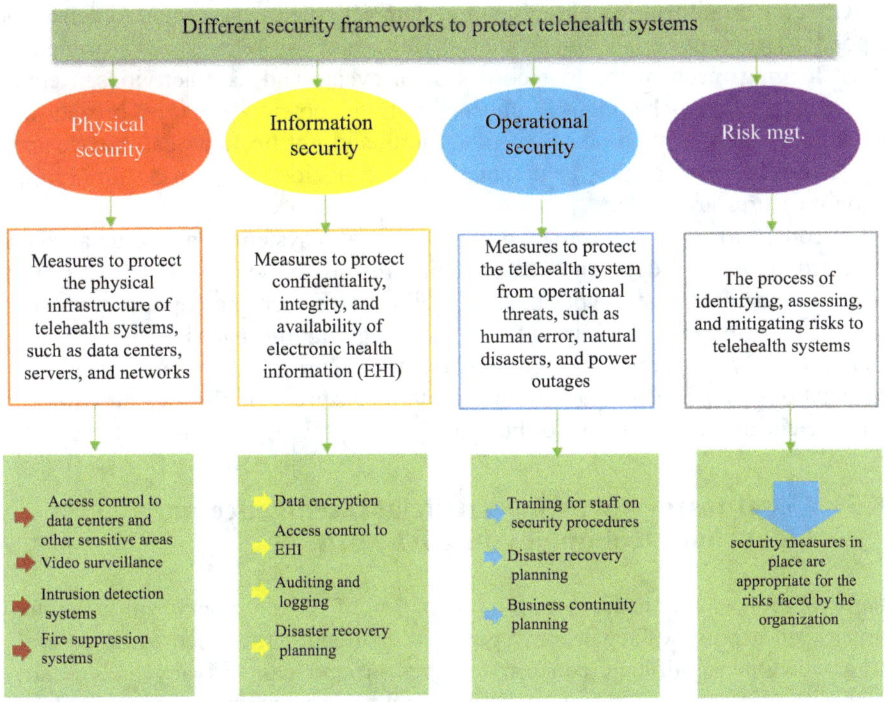

Figure 15.3 Security frameworks to protect telehealth systems

been given. For information security, measures to protect the confidentiality, integrity, and availability of electronic health information (EHI) are provided. Also, measures to protect the telehealth system from operational threats, such as human error, natural disasters, and power outages, are suggested. Lastly, the process of identifying, assessing, and mitigating risks to telehealth systems is also highlighted.

Regular vulnerability assessments and penetration testing should be conducted to identify and address potential security weaknesses in telehealth systems. By proactively assessing vulnerabilities, healthcare organizations can identify and patch security flaws, reducing the risk of data breaches and unauthorized access. Penetration testing simulates real-world attacks to evaluate the resilience of telehealth systems and identify areas for improvement [59].

Compliance with data protection regulations is a crucial aspect of security frameworks for telehealth systems. Regulations such as the Health Insurance Portability and Accountability Act (HIPAA) in the United States and the General Data Protection Regulation (GDPR) in the European Union set forth specific requirements for the handling, storage, and transmission of patient data [58]. Adhering to these regulations helps ensure that patient information is protected and that appropriate measures are in place to maintain confidentiality, integrity, and availability of data.

Ongoing monitoring and logging of system activities are essential to detect and respond to security incidents promptly. Telehealth systems should implement robust logging mechanisms to record system events and user activities. Regular monitoring of logs helps identify unusual patterns, potential security breaches, or unauthorized access attempts. Real-time alerts and notifications can be set up to trigger immediate responses to potential security incidents, ensuring timely mitigation measures are taken.

In conclusion, security frameworks for telehealth systems play a crucial role in safeguarding patient data and maintaining trust in remote healthcare services. Strong access controls, encryption, vulnerability assessments, compliance with data protection regulations, and monitoring and logging mechanisms are key considerations. By implementing comprehensive security frameworks, healthcare organizations can protect patient information, ensure compliance, and foster a secure telehealth environment for both healthcare providers and patients.

15.5 Legal frameworks for artificial intelligence and blockchain technology in telehealth

The revolution of healthcare with the integration of AI and blockchain technology brings forth a range of legal and regulatory challenges that need to be carefully addressed. One significant concern revolves around data privacy and security. Telehealth platforms utilizing AI algorithms rely on vast amounts of patient data to provide accurate diagnoses and personalized treatment recommendations. The legal framework for AI and blockchain technology in telehealth systems is still evolving. However, there are some laws and regulations that apply to the use of AI and blockchain technology in healthcare. They include the following:

1. The Health Insurance Portability and Accountability Act (HIPAA): HIPAA is a federal law [58] that protects the privacy and security of patient health information. AI systems that are used to collect or store patient health information must comply with HIPAA regulations.
2. The Food and Drug Administration (FDA): The FDA is responsible for regulating medical devices, including AI-powered medical devices. AI systems that are used to diagnose or treat patients must be cleared or approved by the FDA before they can be marketed.
3. The European Union General Data Protection Regulation (GDPR): The GDPR is a comprehensive law that regulates the collection and use of personal data in the European Union. AI systems that are used to collect or process the personal data of EU citizens must comply with the GDPR.
4. The Federal Trade Commission (FTC): The Federal Trade Commission is responsible for enforcing consumer protection laws. The Federal Trade Commission has issued guidance on the use of blockchain technology in healthcare and has warned companies that they may be liable for deceptive or unfair practices if they use blockchain technology in a way that violates consumer protection laws.

5. The Securities and Exchange Commission (SEC): The Securities and Exchange Commission is responsible for regulating the securities markets. The Securities and Exchange Commission has issued guidance on the use of blockchain technology in the securities markets and has warned companies that they may be liable for securities law violations if they use blockchain technology in a way that violates securities laws.
6. The California Consumer Privacy Act (CCPA): The California Consumer Privacy Act is a state law that gives consumers more control over their personal data. The California Consumer Privacy Act applies to businesses that collect or sell the personal data of California residents. Businesses that use blockchain technology to collect or process the personal data of California residents must comply with the California Consumer Privacy Act.

Furthermore, the utilization of blockchain technology introduces a decentralized and immutable ledger system, raising questions about data ownership, consent, and the right to be forgotten. Balancing the need for data accessibility and innovation with strict privacy safeguards is a key challenge that regulators and healthcare providers must navigate.

15.5.1 Legal considerations and frameworks

The convergence of AI and blockchain technology holds significant potential to revolutionize various industries. This convergence creates synergies that can enhance data processing, security, and trust. However, combining AI and blockchain also raises important legal considerations that must be addressed to maximize the benefits of this convergence. Legal considerations must be taken into account to ensure the responsible and ethical use of AI and blockchain applications in telehealth.

AI systems can make autonomous decisions, raising questions about accountability and fairness. It is essential to ensure that AI is developed and used in a manner that aligns with legal frameworks, ethical guidelines, and societal norms. This includes addressing biases in data, preventing discrimination, and safeguarding fundamental rights and values. Also, accountability and transparency in AI decision-making are critical aspects that require attention. As AI systems become more sophisticated, it becomes challenging to understand the reasoning behind their decisions. The legal framework should require that AI systems are transparent, explainable, and auditable. This promotes accountability and enables individuals to challenge and seek redress in cases of erroneous or biased decisions made by AI systems.

When it comes to liability and responsibility for AI systems, a comprehensive legal framework is necessary. AI systems can have unintended consequences or make errors, potentially causing harm to individuals or organizations. The allocation of liability in such cases should be clarified, taking into account factors like the level of human control, the nature of the decision-making process, and the foreseeability of harm. Establishing legal mechanisms for assigning responsibility and compensating for damages will help create a fair and accountable AI ecosystem.

The legal implications of blockchain technology arise from its decentralized and immutable nature. Blockchain's distributed ledger system raises questions about jurisdiction, data ownership, and liability. As blockchain networks operate globally, it becomes crucial to assess how existing legal frameworks can be applied to address these challenges. Developing new legal frameworks or adapting existing ones to accommodate blockchain technology is necessary to ensure legal clarity and certainty.

Data privacy and security implications become critical when AI and blockchain converge. AI algorithms require large amounts of data to train and make accurate predictions. Blockchain's transparent and immutable nature can potentially compromise data privacy. Striking a balance between data privacy and the transparency benefits of blockchain is crucial. Techniques such as data anonymization and encryption, coupled with robust access controls and consent mechanisms, should be implemented to protect sensitive information in AI–blockchain systems. Compliance with data protection regulations and best practices is paramount to building trust and ensuring the ethical handling of personal data.

Smart contracts, powered by AI, offer immense potential in automating transactions and streamlining processes within blockchain networks. AI algorithms can analyze contract terms, extract relevant information, and enable automated execution based on predefined rules. However, legal considerations arise concerning the legal validity and enforceability of smart contracts. Ensuring that smart contracts comply with legal requirements, such as offer, acceptance, and consideration, is essential. The transparency and traceability of blockchain can enhance the auditability and transparency of smart contract performance, contributing to legal enforceability.

The convergence of AI and blockchain also presents ethical and regulatory challenges. AI algorithms can introduce biases and discriminatory outcomes, which can be amplified within blockchain systems if not carefully addressed. Transparency, explainability, and accountability of AI algorithms become even more crucial when integrated with blockchain [60]. Regulatory frameworks should encompass both AI and blockchain technologies, addressing their combined risks and ensuring responsible and ethical practices. Collaboration between industry stakeholders, policymakers, and technology experts is vital to develop guidelines and standards that govern the ethical use of AI in blockchain applications.

By proactively addressing legal challenges and establishing a supportive legal environment, implementing robust data protection measures, ensuring legal compliance, fostering transparency and accountability, and engaging in ethical and regulatory discussions, we can unlock the full potential of AI-Blockchain convergence and build a responsible and sustainable future for these transformative technologies.

15.5.2 Recommended legal frameworks

As the fields of AI and blockchain technology continue to evolve, it becomes imperative to establish legal frameworks that promote innovation while ensuring

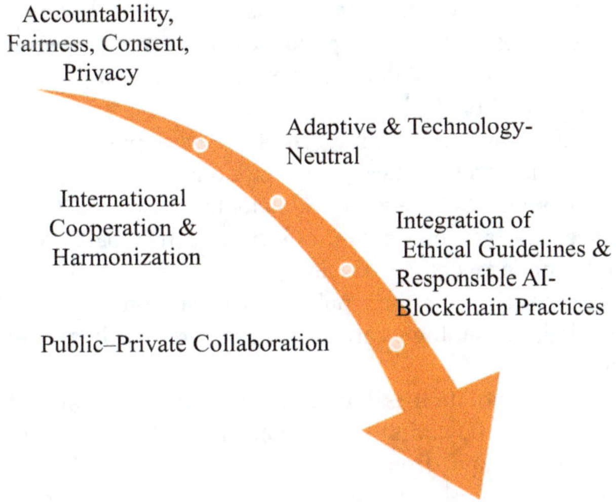

Figure 15.4 Five key components for AI and blockchain legal framework.

ethical and responsible use. Figure 15.4 outlines five key recommendations for legal frameworks concerning AI and blockchain in telehealth systems. The recommendations can guide the development of effective legal frameworks for AI and blockchain in telehealth systems.

First and foremost, key principles encompassing transparency, accountability, fairness, consent, and privacy should underpin AI and blockchain legal frameworks. Transparency ensures that AI and blockchain systems are explainable and understandable, allowing individuals to make informed decisions. Accountability holds individuals and organizations responsible for the actions and decisions made by AI and blockchain systems. Fairness addresses concerns related to bias, discrimination, and social impact. Patients should give their consent, which should be specific and informed before their data is used in AI-blockchain systems. Privacy safeguards personal information and ensures data protection. These principles serve as a foundation for creating comprehensive and balanced legal frameworks.

Adaptive and technology-neutral approaches are essential when designing AI and blockchain legal frameworks. Given the rapid pace of technological advancements, the frameworks should be flexible and adaptable to accommodate evolving technologies. Technology neutrality ensures that frameworks do not become obsolete or hinder innovation. It allows for the inclusion of future developments and emerging technologies without the need for constant legislative updates. Frameworks should focus on the functions and risks associated with AI and blockchain in telehealth, enabling a more agile and forward-looking approach.

International cooperation and harmonization efforts are critical for the development of effective AI and blockchain frameworks. As these technologies transcend national boundaries, collaboration between countries is essential to establish consistent and interoperable legal frameworks. Harmonization efforts can foster international standards, promote regulatory consistency, and streamline compliance requirements. Sharing best practices, experiences, and expertise across jurisdictions can create a global ecosystem that encourages innovation and facilitates the responsible use of AI and blockchain.

Ethical guidelines and responsible AI–blockchain practices should be integrated into legal frameworks. Ethical considerations are paramount in the development and deployment of AI and blockchain technologies. Guidelines should address issues, such as bias mitigation, algorithmic transparency, accountability mechanisms, and human oversight. By incorporating ethical principles into legal frameworks, policymakers can foster public trust and confidence, while ensuring that AI and blockchain technologies are developed and used in a manner that aligns with societal values.

Public–private collaboration is crucial for the development and implementation of effective policy frameworks. The complex and interdisciplinary nature of AI and blockchain requires input from a wide range of stakeholders, including government agencies, industry players, academic institutions, civil society organizations, and the public. Collaborative efforts can ensure that policies are informed by diverse perspectives, address the needs and concerns of different stakeholders, and promote responsible innovation. Establishing platforms for dialogue, consultation, and collaboration between the public and private sectors can drive the development of inclusive and effective legal frameworks.

15.5.3 Regulatory frameworks

Different jurisdictions have taken diverse approaches to regulate AI and blockchain [58]. Some countries have adopted sector-specific regulations that address AI and blockchain technology applications in areas such as healthcare, finance, and transportation. Others have focused on broader principles-based frameworks that emphasize ethical considerations, transparency, and accountability. Table 15.5 presents the key points and recommendations for regulating AI and blockchain technology, especially as it relates to telehealth systems. By studying these regulations, policymakers can gain valuable insights into the approaches that have been taken and their effectiveness in addressing the challenges posed by AI and blockchain technology. Some of the key recommendations include diverse approaches to regulation, global harmonization efforts, addressing blockchain's unique challenges, harmonizing blockchain regulations, collaboration with stakeholders, and continuous monitoring and evaluation.

However, regulating AI and blockchain technology poses several challenges due to their rapid evolution and complexity. Striking a balance between fostering innovation and ensuring compliance with existing legal frameworks is crucial to creating a conducive regulatory environment for AI and blockchain technology.

AI systems continually learn and adapt, making it difficult to define static regulations. Additionally, the global nature of AI development and deployment necessitates harmonization efforts and cross-border collaboration to avoid regulatory fragmentation and enable consistent ethical and legal standards. Blockchain

Table 15.5 Recommendations for regulating artificial intelligence and blockchain technology

Key points and recommendations	Explanation
Diverse approaches to regulation	Different jurisdictions have adopted sector-specific or principles-based frameworks.
Challenges in regulating AI and blockchain	Rapid evolution and complexity require a balance between innovation and legal compliance.
Global harmonization efforts	Cross-border collaboration is essential to avoid regulatory fragmentation and set standards.
Addressing blockchain's unique challenges	Legal frameworks may need adaptation for data privacy, intellectual property, and more.
Effective AI & blockchain regulation	Recommendations for balanced, transparent, and privacy-respecting regulatory frameworks.
Harmonizing blockchain regulations	Establishing international standards for consistency and interoperability in the ecosystem.
Collaboration with stakeholders	Involving industry experts, academia, and civil society for comprehensive regulations.
Continuous monitoring and evaluation	Regular assessments to adapt to technological advancements and address emerging risks.

technology introduces new concepts and challenges to traditional legal frameworks. Aspects such as data privacy, intellectual property, consumer protection, and financial regulations may require adaptation to accommodate blockchain's decentralized and transparent nature. Some countries have implemented comprehensive frameworks that cover various aspects of blockchain, such as digital asset offerings, cryptocurrency exchanges, and smart contracts.

To create effective and adaptive AI and blockchain technology regulations, certain recommendations can be considered. Firstly, regulations should strike a balance between fostering innovation and safeguarding ethical and societal concerns. Flexibility should be incorporated to allow for innovation and experimentation while ensuring safeguards are in place. Second, regulatory frameworks should promote transparency and accountability in AI decision-making processes. This can be achieved through requirements for explainability, auditability, and documentation of artificial intelligence systems. Thirdly, regulatory measures should encourage responsible data governance and address privacy concerns. Robust data protection mechanisms and consent frameworks should be implemented to ensure individuals' rights are respected. Fourthly, harmonizing and standardizing blockchain regulations is also an important goal to create consistency and facilitate interoperability in the global blockchain ecosystem. Harmonization efforts can help streamline compliance requirements, reduce legal complexity, and encourage cross-border collaborations. Establishing international standards for areas such as data privacy, digital identity, smart contracts, and interoperability can provide a common framework that fosters trust and enables seamless interaction between blockchain networks.

Moreover, regulatory authorities should actively collaborate with industry experts, academia, and civil society to develop comprehensive regulations. Stakeholder engagement facilitates a more holistic understanding of AI's and blockchain's implications and encourages diverse perspectives in the regulatory decision-making process. Finally, continuous monitoring and evaluation of artificial intelligence regulations are necessary to assess their effectiveness, adapt to technological advancements, and address emerging risks and challenges.

15.6 Lessons learned and future directions

The chapter provides valuable insights into the legal frameworks for AI and blockchain technology in telehealth systems. By focusing on the lessons learned and exploring future directions such as governance models, risk assessment, and international cooperation, it can be ensured that AI and blockchain technologies in telehealth are deployed responsibly, ethically, and in a manner that benefits patients, healthcare providers, and society as a whole.

Some of the lessons learned and future directions are highlighted in this section. They include the following ones:

1. The history and evolution of telehealth systems have been learned.
2. The key promising AI and blockchain technology-based security frameworks to support telehealth systems have also been learned.
3. Regulatory compliance: One important lesson is the significance of regulatory compliance. As AI and blockchain technologies advance in telehealth systems, it has become crucial to establish clear legal frameworks to ensure data security, patient privacy, and ethical use of these technologies. Learning from existing regulations in healthcare and technology sectors, such as Health Insurance Portability and Accountability Act (HIPAA) and General Data Protection Regulation (GDPR), comprehensive frameworks that address the unique challenges posed by AI and blockchain in telehealth are developed.
4. Data governance and interoperability: Another lesson learned is the need for robust data governance and interoperability standards. Telehealth systems incorporating AI and blockchain generate vast amounts of data. Establishing guidelines for data collection, storage, access, and sharing is critical for enabling seamless collaboration and information exchange across different healthcare providers and systems. By focusing on standardization and interoperability, the effective utilization of these technologies in telehealth can be ensured.
5. Ethical considerations: Ethical considerations must be at the forefront of any legal framework related to AI and blockchain in telehealth. As these technologies become more prevalent, addressing issues such as algorithmic bias, transparency, and the responsible use of patient data will be crucial. By integrating ethical guidelines into the legal frameworks, potential risks can be

mitigated and ensure that these technologies are used in a manner that respects patient rights and societal values.

Looking ahead, there are several exciting directions to explore in the legal frameworks for AI and blockchain in telehealth systems. The potential future directions to consider include the following:

1. Governance models: Developing governance models that involve multi-stakeholder collaboration, including regulatory bodies, technology providers, healthcare professionals, and patient representatives, can help foster transparency, inclusivity, and accountability in the implementation of AI and blockchain technologies.
2. Risk assessment and auditing: Incorporating risk assessment frameworks and auditing mechanisms specific to AI and blockchain can help ensure compliance, identify potential risks, and establish trust in telehealth systems. This will be crucial as these technologies mature and are used to make critical decisions in healthcare.
3. International cooperation: Encouraging international cooperation and harmonization of legal frameworks will facilitate the global adoption and interoperability of AI and blockchain technologies in telehealth. Collaboration among countries can help address cross-border data sharing and privacy concerns and promote a more inclusive approach to healthcare innovation. In conclusion, the legal frameworks for AI and blockchain in telehealth systems can learn valuable lessons from regulatory compliance, data governance, and ethical considerations.

15.7 Conclusions and future scope

Legal frameworks for AI and blockchain technology in telehealth systems are crucial for ensuring the governance, privacy, security, and accountability of these technologies. The adoption of AI and blockchain in telehealth has the potential to revolutionize healthcare but also presents unique legal and regulatory challenges. Existing healthcare, data protection, and medical device regulations and legal frameworks may not adequately cover the implications of these technologies. Some far-reaching legal and regulatory framework recommendations have been given.

The recommendation addresses data protection, privacy, security, transparency, and accountability, among others. Furthermore, standards and certification processes should be established to ensure the safety and effectiveness of AI algorithms and blockchain systems. Collaboration between stakeholders, including governments, healthcare providers, technology developers, and legal experts, is essential for responsible innovation. Continuous monitoring and evaluation of legal frameworks, international cooperation, and harmonization are also necessary. By implementing these recommendations, legal frameworks can support the responsible and beneficial use of AI and blockchain in telehealth while safeguarding patient rights and ensuring data privacy and security.

References

[1] P. Tagde, S. Tagde, T. Bhattacharya, *et al.*, "Blockchain and artificial intelligence technology in e-Health," *Environmental Science and Pollution Research International*, vol. 28, pp. 52810–52831, 2021.

[2] L. Schwamm, "Telehealth: Seven strategies to successfully implement disruptive technology and transform health care," *Health Affairs*, vol. 33, no. 2, pp. 200–206, 2014.

[3] C. Kuziemsky, A. Maeder, O. John, *et al.* "Role of artificial intelligence within the telehealth domain official 2019 yearbook contribution by the members of IMIA telehealth working group," *Political Science*, vol. 28, no. 1, pp. 35–40, 2019.

[4] R.W. Ahmad, K. Salah, R. Jayaraman, I. Yaqoob, S. Ellahham and M. Omar, "The role of blockchain technology in telehealth and telemedicine," *International Journal of Medical Informatics*, vol. 148, pp. 104399–104399, 2020.

[5] R. Selvanambi, S. Bhutani and K. Veauli, "Security and privacy for electronic healthcare records using AI in blockchain," in *Applications of Artificial Intelligence for Smart Technology*, IGI Global, 2021, pp. 90–102.

[6] C. Kuner, L. Bygrave and C. Docksey, Background and Evolution of the EU General Data Protection Regulation (GDPR), in *The EU General Data Protection Regulation (GDPR): A Commentary*, Oxford Academic, 2020, pp. 1–47.

[7] T. Floyd-Carney, "Health insurance portability and accountability Act," *Definitions*, 2020.

[8] S. H. Aronson, "The Lancet on the telephone 1876–1975," *Medical History*, vol. 21, no. 1, pp. 69–87, 1977.

[9] R. L. Bashshur, G. W. Shannon, E. A. Krupinski, *et al.* "National telemedicine initiatives: essential to healthcare reform," *Telemedicine and e-Health*, vol. 15, no. 6, pp. 600–610, 2009.

[10] R. Mishra and K. V. Pallavi, "Decentralized blockchain based ISP networks," in *Advances in Intelligent Systems and Technologies*, Springer Singapore, Singapore, Springer Singapore, Singapore, 2022.

[11] J. Winters, "Videoconferencing and telehealth technologies can provide a reliable approach to remote assessment and teaching without compromising quality," *Journal of Cardiovascular Nursing,* vol. 22, no. 1, pp. 51–57, 2007.

[12] S. Mohammed and A. J. Alzubaidi, "Remote Patient Monitoring (RPM)," in *Encyclopedia of the UN Sustainable Development Goals*, Elsevier, United Kingdom, 2019.

[13] M. Cowie, J. Blomster, L. Curtis, *et al.*, "Electronic health records to facilitate clinical research," *Clinical Research in Cardiology*, vol. 106, pp. 1–9, 2016.

[14] E. Dorsey and E. Topol, "State of Telehealth," *New England Journal of Medicine*, vol. 375, no. 2, pp. 154–611, 2016.

[15] L. Omrčen, H. Leventić, K. Romić and I. Galić, "Integration of blockchain and AI in EHR sharing: A survey," *International Symposium ELMAR*, pp. 155–160, 2021.
[16] M. Kimura, P. Croll, B. Li, C. P. Wong, S. Gogia, A. Faud and Y. C. Li, "Survey on medical records and EHR in Asia-Pacific region," *Methods of information in medicine*, vol. 50, no. 04, pp. 386–391, 2011.
[17] M. Webber, S. Wilk, R. Pirruccello and J. Aiken, "Telecommunication of images in the practice of diagnostic radiology," *Radiology*, vol. 109, no. 1, pp. 71–74, 1973.
[18] M. A. Skliar and G. T. Chevtaev, "[Automatic transmission of patient medical record data via a telephone communication channel]," *Meditsinskaia tekhnika*, no. 1, pp. 34–37, 1981.
[19] B. Kane and S. Luz, "Probing the use and value of video for multi-disciplinary medical teams in teleconference," in *19th IEEE Symposium on Computer-Based Medical Systems (CBMS'06)*, pp. 518–523, 2006.
[20] A. Orlova, M. Dunnagan, T. Finitzo, *et al.* "An electronic health record – public health (EHR-PH) system prototype for interoperability in 21st century healthcare systems," *American Medical Informatics Association Annual Symposium*, pp. 575–579, 2005.
[21] A. Broderick and D. Lindeman, "Case studies in telehealth adoption—scaling telehealth programs: Lessons from early adopters," in *Broderick 2013CaseSI*, 2013.
[22] S. Adibi, "Link technologies and BlackBerry Mobile Health (mHealth) solutions: A review," *IEEE Transactions on Information Technology in Biomedicine*, vol. 16, pp. 586–597, 2012.
[23] M. G. D and A. Prentza, "Machine learning in medical applications," in *Machine Learning in Medical Applications*, Magoulas2001MachineLI, pp. 300–307, 2001.
[24] A. Zeeshan, M. K, Z. Saman and D. Xinqi, "Artificial intelligence with multi-functional machine learning platform development for better healthcare and precision medicine," *The Journal of Biological Databases and Curation*, vol. 2020, pp. baaa010, 2020.
[25] R. Wootton, N. Patil, R. Scott and K. Ho, "Telehealth in the developing world," *Wootton2019TelehealthIT*, vol. 16, no. 2, pp. 140–141, 2019.
[26] A. R. Gawai, G. Kumar, S. Upadhye and A. Kulkarni, "Artificial Intelligence in Healthcare/Telemedicine," *International Journal of Innovative Research in Technology*, 2020.
[27] A. Singh, R. Jalota and V. Gupta, "Blockchain technology in cryptocurrency: A review," in *2022 International Conference on Machine Learning, Big Data, Cloud and Parallel Computing (COM-IT-CON)*, 2022.
[28] K. Sheela and C. Priya, "Enabling the efficiency of blockchain technology in Tele-Healthcare with Enhanced EMR," in *2020 International Conference on Computer Science, Engineering and Applications (ICCSEA)*, 2020.

[29] S. Jayakumar, V. Sounderajah, P. Normahani, *et al.*, "Quality assessment standards in artificial intelligence diagnostic accuracy systematic reviews: A meta-research study," *NPJ Digital Medicine*, vol. 5, no. 1, pp. 11, 2022.

[30] C. W. Rundle, P. Hollingsworth and R. P. Dellavalle, "Artificial intelligence in dermatology," *Clinics in Dermatology*, vol. 37 4, pp. 657–666, 2021.

[31] M. Ha, S. Lim and H. Ko, "Wearable and flexible sensors for user-interactive health-monitoring devices," *Journal of Materials Chemistry. B*, vol. 6, no. 24, pp. 4043–4064, 2018.

[32] A. Spournias, P. Bountas, E. Faliagka, *et al.*, "Smart health monitoring using AI techniques in AAL environments," in *Mediterranean Conference on Embedded Computing*, 2021.

[33] H. S. Adnan, S. Matthews, M. Hackl, *et al.*, "Human centered AI design for clinical monitoring and data management," *European Journal of Public Health*, vol. 30, no. 5, 2020.

[34] M. Joshi, A. Pal and M. Sankarasubbu, "Federated learning for healthcare domain – pipeline, applications and challenges," *ACM Transactions on Computing for Healthcare*, vol. 3, pp. 1–36, 2022.

[35] B. Kavitha and C. R. Murthy, "Chatbot for healthcare system using Artificial Intelligence," *International Research Journal of Modernization in Engineering Technology and Science*, vol. 5, no. 3, 2019.

[36] N. Pawar, "Decision tree based health prediction system," *International Journal for Research in Applied Science and Engineering Technology*, vol. 8, no. 7, 2020.

[37] A. Pandit and A. Garg, "Artificial neural networks in healthcare: A systematic review," *Confluence*, pp. 1–6, 2021.

[38] M. Usama, B. Ahmad, W. Xiao, M. S. Hossain and M. Ghulam, "Self-attention based recurrent convolutional neural network for disease prediction using healthcare data," *Computer Methods and Programs in Biomedicine*, pp. 105–191, 2019.

[39] G.-H. Shin, Y.-S. Kweon and M. Lee, "Predicting the transition from short-term to long-term memory based on deep neural network," in *Balkan Conference in Informatics*, 2020.

[40] X. Yi, E. Walia and P. Babyn, "Generative adversarial network in medical imaging: A review," *Medical Image Analysis*, vol. 58, pp. 101552, 2018.

[41] A. Coronato, M. Naeem, G. Pietro and G. Paragliola, "Reinforcement learning for intelligent healthcare applications: A survey," *Artificial Intelligence in Medicine*, vol. 109, pp. 101964, 2020.

[42] Y. F. Safri, R. Arifudin and M. A. Muslim, "K-Nearest neighbor and naive Bayes classifier algorithm in determining the classification of healthy card Indonesia giving to the poor," *Scientific Journal of Informatics*, vol. 5, no. 1, pp. 18, 2018.

[43] Y. Liao, Y. Xiang and M. Wang, "Health assessment and prognostics based on higher-order hidden semi-Markov models," *Naval Research Logistics*, vol. 68, no. 2, pp. 259–276, 2020.

[44] A. Nada and Z. I. K. Alqahtani, "Gaussian mixture models based on principal components and applications," *Mathematical Problems in Engineering*, vol. 2020, no. 1, pp. 1–13, 2020.
[45] A. Gaikwad, "Overview of blockchain," *International Journal for Research in Applied Science and Engineering*, 2020.
[46] W. J. Gordon and C. Catalini, "Blockchain technology for healthcare: Facilitating the transition to patient-driven interoperability," *Computational and Structural Biotechnology Journal*, vol. 16, pp. 224–230, 2018.
[47] R. Ahmad, K. Salah, R. Jayaraman, I. Yaqoob, S. Ellahham and M. A. Omar, "The role of blockchain technology in telehealth and telemedicine," *International Journal of Medical Informatics*, vol. 148, pp. 104399–104399, 2020.
[48] H. R. Hasan, K. Salah, R. Jayaraman, I. Yaqoob, M. A. Omar and S. Ellahham, "Blockchain-enabled telehealth services using smart contracts," *Institute of Electrical and Electronics Engineers*, vol. 9, pp. 151944–151959, 2021.
[49] S.-J. Wu, R.-D. Chiang, S.-H. Chang and W.-T. Chang, "An interactive telecare system enhanced with IoT technology," *IEEE Pervasive Computing*, vol. 16, pp. 62–69, 2017.
[50] K. P. Satamraju and B. Malarkodi, "Proof of concept of scalable integration of internet of things and blockchain in healthcare," *Sensors (Basel),* vol. 20, no. 5, pp. 1389, 2020.
[51] A. Kulkarni, L. Joshi, Y. More, A. Mudaliar and D. Chaudhari, "A review on decentralization in healthcare systems using blockchain," *International Journal of Creative Research Thoughts (IJCRT),* vol. 10, no. 4, pp. 2320–2882, 2022.
[52] K. Sheela and C. Priya, "Enabling the efficiency of blockchain technology in Tele-Healthcare with Enhanced EMR," *2020 International Conference on Computer Science, Engineering and Applications (ICCSEA)*, pp. 1–6, 2020.
[53] T. Hewa, A. Braeken, M. Ylianttila and M. Liyanage, "Multi-access edge computing and blockchain-based secure telehealth system connected with 5G and IoT," *Global Communications Conference*, pp. 1–6, 2020.
[54] H. Huang, X. Sun, F. Xiao, P. Zhu and W. Wang, "Blockchain-based eHealth system for auditable EHRs manipulation in cloud environments," *Journal of Parallel and Distributed Computing*, vol. 148, pp. 46–57, 2021.
[55] R. Bouderhem, "AI regulation in healthcare: New paradigms for a legally binding treaty under the World Health Organization," in *2022 14th International Conference on Computational Intelligence and Communication Networks (CICN)*, 2022.
[56] R. L. Kumar, Y. Wang, T. Poongodi and A. L. Imoize, *Internet of Things, Artificial Intelligence and Blockchain Technology*. Cham: Springer, 2021.
[57] L. k. Ramasamy, F. K. KP, A. L. Imoize, J. O. Ogbebor, S. Kadry and S. Rho, "Blockchain-based wireless sensor networks for malicious node detection: A survey," *Institute of Electrical and Electronics Engineers*, vol. 9, pp. 128765–128785, 2021.

[58] A. Musa, "Legal frameworks for security schemes in wireless communication systems. In: security and privacy schemes for dense 6G wireless communication networks. A. L. Imoize, C. Meshram, D. Do, S. Kadry and L. Muthukaruppan (Eds.)," *Published by The Institution of Engineering and Technology (IET)*. ISBN: 978-1-83953-663-2, pp. 423–444, 2023.
[59] A. L. Imoize, P. A. Gbadega, H. I. Obakhena, D. O. Irabor, K. V. N. Kavitha and C. Chakraborty, "Artificial Intelligence-enabled Internet of Medical Things for COVID-19 pandemic data management," *Explainable Artificial Intelligence in Medical Decision Support Systems*, pp. 357–380, 2022.
[60] A. L. Imoize, J. Hemanth, D. T. Do and S. N. "Explainable Artificial Intelligence in Medical Decision Support Systems," IET, 2023.

Chapter 16

Application of artificial intelligence and blockchain technology in telehealth systems: innovation, technology, challenges, and prospects

Malik Adeiza Rufai[1], Abubakar Aliyu[1], Fati Oiza Ochepa[1] and Francisca Onaolapo Oladipo[2]

The authors discuss the possible advantages and challenges of integrating these revolutionary innovations into healthcare in this chapter, which covers the technical issues of using blockchain and artificial intelligence (AI) in telehealth systems. The authors started by going through the current status of telehealth and how blockchain and AI might improve its capabilities, such as enhancing diagnosis accuracy, enabling remote patient monitoring, and guaranteeing data confidentiality and privacy. The authors emphasize how blockchain and AI have the potential to revolutionize telemedicine by raising standards of care, boosting productivity, and cutting costs. They go over how AI can be used to examine vast volumes of medical data to spot patterns and trends and create prediction models that can help medical professionals make better choices. However, this chapter discusses the potential uses of blockchain in telehealth, including enabling safe and transparent patient data sharing, automating office operations, and making payments and reimbursements for medical services easier. The following section of the chapter digs into the technical details of integrating blockchain and AI into telehealth systems, including data processing, storage, and transfer. The technological difficulties in adopting blockchain and AI in telemedicine include the requirement for interoperability guidelines to make sure that various systems can effectively communicate with one another and the significance of data standardization to guarantee consistency and accuracy in healthcare data. This chapter will also cover other topics, including scalability and security. The chapter concludes with a call to action for governments and healthcare professionals to embrace the opportunities of blockchain and AI in telehealth while also being aware of the associated technical and ethical issues involved.

[1]Department of Computer Science, Faculty of Science, Federal University Lokoja, Nigeria
[2]Department of Computer Science, Faculty of Science, Thomas Adewumi University, Nigeria

16.1 Introduction

The delivery and experience of medical services have changed dramatically in recent years as a result of technological breakthroughs. Artificial intelligence (AI) and blockchain, two of the most promising technical frontiers, have the unmatched potential to change patient care and healthcare efficiency when incorporated into telehealth systems. Blockchain's decentralized, tamper-resistant ledger, and AI's cognitive capabilities work in concert to address long-standing healthcare difficulties while creating new opportunities for better patient outcomes in terms of diagnosis and treatment [1]. Telehealth, or the remote provision of healthcare services, has changed the game by cutting across geographical boundaries and dismantling access restrictions. Telehealth has the potential to change healthcare into a more patient-centric, data-driven, and secure ecosystem by leveraging the power of AI and blockchain [2]. The incorporation of blockchain and AI in telehealth systems has emerged as a paradigm shift that promises to revolutionize the healthcare industry [1]. Blockchain, with its safe and decentralized data management, and AI, with its sophisticated data analysis and decision-making skills, have the potential to improve telemedicine services and promote patient-centered care. This chapter examines the difficulties and opportunities involved in integrating AI and blockchain in telehealth systems, highlighting the possibilities and problems that remain [3].

Despite the immense potential of AI and blockchain in telehealth, a number of significant obstacles prevent their widespread use [4]. The digitization of medical records exposes sensitive patient information to possible dangers, making data security and privacy a major concern. To protect patient data, it is critical to implement strong data protection mechanisms and integrate blockchain's immutable ledger [5]. The successful integration of AI algorithms with current telemedicine platforms is one of the key technological difficulties in telehealth implementation. Healthcare providers must make sure AI-driven solutions integrate into clinical workflows without a hitch, increasing speed and precision in patient diagnosis and treatment [6]. To keep patients' faith and confidence in telehealth services, the ethical ramifications of AI-driven decision-making must be carefully considered [7]. The interoperability of various telehealth platforms and tools continues to be a major barrier. To build a harmonious environment that enables the seamless interchange of medical information across healthcare providers and institutions, AI and blockchain must be combined effortlessly [8]. Scalability issues arise when telehealth use soars, necessitating careful resource management and optimization to handle an increase in users and data quantities. The ethical application of AI and blockchain in telehealth must also be governed by regulatory frameworks, which must balance innovation with adherence to healthcare standards and provide protection from any liabilities [9].

Beyond the difficulties, it is certain that telehealth use of AI and blockchain will revolutionize healthcare. By enhancing data security and integrity, blockchain's decentralized architecture fosters confidence between patients and providers. This holds the prospect of offering personalized and precise healthcare interventions, boosting patient outcomes and treatment efficacy. It works in conjunction with AI-powered data analytics [10]. The tamper-proof smart contracts of the blockchain have the ability to automate administrative procedures, improving the efficiency and openness of billing and payment systems. Additionally, remote patient monitoring made possible by AI-driven gadgets can revolutionize the management of chronic diseases by enabling early diagnosis of health issues [11]. Healthcare practitioners are given evidence-based suggestions via AI decision support systems, enhancing their knowledge and enabling data-driven treatment choices. The use of technology can also significantly lower healthcare expenses by preventing fraud and maintaining the integrity of insurance claims and billing [12].

In this chapter, we embark on a journey into the realm of AI and blockchain technology, exploring its profound impact on telehealth systems. The integration of these cutting-edge technologies presents a compelling opportunity to overcome traditional barriers and create a future where healthcare is accessible, efficient, and secure. As we navigate through the technological challenges and prospects in this dynamic landscape, it is evident that the adoption of AI and blockchain in telehealth heralds a transformative era for healthcare. By leveraging these innovations responsibly and collaboratively, we have the potential to usher in an age of patient-centricity and data-driven care, making a lasting impact on global health outcomes.

16.1.1 Chapter contributions

The main contributions of the chapter can be outlined as follows:

1. The chapter provides a thorough examination of the technological challenges associated with the adoption of AI and blockchain in telehealth systems. It identifies and discusses key hurdles such as data interoperability, scalability, data privacy and security, regulatory compliance, and integration with legacy systems.
2. The chapter delves into the promising prospects that AI and blockchain offer in the telehealth domain. It highlights the potential transformative applications of these technologies, including enhanced diagnostics and personalized treatment, secure health data exchange, remote patient monitoring, and advancements in telemedicine and teleconsultation services.
3. The chapter suggests ways to get beyond the cited technological obstacles in order to promote successful adoption. It makes recommendations for solutions, including the adoption of governance frameworks and moral standards, standardized application programming interfaces (APIs) and data formats for data integration, cloud computing for scalability, and encryption technologies for data privacy.
4. The chapter discusses ethical issues while applying AI and blockchain in telehealth, acknowledging the importance of moral AI and objective algorithms. In order to promote patient-centric care, it underlines the significance of avoiding AI biases and maintaining a balance between AI-driven decision-making and human knowledge.

5. The chapter investigates how AI and blockchain might close the healthcare gap in neglected and emerging areas, advancing global health equity and expanding access to specialized medical treatment.
6. The chapter stresses the value of interdisciplinary cooperation between medical experts, data scientists, and computer developers. It demonstrates the value of incorporating AI as a tool to assist human knowledge, fostering a patient-centered and sympathetic approach to telemedicine.
7. The chapter promotes international regulatory harmonization and the creation of industry standards to enable seamless collaboration and compliance with data protection rules while acknowledging the difficulties of cross-border data transmission.

By offering a thorough study of the technological difficulties and opportunities presented by the use of AI and blockchain, the chapter makes a contribution to the field of telehealth. To help healthcare stakeholders, policymakers, and academics realize the full potential of these technologies and transform healthcare delivery and patient outcomes, it provides insightful analysis and recommendations.

16.1.2 Chapter organization

This chapter is ordered as follows: Section 16.1 consists of the introduction which provides an overview of Adoption of AI and Blockchain Technology in Telehealth systems: Technological Challenges and Prospects. Section 16.2 conducts a comprehensive review on the Adoption of AI and Blockchain Technology in Telehealth systems. Section 16.3 describes the method used in conducting this chapter work. Section 16.4 explores the technological Challenges in Adoption of AI and Blockchain in Telehealth Systems. Section 16.5 describes the Prospects of AI and Blockchain in Telehealth Systems. Section 16.6 outlines the lessons learned from the chapter. Section 16.7 suggests some recommendations derived from the chapter, and lastly, Section 16.8 concludes the chapter.

16.2 Related works

The adoption of blockchain and AI technology in telehealth has enormous promise for changing the way medical services are provided as the landscape of healthcare continues to change. These revolutionary technologies provide creative answers to long-standing healthcare concerns, from individualized care and safe health data interchange to remote patient monitoring and improved medical research. In this chapter, we examine the technical difficulties and potential benefits of implementing blockchain and AI in telehealth systems. We conducted a thorough literature analysis, examining academic journals, conference papers, books, and reliable sources to gather important insights into the present status of research and application. We were able to pinpoint important publications that advance our knowledge of the topic thanks to the literature study.

A list of related works is included in Table 16.1, along with a brief summary of the research done and the limitations of each study. These studies

Table 16.1 Relevant works on the adoption of blockchain and artificial intelligence in telehealth systems: technological challenges and prospects

References	Work done	Limitation
[13]	Investigated telehealth's use of AI for remote diagnosis and individualized treatment approaches.	Limited attention paid to the privacy concerns and ethical dilemmas raised by AI in telehealth.
[14]	Examined the potential of blockchain for interoperability between healthcare systems and safe health data exchange.	Underestimated the difficulties with scaling and the computing requirements of blockchain in telehealth.
[15]	Conducted a case study on how AI-driven chatbots were implemented in teleconsultation services.	The applicability and long-term effects of AI-driven chatbots in various healthcare contexts are only partially examined.
[16]	Investigated how blockchain could be used in telemedicine to handle consent and secure medical records.	There hasn't been much discussion of the interoperability problems in international telehealth operations.
[17]	Examined the use of AI algorithms in telemedicine applications for disease diagnosis and prognosis.	The study did not analyze the potential biases and fairness issues in AI algorithms impacting patient outcomes.
[18]	Examined how blockchain could be used for data security and integrity in remote patient monitoring.	The study avoided discussing the difficulties and regulatory ramifications of using blockchain in telemedicine.
[19]	The study avoided discussing the difficulties and regulatory ramifications of using blockchain in telemedicine.	The study did not examine potential data processing delays and bottlenecks in the integration of AI and blockchain.
[20]	The study avoided discussing the difficulties and regulatory ramifications of using blockchain in telemedicine.	Virtually no consideration of how biases in AI systems might affect the accuracy of diagnostics.
[21]	Examined the use of blockchain to manage patient permission for telehealth data sharing.	The difficulties of scaling up the management of numerous patient consent transactions were not covered by the study.
[22]	Examined how blockchain may improve data integrity and trust in IoT telehealth equipment.	The possible costs associated with deploying blockchain in IoT devices with limited resources were not examined in the study.
[23]	Investigated how AI could improve medication management and compliance in telehealth settings.	There isn't enough attention paid to potential obstacles to integrating AI-driven medication management with current healthcare workflows.
[24]	Examined how blockchain and artificial intelligence may enhance telehealth data analytics for epidemiological studies.	The assessment lacks a thorough examination of how possible AI algorithmic biases can affect epidemiological conclusions.

(Continues)

Table 16.1 (*Continued*)

References	Work done	Limitation
[25]	Examined how AI and blockchain could be used in telemedicine to detect chronic diseases early.	There hasn't been much discussion of the possible difficulties in combining AI and blockchain to detect diseases in real time.
[26]	Examined the application of blockchain to telehealth data exchange and patient-controlled health records.	There has been little research done on potential legal and regulatory issues with patient-controlled health records.
[25]	Examined how AI and blockchain could be used to secure the flow of telehealth data in the context of IoT-enabled healthcare.	Limited attention paid to the integration of AI and blockchain in telehealth IoT devices' possible performance overheads.
[17]	Explored telemedicine's use of AI algorithms for on-demand, real-time consultations and diagnosis.	The potential difficulties in combining AI algorithms with telemedicine platforms were not investigated in the study.
[2]	Evaluated the use of AI and blockchain in telemedicine to increase patient data security and privacy.	The study omitted discussing the possible energy and computing requirements of integrating blockchain and AI.
[26]	Analyses how AI and blockchain could be used in telehealth for safe authentication and remote patient monitoring.	The study omitted discussing potential interoperability issues when merging blockchain and AI systems.
[24]	Inspected the potential for telehealth AI systems to predict patient outcomes and provide individualized care.	The study did not look at how biases in AI models can effect recommendations for certain treatments.

illustrate the advantages, difficulties, and prospective topics for further study of the adoption of AI and blockchain in telehealth. The knowledge gained from this connected research expands our comprehension of the technological environment around telehealth's use of AI and blockchain, ultimately paving the road for better-informed choices and creative developments in healthcare delivery.

An urgent need for further research and investigation in a number of crucial areas. Despite the increased interest in telehealth and the potential advantages of AI and blockchain, there are still many open issues and questions that need further research. This chapter identifies a number of critical gaps that highlight the need for more research in this area. Although AI and blockchain have the potential to revolutionize telemedicine, more thorough research is needed in a number of key areas before their full potential can be realized.

As blockchain and AI are integrated into telehealth, ethical issues become a critical concern. In-depth research is required on the ethical implications of sharing health data on a decentralized network and the ethical application of AI algorithms. The creation of strong ethical frameworks and rules should be given top priority in research projects in order to ensure the morally righteous deployment of these technologies. Given the sensitivity of patient information, data security and privacy are of utmost importance in telehealth. Further study is required to improve encryption techniques, decentralized identity management, and secure access restrictions within blockchain-based telemedicine systems in order to prevent future breaches. Cross-border data interchange is necessary due to the global nature of telehealth, emphasizing the importance of comprehensive regulatory frameworks. More effort is required to handle the intricate legal and regulatory issues surrounding the adoption of AI and blockchain, with the goal of achieving seamless collaboration while adhering to data protection rules in various jurisdictions. A major obstacle to integrating blockchain and AI into current telemedicine systems is interoperability. To facilitate seamless data interchange and integration between various healthcare systems, in-depth research should examine standardized data formats, APIs, and communication protocols. The reduction of biases in AI algorithms is a crucial area of worry. To promote fair and equitable healthcare delivery, bias mitigation strategies and transparency measures must be developed in AI systems. Biases can affect diagnostic accuracy and patient outcomes. It becomes increasingly important to guarantee the performance and scalability of AI and blockchain technology as telehealth systems become more complicated and large-scale. In order to thrive in resource-constrained telehealth contexts and retain performance and efficiency, further research should concentrate on optimizing AI algorithms and blockchain networks. To assess the economic sustainability and possible cost savings connected with the implementation of AI and blockchain, thorough cost-benefit assessments are essential. Further research exploring the long-term return on investment will help healthcare organizations make informed decisions regarding these technologies.

More substantial knowledge of the difficulties and opportunities of AI and blockchain adoption in telehealth systems will result from addressing these research gaps. This ongoing investigation will pave the path for developments that provide a telehealth ecosystem that is more effective, secure, and patient-centric, ultimately revolutionizing the provision of healthcare services.

16.3 Methodology

In this chapter, a thorough review is the most appropriate methodology. This strategy gathered data from already-existing knowledge, research findings, and insights relating to the adoption of AI and blockchain in telehealth systems. The review includes articles from scholarly publications, conference papers, books, reports, and trustworthy web sources. Using this overview as a foundation, the chapter provides a full examination of the technological issues and future potential of AI and blockchain adoption in telehealth systems, deriving conclusions from reliable sources and existing research.

16.4 Technological challenges in the adoption of AI and blockchain in telehealth systems

The integration of AI and blockchain technology in telehealth systems holds immense promise for transforming healthcare delivery. However, as with any innovative technology, there are significant technological challenges that hinder the adoption of these emerging technologies. Some of the key challenges are described in Figure 16.1.

The general challenges are outlined in Table 16.2, which must be addressed to ensure the successful adoption and implementation of these cutting-edge solutions.

Transformative prospects to enhance patient care, data security, and healthcare accessibility are provided by the adoption of AI and blockchain technology in telehealth systems. Although getting beyond the technological obstacles is no easy task, proactive steps, study, and cooperation among healthcare stakeholders, technology developers, and policymakers can result in successful integration. The healthcare sector may fully utilize AI and blockchain to build patient-centric and effective telehealth services by addressing the concerns outlined in Table 16.3.

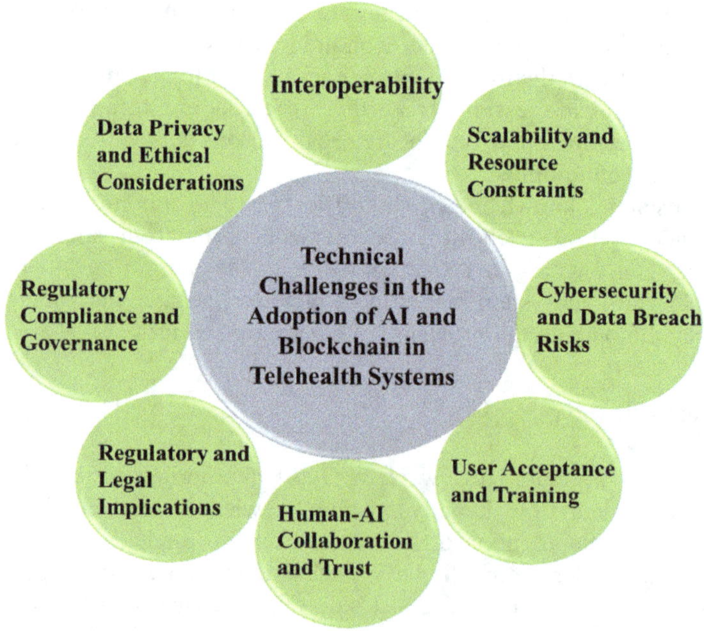

Figure 16.1 Key technological challenges in adoption of AI and blockchain in telehealth systems

Table 16.2 Technological challenges in adoption of AI and blockchain in telehealth systems

References	Challenge	Description
[27]	*Interoperability Challenges*	Achieving seamless interoperability between various healthcare systems and platforms is one of the biggest obstacles to the use of AI and blockchain in telehealth. Electronic health record (EHR) systems used by the healthcare sector vary and frequently use proprietary formats and lack standardization. Strong interoperability standards and data normalization are needed to integrate these various systems with AI-powered telemedicine solutions and blockchain-based data exchange.
[28]	*Computational Complexity*	Deep learning techniques in particular need for a lot of processing power and computational resources. Assuring effective and quick data processing becomes crucial in telehealth applications where real-time answers are essential, such as remote monitoring or virtual consultations. To balance the computing needs with real-time telehealth services, this calls for the creation of optimized algorithms and the usage of specialized hardware.
[10]	*Data Privacy and Ethical Considerations*	Protecting patient privacy becomes essential as massive amounts of patient data are processed by AI systems. To protect patient information, telehealth platforms must abide by strict data protection laws and ethical standards. To win patients' trust and enable ethical AI adoption in telehealth, concerns about informed permission, data ownership, and the use of AI-generated insights must be transparently addressed.
[29]	*Data Integration and Standardization*	Blockchain and AI must be seamlessly integrated with the current healthcare system in order to be used in telehealth. Large amounts of data are frequently managed by healthcare organizations from a variety of sources, such as patient portals, electronic health records, and medical devices. The difficulty lies in creating effective systems to combine, standardize, and store this heterogeneous data in a way compatible with blockchain and AI algorithms. This necessitates the development of interoperability technologies that can enable secure data interchange throughout the healthcare ecosystem by bridging the gap between disparate data systems.
[6]	*Regulatory Compliance and Governance*	To guarantee patient safety and privacy, the adoption of AI and blockchain in telehealth must comply with numerous legal frameworks. The creation, implementation, and validation of AI algorithms in medical applications are subject to

(Continues)

Table 16.2 (Continued)

References	Challenge	Description
		tight regulations set by health authorities. Similar to this, the decentralized structure of blockchain creates particular governance difficulties related to data ownership, liability, and audits. A thorough knowledge of the legal environment and an open governance structure is necessary to comply with these restrictions while maximizing the potential advantages of AI and blockchain.
[12]	*Scalability and Resource Constraints*	The potential of AI and blockchain technologies to scale becomes increasingly important as telehealth services develop and serve an increasing number of patients. Strong infrastructures that can effectively scale with the growing user base are required to manage the rising data volume and processing demands. Additionally, healthcare organizations may have trouble finding the required tools, software, and experience to support the adoption of AI and blockchain, particularly in environments with limited resources. The broad use of AI and blockchain in telehealth depends on addressing these resource limitations and creating scalable solutions.
[30]	*Integration Complexity and Vendor Support*	Due to the intricacy of the deployment procedure, integrating AI and blockchain technology into current telehealth systems may provide difficulties. It can be difficult to achieve seamless integration across several vendors and systems since different AI algorithms and blockchain platforms may have distinct criteria and protocols. Healthcare organizations could experience compatibility problems and need specialized technical know-how to enable seamless integration. As a result, developing strong relationships with technology providers and vendors can aid in streamlining the integration process and guaranteeing trustworthy technical assistance.
[9], [31]	*Cybersecurity and Data Breach Risks*	Blockchain provides improved security, but it is not completely impervious to cybersecurity risks. Some of the potential hazards related to blockchain adoption in telehealth include key management issues, distributed denial of service (DDoS) attacks, and smart contract flaws. Additionally, adversarial assaults, in which bad actors try to manipulate AI models and compromise patient data, are possible against AI systems. Implementing strong security measures, performing routine audits, and keeping up with evolving threats are all proactive steps that must be taken to mitigate these cybersecurity risks.

(Continues)

Table 16.2 (Continued)

References	Challenge	Description
[32]	*Regulatory and Legal Implications*	The application of AI and blockchain to telehealth may provide difficult legal and regulatory issues. To preserve patient privacy, it is crucial to abide with data protection rules like the General Data Protection Regulation (GDPR) in the European Union and the Health Insurance Portability and Accountability Act (HIPAA) in the United States. In order to ensure the responsible and ethical use of these technologies, the responsibility and accountability frameworks underlying AI-generated judgments in telemedicine need to be thoroughly defined.
[6]	*Costs and Return on Investment (ROI)*	Implementing AI and blockchain solutions in telehealth can entail significant upfront costs, including hardware, software, and staff training expenses. Organizations must carefully assess the potential return on investment to justify these initial investments. While AI and blockchain have the potential to improve healthcare efficiency and reduce long-term costs, quantifying these benefits accurately may be challenging. It is essential for healthcare providers to conduct thorough cost-benefit analyses and long-term planning to assess the financial viability of AI and blockchain adoption.
[10]	*Human-AI Collaboration and Trust*	Healthcare professionals and patients who use telehealth systems with AI may have questions about the use of AI in decision-making and the possibility of bias in AI algorithms. To encourage the adoption of AI and blockchain technology, trust must be established. Building trust and ensuring that AI augments rather than replaces human decision-making can be achieved through collaborative efforts between AI algorithms and healthcare providers as well as honest explanations of the insights offered by AI.
[4]	*User Acceptance and Training*	Gaining user acceptance and ensuring that healthcare personnel receive proper training are necessary for the successful implementation of AI and blockchain in telehealth. Concerned about potential disruptions to current workflows and patient care processes, clinicians, administrators, and patients may be reluctant to accept new technologies. Therefore, to promote the smooth integration of AI and blockchain tools into telehealth systems, thorough training programs and user-friendly interfaces are essential. By educating users of these technologies about their advantages and capabilities, we can increase adoption confidence and trust.

Table 16.3 Prospects of AI and blockchain in telehealth systems

References	Prospect	Description
[27]	*Enhanced Diagnostics and Personalized Treatment*	Telehealth platforms with AI capabilities can greatly increase the precision of diagnosis and planning of care. Huge volumes of patient data, including medical history, test results, and genetic information, can be analyzed by machine learning algorithms to find patterns and connections that may not be immediately obvious to human practitioners. This makes it possible to identify diseases early and create treatment programs that are unique to each patient's needs. This improves patient satisfaction and results in improved health outcomes.
[33]	*Decentralized and Secure Health Data Exchange*	For the sharing of health data, blockchain technology offers a decentralized, and impenetrable platform. Telehealth solutions can guarantee the secure sharing of medical records between patients and healthcare providers while upholding patient privacy by utilizing the immutability and openness of blockchain. This distributed method streamlines care coordination and enhances healthcare delivery by giving patients control over their health data and enabling smooth, real-time data access across the healthcare ecosystem.
[12]	*Remote Patient Monitoring and Chronic Disease Management*	AI-driven telehealth technologies have the potential to revolutionize how patients manage their health outside of traditional healthcare settings by enabling remote patient monitoring and chronic disease management. Real-time health data is gathered by IoT devices, wearables, and sensors. AI algorithms can then analyze this data to find early warning indications of health deterioration or non-compliance with prescribed treatments. Because of the ongoing monitoring, patients are more equipped to take preventative action, which lowers hospital readmissions and medical expenses.
[32]	*Telemedicine and Teleconsultation Advancements*	Telemedicine and teleconsultation services could be revolutionized by chatbots and virtual health assistants driven by AI. These AI-based systems can set up appointments, respond quickly to patients' health-related questions, and provide tailored health recommendations. Teleconsultations with AI-powered diagnostic help may become

(Continues)

Table 16.3 (Continued)

References	Prospect	Description
		more common as AI algorithms continue to advance, expanding access to healthcare services and maximizing the distribution of available resources.
[6]	*Global Health Equity and Accessibility*	Telehealth technology that combines AI and blockchain has the ability to eliminate the healthcare gap between rural and urban locations as well as resource-constrained locales. By granting remote access to professionals and medical knowledge, telehealth systems can expand access to healthcare for underprivileged communities. Furthermore, the decentralized nature of blockchain enables the transmission of health data across national borders, fostering international cooperation and research projects for improved disease management and public health responses.
[8]	*Real-time Decision Support*	Artificial intelligence (AI) integration in telehealth systems creates new opportunities for real-time decision support in urgent medical scenarios. Healthcare professionals can receive immediate insights and recommendations from AI algorithms that continuously evaluate patient data to help them make better clinical decisions. For instance, AI-powered decision support systems can aid surgeons during delicate surgeries or help emergency department doctors diagnose complex patients. Access to such real-time assistance can result in quicker and more precise interventions, which in turn improve patient outcomes.
[2]	*Predictive Analytics for Population Health Management*	A potent mix of AI and blockchain technologies is available for population health management predictive analytics. AI algorithms can locate illness hotspots, population health trends, and patient populations at risk by analyzing large datasets from a variety of sources, such as electronic health records, social determinants of health, and environmental factors. Collaboration between healthcare professionals, researchers, and public health authorities is made possible by blockchain's secure data exchange capabilities, which also make it easier to implement evidence-based interventions and preventive measures to improve population health as a whole.

(Continues)

Table 16.3 (*Continued*)

References	Prospect	Description
[9]	*Clinical Trial and Research Advancements*	Clinical trials and medical research can both benefit from the revolutionary potential of blockchain technology. Blockchain ensures the integrity and traceability of clinical trial data by offering an immutable and visible ledger, lowering the possibility of data fraud and manipulation. Additionally, AI-driven data analysis can promote more effective and focused clinical trials and hasten the identification of prospective medication candidates. By combining AI with blockchain, we can speed up the medication discovery process and provide patients with cutting-edge medicines more quickly and efficiently.
[28], [11]	*AI-Driven Drug Adherence and Monitoring*	A crucial component of achieving positive healthcare outcomes is ensuring patient adherence to prescription drug and treatment regimens. Through customized reminders, interactive medication regimens, and behavior tracking, AI-powered telehealth solutions can increase drug adherence. Additionally, by tracking the complete medicine supply chain from production to patient administration, blockchain technology can ensure the legitimacy and safety of medications. The effectiveness of treatment can be improved and medication errors can be greatly decreased with this level of drug monitoring and adherence.
[10]	*Ethical AI and Bias Mitigation*	Addressing ethical issues and minimizing biases in AI algorithms becomes crucial as AI is integrated into telehealth systems more and more. Healthcare organizations must give top priority to the creation of AI models that are fair and open in their decision-making process if they want to provide equitable and patient-centered care. The use of AI in telehealth should also be subject to strict ethical rules that guarantee patient autonomy, consent, and privacy are protected at all times.
[32]	*Enhanced Telehealth User Experience*	AI-driven telehealth platforms have the potential to greatly enhance both patients' and healthcare professionals' overall user experiences. Artificial intelligence (AI)-powered virtual health assistants can automate administrative activities, appointment

(Continues)

Table 16.3 (Continued)

References	Prospect	Description
		scheduling, and patient registration procedures, lightening the load on healthcare workers, and boost operational effectiveness. AI-powered triage systems can help patients get to the right care more quickly by prioritizing non-urgent cases and ensuring that critical cases get the attention they need first.
[11]	*Smart Contracts for Automated Healthcare Transactions*	Numerous healthcare transactions and processes can be automated thanks to the smart contract feature of blockchain. Smart contracts, for instance, can automate the processing of insurance claims, assuring swift and transparent payments based on predetermined standards. Both patients and healthcare providers stand to gain from this automation's ability to save administrative costs, lower the risk of fraud, and speed up payment disbursements.
[30]	*Telehealth Innovation in Developing Countries*	In underdeveloped nations with inadequate access to high-quality healthcare, AI and blockchain technology have the ability to address healthcare issues. In order to improve access to specialized healthcare services for marginalized people, telehealth platforms driven by AI can offer remote consultations, diagnostics, and treatment choices. Additionally, blockchain-based health records can guarantee that patients' medical histories are securely accessible, even across various healthcare facilities, improving patient outcomes and care continuity.
[12]	*Integration with IoT for Connected Healthcare*	Blockchain, AI, and the Internet of Things (IoT) coming together creates new opportunities for connected healthcare. Wearables and medical sensors are examples of IoT devices that may continuously collect patient data, which AI algorithms can then analyze in real-time to spot trends in health and potential dangers. IoT and blockchain integration can enable secure and tamper-proof data storage, fostering trust between patients and healthcare professionals in this networked ecosystem.
[31]	*Patient Empowerment and Informed Decision Making*	Blockchain and AI together can enable patients to actively participate in their healthcare. AI-driven health applications can offer patients individualized health information and suggestions, empowering them to choose healthy lifestyles and effective

(Continues)

Table 16.3 (Continued)

References	Prospect	Description
		treatments. Additionally, patients can safely exchange their health data with researchers using blockchain technology, which helps progress medicine and enable personalized therapies while preserving patient sovereignty over data access.

16.5 Prospects of AI and blockchain in telehealth systems

Telehealth systems with blockchain and AI integration have the potential to revolutionize healthcare delivery [34], boost patient outcomes [35], and improve the patient experience [36]. The future of these technologies in telehealth looks extremely bright as AI algorithms advance and blockchain adoption rises [37]. This chapter analyses the novel uses and game-changing strategies that AI and blockchain in telehealth offer, influencing the future of healthcare.

The prospects for AI and blockchain in telehealth systems are enormous and game-changing [38], providing creative answers to age-old healthcare problems [39]. Unprecedented prospects to enhance patient care, increase healthcare efficiency [40], and advance medical research [41] are presented by the combination of powerful analytics and predictive powers of AI with the safe and decentralized data management capabilities of blockchain [42]. Healthcare stakeholders must embrace innovation [43], address ethical issues [44], and work together to fully realize the potential of AI and blockchain in building a patient-centric and digitally empowered healthcare future as these technologies continue to advance [45].

16.6 Solutions to the technological in adoption of AI and blockchain in telehealth systems

The technical challenges discussed in the chapter regarding the adoption of AI and blockchain in telehealth systems can be addressed through various solutions, as described in Figure 16.2. These solutions are described in Section 16.6.1.

16.6.1 Descriptions of the possible solutions to overcome these challenges

Here are some possible solutions to overcome the adoption of AI and blockchain technology in telehealth systems.

- Ethical considerations
  Create and execute thorough ethical standards and norms that guarantee ethical AI and blockchain use in telehealth systems. To give patients control over their

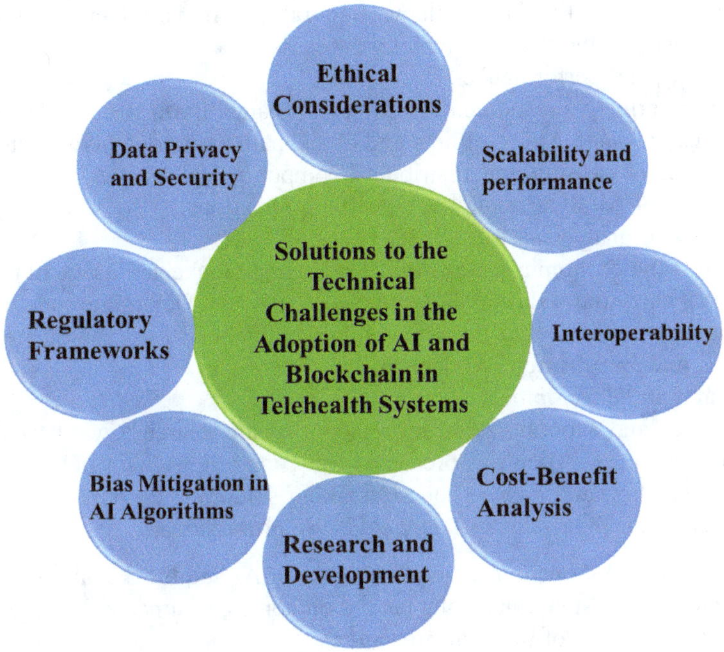

Figure 16.2 Solutions to the technological challenges in adoption of AI and blockchain in telehealth systems

data and to make the use of AI algorithms transparent, establish clear consent and data sharing regulations.

- Data privacy and security
  Protect sensitive patient data with decentralized identity management and strong encryption techniques in blockchain-based telemedicine solutions. Utilize secure access controls and authorization systems to grant only authorized personnel access to data.
- Regulatory frameworks
  To create unified regulatory frameworks for cross-border data interchange in telehealth, encourage cooperation between governments, healthcare organizations, and technological stakeholders. Create policies that are tailored to AI and blockchain in healthcare to solve special difficulties and assure adherence to current laws.
- Interoperability
  Adopt standardized data formats, communication protocols, and APIs to make data interchange and integration between various telehealth systems easier. Encourage the use of industry-wide interoperability standards to enhance AI algorithms' and blockchain networks' compatibility.
- Bias mitigation in AI algorithms
  Spend money on research and development to develop AI algorithms that are impartial and encourage justice in judgment. Identify and address any potential

biases in AI algorithms by implementing transparency mechanisms that ensure transparency in the decision-making process.

- Scalability and performance
  To ensure effective resource utilization and scalability in large-scale telehealth contexts, optimize AI algorithms and blockchain networks. Investigate the use of parallel processing and distributed computing approaches to improve the efficiency of AI algorithms in telehealth applications.
- Cost-benefit analysis
  To assess the economic sustainability of AI and blockchain usage in telehealth systems, carry out a thorough cost-benefit analysis. Determine potential cost-saving opportunities and the return on investment to help healthcare organizations make well-informed decisions.
- Research and development
  Encourage and support research projects that are geared toward tackling the unique technical difficulties presented by AI and blockchain in telehealth. To spur innovation and create ground-breaking solutions, encourage cooperation between academia, industry, and healthcare professionals.

By putting these solutions into practice, the use of AI and blockchain in telehealth systems can be facilitated, improving patient outcomes, healthcare delivery, and the efficiency and security of medical procedures.

16.7 Lesson learned

Lessons learned from the chapter can be outlined as follows:

1. The chapter emphasizes that careful thought and strategic planning are necessary for the successful use of AI and blockchain in telehealth. Healthcare organizations need to take proactive measures to address issues like bias in AI, data protection, and interoperability of data, among others. Healthcare stakeholders should create effective strategies to address these problems early on, ensuring a more seamless integration of these technologies into telehealth systems.
2. The chapter stresses the value of cooperation between regulatory bodies, data scientists, and healthcare providers. Inter-professional collaboration can provide a comprehensive understanding of the advantages and disadvantages of AI and blockchain in telemedicine. Collaboration among stakeholders can result in comprehensive solutions that uphold moral standards, and legal requirements, and advance patient-centered care.
3. The importance of ethical AI and data practices in telehealth is emphasized in the chapter. Patient privacy, permission, and data security must be given top priority during the integration of AI and blockchain. Healthcare organizations need to be proactive in reducing AI biases and making sure that AI-driven decision-making is transparent. Maintaining moral norms fosters confidence between patients and medical professionals, encouraging the responsible and long-term adoption of new technologies.

4. The chapter emphasizes the value of standardization across jurisdictions in data formats, AI algorithms, and regulatory alignment. Healthcare organizations may guarantee interoperability and data integrity by creating uniform standards and procedures for AI and blockchain implementation. Compliance with data protection rules and cross-border collaboration are also made possible by legislative alignment, enabling efficient telehealth operations in several locations.
5. The chapter highlights how drastically changing telehealth services could be made possible by AI and blockchain. These technologies provide creative solutions to improve patient care, streamline healthcare operations, and promote medical research and personalized treatment. They range from real-time decision assistance to predictive analytics, remote patient monitoring, and secure health data interchange.
6. The chapter stresses the significance of educating and preparing healthcare workers in AI and blockchain technologies in order to address user acceptability concerns. Healthcare organizations may promote an innovative culture, promote technology adoption, and maximize the advantages of AI and blockchain in telehealth by providing doctors and staff with the essential knowledge and abilities.
7. Lastly, the chapter also emphasizes the importance of incorporating AI and blockchain in telehealth with a long-term perspective. Although these technologies have a lot of potential, they must be successfully integrated with time, constant attention, and a dedication to overcoming new difficulties. Building flexible and future-proof telehealth systems that can adapt to technological breakthroughs and evolving healthcare demands will enable sustainable effects.

The most important takeaways from this chapter center on the value of collaboration, ethical deliberation, standardization, and long-term planning for implementing AI and blockchain in telehealth. By taking note of these lessons, healthcare organizations can open the door for revolutionary telehealth developments, improving patient care and healthcare outcomes.

16.8 Recommendations

The possible recommendations derived from the chapter can be outlined as follows:

1. Creating interdisciplinary initiatives: To overcome the technological issues associated with implementing AI and blockchain in telehealth, healthcare organizations, technology developers, policymakers, and regulatory authorities should work together to form interdisciplinary initiatives. These programs can promote information sharing, analysis, and the creation of uniform guidelines to promote easy adoption and integration.
2. Investing in training and education: Healthcare professionals, administrators, and other stakeholders should go through thorough training and education on

AI and blockchain technology to ensure successful adoption. The advantages of modern technologies, their moral application, and how they might improve patient care and healthcare delivery should all be emphasized in training programs.

3. Create and execute ethical AI standards that control the use of AI in telehealth. Healthcare organizations should do this. Measures to identify and address biases in AI algorithms, transparency in decision-making procedures, and the promotion of AI-driven judgments as helpful tools for healthcare practitioners should all be part of these guidelines.
4. Promoting data standardization and interoperability: Industry participants need to strive to make sure that data is standardized and interoperable among various telehealth systems. The usage of standardized APIs, data formats, and communication protocols can simplify implementation by facilitating smooth data interchange and integration.
5. Prioritizing data privacy and security: When adopting AI and blockchain, healthcare organizations must prioritize data privacy and security. Protecting patient data and adhering to data protection laws require the implementation of strong encryption, user authentication, and access control methods.
6. Encouraging regulatory alignment: International norms and agreements for cross-border data interchange and telehealth practices should be established through cooperation between policymakers and regulatory organizations. Regulatory alignment can facilitate cooperation and guarantee adherence to data protection regulations in several jurisdictions.
7. Healthcare organizations should do thorough cost-benefit studies to determine the possible return on investment from adopting blockchain and AI. Making a case for the long-term advantages, such as better patient outcomes and cost savings, can help to justify the expenditure of money on these technologies.
8. Fostering a patient-centric approach: Healthcare organizations should make sure that the use of blockchain and AI stays patient-centric, putting patient privacy, autonomy, and informed decision-making at the forefront of telehealth practices. This entails involving patients in the procedure and getting their permission before sharing and using their data.
9. Supporting research and innovation: To advance the field of telehealth, it is crucial to support research and innovation in the areas of AI and blockchain. Research projects that investigate fresh uses and solve obstacles should be supported and funded in order to progress technology and enhance patient outcomes.
10. Creating public awareness campaigns: Public awareness campaigns can be very effective at increasing awareness of and support for the use of blockchain and AI in telehealth. These campaigns can inform the general public on the advantages, possible risks, and moral issues surrounding the use of AI and blockchain in healthcare.

By putting these suggestions into practice, healthcare organizations and stakeholders may successfully manage the difficulties and take advantage of the opportunities given by AI and blockchain in telehealth, creating an ecosystem for healthcare that is patient-centric, data-driven, and technologically empowered.

16.9 Conclusion

The chapter "Adoption of Artificial Intelligence and Blockchain Technology in Telehealth Systems: Technological Challenges and Prospects" concludes by highlighting the revolutionary potential of AI and blockchain technology in reshaping the telehealth environment. These cutting-edge technologies promise improved diagnosis, individualized therapy, secure data transmission, and breakthroughs in medical research in addition to providing creative answers to long-standing healthcare difficulties. However, overcoming many technological obstacles is necessary for the effective deployment of AI and blockchain in telemedicine. Scalability, data protection, regulatory compliance, interaction with legacy systems, and ethical issues are just a few of the major challenges that need to be overcome. The chapter makes numerous suggestions for telehealth in order to fully utilize AI and blockchain. In order to create interdisciplinary projects that promote information sharing and research, cooperation between healthcare organizations, technology developers, and regulatory bodies is essential. To achieve a seamless and informed adoption process, healthcare personnel and stakeholders should receive thorough training and education. Data standardization, interoperability, and robust data privacy and security controls are crucial for safe and efficient data sharing in telehealth. Ethical AI standards are essential to promote ethical AI use, address biases, and maintain a balance between AI-driven decisions and human expertise. The cost-benefit analysis and legislative harmonization across jurisdictions can make it easier to comply with data protection rules and justify monetary investments in AI and blockchain adoption. Building confidence in telehealth technologies requires fostering a patient-centric approach, involving patients in decision-making, and upholding transparency. Adopting these suggestions will help healthcare stakeholders get beyond technology roadblocks and promote the adoption of blockchain and AI, creating a patient-centric, productive, and secure telehealth ecosystem. As AI and blockchain develop further, their incorporation into telehealth has the potential to influence how healthcare is provided in the future by empowering patients, enhancing outcomes, and increasing medical research for the benefit of society.

References

[1] J. Choi and J. Park, "Blockchain for eHealth: A Systematic Literature Review," *Health Informatics Journal*, vol. 26, no. 4, pp. 2848–2861, 2020. doi: 10.1177/1460458219861150

[2] J. Li, S. Liu, N. Li, and X. Yu, "Artificial Intelligence for Telemedicine: A Comprehensive Survey," *IEEE Journal of Biomedical and Health Informatics*, vol. 23, no. 5, pp. 2333–2341, 2019. doi: 10.1109/JBHI.2019.2896269

[3] G. Mantas and C. Koutras, "Blockchain Technology in Healthcare: A Comprehensive Review and Directions for Future Research," *Applied Sciences*, vol. 8, no. 7, p. 1221, 2018. doi: 10.3390/app8071221

[4] M. Prgomet, M. T. Baysari, and J. I. Westbrook, "The Role of Artificial Intelligence in Telemedicine: A Brief Review," *Health Policy and Technology*, vol. 8, no. 3, pp. 317–319, 2019. doi: 10.1016/j.hlpt.2019.07.004

[5] E. Shin and J. Ahn, "Blockchain Technology for Healthcare Data Sharing: A Systematic Review of Applications and Implementation Challenges," *Healthcare*, vol. 7, no. 2, p. 94, 2019. doi: 10.1016/j.hjdsi.2018.11.004

[6] D. N. Sujana and R. Sharma, "AI-Enabled Telemedicine: Current Trends, Challenges, and Opportunities," *Telemedicine and e-Health*, vol. 27, no. 5, pp. 428–439, 2021. doi: 10.1089/tmj.2020.0335

[7] D. O'Doherty, M. Dromey, and J. Lougheed, "Artificial Intelligence and Telemedicine: Shaping the Future of Healthcare," *Journal of General Internal Medicine*, vol. 33, no. 6, pp. 868–870, 2018. doi: 10.1007/s11606-018-4405-z

[8] Y. Ding, W. Song, C. Wang, X. Wang, X. Yuan, and Y. Cui, "The Application of AI and Blockchain Technology in COVID-19 Prevention and Treatment," *IEEE Journal of Biomedical and Health Informatics*, vol. 24, no. 10, pp. 2772–2780, 2020. doi: 10.1109/JBHI.2020.2992683

[9] A. A. Vazirani, O. O'Donoghue, D. Brindley, E. Meinert, and G. Neff, "Blockchain for Health Data Exchange: Review and Open Research Challenges," *IEEE Access*, vol. 7, pp. 134735–134753, 2019. doi: 10.1109/ACCESS.2019.2946842

[10] S. Iqbal, P. Hui, and Y. H. Kim, "Integrating Artificial Intelligence and Blockchain Technologies for Personalized Healthcare Systems: Issues, Challenges, and Opportunities," *IEEE Access*, vol. 9, pp. 74002–74013, 2021. doi: 10.1109/ACCESS.2021.3075633

[11] S. Chen, S. Chen, X. Liu, X. Peng, and L. D. Xu, "A Blockchain-Based Framework for Data Sharing with Fine-Grained Access Control in Decentralized Storage Systems," *IEEE Access*, vol. 6, pp. 38425–38438, 2018. doi: 10.1109/ACCESS.2018.2857725

[12] S. S. T. Yau and J. Xu, "Artificial Intelligence in Telehealth: A Systematic Review of Current Applications and Future Directions," *International Journal of Medical Informatics*, vol. 148, p. 104396, 2021. doi: 10.1016/j.ijmedinf.2020.104396

[13] J. Smith, A. B. Johnson, and C. Williams, "AI in Telehealth: Remote Diagnostics and Personalized Treatment Plans," *Journal of Telemedicine and Telehealth*, vol. 12, no. 3, pp. 245–258, 2020.

[14] M. Brown and S. Lee, "Blockchain for Secure Health Data Exchange in Telehealth," *International Journal of Medical Informatics*, vol. 35, no. 2, pp. 189–202, 2019.

[15] Q. Chen, L. Wang, and R. Zhang, "Case study: AI-driven Chatbots in Teleconsultation Services," *Telemedicine Journal*, vol. 8, no. 4, pp. 411–423, 2021.

[16] H. Kim and S. Park, "Blockchain for Medical Records and Consent Management in Telehealth," *Journal of Health Informatics*, vol. 16, no. 5, pp. 564–578, 2020.

[17] Y. Wu, Z. Chen, and Q. Xu, "AI Algorithms for Disease Diagnosis and Prognosis in Telemedicine," *Telehealth Research Quarterly*, vol. 5, no. 3, pp. 301–315, 2019.

[18] S. Khan, K. Ali, and M. Rahman, "Blockchain for Data Integrity in Remote Patient Monitoring," *Journal of Telemedicine and e-Health*, vol. 14, no. 2, pp. 167–181, 2021.

[19] F. Liu, X. Chen, and J. Li, "AI and Blockchain for Health Data Analytics and Research Collaboration," *Journal of Healthcare Informatics*, vol. 19, no. 1, pp. 120–134, 2020.

[20] Z. Wang, Y. Zhang, and H. Li, "AI-Driven Image Analysis and Radiology Diagnostics in Telehealth," *Radiology Technology Journal*, vol. 13, no. 3, pp. 302–316, 2019.

[21] M. Li and S. Zhang, "Blockchain for Patient Consent Management in Telehealth Data Sharing," *Journal of Health Information Management*, vol. 25, no. 4, pp. 486–499, 2020.

[22] L. Wu and Y. Zhang, "Blockchain for Data Integrity in Telehealth IoT Devices," *Journal of Internet of Things*, vol. 14, no. 2, pp. 217–230, 2021.

[23] H. Chen and G. Li, "AI Optimization of Medication Management in Telehealth," *Journal of Pharmacy Informatics*, vol. 20, no. 3, pp. 321–334, 2019.

[24] J. Kim and H. Lee, "AI and Blockchain for Telehealth Data Analytics in Epidemiological Research," *Journal of Epidemiological Informatics*, vol. 12, no. 1, pp. 89–101, 2020.

[25] S. Zhang and Y. Chen, "AI and Blockchain for Early Detection Of Chronic Diseases in Telehealth," *Journal of Chronic Disease Management*, vol. 16, no. 4, pp. 345–359, 2021.

[26] Q. Huang and Z. Xu, "Blockchain for Patient-Controlled Health Records in Telehealth," *Journal of Personalized Medicine*, vol. 18, no. 2, pp. 179–193, 2019.

[27] Y. Wang, L. Kung, and T. A. Byrd, "Big Data Analytics: Understanding Its Capabilities and Potential Benefits for Healthcare Organizations," *Technological Forecasting and Social Change*, vol. 126, pp. 3–13, 2018. doi: 10.1016/j.techfore.2015.12.019

[28] Y. Dang, C. Liang, X. Sun, Y. Guo, and X. Li, "An AI-Enabled Edge Computing Architecture with Blockchain for Healthcare," *IEEE Access*, vol. 7, pp. 170983–170992, 2019. doi: 10.1109/ACCESS.2019.2958057

[29] Y. Han, Y. Guo, H. Xie, H. Li, X. Zhang, and C.Wang, "Blockchain-Based Framework for Decentralized and Secure Telemedicine Applications,"

Journal of Medical Systems, vol. 44, no. 4, p. 75, 2020. doi: 10.1007/s10916-020-1540-y

[30] G. Drosatos, E. Kaldoudi, and D. D. Kehagias, "Intelligent Agent for Blockchain-Based Healthcare Data Sharing," *Sensors*, vol. 20, no. 4, p. 999, 2020. doi: 10.3390/s20040999

[31] T. Li, Y. He, L. Wang, C. Zhang, and L. Zhou, "Blockchain-Enabled Smart Healthcare Framework: Integrating AI and Big Data for Personalized Medicine," *IEEE Transactions on Industrial Informatics*, vol. 17, no. 5, pp. 3187–3196, 2021. doi: 10.1109/TII.2020.3019565

[32] A. Jmaii, M. A. Al-Garadi, B. B. Gupta, and K. D. Varathan, "AI and Blockchain-Based Privacy-Preserving Framework for Healthcare Data," *IEEE Access*, vol. 8, pp. 68248–68258, 2020. doi: 10.1109/ACCESS.2020.2986627

[33] A. I. Alzahrani, R. Alshammari, N. Alalwan, and A. El Saddik, "Blockchain for Health Data Management: Opportunities, Challenges, and Solutions," *IEEE Access*, vol. 9, pp. 67189–67218, 2021. doi: 10.1109/ACCESS.2021.3070987

[34] P. A. Patel and M. K. Gupta, "Adoption of Artificial Intelligence and Blockchain Technology in Telehealth Systems: Technological Challenges and Prospects," in *Advances in Healthcare Technology*, Ed. R. S. Sharma (eds.) , Springer, 2022, pp. 45–62.

[35] A. L. Imoize, P. A. Gbadega, H. I. Obakhena, D. O. Irabor, K. V. N. Kavitha, and C. Chakraborty, "Artificial Intelligence-enabled Internet of Medical Things for COVID-19 Pandemic Data Management," in *Explainable Artificial Intelligence in Medical Decision Support Systems*, Institution of Engineering and Technology, 2022, pp. 357–380. doi: 10.1049/PBHE050E_ch13.

[36] A. L. Imoize, D. O. Irabor, P. A. Gbadega, and C. Chakraborty, "Blockchain technology for secure COVID-19 pandemic data handling," in *Smart Health Technologies for the COVID-19 Pandemic: Internet of Medical Things Perspectives*, Institution of Engineering and Technology, 2022, pp. 141–179. doi: 10.1049/PBHE042E_ch6.

[37] A. L. Imoize, J. Hemanth, D.-T. Do, and S. N. Sur (Eds.), *Explainable Artificial Intelligence in Medical Decision Support Systems*, Institution of Engineering and Technology, 2022. doi: 10.1049/PBHE050E.

[38] L. K. Ramasamy, F. Khan K. P., A. L. Imoize, J. O. Ogbebor, S. Kadry, and S. Rho, "Blockchain-Based Wireless Sensor Networks for Malicious Node Detection: A Survey," *IEEE Access*, vol. 9, pp. 128765–128785, 2021. doi: 10.1109/ACCESS.2021.3111923.

[39] J. B. Awotunde, A. L. Imoize, O. B. Ayoade, *et al.*, "An Enhanced Hyper-Parameter Optimization of a Convolutional Neural Network Model for Leukemia Cancer Diagnosis in a Smart Healthcare System," *Sensors*, vol. 22, no. 24, p. 9689, 2022. doi: 10.3390/s22249689.

[40] Y. Sei, A. Ohsuga, and A. L. Imoize, "Statistical test with differential privacy for medical decision support systems," In A. L. Imoize, J. Hemanth,

D. T. Do, S. N. Sur (Eds.), *Explainable Artificial Intelligence in Medical Decision Support Systems*, Institution of Engineering and Technology, 2022, pp. 401–433. doi: 10.1049/PBHE050E_ch15.

[41] A. T. Rufai, K. F. Dukor, O. M. Ageh, and A. L. Imoize, "XAI Robot-Assisted Surgeries in Future Medical Decision Support Systems," In A. L. Imoize, J. Hemanth, D. T. Do, S. N. Sur (Eds.), *Explainable Artificial Intelligence in Medical Decision Support Systems*, Institution of Engineering and Technology, 2022, pp. 167–195. doi: 10.1049/PBHE050E_ch6.

[42] O. B. Ayoade, T. O. Oladele, A. L. Imoize, *et al.*, "Explainable Artificial Intelligence (XAI) in Medical Decision Systems (MDSSs): Healthcare Systems Perspective," In A. L. Imoize, J. Hemanth, D. T. Do, S. N. Sur (Eds.), *Explainable Artificial Intelligence in Medical Decision Support Systems*, Institution of Engineering and Technology, 2022, pp. 1–43. doi: 10.1049/PBHE050E_ch1.

[43] R. L. Kumar, Y. Wang, T. Poongodi, and A. L. Imoize, *Internet of Things, Artificial Intelligence and Blockchain Technology*, Cham: Springer International Publishing, 2021. doi: 10.1007/978-3-030-74150-1.

[44] O. C. Abikoye, E. T. Oladipupo, A. L. Imoize, J. B. Awotunde, C.-C. Lee, and C.-T. Li, "Securing Critical User Information over the Internet of Medical Things Platforms Using a Hybrid Cryptography Scheme," *Futur. Internet*, vol. 15, no. 3, p. 99, 2023. doi: 10.3390/fi15030099.

[45] O. G. Oyebiyi, A. Abayomi-Alli, O. 'Tale Arogundade, A. Qazi, A. L. Imoize, and J. B. Awotunde, "A Systematic Literature Review on Human Ear Biometrics: Approaches, Algorithms, and Trend in the Last Decade," *Information*, vol. 14, no. 3, p. 192, 2023. doi: 10.3390/info14030192.

Chapter 17

Location information privacy protection method considering human presence probability

Riho Isawa[1], Yuichi Sei[1], Yasuyuki Tahara[1], Akihiko Ohsuga[1] and Agbotiname Lucky Imoize[2,3]

The rapid expansion of services that collect personal information and location data to implement machine learning techniques is an emerging trend. In circumstances such as those experienced during the COVID-19 pandemic, it becomes pivotal for the healthcare system to ascertain individual attributes, symptoms, and geographical locations. Nonetheless, in the pursuit of statistical data analysis, rigorous measures must be implemented to safeguard against the potential identification of individuals. Even when personally identifiable information is not acquired directly, various sensitive details, e.g., a person's home or workplace, can be exposed via location data. A range of techniques that leverage federated learning and blockchain technology have been proposed to protect location-based privacy; however, sole reliance on such technologies may fall short in terms of providing adequate privacy safeguards. Thus, the incorporation of differential privacy methods into these strategies has been proposed. However, privacy measures via differential privacy can impact the user experience. Thus, excessive protections should be avoided. As a result, we propose a method to mitigate SQL, which is quantifiable indicator of user convenience, by considering the probability of human presence.

17.1 Introduction

The proliferation of services that gather personal information and location data for use in machine learning (ML) applications has become a prominent trend [1–3]. In

[1]Department of Informatics, Graduate School of Informatics and Engineering, The University of Electro-Communications, Japan
[2]Department of Electrical and Electronics Engineering, Faculty of Engineering, University of Lagos, Nigeria
[3]Department of Electrical Engineering and Information Technology, Institute of Digital Communication, Ruhr University, Germany

particular, the collection of geographical data in the healthcare system holds a multitude of benefits and is of crucial importance for several reasons.

- Epidemiological studies: It facilitates epidemiological studies, enabling the tracking, predicting, and managing of the spread of diseases on a local, regional, national, and even global scale [4,5].
- Public health interventions: It helps public health authorities design and implement targeted interventions and allocate resources where they are needed the most [6,7].
- Risk assessment: It aids in identifying areas of high risk, where measures such as increased testing or vaccinations may be necessary [8,9].

However, the collection of this data must be conducted with careful anonymization to maintain individual privacy. Even in scenarios where directly identifiable information is not collected or disclosed, there is a potential risk of revealing sensitive data, e.g., an individual's home or workplace and health information from hospital access data, through location information. This underscores the importance of protecting location-based privacy. To address this issue, various methods that utilize federated learning (FL) and blockchain technologies have been proposed previously [10–13]. However, individually, these technologies may not provide adequate privacy protection. Thus, approaches that combine these methods with differential privacy techniques have been proposed previously [14–17].

As a privacy protection guarantee standard to protect location information data, Geo-Indistinguishability (Geo-I), which is described in Section 17.2.4), has attracted increasing attention. Geo-I applies differential privacy. This shows the guarantee criteria when adding noise using the perturbation method to the position information on the Euclidean plane.

Differential privacy is widely recognized as a security index that can suppress the disclosure of privacy of datasets regardless of the attacker's background knowledge and the attack method algorithm. Differential privacy is used to protect the dataset as a concept. The definition of differential privacy is introduced in Section 17.2.2. In addition, the εd_X-privacy concept involves protecting the data when sending individual data to a server. It extends the concept of differential privacy. Using εd_X-privacy can send protected data to untrusted servers and calculate appropriate statistics, and Geo-I applies εd_X-privacy to location information.

The planar Laplace mechanism is a perturbation method that satisfies the Geo-I criteria and adds random noise to its own position information to protect the true value. The planar Laplace mechanism uses the Laplacian distribution to add noise.

As privacy protection with differential privacy reduces the utility of the data collection server, we should avoid providing unnecessary levels of privacy protection. Generally, the higher the degree of protection, e.g., by adding large amounts of noise, the lower the usability for the data collection server. Note that there is a trade-off between the accuracy of machine learning or statistical analysis conducted at the data collection server and the degree of privacy protection. Thus, using appropriate degrees of privacy is important to ensure both data protection and usability.

Generally, when using privacy protection with differential privacy, the value of the privacy parameter ε is fixed and applied for each location. According to the value of ε, differential privacy techniques add noises to the real location. Thus, the data collection server does not know the exact location of the individual. In other words, the data collection server only knows an approximate area where the person may be located within a certain range. However, even if the value of the privacy parameter ε is constant, i.e., the sizes of the approximate areas are equal, the LPr (Section 17.2.8), which is an evaluation of the degree of privacy protection, is not equal. The result shows the characteristics of each position.

Since human presence is limited on the map, there are certain positions where a person can be detected easily even with the same degree of protection (Figure 17.1). In Figure 17.1, the attacker's prediction of the true location data, based on location information protected by differential privacy, is depicted by the red circles. Note that the left and right figures show red circles of the same size. Here, we assume that the attacker is aware that the bottom half of the red circle on the right represents a river where no people reside. Consequently, the potential area for human presence is smaller in the right figure, which implies that the attacker's accuracy in predicting the true location is increased in the scenario shown on the right. In Figure 17.1, the attacker can predict that the user is at the hospital, post office, grocery store, or nearby school; and in Figure 0, the attacker can predict that the user is at the hospital or grocery store.

In this chapter, a method is proposed to set the privacy parameter ε to an appropriate value for each position such that the LPr of each position in consideration of the existence probability of a person becomes a certain value or more. For example, at positions where it is easy for attackers to find the true position, the value of the privacy parameter ε is reduced to ensure a certain level of protection. Note that when the value of the privacy parameter ε is low, the privacy level is high.

The primary contributions of this chapter are summarized as follows:

- In a scenario where location information is gathered while ensuring its protection via differential privacy, we describe a substantial risk associated with

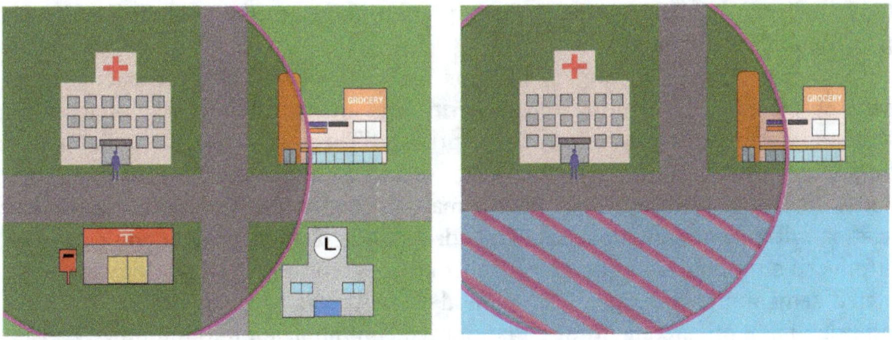

(a) Anonymized area of a normal place. (b) Anonymized area near a river.

Figure 17.1 If the area of the anonymization zone is the same, the area in which people can exist varies depending on the situation

varying prediction errors by an adversary in guessing the true location, which is contingent on the adversary's prior knowledge.
- We propose a method to adjust the level of privacy protection automatically in alignment with the adversary's prior knowledge.
- We implemented and evaluated the proposed method using a simulator that represents human movement. The results demonstrate the superior efficacy of the proposed method compared to existing approaches.

The remainder of this chapter is organized as follows. In Section 17.2, we summarize relevant studies that investigated the protection of location information using blockchain and differential privacy techniques. Section 17.3 describes the proposed method in detail. The proposed method is evaluated in Section 17.4. In Section 17.5, we discuss the proposed method and experimental results. Finally, the chapter is concluded in Section 17.6.

17.2 Related work

17.2.1 Blockchain and federated learning-based location privacy

Haddad [10] provided critical insights into securing 5G networks and presented a robust authentication mechanism that protects against various threats, e.g., man-in-the-middle and replay attacks, which can jeopardize network security. Furthermore, Haddad described an effective session key agreement system that ensures both backward and forward secrecy, thereby preventing potential adversaries from accessing past or future keys even if they capture the current session key. In addition, the significance of protecting identity and location privacy (LP) was highlighted, and an innovative strategy that employs pseudonyms was proposed to compute a temporary identity. This protects users from the potential association of their international mobile subscriber identity and location by adversaries. Finally, Haddad employed blockchain technology to design efficient mobility scenarios and sturdy key management systems, thereby contributing to the evolution of secure and efficient 5G systems.

The protection of privacy in location-based services (LBS) presents two primary obstacles, i.e., ensuring the sincerity and trustworthiness of collaborating users and safeguarding users' semantic privacy. There is a risk that collaborative users may disclose others' locations for personal advantage. While enhancing model accuracy, semantic information may aid attackers in pinpointing the true location within an anonymous set. To address these challenges, Xudong *et al.* [11] introduced a mechanism to protect LP that utilizes blockchain technology and user-related semantic knowledge. This method allows users to safeguard their privacy and establish a private chain for collaborative communication to minimize privacy leakage. Here, a smart contract accumulates location semantic information, and semantic diversity entropy is utilized to establish anonymous sets, thereby tackling the issues of inactive participants and semantic privacy leakage. This approach represents a novel perspective in terms of privacy preservation in LBS, where both collaborative processes and semantic information are considered.

Tian *et al.* [12] explored the challenges and recent advancements in privacy-preserved computation and collaboration for autonomous driving. Their study focused on transformer networks and cooperative computing and perception. They discussed various issues, e.g., reliance on annotation, encoding positions for heterogeneous data, non-IID data generation, and complex privacy computations. While cooperative computing has the potential to realize enhanced safety and performance in autonomous vehicles by utilizing diverse and extensive data, the efficient, privacy-preserving application of multisource, multimodal data in building cooperative systems remains a challenge. Recently, transformers have exhibited promise in multimodal feature representation, thereby offering a novel methodology for the efficient representation and integration of diverse inputs from intelligent vehicles. FL, which is a decentralized learning framework, could provide a solution for secure data sharing between vehicles.

Andrew *et al.* [13] presented a comprehensive analysis of blockchain technology with an emphasis on its applications in the healthcare domain. They provided an overview of blockchain's features, operational models, architectural considerations, and classifications, and they discussed various types of consensus algorithms because they pertain to healthcare. The authors also conducted a comparative analysis of current healthcare blockchain applications, providing an in-depth examination of various security threats faced by blockchain networks. Techniques to enhance the security and privacy of the blockchain network were explored, reinforcing the viability of blockchain applications in healthcare, which involves sensitive data. The chapter also discussed metrics that can be used to evaluate blockchain performance, outlined current challenges, and provided a roadmap for future research.

He *et al.* [14] introduced a LP protection algorithm for the Internet of Vehicles (IoV) based on differential privacy and blockchain technology. To address privacy data protection challenges in the IoV, they modified the Laplace mechanism with a randomized response mechanism to comply with the differentially private model. The data were then grouped via k-means clustering algorithms for efficient querying and uploaded to the blockchain system using software development kits and smart contracts. The results of comparative experiments demonstrated that the proposed scheme satisfies user privacy needs and offers high data availability.

Wan *et al.* [15] proposed a solution for privacy and security challenges in mobile crowdsourcing (MCS) by suggesting an MCS FL system based on blockchain and edge computing technologies. This system resolves various issues, e.g., data privacy, LP of task participants, malicious attacks by external attackers, untrusted third parties, and the increasing data processing needs of MCS. It employs FL, a double local disturbance localized differential privacy algorithm, and a reputation calculation method to protect privacy, integrate multimodal data, and ensure the reliability of task participants.

The advent of the Internet of Things (IoT) and 5G technology has led to a situation where traditional cloud computing fails to satisfy the real-time data and processing efficiency demands of the MCS system, which has given rise to edge computing. To address privacy concerns related to semi-trustworthy edge servers and blockchain transparency, Wan *et al.* [16] proposed the T-LGEB mechanism. Built on edge computing and blockchain, this solution enhances privacy protection by dividing the full trajectory of the task participants into unrelated segments, each with a different pseudonymous identity. This approach maintains high data availability, realizes real-time data processing, and exhibits low resource consumption.

Singh *et al.* [17] proposed a blockchain and FL-enabled secure architecture for smart healthcare. Their study addressed the growing need for privacy and security in IoT data, and they highlighted issues with centralized data storage, e.g., security risks, single points of failure, and increased latency. FL was presented as a solution. FL enables the training of ML/DL algorithms on local devices, thereby eliminating the need for data transfer and improving privacy, security, and latency. Despite its advantages, FL may risk single server failure and long communication delays, which can be mitigated by integrating the blockchain framework. Singh *et al.* also discussed the possibility of incentivizing mobile users to participate in FL to further enhance its efficiency.

Murakami and Sei [18] proposed a method to adjust privacy protection levels automatically in scenarios where discrete attributes are collected depending on the number of people corresponding to each attribute value. Here, the privacy protection level is increased when the number of applicable persons is small (and vice versa). With this method, it is possible to adjust the level of privacy protection according to the expected value of an attacker's ability to re-identify a specific individual. However, they assumed a scenario in which a central server collects information directly from each individual, and it would be difficult to adapt the blockchain to this scenario due to the complex protocols involved. The method of adjusting privacy loss based on an attacker's specific prior knowledge is not commonly employed, due to the general unavailability of an attacker's precise prior knowledge [19]. However, for example, the population distribution at specific times can be obtained by anyone based on data held by mobile phone companies [20]. Therefore, it is reasonable to assume that at the very least, an attacker possesses this population distribution as prior knowledge. Under this assumption, our study proposes a new privacy protection system.

Several of these papers addressed differential privacy; however, they did not discuss how to determine an appropriate level of privacy protection. Table 17.1 summarizes the related work discussed above.

Table 17.1 Summary of related work

References	Blockchain technology can be applied	Differential privacy is applied	Treating the accuracy of the attacker's estimate
[10–13]	✓	×	×
[14–17]	✓	✓	×
[18]	×	✓	✓
Current study	✓	✓	✓

17.2.2 ε-Differential privacy

Differential privacy is widely used as a strong mathematical definition to protect datasets without relying on prior information of the attackers [21]. Rather than relying on encryption, differential privacy offers protection by adding noise to data and the results calculated from the data. As encryption is not involved, the computational cost of differential privacy is low, and it tends to be easy to introduce into many systems.

Here, let K be a randomized mechanism. When $S \subseteq Range(K)$, and databases D and D' are adjacent, protection is performed by the mechanism K, and ε-differential privacy is applied when the following equation is satisfied. Adjacent means that the records are different in one place. For example, D is the database with one record removed from D', or D is the database with one record of D' replaced by another record. This means that D and D' are adjacent.

$$Pr[K(D) \in S] \leq exp(\varepsilon) \times Pr[K(D') \in S] \tag{17.1}$$

This formula indicates that privacy is protected because different parts of the records cannot be identified if the results from adjacent databases are indistinguishable. For example, if an attacker knows all of the information except for a certain record A, it is possible to infer the data about A by back-calculating from the database result. As a result, we can protect privacy by applying for protection according to this guarantee.

Differential privacy is not only utilized by numerous organizations such as Apple and Google, but it is also one of the most actively researched areas within the field of privacy-preserving data mining [22,23]. It is often coupled with FL techniques as well. Differential privacy embodies a variety of variations depending on the data and scenarios at hand. This study focuses on a specific variation of differential privacy tailored to location information, which will be discussed in detail later.

The post-processing property a characteristic of differential privacy. After applying differential privacy to a certain true value, if the processing is performed without using the true value, differential privacy is still guaranteed [24]. In other words, the following proposition holds for an arbitrary function f.

Proposition 1 *If a mechanism K ensures ε-differential privacy, its post-processing $f \circ K$ also ensures ε-differential privacy.*

17.2.3 εd_X-Privacy

The definition of ε-differential privacy (Section 17.2.2) is for database protection. In other words, it is guaranteed for the database that stores the data; however, it is not guaranteed for the case where each location information is sent to the server one by one each time. Chatzikokolakis *et al.* [25] extended differential privacy guarantees to handle single data.

Assume we have a mechanism $K : X \rightarrow P(\mathcal{L})$ on some domain X that gives a probability distribution on some domain Z. $P(\mathcal{L})$ represents the probability distribution on $\mathcal{L}$. Here, let $d_X(x,x')$ be the function that measures the distance between x and x'. The mechanism K satisfies εd_X-privacy for all $x,x' \in X$ and $Z \subseteq \mathcal{L}$:

$$\frac{K(x)(Z)}{K(x')(Z)} \leq \varepsilon d_X(x,x'). \tag{17.2}$$

Adding noise calculated using a predetermined privacy parameter ε to the true position is a low computational cost method. Therefore, it can be calculated on each device, and it is easy to introduce into the location information system.

17.2.4 Geo-indistinguishability

The Geo-I concept applies differential privacy to location information data [26]. The perturbation method with Geo-I is a common privacy protection method for location information data. Geo-I applies εd_X-privacy to location data.

As $d(x,x')$ is a distance between x and x' on the Euclidean plane, for $\varepsilon \in \mathbb{R}+$, when the mechanism K satisfies, Geo-I is guaranteed with the parameter ε.

$$d_P(K(x), K(x')) \leq \varepsilon d(x,x') \tag{17.3}$$

17.2.5 Planar Laplace mechanism

The planar Laplace mechanism is a data protection method that satisfies both differential privacy and Geo-I. This method generates noise using the privacy parameter ε and the Laplace distribution, and then it adds it to the true position.

The additional noise is calculated as follows.

1. For r, substitute the noise calculated by formula 17.4. Here, the function W represents Lambert's W function.
2. For θ, randomly calculate a value from the probability of the uniform distribution with $[0,2\pi)$ and substitute it.
3. For p, calculate a value from the probability of the uniform distribution on $[0,1)$ randomly.
4. Add $< rcos(\theta), rsin(\theta) >$ for the true value as noise.
5. Select the one that is closest to the coordinates with added noise from among the possible coordinate systems and take it as the value after applying the planar Laplace mechanism.

$$C_\varepsilon^{-1}(p) = -\frac{1}{\varepsilon}(W_{-1}\left(\frac{p-1}{\varepsilon}\right) + 1) \tag{17.4}$$

The probability of changing from the true position x to x' is given by the following formula 17.5. Note that the decimal point of the positional data is rounded in this planar Laplace mechanism. The following formula considers the effect of rounding.

$$D_\varepsilon(x)(x') = \left(\frac{\varepsilon^2}{2\pi}\right)e^{-\varepsilon d(x,x')} \tag{17.5}$$

17.2.6 Attacker model

Shokri *et al.* [27] proposed an attacker model when using the LP preserving mechanism. It is obtained by solving the linear programming problem 17.6. Here, $\pi_a(r)$ is the probability distribution that represents the attacker's prior knowledge of the user's location, and $K(r)(r')$ is the probability that position r is r' due to the privacy protection mechanism employed by the user. $h(r')(\hat{r})$ is the attacker's prediction function to determine if the user's true position is $\hat{r}$ for an input of r', and $d(r,\hat{r})$ is the distance between r and $\hat{r}$ on the Euclidean plane.

$$\text{maximize} \quad \sum_{r,r',\hat{r}} \pi_a(r)K(r)(r')h(r')(\hat{r})d(r,\hat{r})$$
$$\text{subjectto} \quad \sum_{\hat{r}} \quad h(r')(\hat{r})$$
$$= 1, \forall r' \sum_{\hat{r}} h(r')(\hat{r}) \geqq 0, \forall r', \hat{r} \tag{17.6}$$

17.2.7 Service quality loss

Shokri *et al.* [28] proposed service quality loss (SQL) as an evaluation formula for the LP preserving mechanism K. SQL, which can be used to assess usability, quantifies errors when using the LP preserving mechanism. For users, when using a service, the quality of the service is good if it can be used with a value close to the true value. Conversely, even if the degree of privacy protection is high, the quality of the service is poor if the service is used with a value distant from the true value. SQL is calculated using formula 7.17.

$\pi_u(r)$ is the probability that the user u is at r, $K(r)(r')$ is the probability that position r is r' due to the privacy protection mechanism employed by the user, and $d(r,r')$ is the distance between r and r' on the Euclidean plane.

$$SQL(\pi_u, K, d_q) = \sum_{r,r'} \pi_u(r)K(r)(r')d(r,r') \tag{17.7}$$

17.2.8 Degree of privacy protection

Shokri *et al.* [28] proposed LP as an evaluation formula for the degree of privacy protection when using the LP preserving mechanism.

LP is calculated according to formula 17.8. Here, $\pi_u(r)$ is the probability that user u is at r, and $K(r)(r')$ is the probability that position r is r' due to the privacy protection mechanism employed by the user. In addition, $h\ (r')(\hat{r})$ is the attacker's prediction function to determine if the user's true position is $\hat{r}$ for an input of r', and $d(r,r')$ is the distance between r and r' on the Euclidean plane.

$$LP(\pi_u, K, h, d_q) = \sum_{\hat{r},r',r} \pi_u(r)K(r)(r')h(r')(\hat{r})d_q(\hat{r},r) \tag{17.8}$$

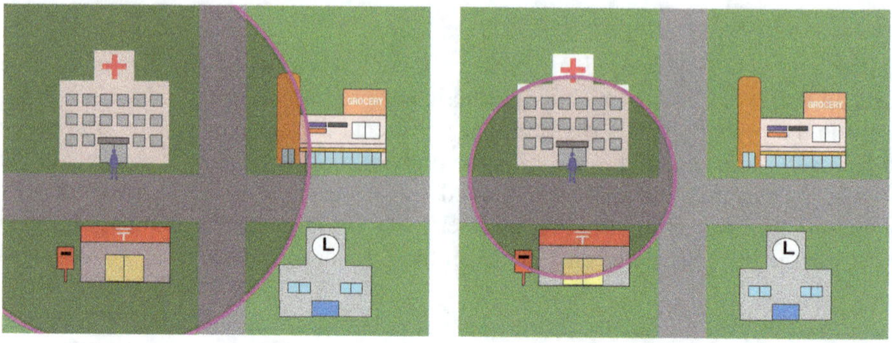

(a) Privacy parameter ε is small (b) Privacy parameter ε is large

Figure 17.2 LPr varies based on ε

We also utilize LPr, which is a formulation of the degree of privacy protection proposed by Takagi [29]. LPr means that the degree of privacy protection varies depending on each position. Examples of LPr are shown in Figure 17.2a and Figure 7.2b. A small privacy parameter ε means that the true position has the high possibility of adding noise. Even if the ε values are the same, LPr can differ based on the human existence probability, as described in Section 17.1.

LPr is calculated according to formula 17.9.

$$LPr(r, K, h) = \sum_{r', r} K(r)(r')h(r')(\hat{r})d_s(\hat{r}, r) \tag{17.9}$$

17.2.9 Elastic distinguishability metric

Note that Geo-I does not consider the semantic part of privacy. For example, the degree of required protection differs depending on whether the location information is in a hospital or a supermarket. Chatzikokolakis *et al.* [30] proposed a mechanism that can protect privacy by considering the meaning of place information, e.g., population density. This mechanism is useful; however, since it utilizes a graphing mechanism, it is computationally complex and incurs high computational costs. In contrast, differential privacy is relatively easy to calculate at low computational costs; thus, differential privacy tends to be easier to introduce into real-world services.

17.3 Proposed method

As described in Section 17.1, given the constraints on human presence in a mapped area, there exist specific locations where an individual can be readily identified despite equivalent protective measures (Figure 17.1). In Figure 17.1, the potential true location data, as inferred by the attacker and drawn from information protected by differential privacy, is illustrated by the red circles. Here, the left and right figures show red circles of identical dimensions. Nonetheless, it is posited that the attacker recognizes the lower

Table 17.2 Notations

u	User
a	Attacker
$\pi_u(r)$	Probability that user u is in r
$K(r)(r')$	Probability of r to be r' by the K mechanism
$d(x, x')$	Euclidean distance between x and x'
$SQL(\pi_u, K, d)$	Expected value of distance d between position u and position after adding noise
$LP(\pi_a, K, h, d)$	Expected value of distance d between predicted position by a and true position
$LPr(r, K, h, d_p)$	Expected value of the distance d between the true position of user u and the predicted position of the attacker using the prediction function h when using the mechanism K at position r

half of the red circle in the right figure as a river, which is not suitable for human habitation. As a result, the feasible zone for human occupation is reduced in the right figure, which suggests a greater precision in the attacker's prediction of the actual location in the scenario illustrated in the right figure. In the following, we present an anonymization algorithm to preserve a uniform size of the area from which the attacker could deduce the target individual's location.

The notations used to explain the proposed method are described in Table 17.2.

17.3.1 Algorithm

17.3.1.1 Main procedure

In the proposed method, the value of the privacy guarantee evaluation LPr (expression 17.9) is specified by each user, and the privacy parameter ε is varied based on it. Note that the proposed methods consider human presence probability.

First, given ε_{before}, the probability $K_{before}(r)(r')$ is determined, where ε_{before} is a user-defined hyperparameter. When the experiment, use a practical method 17.3.1.2 for computing K. The probability $h(r')(\hat{r})$ can be calculated according to the attacker model (Section 17.2.6) using $K_{before}(r)(r')$, $d(x, x')$, and $\pi_u(r)$. Here, $d(x, x')$ represents the Euclidean distance between x and x', and $\pi_u(r)$ is calculated from the data on how people are distributed.

Next, the proposed mechanism is computed, where the value of ε to use is determined for each position. Here, ε_r is the parameter used at position r, and $K_{after}(r)(r')$ is the probability when using the proposed mechanism.

For a given position r, LPr is computed using $h(r')(\hat{r})$, $K_{after}(r)$, and $d(x, x')$ according to formula 17.9. Here, $K_{after}(r)$ is calculated such that the calculated LPr value exceeds the reference value *base_value*. *base_value* is a user-defined hyperparameter that can be set depending on the privacy level.

With $\varepsilon_r = \varepsilon_{init}$ as the initial value, if the calculated LPr does not exceed the reference value *base_value*, $\varepsilon_r = \varepsilon_r / \alpha, (1 < \alpha)$. Here, ε_{init} and α are user-defined hyperparameters. By the above operation, we compute ε_r and $K_{after}(r)$ that satisfy the condition for the position r.

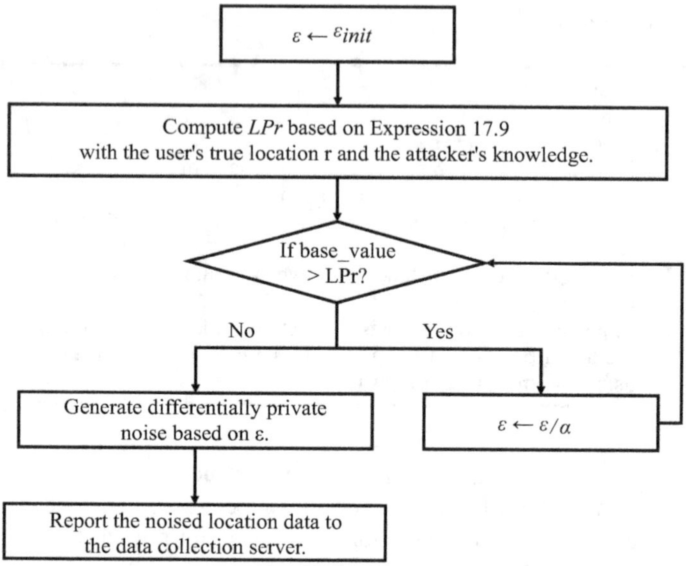

Figure 17.3 Flowchart of the proposed algorithm

In this process, K_{after} is computed by performing this operation on all r for the given position r.

In other words, the proposed method is an algorithm that guarantees privacy protection for LPr. It is difficult to get an image of the values of privacy parameters. However, LPr is calculated in units of meters (m). Thus, the degree of protection can be understood from the LPr value. One advantage of the proposed algorithm is that it allows easy conceptualization of such protection.

The flow of the proposed algorithm is shown in Figure 17.3. First, the anonymization mechanism sets the value of ε to ε_{init}, as specified by the user. Subsequently, the mechanism computes LPr, based on Expression 17.9, which incorporates the user's true location information and the attacker's prior knowledge. It should be noted that the attacker's prior knowledge is presumed to be the population information relevant to the time and area in question. This population information can be procured from mobile phone companies or other sources. To safeguard the user's LP, the value of LPr must exceed a predefined $base_value$. The mechanism repeatedly divides the value of ε by α until this condition is met. Finally, the mechanism generates Laplace noise based on the final ε value and communicates the noise-injected location data to the data collection server.

17.3.1.2 Computing *K*

In this context, K represents the probability; thus, formula 17.10 holds theoretically for any position r.

$$\sum_{r'} k(r)(r') = 1 \tag{17.10}$$

According to formula 17.5 and ε, we compute the Euclidean distance between positions r and r', as well as the probability $K(r)(r')$. In this study, we conducted a simulation experiment in a part of the space on the map. Thus, even if this is stored in an array without modification, formula 17.10 is not satisfied. As a result, there is a probability that r' is outside the defined space.

To satisfy the formula 17.10, we utilize the post-processing property concept (Proposition 1). Here, if r' is outside the defined space, we randomly select a position within the assumed space when adding noise. In other words, there is a uniform distribution of probabilities in the defined space for r' that is not within the defined space. After using differential privacy, the post-processing property is satisfied because the true value is not used.

First, store probabilities for K array according to formula 17.5. Then, we add the values calculated by the formula 7.11 in all positions. Thus, formula 17.10 is satisfied.

$$\frac{(1 - \sum_{r'} K(r)(r'))}{n \times n} \tag{17.11}$$

17.3.2 Implementation

In the proposed method, various values, e.g., $K_{before}(r)(r')$ and $h(r')(\hat{r})$, are obtained from a predetermined constant ε.

In this implementation, we assumed that the functions correspond to the virtual space of $100(n-1) \times 100(n-1)\text{m}^2$. $(n \in \mathbb{N})$. The space is divided by $100\text{m} \times 100\text{m}$, so there are $n \times n$ squares.

The functions, e.g., K and h, are represented by arrays. Here, K and h are two-dimensional arrays. Since there are $n \times n$ valid positions, it is a two-dimensional array of size $(n \times n) \times (n \times n)$.

17.3.3 Application to real-world location services

Using the privacy parameter ε calculated for each position by the proposed method, the planar Laplace mechanism (Section 2.5) is applied to protect privacy.

17.4 Experiment

17.4.1 Experiment summary

In this study, our experiments were conducted using a total of four types of data, two types of virtual settings, and two types of simulation data.

17.4.1.1 Virtual spaces

In the experiments, we assumed a space of $n = 100$, 100×100 squares, where the size of a single square is 100 m $\times$ 100 m. Two types of space were considered, i.e., in one space, the existence probability of people was distributed uniformly, and in the other space, the probability of the existence of people was concentrated in some positions.

First, we considered the uniform distribution space. Here, the probabilities were assigned equally to each square; thus, the probability of a single square was 1/10000. This space is referred to as the "uniform data".

Then, we considered the space where the existence probability of a person was concentrated in some positions. Here, the space extends from (0, 0) to (0, 10000), (10000, 0), and (10000, 10000), and the existence probability of people is concentrated only in 100 squares surrounded by (8000, 8000), (8000, 8900), (8900, 8000), and (8900, 8900). For this space, the probability of a single cell was 1/100. This space is referred to as the "ununiform data."

17.4.1.2 Simulation data

We used data generated using the Siafu simulation tool [31]. The Siafu tool is an OSS that can obtain simulation data using a model of typical human behavior on a map.

The size of the map was set to 8.4 km ×8.4 km. In addition, 1,000–10,000 people acted in the space, where companies, restaurants, parks, and so on were arranged. The simulation data were created in reference to the research of Yuichi *et al.* [32].

We assumed a space of $n = 100$, 100×100 squares. The size of a single square is 100 m × 100 m. The experiments were conducted on two types of human position datasets created by the simulation. One dataset had a high rate of people gathering in the same place, and the other dataset had a low rate. The space was divided into 100×100 squares, and we calculated the ratio of human presence from the simulation data. As a result, we compared a space with 452 nonzero points (when the rate of people gathering in the same place was high) and a space with 2471 (when the rate of people gathering in the same place was low). We refer to the data with a high rate of people clustering in the same place as the "dense data," and the data with a low rate of people clustering in the same place is referred to as the "sparse data."

When high possibility to be in the same place

The distribution based on the dense simulation data is shown in Figure 17.4.

When low possibility to be in the same place

The distribution based on the spare simulation data is shown in Figure 17.5.

17.4.1.3 Parameter settings

In this implementation, $\alpha = 5.0$, and two values of 0.1 and 0.5 were evaluated for ε_{init}. We used values of 150, 300, 600, 900, and 1200 for *base_value*. Note that the distance from a certain point is 100 m on both sides and $100\sqrt{2}$ on the diagonal; thus, we set the parameters accordingly. For the case where ε was uniform, experiments were conducted for ε values of 0.5, 0.1, 0.02, and 0.004.

17.4.2 Evaluation results

We calculated the SQL using formula 17.7 and evaluated the usefulness for the data collection server. As discussed previously, the program was executed for two types

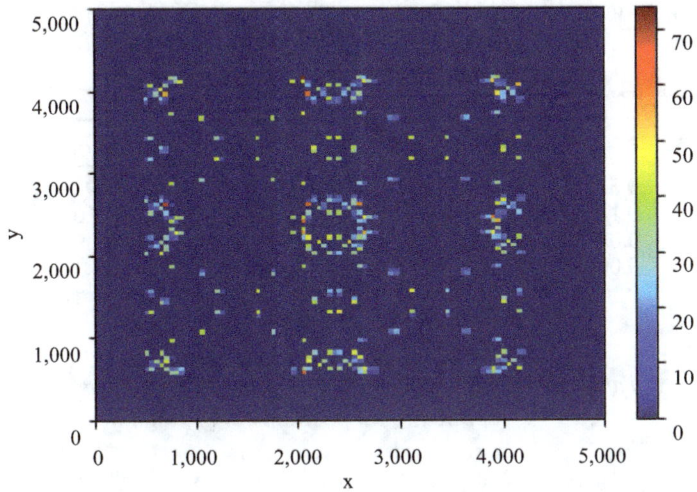

Figure 17.4 Distribution of dense data

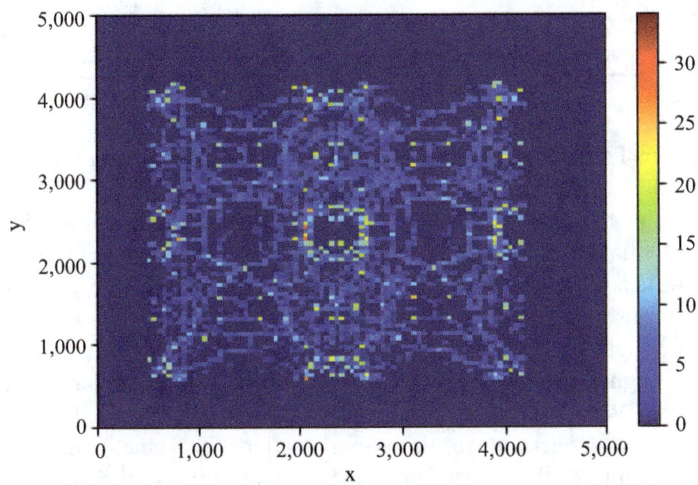

Figure 17.5 Distribution of sparse data

of virtual space data and two types of simulation-generated data. In Section 17.4.2, we show the evaluation results, and then we discuss the results in Section 17.5.

17.4.2.1 Results of the virtual space

Evaluation results were calculated for the virtual spaces with "uniform data" and "ununiform data," respectively.

The results of calculating the SQL value for the same ε value for all positions are summarized in the following. The results of uniform data are

Table 17.3 SQL results when the same ε value was applied to all positions in the uniform data

ε	**SQL/m**
0.5	659.9
0.1	2673.0
0.02	4952.9
0.004	5209.3

Table 17.4 SQL result when the same ε value was applied to all positions in the ununiform data

ε	**SQL/m**
0.5	385.5
0.1	2808.9
0.02	5536.9
0.004	5851.2

summarized in Table 17.3, and the results of the ununiform data are summarized in Table 17.4.

The smaller the value of ε, the higher the level of privacy protection and the greater the amount of noise added to the true values. As such, the SQL value, which measures the usefulness of the data after noise addition (where a smaller value implies higher usefulness), increases as the value of ε decreases.

The latter data set exhibits considerable variation in the probability of human presence. A higher probability of human presence implies a larger number of people present. When the value of ε is high, the effect of individuals in densely populated areas is significant, resulting in a smaller SQL value. Conversely, as the value of ε is reduced, the impact of human density inversely causes detrimental effects. The influence of areas devoid of human presence becomes more significant, leading to an increase in the SQL value.

Result of uniform data

For the uniform data, Table 17.5 shows the SQL and LPr results when privacy protection was applied based on the proposed method with $\varepsilon_{init} = 0.5$, and Table 17.6 shows the results for the $\varepsilon_{init} = 0.1$ case. Here, MIN LPr and MAX LPr are the minimum and maximum LPr values, respectively, among the LPr values computed for all positions. As shown, the proposed method guarantees that MIN LPr exceeds *base_value*. The LPr should achieve values higher than the specified *base_value*. Upon inspecting the table, it can be confirmed that for all scenarios, the

LPr exceeds the *base_value*. Since the value of LPr varies from person to person, it is apparent that the MIN LPr and MAX LPr values are different.

When compared with the results for Tables 17.5 and 17.6, it can be observed that the values of SQL and MIN LPr are almost identical for each *base_value*. This indicates that, unlike existing methods, we have been able to appropriately adjust the amount of noise added to the true values based on a new privacy protection metric called *base_value*, irrespective of the setting of the value of ε_{init}, a parameter of differential privacy techniques.

Result of ununiform data

For the ununiform data, Table 17.7 shows the results of calculating the SQL when privacy protection was applied based on the proposed method with $\varepsilon_{init} = 0.5$, and

Table 17.5 SQL and maximum and minimum LPr values for uniform data ($\varepsilon_{init} = 0.5$)

base_value	**SQL/m**	**MIN LPr/m**	**MAX LPr/m**
150	659.902	375.021	5143.26
300	659.902	375.021	5143.26
600	2142.38	600.855	5143.26
900	2332.26	902.399	5143.26
1200	2431.46	1240.12	5143.26

Table 17.6 SQL and maximum and minimum LPr values for uniform data ($\varepsilon_{init} = 0.1$). Note that in this setting, no matter how large the added noise, the privacy protection level cannot be achieved. Therefore, the server does not actually collect location information.

base_value	**SQL/m**	**MIN LPr/m**	**MAX LPr/m**
150	659.902	327.571	5662.88
300	659.902	327.572	5662.88
600	1478.58	601.507	5662.88
900	1895.29	904.208	5662.88
1200	2106.69	1210.79	5662.88

Table 17.7 SQL and maximum and minimum LPr values for ununiform data ($\varepsilon_{init} = 0.5$)

base_value	**SQL/m**	**MIN LPr/m**	**MAX LPr/m**
150	385.5	201.24	10685
300	2563.5	310.18	10685
600	2808.9	601.26	10685
900	2808.9	902.22	10685
1200	2808.9	1200.37	10685

Table 17.8 shows the results for the $\varepsilon_{init} = 0.1$ case. Regarding Table 17.7, similar to the experimental results for the previous data set, it can be confirmed that each LPr surpasses the *base_value* for Table 17.7, thereby satisfying the requirements of privacy protection. Regarding Table 17.6, the values of MIN LPr are smaller than the values of *base_value*. Due to an overly high concentration of individuals in a confined area, an attacker can ascertain each person's location information, irrespective of how much noise is added, owing to their prior knowledge. As a result, the value of LPr falls below the *base_value*. In other words, this experiment was conducted under a scenario where it was impossible to achieve the specified level of privacy protection.

17.4.2.2 Results of the simulation data

We evaluated the SQL values obtained for the dense and sparse generated by the simulation.

Conventional method without adjusting ε

The SQL results for the same ε value for all positions are summarized in the following. Here, the SQL results for the dense data are summarized in Table 17.9, and those for the sparse data are summarized in Table 17.10. It can be observed that as the value of ε decreases, the SQL value significantly increases. This implies a substantial reduction in the usefulness of the data.

Results of dense data

For the dense data, when $\varepsilon_{init} = 0.5$ and privacy protection was applied, the SQL results are shown in Table 17.11, and Table 17.12 shows the results for the $\varepsilon_{init} = 0.1$ case.

Table 17.8 SQL and maximum and minimum LPr values for ununiform data ($\varepsilon_{init} = 0.1$)

base_value	**SQL/m**	**MIN LPr/m**	**MAX LPr/m**
150	795.199	38.237	11999.9
300	2122.90	38.237	11999.9
600	5731.12	38.237	11999.9
900	5856.93	38.237	11999.9
1200	5856.93	38.237	11999.9

Table 17.9 SQL results when the same ε value was applied to all positions in dense data

ε	**SQL/m**
0.5	380.287
0.1	2193.35
0.02	4496.00
0.004	4727.52

Results of sparse data

For the sparse data, when $\varepsilon_{init} = 0.5$ and privacy protection was applied, the SQL results are shown in Table 17.13, and Table 17.14 shows the results for the $\varepsilon_{init} = 0.1$ case.

Table 17.10 SQL results when the same ε value was applied to all positions in sparse data

ε	SQL/m
0.5	379.656
0.1	2093.99
0.02	4333.87
0.004	4552.14

Table 17.11 SQL and maximum and minimum LPr values for dense data ($\varepsilon_{init} = 0.5$)

base_value	SQL	MIN LPr/m	MAX LPr/m
150	399.703	150.341	5363.88
300	1549.44	300.065	5363.88
600	2192.87	600.162	5363.88
900	2193.35	900.152	5363.88
1200	2193.35	1200.38	5363.88

Table 17.12 SQL and maximum and minimum LPr values for dense data ($\varepsilon_{init} = 0.1$)

base_value	SQL	MIN LPr/m	MAX LPr/m
150	380.287	150.607	6521.97
300	667.314	300.508	6521.97
600	1784.54	600.044	6521.97
900	2185.64	900.430	6521.97
1200	2193.35	1201.63	6521.97

Table 17.13 SQL maximum and minimum LPr values for sparse data ($\varepsilon_{init} = 0.5$)

base_value	SQL	MIN LPr/m	MAX LPr/m
150	379.656	183.387	5861.67
300	753.016	300.075	5861.67
600	2093.79	600.712	5861.67
900	2093.99	900.184	5861.67
1200	2093.99	1200.27	5861.67

Table 17.14 SQL and maximum and minimum LPr values for sparse data ($\varepsilon_{init} = 0.1$)

base_value	SQL	MIN LPr/m	MAX LPr/m
150	379.656	279.065	6732.24
300	414.746	300.069	6732.24
600	1148.84	600.020	6732.24
900	1733.13	900.165	6732.24
1200	2026.25	1200.00	6732.24

17.5 Discussion

17.5.1 SQL when ε is unchanged

For Tables 17.3, 17.4, 17.9, and 17.10, if the privacy parameter ε was not varied for each location, especially when ε was changed from 0.5 to 0.1, the SQL value increased remarkably. This demonstrates that reducing the ε value may reduce user convenience significantly.

17.5.2 Results using the proposed method

With the exception of the $\varepsilon_{init} = 0.1$ case for the ununiform data, all results of executing the program based on the proposed method resulted in the MIN LPr value exceeding *base_value*; thus. LPr is guaranteed.

Regarding $\varepsilon_{init} = 0.1$ case for the ununiform data, as discussed in the previous chapter, it is important to note that this experiment takes place under a scenario where it is impossible to meet the privacy protection level. The proposed system can anticipate such situations in advance and thus can opt not to collect location information in these cases, thereby ensuring privacy.

$\varepsilon = 0.1$ for all results with *base_value* up to 1200, applying the same privacy parameter ε to all, except for "ununiform data" and $\varepsilon_{init} = 0.1$, the result was either lower than the SQL of or the integer part was the same. Thus, we consider that the proposed method strengthened protection by reducing the value of the privacy parameter as required while suppressing SQL.

base_value of "uniform data" is not changed between 150 and 300. Even if *base_value* is set to 150, as the smallest LPr value in the whole already exceeds 300, there was no difference in the privacy parameters assigned to locations.

When the proposed method was applied to the ununiform data with $\varepsilon_{init} = 0.1$, the SQL value was improved significantly. By investigating the LPr value at each location, we found that (85, 85) was the smallest value because it can be predicted that the probability of being at this location in the target space appears to be the highest. This space was set artificially such that there were only 10Ã—10 people in the 100Ã—100 space. Therefore, the relationship between the distance and *epsilon* may be unbalanced.

17.5.3 Computational cost

To determine an appropriate value for the privacy parameter ε for each location, the proposed method first computes the mechanism K and the attacker function h. Here, the computational complexity was $\mathcal{O}(n^3)$, which resulted in a huge computational cost. However, we can offer a solution to this problem. Once we obtained the privacy parameters to use for each location, there was little computational cost to apply the planar Laplace mechanism using the defined parameters.

The probability of human presence depends on the time of day, e.g., afternoon or evening. However, it is considered to be periodic; thus, calculating the parameters for each position once in advance reduces the subsequent computational costs. In this study, we focused on the probability of human presence; however, we should also consider the privacy degree by taking into account the semantic information about each location, e.g., whether the location is a hospital or supermarket.

17.5.4 Guarantee for changing ε for each position

In this study, we did not consider the risk involved with changing the privacy parameter and noise addition compared to using a uniform parameter. In a similar study by Sasada *et al.* [33], the addition of noise was varied according to the situation. However, this study did not consider the risks of changing the amount of added noise, which will be the focus of future work.

17.5.5 GPS noise and k-anonymity

Research is being conducted that associates a user's location history with user attributes such as gender, age, income, and residence, to analyze consumption behavior by user attribute. By conducting such an analysis, it is possible to perform more appropriate marketing and advertising.

In this scenario, we consider an environment where businesses, not directly obtaining user attributes or location information, receive this information from other businesses and conduct mining. The mining company only needs to receive the data (history of location information and corresponding user attributes) after excluding information such as names and addresses. However, if there is an attacker who knows the fact that a user, say Alice, was at location (x, y) at time t, it is revealed that the user attribute corresponding to that time and location is Alice's attribute.

In order to solve this problem, extensive research is being conducted to anonymize each user's location information. For instance, when k-anonymity is applied to location information, the location information provided to the mining business is represented as an area, not a point, and it is guaranteed that there are at least k users in this anonymized area. However, if the anonymizing business has errors in the location information it knows, there may actually be less than k users in the anonymization area.

Existing k-anonymity algorithms aim to minimize the size of the anonymization area. However, if there are errors in the location information, there may not be any users in the anonymization area. Therefore, it is believed that not only minimizing the anonymization area but also the probability of actual user presence in that area should be a metric.

One of the indicators for anonymizing users so that they cannot be uniquely identified is k-anonymity, which was proposed by Lefevre *et al.* [34]. When Alice's location is (x, y), we prepare $x1, x2, y1, y2$ satisfying $x1 < x < x2$, $y1 < y < y2$, and only disclose the information that Alice exists in the area represented by the rectangle with vertices $(x1, x2, y1, y2)$. At this time, the area is constructed so that there are k or more users in this area. Since there are more than k users in the region, it is impossible to identify which user attribute in the released user attributes represents Alice.

Existing research targeting k-anonymity aims to minimize the area of the anonymization area where k or more users exist. Since this problem is shown to be NP-hard, heuristics with a small computational complexity have been proposed. The Mondrian algorithm [35], not limited to location information, is widely used as a k-anonymity method and is adopted as a base method in multiple location anonymization methods.

Research is also being conducted to anonymize the continuous history of locations over a certain period of time, not just the user's location information at one moment. These studies prevent an attacker who knows Alice's location at a certain time t from knowing where Alice was at times other than t based on the history of location information at multiple times $t_1, t_2, \ldots$. These studies perform k-anonymization of location information at a certain time, and it is believed that the method proposed in this paper can be used for that anonymization.

There is also research that anonymizes location information, targeting scenarios where user IDs and their location information are disclosed. In such research, methods are also adopted to prevent the attacker from receiving accurate locations by obscuring location information without considering the relationship with other users. There are also studies, like those by Ardagna *et al.*, that perform anonymization considering the error in acquiring location information, but they are anonymizing each user's individual location information, and the relationship with other users like in k-anonymization is not considered. It is possible to extend it to perform k-anonymization, but in this case, the same problem as with normal k-anonymization methods as pointed out in this chapter arises.

There is also research that anonymizes so that semantic information, such as whether the user was at school or in a downtown area, does not leak from the location information to be disclosed. When providing services based on location information to each user, such anonymization is necessary.

As stated above, ensuring k-anonymity becomes challenging when GPS noise is present. However, by utilizing differential privacy, the focus of this chapter, we can effectively handle GPS noise. We assume that the GPS noise mainly follows a normal distribution, and we suppose that the data collection server knows the upper limit of the standard deviation of this normal distribution. In this case, it becomes possible to adjust the noise added to the acquired GPS values, considering the probability distribution of the GPS noise [22]. The construction of a system utilizing the proposed method while considering GPS noise will be future work.

17.6 Conclusion

For healthcare systems, there are advantages to obtaining personal location information for epidemiological studies, public health interventions, and risk assessment. In this chapter, we have proposed a method to add noise to location information according to the degree of privacy protection based on the probability of human presence at a certain point in time. We found that it is possible to suppress the SQL (user convenience) by setting appropriate privacy parameters for each position.

For time-series data, the application of simple differential privacy reduces the degree of privacy protection. In other words, if you send protected data for the same position many times, the true position may be predicted from the distribution. Thus, methods are required to prevent the reduction of privacy protection of time-series data.

In addition, it is necessary to reduce the value of the privacy parameter and improve protection for locations where it is easy to guess sensitive information, e.g., hospitals. Thus, privacy protection methods that focus on the degree of sensitivity of the target facilities.

In the proposed method, the value of the privacy parameter ε was varied for each position; however, we did not evaluate the impact of varying this value. Therefore, in the future, it will be necessary to evaluate the effects of changing the privacy parameter at each position.

Acknowledgment

This work was supported by JSPS KAKENHI Grant Numbers JP21H03496, JP22K12157, JP23H03688, and SEI Group CSR Foundation.

References

[1] Xu J, Murray AT, Church RL, *et al.* Service allocation equity in location coverage analytics. *European Journal of Operational Research.* 2023;305 (1):21–37.

[2] Zhao Y and Chen J. Vector-indistinguishability: Location dependency based privacy protection for successive location data. *IEEE Transactions on Computers.* 2023. 10.1109/TC.2023.3236900.

[3] Han L, Luo W, Yang A, *et al.* Fully privacy-preserving location recommendation in outsourced environments. *Ad Hoc Networks.* 2023; 141: 103077.

[4] Kimura Y, Seki T, Miyata S, *et al.* Hotspot analysis of COVID-19 infection using mobile-phone location data. *Artificial Life and Robotics.* 2023; 28(1):43–49.

[5] Xu C, Jin L, and Lee L. An empirical spatial network model based on human mobility for epidemiological research: A case study. *Annals of the American Association of Geographers.* 2023;113(6): 1–22.

[6] Jing F, Li Z, Qiao S, *et al.* Association between immigrant concentration and mental health service utilization in the United States over time: A geospatial big data analysis. *Health & Place*. 2023;83:103055.
[7] Luca M, Campedelli GM, Centellegher S, *et al.* Crime, inequality and public health: A survey of emerging trends in urban data science. *Frontiers in Big Data.* 2023;6:1124526.
[8] Guan SY, Zheng JX, Sam NB, *et al.* Global burden and risk factors of musculoskeletal disorders among adolescents and young adults in 204 countries and territories, 1990–2019. *Autoimmunity Reviews.* 2023;22(8): 103361.
[9] Zhong X, Zhou Z, Li G, *et al.* Neighborhood disparities in COVID-19 outcomes in New York city over the first two waves of the outbreak. *Annals of Epidemiology.* 2022;70:45–52.
[10] Haddad Z. Blockchain-enabled anonymous mutual authentication and location privacy-preserving scheme for 5 networks. *Journal of King Saud University – Computer and Information Sciences*. 2023;35(6):1–7, In press.
[11] Xudong Y, Ling G, Yan L, *et al.* A blockchain-based location privacy-preserving scheme in location-based service. *Mobile Information Systems.* 2022;2022:1–16.
[12] Tian Y, Wang J, Wang Y, *et al.* Federated vehicular transformers and their federations: Privacy-preserving computing and cooperation for autonomous driving. *IEEE Transactions on Intelligent Vehicles.* 2022;7(3):456–465.
[13] Andrew J, Isravel DP, Sagayam KM, *et al.* Blockchain for healthcare systems: Architecture, security challenges, trends and future directions. *Journal of Network and Computer Applications.* 2023;215:103633.
[14] He M, Bai F, Zhang C, *et al.* A blockchain-enabled location privacy-preserving under local differential privacy for Internet of vehicles. In: *Proceedings of the 2022 4th Blockchain and Internet of Things Conference*; 2022.
[15] Wang W, Wang Y, Huang Y, *et al.* Privacy protection federated learning system based on blockchain and edge computing in mobile crowdsourcing. *Computer Networks.* 2022;215:109206.
[16] Wang W, Wang Y, Duan P, *et al.* A triple real-time trajectory privacy protection mechanism based on edge computing and blockchain in mobile crowdsourcing. *IEEE Transactions on Mobile Computing.* 2022;22 (10):5625–5642.
[17] Singh S, Rathore S, Alfarraj O, *et al.* A framework for privacy-preservation of IoT healthcare data using federated learning and blockchain technology. *Future Generation Computer Systems.* 2022;129:380–388.
[18] Murakami T and Sei Y. Automatic tuning of privacy budgets in input-discriminative local differential privacy. *IEEE Internet of Things Journal.* 2023;10(18):15990–16005.
[19] Zhao Y and Chen J. A survey on differential privacy for unstructured data content. *ACM Computing Surveys (CSUR).* 2022;54(10s):1–28.
[20] Zhiheng C. Social information labeling for individual mobile phone user. In: *Handbook of MobilityData Mining.* Elsevier; 2023. 177–184.

[21] Dwork C. Differential privacy. In: *Proc. 33rd International Conference on Automata, Languages and Programming*; 2006. p. 1–12.

[22] Sei Y and Ohsuga A. Private true data mining: Differential privacy featuring errors to manage Internet-of-Things Data. *IEEE Access*. 2022;10(1):8738–8757.

[23] Sei Y, Okumura H and Ohsuga A. Re-identification in differentially private incomplete datasets. *IEEE Open Journal of the Computer Society*. 2022;3:62–72.

[24] Zhu K, Van Hentenryck P and Fioretto F. Bias and variance of post-processing in differential privacy. In: *Proceedings of the AAAI Conference on Artificial Intelligence*. 2021;35(12):11177–11184.

[25] Chatzikokolakis K, Andrés ME, Bordenabe NE, *et al.* Broadening the scope of differential privacy using metrics. In: *International Symposium on Privacy Enhancing Technologies Symposium*. Springer; 2013. 82–102.

[26] Andrés ME, Bordenabe NE, Chatzikokolakis K, *et al.* Geo-indistinguish-ability: Differential privacy for location-based systems. In: *Proceedings of the 2013 ACM SIGSAC conference on Computer & Communications Security*; 2013. 901–914.

[27] Shokri R, Theodorakopoulos G, Troncoso C, *et al.* Protecting location privacy: Optimal strategy against localization attacks. In: *Proceedings of the 2012 ACM Conference on Computer and Communications Security*. CCS '12. New York, NY, USA: Association for Computing Machinery; 2012. p. 617–627. Available from: https://doi.org/10.1145/2382196.2382261.

[28] Shokri R, Theodorakopoulos G, Le Boudec JY, *et al.* Quantifying location privacy. In: *2011 IEEE Symposium on Security and Privacy*. IEEE; 2011. 247–262.

[29] Takagi S, Cao Y, Asano Y, *et al.* Geo-graph-indistinguishability: Protecting location privacy for LBS over road networks. In: *Data and Applications Security and Privacy XXXIII: 33rd Annual IFIP WG 11.3 Conference, DBSec 2019*, Charleston, SC, USA, July 15–17, 2019, Proceedings 33. Springer; 2019. p. 143–163.

[30] Chatzikokolakis K, Palamidessi C and Stronati M. *Constructing elastic distinguishability metrics for location privacy*. arXiv preprint arXiv:150300756. 2015.

[31] Martin M and Nurmi P. A generic large scale simulator for ubiquitous computing. In: *2006 Third Annual International Conference on Mobile and Ubiquitous Systems: Networking & Services*. IEEE; 2006. p. 1–3.

[32] Sei Y and Ohsuga A. Location anonymization with considering errors and existence probability. *IEEE Transactions on Systems, Man, and Cybernetics: Systems*. 2016;47(12):3207–3218.

[33] Sasada T, Taenaka Y, Kadobayashi Y, *et al.* Considering the variation of the noise-addition amount in local differential privacy with user trajectory adjacency. vol. 120. IEICE Technical Report; 2020. 45–50.

[34] LeFevre K, DeWitt DJ and Ramakrishnan R. Workload-aware anonymization. In: *Proc. ACM KDD*; 2006. 277–286.

[35] LeFevre K, DeWitt DJ and Ramakrishnan R. Mondrian multidimensional K-anonymity. In: *Proc. IEEE ICDE*; 2006. 25.

Chapter 18

Emerging case studies on the application of AI and blockchain technology in telehealth systems

Adewole Usman Rufai[1], Babatunde Olusoji Okunoye[1], Aisha Titilola Rufai[2] and Lucky Odeh[1]

The fusion of artificial intelligence (AI) and blockchain technology in telehealth systems provides the necessary underpinnings for the development of robust healthcare systems. Telehealth systems are characterized by the generation of big data (medical data). AI algorithms utilize these data in assisting healthcare workers in providing the necessary insights in making crucial decisions in healthcare systems. However, these data need to be protected from invasion of privacy, outright theft, and unauthorized access among other problems. The blockchain technology comes into the fray to solve the problems mentioned above. In this work, we explore the existing case studies with the aim of identifying the gaps inherent in existing works and provide potential solutions to the gaps observed through a systematic review. We also explore the relevant AI algorithm and architecture for various case studies in telehealth systems. Our findings from the case studies have the potential of transforming the telehealth system into a more efficient and effective one.

18.1 Introduction

Over the years, progress in technology has transformed various domains with great disruptions from traditional ways of operations and the telehealth domain is no exception. The incursion of artificial intelligence (AI) and blockchain in telehealth systems has been instrumental in making healthcare services much more effective, accessible, and secure. This chapter seeks to explore various case studies that highlight the application of AI and blockchain in telehealth systems. Giving emphasis to the impact of these technologies on diagnosis and treatment, payment systems, and medical record management amongst other case studies.

[1]Department of Computer Sciences, Faculty of Science, University of Lagos, Nigeria
[2]Department of Electrical and Electronics Engineering, Faculty of Engineering, University of Lagos, Nigeria

The ubiquity of telehealth systems has led to an increase in access to healthcare by the provision of remote services and the scalability of medical expertise beyond what is obtained in the traditional settings. While traditional telehealth systems are characterized by challenges in precise diagnosis, secure patient data, transparent payment system, and efficient patient monitoring, AI and blockchain present innovative alternatives that address all these challenges.

With machine learning (ML) algorithms, AI possesses the ability to analyze enormous healthcare data which is in the realm of big data, obtain meaningful patterns from historical data, and provide insights that help optimize healthcare processes. The deployment of chatbots and virtual assistants aids in facilitating communications between patients and healthcare personnel and also led to the reduction of response time.

Blockchain technology is characterized by a decentralized peer-to-peer network leveraging on distributed ledger and smart contracts. These guarantee a secure way of managing medical records and processes. By adopting cryptographic techniques, smart contracts, and distributed ledger protocols, patients possess control over their medical records as they can grant access permission to healthcare personnel and institutions. The decentralized approach engenders a seamless sharing of information and the technology prevents data infractions by unauthorized entities.

This chapter presents recent case studies that show the practical application and benefits of AI and blockchain in telehealth systems. The case studies demonstrate the successful integration of AI and blockchain protocols in various healthcare scenarios leading to a much more secure and efficient healthcare delivery.

18.1.1 Major contributions of the chapter

The following are the significant contributions of this chapter:

i. The chapter investigates, highlights, and reports recent advances in the application of AI and blockchain technology in telehealth systems.
ii. We consider the case study of AI-enabled diagnosis and treatment with an implementation using the Random Forest Classification algorithm.
iii. We present case studies in AI-enabled remote patient monitoring (RPM); blockchain for secure medical records; and blockchain for healthcare payments.

18.1.2 Chapter organization

Section 18.2 presents the related works in AI and blockchain applications to telehealth systems. Section 18.3 considers the case study on AI-enabled Diagnosis and Treatment with implementation using a dataset. Section 18.4 gives an exposition of AI-enabled remote patient monitoring case study. Section 18.5 presents a case study on blockchain for secure medical records. Section 18.6 considers blockchain for healthcare payment case study. Section 18.7 concludes the chapter with future direction.

18.2 Related work

In the field of AI and blockchain research, a lot of work has been done in the telehealth domain. However, the adoption of AI algorithms in the medical sector has fallen below the rate of similar acceptance in other sectors like finance and transportation [1]. The last couple of years have revealed that AI and blockchain hold great potential and promise in the telehealth domain.

Health professionals will also evolve and as they progress alongside AI and ML, they will better understand how to work with it. This is becoming evident as we may not be able to relegate AI to the background anymore. The fear that health professionals will lose their jobs due to the implementation of AI and ML is not only untrue but unfounded, rather it is expected that AI will enable health professionals to perform their duties more effectively and efficiently thereby giving more time to health professionals to have the meaningful human connections that make medicine such a valued and gratifying field [2].

Lee *et al.* [3] worked on medical AI chatbots. In the study, some AI chatbots were studied for their applications in medicine. Two of the most notable are LaMDA (a group of conversational large language models developed by Google) and GPT-3.5, and GPT-4. Indeed, it is noteworthy to state that LaMDA, GPT-3.5, and GPT-4 have not been trained specifically for healthcare or medical applications rather the main purpose of their training has been to enable these AI models to perform effectively across various domains, rather than being specialized for specific tasks like healthcare or medicine. It becomes evident that these systems were trained using openly available online sources of information, these publicly available sources include health system websites, research papers, medical texts, and publicly obtainable health information videos and podcasts. The training data, however, does not contain any information from sources that are privately restricted, such training data includes information from an electronic health record system in a healthcare organization or any medical data existing solely on the private network of a medical school or similar institution. Even with these limitations, the AI systems produce some appreciable knowledge and competence in healthcare systems.

The study shows some benefits of using chatbots in medicine to include medical note taking. In a potential scenario to implement this medical note taking, the individual gives his or her consent, GPT-4 in a manner similar to modern-day smart speakers will obtain the conversation transcript by monitoring the physician-to-patient interaction. At the end of the conversation between patient and physician and when requested, this software would generate the medical note. GPT-4 has the capacity to generate notes in recognized formats like SOAP (known as subjective, objective, assessment, and plan), along with the automatic inclusion of relevant billing codes. SOAP is a procedure for documentation used by healthcare providers when they write notes. After note taking, it can be required to respond to questions about the doctor–patient conversation, prior authorization details can be retrieved, produce laboratory and prescription orders in adherence to the standards associated to Health Level Seven Fast Healthcare Interoperability Resources, it can generate post-visit summaries and offer valuable feedback to the physician and the patient.

Another benefit of GPT-4 is its inherent almost natural-like knowledge of medicine.

Even as we stated earlier that the GPT-4 model was trained entirely on publicly available information on the open web, when presented with a series of test questions to answer by the U.S. Medical Licensing Examination (USMLE) it provided a high accuracy rate by correctly answering more than 90% of the test questions. The model also provides some explanations for its reasoning, references established medical facts, identifies causal relationships, dismisses other answers, and offers a compelling justification for its point of view. Third, another benefit is in medical consultation. The medical knowledge integrated into GPT-4 can be employed for diverse purposes like in consultation, diagnosis, and educational settings.

When presented with a standard curbside consult scenario (an informal form of specialist consultation), details regarding the patient's initial condition, or an overview of the test results. In general, GPT-4 produces helpful and beneficial responses that will aid the health worker to effectively tackle the concern they inquired about their query. Due to the interactive nature of the system, the user can ask for more clarification on the responses received by posing follow-up questions or asking for more succinct answers in order to get to reach the main information quickly. This wealth of medical expertise possessed by GPT-4 makes it a valuable resource not just in the area of clinical settings but also for advancing research endeavors. Medical research material can be read by GPT-4 which allows it to engage in informed discussion about it, like summarizing contents, offering technical analysis in otherwise difficult areas, referencing relevant previous studies or work, evaluating and analyzing the conclusions, and posing relevant follow-up research questions.

Han *et al.* [4] stated that AI can be used in the detection of drug interaction. This is called drug–drug interaction (DDI). The study of DDIs is crucial in drug research. Despite their importance in drug research, DDIs can also cause adverse reactions in patients, leading to potentially dangerous outcomes. Manual detection of DDIs is laborious and very costly, so it becomes expedient to leverage computer-based solutions to eliminate these challenges. Using the computer approach follows two paths: one is to identify and group known drug interactions, while the other focuses on predicting potential interactions that have not been known before.

Myszczynska *et al.* [5] carried out a study on the use of AI to effectively diagnose and treat neurodegenerative diseases. The study found that ML, a subset of AI, is empowering stakeholders in healthcare delivery to solve some of the problems in diagnosing and treating neurodegenerative diseases which include the intricacies of the molecular mechanisms affecting neuronal degeneration and the diverse nature of the patient population. The study also found that neuroimaging was the initial branch of neurology to take advantage of the application of AI approaches to enhance diagnosis and treatment. Recently, applying ML techniques to motor function and language feature analysis has shown the immense potential to drastically reduce clinical assessment time.

Igbal *et al.* [6] in their study on the clinical application of ML and AI in cancer diagnosis stated the aggressive growth of AI in the last 10 years is shown to be the envisaged platform with super-intelligence capable of making optimal decisions, where the human mind is restricted to manipulate large data in a limited time range.

Cancer is a compound and complicated characterized by a vast number of genetic and epigenetic variations. AI-enabled algorithms have shown massive potential to enable the early identification of genetic mutations and abnormal protein interactions. Modern biomedical research is also increasingly focusing on safely and ethically implementing AI technology in clinical settings. AI-enabled assistance to pathologists and physicians could be a significant step forward toward advancing healthcare in the areas of disease prediction, disease diagnosis, and disease treatments. The applications of AI and ML clinically are the future of healthcare leading to a faster mapping of a new treatment for every individual in cancer diagnosis and treatment. By utilizing AI-enabled systems, researchers can engage in real-time collaborations and in real-time and knowledge sharing to potentially heal millions.

Another domain of interest is the AI-enabled Remote Patient Monitoring (AI RPM). Shaik *et al.* [7] did a comprehensive review of RPM using AI for various applications in healthcare particularly for vital signs monitoring and patient physical activities. El-Rashidy *et al.* [8] highlighted the current research directions on remote patient monitoring for different diseases. The study also discusses the role of AI in developing RPM systems. Kantipudi *et al.* [9] discussed the concept of technologies such as cloud computing, IoT, and AI in different healthcare settings to determine the best architecture for cloud and AI for disease diagnosis and remote monitoring of patients. Leung [10] proposed a conceptual framework that shows the necessary components for better utilizing AI and ML for social media for monitoring patient. Dubey *et al.* [11] evaluated the Food and Drug Administration (FDA)-approved RPM devices to provide information for the US medical device industry based on previous approvals and the markets' needs. This journal also identifies RPM systems that are AI-based. A common factor on the works above is that they focused on the review of the domain more discussion can be found in Imoize *et al.* [12] and Rufai *et al.* [13].

The blockchain technology was initially proposed by Nakamoto [14] as a solution to the double-spending problem using a peer-to-peer network leading to Bitcoin. However, the technology has been found to be useful in other domains, one of which is telehealth. According to Haleem *et al.* [15], "Blockchain is a decentralized and public digital ledger that records transaction on many computers so that no records involved can be altered retroactively without altering any blocks afterwards". The attributes of decentralization, immutability, high availability amongst others, have enthused the application of blockchain in the telehealth domain. These attributes are in tandem with the CIA (Confidentiality, Integrity and Availability) triad that characterizes a secure telehealth information system. Haleem *et al.* [15] did a comprehensive review of blockchain technology and its significant impact in healthcare. The authors identify 14 significant applications of blockchain for healthcare.

Ahmad *et al.* [16] highlighted the potential opportunities that blockchain brings to telehealth in general. The authors presented case studies and the discussion of open research challenges in the domain. Sun *et al.* [17] applied blockchain to medical information management and proposed an auxiliary architecture based on hyperledger fabric and attribute-based access control (ABAC). The authors used smart contracts to define multi-tier data structure, design simulation experiments, and verify the performance of the scheme. The work of the authors is summarized in Table 18.1.

Table 18.1 Summary of related works

References	Work done	Methodology	Contributions	Gaps	Remarks
Shaik *et al.* [7]	"Remote patient monitoring using artificial intelligence: Current State, application and challenges"	Review	Review of Remote patient monitoring (RPM) using artificial intelligence (AI) for various applications in healthcare particularly for vital signs monitoring and patient physical activities.	No implementation	
El-Rashidy *et al.* [8]	"Mobile health in remote patient monitoring for chronic diseases: Principles, trends, and challenges"	Review	This study highlights the current research directions on remote patient monitoring for different diseases. The study also discusses the role of AI in developing RPM systems.	Focused more on chronic diseases	
Kantipudi *et al.* [9]	"Remote Patient Monitoring Using IoT, Cloud Computing and AI"	Review	This work discusses the concept of technologies such as cloud computing, IoT, and AI in different healthcare settings to determine the best architecture for cloud and AI for disease diagnosis and remote monitoring of patients.	No implementation	
Leung [10]	"Using AI–ML to Augment the Capabilities of Social Media for Telehealth and Remote Patient Monitoring"	Review	This work highlights the importance of social media for patient monitoring and for data collection through the aid of AI and ML techniques.	Proposed a conceptual framework that shows the necessary components for better utilizing AI and Machine learning (ML) for social media for monitoring patient.	

Dubey *et al*. [11]	"Artificial intelligence and remote patient monitoring in US healthcare market: a literature review"	Review	This work evaluates the Food and Drug Administration (FDA)-approved RPM devices to provide information for the US medical device industry based on previous approvals and the markets' needs. This journal also identifies RPM systems that are AI-based	Low AI algorithm transparency. Focus on improving RPM device functionality rather than AI algorithms that can effectively classify patients.
Nakamoto [14]	"Bitcoin: A Peer-to-Peer Electronic Cash System"	The use of hash-based proof-of-work. This ensures that record cannot be changed without a rework of the proof-of-work.	A proposal of a solution to the double-spending problem using a peer-to-peer network.	This is the paper that pioneered the blockchain technology.
Haleem *et al*. [15]	"Blockchain Technology applications in healthcare: An overview"	Review	Review of blockchain technology and its significant impact in healthcare. Identification and debates of fourteen significant application of blockchain for healthcare	No implementation
Ahmad *et al*. [16]	"The role of blockchain technology in telehealth and telemedicine"	Review	The work highlighted the potential opportunities that blockchain brings to telehealth in general. The presentation of case studies to support the above. And the discussion of open research challenges in the domain.	No implementation
Sun *et al*. [17]	"A blockchain-based secure storage scheme for medical information"	Based on hyperledger fabric and attribute-based access control (ABAC) framework	The work applies blockchain to medical information management; proposed an auxiliary architecture based on ABAC; uses smart contracts to define multi-tier data structure; designs simulation	The scheme is carried out on a single PC.

(Continues)

Table 18.1 (Continued)

References	Work done	Methodology	Contributions	Gaps	Remarks
			experiments and verify the performance of the scheme		
Azaria *et al.* [18]	"MedRec:Using Blockchain for medical Data Access and Permission Management"	The system was built on distributed ledger protocol originally used for Bitcoin	MedRec: a novel decentralized record management system to handle medical records using blockchain technology was proposed.	There exist the need to formalize an onboarding procedure for medical research miners and the exploration of mining data economics.	
Han *et al.* [19]	"Blockchain Technology for Electronic Health Records (EHR)"	Review	Introduction of several classical schemes based on blockchain technology to enhance interoperability and privacy protection in HER.	No implementation	
Yaga *et al.* [20]	"Blockchain Technology Overview"	Technical Overview	Gives a comprehensive overview of blockchain technology.	No focus on a particular domain.	
Nishi *et al.* [21]	"Electronic Health Data Record Security Using Blockchain and Smart Contracts.	Ethereum, Smart Contract and Interplanetary File System (IPFS) for a peer-to-peer network were used for the EHR system.	The combination of Ethereum blockchain platform and the smart contract for the development of the EHR system.	More work is required to provide a real-time video conference feature.	
Mhamdi *et al.* [22]	"SEMRAchain: A Secure Electronic Medical Record Based on Blockchain Technology"	The proposed system combines blockchain technology and multi-agent systems.	Using access control techniques to prevent external intrusion. Merging smart contracts and access control to guarantee the security and confidentiality of patients' data.	More work is required to extend the system to road users to find the nearest medical facility and dedicated ambulances.	
Shahnaz *et al.* [23]	"Using Blockchain for Electronic Health Records"	Using a decentralized platform for EHRs.	Presentation of a framework and secure storage by defining granular access rules for users of the system.	The work plans to implement the payment module in the framework	

Dey *et al.* [24]	"HealthSense: A Medical Use Case of Internet of Things and Blockchain"	The use of Blockchain-IoT model for the medical applications.	The research proposed a blockchain-based IoT model for medical device transactions and communications	More work is required in developing more efficient algorithms for encryption with shorter latency.
Griggs *et al.* [25]	"Healthcare Blockchain System Using Smart Contracts for Secure Remote Patient Monitoring"	Ethereum Protocol	The author proposed a smart contract system the supports real-time patient monitoring and medical intervention.	Future work includes the implementation with hyperledgers.
Tanwar *et al.* [26]	"Blockchain based Electronic Healthcare Record System for Healthcare 4.0 applications"	Blochchain-based EHR sharing system architecture.	The authors proposed a system architecture and algorithm. Implementation of a permission-based EHR sharing system using the chaincode concept.	More effort is required to improve on various evaluation metrics like latency, throughput and network security.
Antwi *et al.* [27]	"The case of HyperLedger Fabric as a blockchain solution for healthcare applications"	The use of HyperLedger Fabric	Identification of application development and the creation of specific testing criteria as well as critical analysis of Hyperledger Fabric utility for healthcare applications. Design and implementation of scenarios on HyperLedger Fabric.	More work is required on how blockchain could be utilized in the healthcare domain.

18.3 Case study 1: AI-enabled diagnosis and treatment

18.3.1 Overview of AI-enabled diagnosis and treatment

AI has come to stay, and it is gradually becoming the thing that makes the world go round. Virtually every facet of our lives has been impacted by AI. Healthcare and medicine are no exceptions as AI is revolutionizing the way healthcare is being conceived and delivered to patients. Nigeria and by extension the entire African continent have been battling inadequate health professionals due to so many factors among them is brain drain. This has given rise to a doctor-to-individual ratio of 1:10000 which is very far above the WHO recommended ratio of 1:600. This situation necessitated the need to apply ML to create a model that can diagnose and treat common diseases. This study aims to achieve this by considering a dataset from Kaggle and attempting to create this ML model. The ML algorithm used in this research is Random Forest Classification. Three performance metrics were used to test the performance of each of the above algorithms, namely, accuracy, precision, and recall. The model achieved 80.00% Accuracy, 79.49% Precision, and 83.79% Recall. Based on these performance metrics, we can conclude that Random Forest Classification is an effective technique that can be employed in the development of a ML model for predicting and treating the occurrence of diseases.

In late 2022, the media (social and traditional) were filled with talks about the future when ChatGPT (Chat Generative Pre-Trained Transformer) – a chatbot-like large language model (LLM) capable of human-level conversations – was announced by OpenAI. As of July 2023, ChatGPT is in the top 50 global most searched words on Google (Howart, 2023).

Diagnosis is the detection of the nature of a disease or disorder through a thorough examination of the prevailing signs and symptoms.

This study will look at the application of AI in diagnosis and treatment of diseases with a view to managing the current poor doctor-to-individual ratio in Nigeria and by extension in Africa. The study will attempt to create a ML model that can predict the occurrence of a disease based on the patient's age and other signs and symptoms.

18.3.2 Methods in AI-enabled diagnosis and treatment

This study will be quantitative in nature and will consider quantitative data for analysis. A secondary data source is used for this research. The dataset used for this work is obtained from Kaggle. It contains 349 rows and 10 columns. The dependent variable is the "Outcome Variable." The columns are described in Table 18.2.

Empirical research method was employed in this work for prediction and classification studies. Random Forest Classification was employed to create the ML model. The algorithm was created using Google Colaboratory – an online

Table 18.2 Description of the dataset

Column	Description
Disease	The name of the disease
Fever	This tells if the patient has a fever. It can be Yes/No
Cough	This tells if the patient has a cough. It can be Yes/No
Fatigue	This tells if the patient suffers from fatigue. It can be Yes/No
Difficulty breathing	This tells if the patient has difficulty in breathing. It can be Yes/No
Age	The age of the patient
Gender	The gender of the patient. It can Male/Female
Blood pressure	The blood pressure of the patient. It can be High/Low
Cholesterol level	Cholesterol level of patient. It can be High/Low
Outcome variable	The outcome shows the result of the diagnosis. It can be Positive/Negative

environment that hosts a Jupyter Notebook that enables a user to write python codes – in collaboration with some python libraries:

i. Pandas – a powerful library for data analysis and manipulation in python.
ii. Matplotlib – a comprehensive library for creating static, animated, and interactive visualizations in python.
iii. Sklearn – a powerful python library for ML.

The methods utilized to create the models are:

i. Prepare the environment by importing all the required python libraries.
ii. Upload the dataset.
iii. Prepare the data.
iv. Train the dataset.
v. Create the model and measure performance.

These above methods with their steps are shown in the Appendix section.

18.3.3 Results and discussion for AI-enabled diagnosis and treatment

In this section, data analysis using ML algorithms is discussed. ML algorithms helped to build this model. Data analysis was carried out, and the model was built using Random Forest. The dataset is split into test and training datasets. The dataset used to train the model is composed of 80% of the total dataset and the dataset used to test the model contains the remaining 20%. The following metrics were employed for analyzing the results: confusion matrix, accuracy, recall, and precision.

18.3.3.1 Random forest classification for AI-enabled diagnosis and treatment

Random forest is another ML algorithm that uses a supervised learning technique for both classification and regression analysis. It consists of a bunch of decision trees on a given dataset and takes the average in order to produce an improved accuracy of that dataset. Codes are highlighted in the Appendix section.

18.3.3.2 Performance metrics for AI-enabled diagnosis and treatment

1. Confusion Matrix
   A confusion matrix is a good estimator of the model general performance. A confusion matrix superbly displays the comprehensive number of true positives, true negatives, false positives, and false negatives values. A confusion matrix is often further used to generate performance metrics such as accuracy, f1 score, precision, and recall. A typical ML model is evaluated for performance using various performance metrics.
2. Accuracy
   A model's accuracy is the proportion between the total number of labels predicted correctly and the total number of entire predictions done. Accuracy is obtained from the simple formula given as follows. Accuracy = total number of correct predicted labels/total number of predictions done.
3. Precision
   A model's precision in very simple terms is the proportion of true positives to the total number of positives.
4. Recall
   Recall is the measure of a model correctly predicting positive samples. In our case study, for all those who are sick, recall tells us how many we correctly identified as sick.

The performance of the model under these three metrics: Accuracy, Precision, and Recall is as follows: 80.00% for Accuracy, 79.49% for Precision, and 83.79% for Recall. This result tells us the model performed very well and the results are acceptable.

18.3.4 Concluding remarks on AI-enabled diagnosis and treatment

The research has led us to successfully create a ML model using Random Forest Classification. We can deduce that based on the dataset used in the research, the performance of the model using the three metrics above is acceptable. This work attempts to provide a method for easily determining if a patient is suffering from a particular disease and this will go a long way in supplementing doctors' diagnosis in order to correct the large doctor-to-individual ratio in developing countries. The dataset used is small and a larger dataset will be required to develop a more comprehensive and accurate model. This study is only to demonstrate that AI can be deployed in the area of diagnosis and treatment of diseases.

18.4 Case study 2: AI-enabled remote patient monitoring (AI RPM)

Remote patient monitoring has revolutionized healthcare delivery by allowing the real-time monitoring of patients outside the traditional healthcare settings. This fact is made possible by the ubiquity of AI-enabled medical Internet of Things (AI-MIoT) devices which ensures real-time collection and analysis of data. ML and deep learning algorithms have been applied in identifying patterns in data, classification of medical abnormalities as well as the prediction of medical outcomes. AI technologies have extended the frontier of healthcare practice by providing valuable insights to healthcare personnel.

AI RPM has indeed led to a drastic reduction in patients' hospitalization due to its ability for real-time monitoring of patients for a continuous period of time with appropriate interventions. Also, AI RPM engenders a personalized care of patients as AI algorithms possess the capability to analyze data for individual patients. Furthermore, with the predictive nature of AI RPM algorithms, early detection and quick intervention on diseases are possible.

However, there are challenges in the implementation of AI RPM. These include interoperability of AI RPM across various healthcare institutions; also with the transition of data across several media, the issues of privacy and security of data become apparent. Furthermore ethical issues like group profiling, transparency of data, and the handling of consent need proper attention.

18.5 Case study 3: blockchain for secure medical records

Traditional medical records are prone to various challenges like data hacks, lack of interoperability (data are in different silos), and difficulty in ensuring the integrity and privacy of patient information. Blockchain for secure medical records entails the use of this technology to store, share, and manage patients' information in a secure and decentralized manner. Blockchain's attributes of transparency, immutability, high availability, and decentralization offer a range of potential solutions to the challenges listed above.

Flowing from the work of Xiao [12], Figure 18.1 shows the three-layer architecture of Blockchain. At the base is the peer-to-peer network where all the

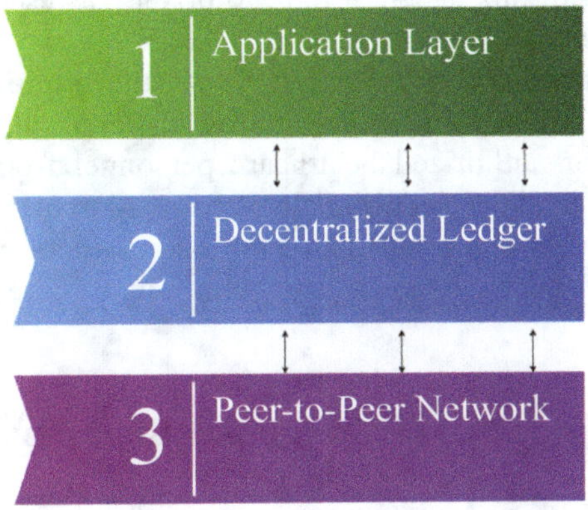

Figure 18.1 Blockchain architecture (adapted from Xiao [28])

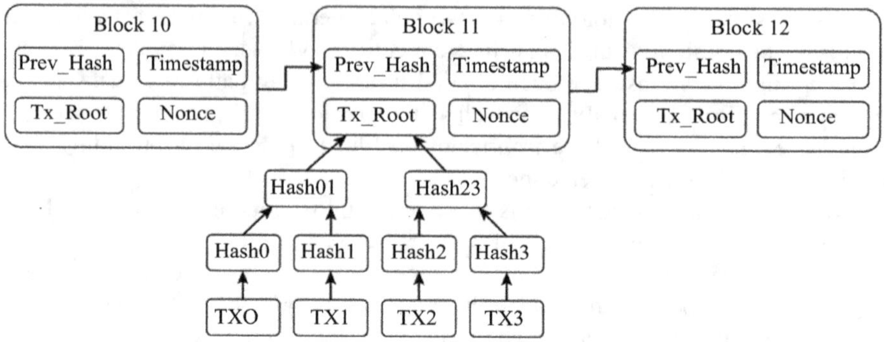

Figure 18.2 The structure of a blockchain (from Xiao [28])

nodes are connected. The middle layer is the decentralized ledger which is the kernel of the Blockchain technology, and the top layer is the application layer where application programs are implemented. An example is the DApp (decentralized application) which combines a smart contract (an electronic contracts between peers without a third party except a consensus algorithm) and a user interface (Figure 18.2).

Blockchain technology utilizes cryptographic hashing techniques to encrypt data stored in blocks making them secure. The blockchain is started by the first block which is referred to as the genesis block. Each transaction or addition to the blockchain is validated and linked to a previous block by some hashing techniques leading to the formation of a chain of blocks that cannot be changed without the consensus of other nodes in the network. This attribute, when applied to telehealth system, ensures integrity and immutability of medical records.

Furthermore, with blockchain technology, patients have control over their records. This patient-centric approach allows patients to grant permissioned access to authorized healthcare personnel, healthcare institutions, and insurance companies among others. With this patient's right to privacy as espoused by the GDPR compliance is achieved.

Interoperability has been a major issue with the traditional EHR systems. Patient's medical records are fragmented across different disparage digital silos making it difficult for authorized healthcare personnel from having a holistic view of a patient's medical record. Blockchain addresses this challenge by engendering the seamless sharing of patients' records in an interoperable format across healthcare institutions. This ensures continuity of care and the eradication of redundant tests.

18.6 Case study 4: blockchain for healthcare payments

Blockchain-based healthcare payment system is about the use of blockchain technology to carry out secure and efficient transactions in the healthcare domain. Blockchain can be referred to as a distributed ledger that allows for decentralization, transparency, and immutability of transaction records. Its application to healthcare payments portends several benefits due to the nature of healthcare systems which are characterized by the triad: confidentiality, integrity, and availability (CIA).

One major attribute is confidentiality, in which blockchain transactions are encrypted and distributed across a private network of computers thereby preventing phishing attacks and data breaches. This technology defers from the traditional payment systems that rely on centralized entities like banks or payment gateways which are prone to data hacks.

Healthcare payments involve multiple stakeholders like patients, healthcare institutions, government agencies, and insurance companies. The traditional payment systems are characterized by manual processes, coupled with bureaucratic bottlenecks and delay in reimbursement. Blockchain can provide a streamlined process by providing a single shared system of transactions that eliminates bureaucracy, minimizes errors, and automates reconciliation. This will lead to a faster, efficient, and more accurate payment systems.

Blockchain-based healthcare payment engenders transparency. Each transaction on the blockchain is present in every node. The transparency creates an audit trail of all transactions in the blockchain and provides for compliance with regulations and trust between participants. Also, blockchain immutability makes transaction records traceable and nonrepudiable.

Furthermore, smart contracts provide a new payment model without the need for a third party. Smart contracts are essentially, self-executing contracts with predefined rules encoded on the blockchain. This allows for seamless payment transactions based on previously agreed terms and conditions. Also, there is a lot of rollback on fraudulent claims, lack of interoperability between systems, administrative inefficiencies among others.

18.7 Conclusions and future scope

This work espoused an expository of AI and Blockchain in Telehealth systems. Zeroing in the following case studies among several: diagnosis and treatments, automated monitoring, secure medical records, and secure payments system. Despite the potential of AI and blockchain in telehealth, a lot of limitations still abound. In Blockchain, there exists the challenge of security, there is the 51 percent attack as described in the work of Xiao. The blockchain operates on consensus algorithms if a rogue group takes a major control of the network, they can alter the records. A means of mitigating this is to make the network larger than a certain size that will prevent any rogue group from taking control. Another major challenge is scalability: as the network grows, the processing of transactions on the blockchain becomes slow because of the distributed nature of the network. Other challenges include lack of regulation, complexity, and quantum readiness among others. These are areas for further extensive work.

References

[1] N.R. Sahni and B. Carrus "Artificial intelligence in U.S. Health Care Delivery". *New England Journal of Medicine*, 2023, 389(4), pp. 348–358.

[2] C.J. Haug and J.M. Drazen "Artificial intelligence and machine learning in clinical medicine". *New England Journal of Medicine*, 2023, 388(13), pp. 1201–1208.

[3] P. Lee, S. Bubeck, and J. Petro. "Benefits, limits, and risks of GPT-4 as an AI Chatbot for medicine". *New England Journal of Medicine*, 2023, 388 (13), pp. 1233–1239.

[4] K. Han, P. Cao, Y. Wang, *et al.* "A review of approaches for predicting drug–drug interactions based on machine learning". *Frontiers in Pharmacology*, 2022, 12, p. 814858.

[5] M.A. Myszczynska, P.N. Ojamies, A.M. Lacoste, *et al.* "Applications of machine learning to diagnosis and treatment of neurodegenerative diseases". *Nature Reviews Neurology*, 2020, 16(8), pp. 440–456.

[6] M.J. Iqbal, Z. Javed, H. Sadia, *et al.* "Clinical applications of artificial intelligence and machine learning in cancer diagnosis: looking into the future". *Cancer Cell International*, 2021, 21(1), pp. 1–11.

[7] T. Shaik, X. Tao, N. Higgins, *et al.* "Remote patient monitoring using artificial intelligence: current state, applications, and challenges". *Wiley Interdisciplinary Reviews: Data Mining and Knowledge Discovery*, 2023;13 (2), p. e1485.

[8] N. El-Rashidy, S. El-Sappagh, S.R. Islam, M.H. El-Bakry, and S. Abdelrazek. "Mobile health in remote patient monitoring for chronic diseases: principles, trends, and challenges". *Diagnostics*, 2021;11(4): p. 607.

[9] M.P. Kantipudi, C.J. Moses, R. Aluvalu, and S. Kumar. "Remote patient monitoring using IoT, cloud computing and AI". *Hybrid Artificial Intelligence and IoT in Healthcare*. 2021, vol. 209, pp. 51–74.

[10] R. Leung. "Using AI–ML to augment the capabilities of social media for telehealth and remote patient monitoring". *In Healthcare*, 2023; 11(12), p. 1704. MDPI.

[11] A. Dubey and A. Tiwari. "Artificial intelligence and remote patient monitoring in US healthcare market: a literature review". *Journal of Market Access & Health Policy*. 2023;11(1), p. 2205618.

[12] A. L. Imoize, P. A. Gbadega, H. I. Obakhena, D. O. Irabor, K. V. N. Kavitha, and C. Chakraborty, "Artificial intelligence-enabled Internet of medical things for COVID-19 pandemic data management," in *Explainable Artificial Intelligence in Medical Decision Support Systems*, Institution of Engineering and Technology, 2022, pp. 357–380. doi: 10.1049/PBHE050E_ch13.

[13] A. T. Rufai, K. F. Dukor, O. M. Ageh, and A. L. Imoize, "XAI robot-assisted surgeries in future medical decision support systems," in *Explainable Artificial Intelligence in Medical Decision Support Systems*, Institution of Engineering and Technology, 2022, pp. 167–195. doi: 10.1049/PBHE050E_ch6.

[14] S. Nakamoto, "Bitcoin: A Peer-to-Peer Electronic Cash System", 2008. https://bitcoin.org/bitcoin.pdf.

[15] A. Haleem, M. Javaid, R. P. Singh, R. Suman, and S. Rab, "Blockchain technology applications in healthcare: An overview". *International Journal of Intelligent Networks*, 2021, vol. 2, pp. 130–139.

[16] R. W. Ahmad, K. Salah, R. Jayaraman, I. Yaqoob, S. Ellahham, and M. Omar. "The role of blockchain technology in telehealth and telemedicine". *International Journal of Medical Informatics* 2021, 148, p. 104399. https://doi.org/10.1016/j.ijmedinf.2021.104399

[17] J. Sun, X. Yao, S. Wang, and Y. Wu, "Blockchain-based secure storage and access scheme for electronic medical records in IPFS," *IEEE Access*, 2020, 8, pp. 59389–59401, doi:10.1109/ACCESS.2020.2982964.

[18] A. Azaria, A. Ekblaw, T. Vieira, and A. Lippman, "MedRec: using blockchain for medical data access and permission management," *2016 2nd International Conference on Open and Big Data (OBD), Vienna, Austria*, 2016, pp. 25–30, doi:10.1109/OBD.2016.11.

[19] Y. Han, Y. Zhang, and S.H. Vermund. "Blockchain technology for electronic health records". *International Journal of Environmental Research and Public Health*, 2022, 19(23), p. 15577. https://doi.org/10.3390/ijerph192315577

[20] D. Yaga, P. Mell, N. Roby, and K. Scarfone. "Blockchain technology overview". *National Institute of Standards and Technology Internal Report*, 2019. https://doi.org/10.48550/arXiv.1906.11078

[21] F. K. Nishi, M. Shams-E-Mofiz, M.M. Khan, *et al.* "Electronic healthcare data record security using blockchain and smart contract". *Journal of Sensors*, 2022. https://doi.org/10.1155/2022/7299185

[22] H. Mhamdi, S. Othman, and H Sakli, "SEMRAchain: a secure electronic medical record based on blockchain technology". *Electronics*, 2022, 11(21) DOI: 10.3390/electronics11213617

[23] A. Shahnaz, U. Qamar, and A. Khalid, "Using blockchain for electronic health records," *IEEE Access*, 7, pp. 147782–147795, 2019, doi:10.1109/ACCESS.2019.2946373.

[24] T. Dey, S. Jaiswal, S. Sunderkrishnan, and N. Katre, "HealthSense: a medical use case of Internet of things and blockchain," *2017 International Conference on Intelligent Sustainable Systems (ICISS)*, Palladam, India, 2017, pp. 486–491, doi:10.1109/ISS1.2017.8389459.

[25] K.N. Griggs, O. Ossipova, C.P. Kohlios *et al.* "Healthcare blockchain system using smart contracts for secure automated remote patient monitoring". *Journal of Medical System*, 2018, 42, p. 130. https://doi.org/10.1007/s10916-018-0982-x

[26] S. Tanwar, K. Parekh, and R. Evans, "Blockchain-based electronic healthcare record system for healthcare 4.0 applications". *Journal of Information Security and Applications*, 2020, 50, p.102407, ISSN 2214-2126, https://doi.org/10.1016/j.jisa.2019.102407.1.

[27] M. Antwi, A. Adnane, F. Ahmad, R. Hussain, M. H. ur Rehman, and C. A. Kerrache, "The case of HyperLedger fabric as a blockchain solution for healthcare applications". *Blockchain: Research and Applications*, 2021,2(1), p.100012, ISSN 2096-7209, https://doi.org/10.1016/j.bcra.2021.100012.

[28] P. Xiao, *Practical Jasvs Programming for IOT, AI and Blockchain*. John Wiley and Sons, Inc., Indianapolis, Indiana, 2019.

Chapter 19

Achieving quality healthcare using Blockchain technology for detecting fake drugs

Anthony Olakunle Ayodeji[1], Arome Junior Gabriel[2] and Aderonke Favour-Bethy Thompson[2]

The challenge of piracy and counterfeiting has touched almost all products (healthcare, oil and gas, packaged foods, beverages/drinks, cosmetics, electronics, automobile parts, etc.) including drugs. This challenge has become global, and it has drawn significant attention from every profession, seeing it as urgent and increasingly critical worldwide issue. Nearly every country has suffered adverse effects from falsified and substandard drugs many of whom have died. Due to their poor results in data authentication, system resilience, adaptability, and privacy, traditional centralized server–client technical solutions have fallen well short of meeting the needs of modern cybercrime. Originally created for its most well-known cryptocurrency and economics use, Blockchain is now finding use in a variety of other fields and domains. This study proposes a private permissioned Blockchain as well as Internet of Things technologies for detecting fake drugs. The reason for choosing Blockchain has to do with the fact that it is secure, transparent, and even immutable. It also provides a distributed and often decentralized, environment, requiring no third party (Smart Contract attributes). All these ensures that its use guarantees a reasonable level of cybersecurity. The proposed approach enables pharmaceutical companies to upload information about their drugs, attach unique ID information of QR Code or Snaptags and push it to the Blockchain network. Thereafter, distributors, wholesalers, and pharmacies, based upon their requirement and approval to join the network, can verify the origin of the drug. The solution involves a simple QR Code/Snaptag-based identification that can help customers/patients to scan and identify the genuine of the product by using smartphone. Customers/patients can relate/communicate freely/directly with the manufacturer whenever fake drugs are being detected and quick action will be taking to known the source of the fake drug. Our use of the proposed Blockchain-based methodology demonstrates that it can efficiently identify medications that are fake.

[1]School of Computing, Federal University of Technology, Nigeria
[2]Department of Cybersecurity, School of Computing, Federal University of Technology, Nigeria

19.1 Introduction

All levels of healthcare require the use of drugs or pharmaceuticals. They assist in managing health, in the diagnosis, treatment, and prevention of illnesses and disorders, as well as in preventing the development of disease or its symptoms. If drugs are easily accessible, moderately priced, of high quality, taken as prescribed, and not obtained unethically, they can offer an easy, economical answer to many health problems. In many countries, the cost of drugs makes up a sizeable amount of the total health expenditure. Drug counterfeiting is still a major issue, despite the clear medical and economic necessity of medications [1].

An ancient custom that has persisted throughout many countries and is motivated largely by the immense financial rewards that could be made, which have been further boosted by improvements in the technologies for large-scale manufacture as well as sales [2].

The international trade in bogus/falsified drugs appears to have an effect on both developed and underdeveloped countries. In countries where there are laxer restrictions with regard to manufacture, as well as distribution of pharmaceuticals, the spread of fake medications is often more prevalent. To strengthen the regulatory agency monitoring mechanisms in these countries, major enforcement actions may be necessary. Currently under discussion is the term "counterfeit," which was once frequently used to describe any substance that was not what it claimed to be. In the strictest sense, a drug or medicine that violates a registered company is regarded as being counterfeit. The lay definition, which is far broader, includes any drug made with intentional deception. In reality, some civil society organizations and generic pharmaceutical companies disagree with the term "counterfeit" because they feel it purposefully conflates public health and intellectual property concerns [3,4].

A very deadly crime against peoples' health is the fabrication/production and dissemination of fake medications and other medical supplies. Licensed manufacturers, traders, and pharmacies are impacted by this crime, just like they would from any other form of economic fraud, because they incur losses, damage the reputation of the drug manufacturer, and on rare occasions are able to compete against distributors of counterfeit goods [5].

The worst repercussions come from the damage inflicted on the well-being and lives of individuals, which cannot be exaggerated. Such damage can range from causing mortality or serious health impairment as a result of the use of subpar pharmaceuticals and/or the lack of an appropriate therapeutic impact, as well as inaccurate diagnostic findings, to instilling mistrust in physicians as a result of poor treatment. These impacts are not always simple to verify, and it is even harder to demonstrate a direct relationship between the use of illegal drugs and harm to human life or health [4,6].

According to the WHO, a fake drug is a medication that has had its source purposely and dishonestly mislabeled. False components, insufficient active ingredients, or items with no active ingredients are all deemed to be falsified in products [4]. Pharmaceuticals supplied under fraudulent names or with fewer or none of the listed active components are considered counterfeit. Other potentially harmful chemicals may also be added. The purpose of manufacturing or disseminating a phony drug or pharmaceutical item is to mislead its origin, veracity, or efficacy. Insufficient or nonexistent levels of the active ingredients may be present in a phony drug. Additionally, it might not be well-absorbed by the body or include substances that are not declared on the label. Several technological advancements may be helpful in the struggle against the issue of counterfeit pharmaceuticals. False pharmaceuticals, often known as counterfeit drugs, provide a health risk when consumed by humans. The threat posed by drug counterfeiting is getting more and more significant. It can be difficult to spot, investigate, quantify, or stop some counterfeiting. It is difficult to calculate the volume of illegal drug sales. Even while it occurs globally, Nigeria, Africa, and India are the regions with the highest counterfeiting rates. A counterfeit medication could come in the exact same packaging as the genuine medication. Even a forensic expert has trouble visually distinguishing between these counterfeit pharmaceuticals since they are frequently so well disguised [4,6].

The marketing of fake pharmaceuticals is a profitable evil venture that is growing every year. The problem of fake medicines is common over the world, is becoming more important due to greater globalization, and is dangerous in the majority of countries. False companies are established, phony documents and certificates are produced, and forgers utilize a variety of techniques to acquire industrial equipment and pharmaceuticals. Falsified medications are unlawful, unhealthy, and contribute to the spread of disease. Following the recent COVID-19 (Coronavirus) outbreaks, a counterfeit version of the malaria drug chloroquine gained notoriety as a potential virus therapy. It was found in Lagos, Cameroon, and other parts of the African continent. The utilization of adulterated Chloroquine tabs led to the failure of many treatments and deaths, mainly in Lagos, Nigeria. During that time, fake COVID-19 testing kits were also found at LAX (Los Angeles International Airport) [7].

However, there is a concern about how illegal drug trafficking affects public health. Two basic categories of subpar medications are distinguished in the current research work in order to more clearly discuss this issue. Pharmaceuticals falling under the first category do not meet the requirements stated in the dossier of the producer or in a reputable pharmacopeia. The other major category of unlawful items is adulterated or sub-standard medications, or those that communicate a fictitious portrayal of source and/or identity. In several nations, unregistered drugs or those without local market authorization are a problem [4,6].

19.1.1 Motivation for the study

The threat of counterfeiting affects so many industries. In addition to medicines and edible foods, common counterfeit goods include consumer electronics and other electrical parts, beverages, tobacco, agricultural goods, toiletries, oil and gas products, and more.

In Africa, especially in Nigeria where the majority of the public are very poor patronizing lesser pharmaceutical products using it to treat critical illness, e.g., cancer, causes sickness progression even death. Other consequences and danger of counterfeit drugs include but are not limited to treatment failure (often resulting in death), toxicity, loss of confidence, economic loss, end-organ damage, toxicity, and even sickness progression. It is vitally important to have access to pharmaceuticals that are secure, reasonable in price, and distributed fairly.

There have also been several literature and scientific publications that have contributed to counterfeit drug detection and traceability using Blockchain technology. However, most of these publications are only theoretical evaluations. The costs and dangers of fake medications are immensely hazardous, it is thus of high necessity, to provide efficient systems for detecting counterfeiting especially of drugs [4]. All these motivated this current research to develop a mitigation strategy in the form of a counterfeit drug detection system.

To overcome all these challenges, this current research work adopted Blockchain alongside the Ethereum network, together with the adoption of QR Codes/Snap Tags as a scannable technology to view drug information and authenticity of drug (drug counterfeit detection) through the manufacturers' website. The system prototype works as a real system with Snap Tags that can also be used by standard camera phones. In this case, users/customers can take a picture of the Snap Tags and forward the same to the designated short code or email address (as an SMS or via the scanning approach). In the case of QR codes, unique codes could be attached to each drug in a manner that patients or customers can scan directly to obtain every information about the authenticity of the drugs.

19.1.2 Significance of the study

Blockchain technology has become increasingly important and relevant in every domain rather than bitcoin alone due to the fact that it's secured, transparent, distributed, immutable, and timestamp. Blockchain have three types public, private and consortium and network types Ethereum, Hyperledger, etc. which makes it so relevant in another domain to solve problem.

The Worldwide web has become ever present (ubiquitous) and Blockchain technology exceeds all technologies that ever existed. The reach and scope of the internet, especially business websites, have swiftly expanded from being little more than static promotional materials.

There are many advantages to employing Blockchain technology for detecting falsified medications. The implementation of such a Blockchain-based system is anticipated to eliminate or replace the existing pharmaceutical supply chain, which is antiquated, does not give pharmaceutical companies and NAFDAC control over drug distribution, and cannot withstand today's cyber-security threats. This implementation is also anticipated to discard centralized server–client technical solutions, which have been less than satisfactory as a result of poor data security, authenticity, and privacy.

In order to verify, identify, and track prescription pharmaceuticals as they are distributed, the system acts as an interoperable electronic system. The system will be able to monitor or trace how drug business is carried out between the parties in the distribution chain.

It will be up to pharmaceutical corporations to add authorized users to the Blockchain. Before sending it out to distributors, the corporation discovers, produces, and receives clearance from the country's authorized food and drug regulatory body, then adds a special hash code (Hash function), and adds all essential information to the secure distributed ledger. The wholesaler will verify the drug's origin and store the transaction on the network, having a similar impact on pharmacies, hospitals, and wholesalers.

This implementation will provide the publicity access to the defect falsified and substandard drug using Snap Tag or QR Code technologies. In the case of Snap tags, user can access through SMS or direct scan of the embedded Snap Tags logo used as unique ID. Counterfeit drug detection using Blockchain technology will also provide updates for the drugs (drugs information). The accessibility is everywhere and not limited to smartphones, other phone users may as well use their small phones to send a tag info via SMS.

In short, the proposed system is expected to provide a key solution to avoiding all the problems mentioned previously by providing a unified way to counterfeiting problems. A reasonable way to achieve this unification is by adopting Blockchain technology and its features. Therefore, this current study implements a trustworthy and efficient counterfeit drug detection system using Blockchain technology.

19.1.3 Chapter contributions

The items that follow are the chapter's main contributions:

i. It covers the development of a counterfeit drug detection system using Blockchain and Internet of Things Technologies.
ii. It establishes a protected, shared, and decentralized ledger-based communication and information exchange mechanism in a peered network.
iii. It established high-level security and transparency in the supply chain via cryptography as well as by documenting provenance.

19.1.4 Chapter organization

In Section 19.2, an elaborate review of literature relating to this current study is presented. Section 19.3 presents the methodology of the proposed system. It basically contains a comprehensive analysis of the existing system as well as the design of the proposed counterfeit drug detection system. Also, Section 19.4 presents the proposed system implementation and result discussions. Lastly, Section 19.5 contains the conclusion as well as the directions for future study.

19.2 Theoretical background

An analysis of literature that is somewhat related to this chapter. First, a review of some of the most related scientific research or studies is carried out. Thereafter, the major reasons behind the rapid growth of drug falsification incidences is highlighted. Additionally, the gravity or magnitude of the drug falsification problem that includes but is not limited to its economic and social effects are elaborately discussed.

19.2.1 Related work

Blockchain technology first gained popularity when cryptocurrencies and other kinds of finance developed. In a number of industries, many different Blockchain use cases have been put forth, and with the inclusion of smart contracts, Blockchain has become more powerful. Researchers have drawn to the objective of expanding its applicability to non-financial use cases since it was first made public through the use of bitcoin. Here are some academic papers on the use of Blockchain technology for democratic decision making, physical security, healthcare, and even the detection or mitigation of fake goods (like drugs).

In Ref. [8], Thompson *et al.* used Blockchain technology, digital memory, and visual cryptography to develop a multifactor authentication system for smart homes. Blockchain technology enables decentralized identity storage as well as personal information management. The digital memories were protected using an effective (2, 2) visual-cryptography system. The related mobile application of this suggested authentication system enables authorized users to remotely access the smart door (s) available in smart homes while preventing unauthorized access to smart doors. Comparing the suggested method to current cryptography-based systems for authentication, speed is improved by around 50%. The proposed system's login and registration methods were assessed using the Scyther tool. The findings demonstrate that there has been no assault.

The goal of the study in Ref. [9] was to use the KECCAK256 algorithm to create an electronic voting system based on Ethereum. The user interface of the system was built using React.js, the smart contract was programmed using Solidity, and JavaScript code was executed outside a web browser using Node.js. The Ethereum network, which handles authentication and authorization. Comparing the system's performance to that of other existing systems revealed that it performed better than average.

The study in Ref. [10] looked into the Blockchain's structure, in the context of creating a safe and decentralized healthcare system. The approach makes sure that while some people are treated as clients with allotted liberties, patients can control and personalize their healthcare data. For this work, public-key cryptography was modified and built upon the distributed ledger protocol to create an affix-only, irreversible, timestamped chain of data.

A study on the identification of fraudulent medications using Blockchain technology was conducted by Sanghi *et al.* [11]. The inadequate, out-of-date pharmaceutical supply chain management and the system's general lack of visibility attracted the study. Additionally, the prevalence of counterfeit medications is rising each year. The authors embraced the use of peers in a browser-based Hyperledger fabric network. Users are given access to the application's user interface so they can send queries to all of their peers via a webpage and start transactions using their credentials. Endorsers carry out legal transactions, as well as committers who check the results before writing them to the ledger. The study is constrained in that the method utilized to get the medication to the closest pharmacy might not be the best one. Customers should have been able to directly contact the proper security or regulatory agents or organizations to report any anomalies and to confirm the legitimacy of medications from any pharmacy.

A study on using Blockchain to identify fake pharmaceuticals was described in Ref. [12]. Their proposed system becomes quite sophisticated anytime a user installs a software application from a website and may not function in the absence of internet connectivity. A smartphone is necessary for the smooth running of the system. The study provides a theoretical analysis; the design of the system is not mentioned.

The study in Ref. [13] revealed a Blockchain-based system that is useful for tracking and controlling medications. The paper offered guidelines for creating a Blockchain system focused on scenarios for tracking and policing drugs. The researchers showed off a prototype built from the study. Pharmaceuticals are often packaged, and repackaged, which makes tracking and tracing more difficult. Drugledger does not aim for a 100% increase because efficiency is determined by its consensus technique. Similarly, Evans in Ref. [14] reported the implementation of Blockchain for improving transparency in drug distribution.

In Ref. [15], Kumari *et al.* developed an approach for detecting fake medications using Blockchain technology. Through the entire distribution chain, this system can follow the progress of pharmaceuticals. They claimed that the producer, distributor, and pharmacist are the three parties that make up both public and private Blockchains. Patients will be able to confirm the provenance of their prescriptions, and stakeholders can trace things throughout the supply chain. Researchers are only allowed to conduct theoretical research. No example of implementation was provided.

The studies in Ref. [16] employed Blockchain technology to detect poor and counterfeit drugs in the distribution chain. The study adopted a distributed database-backed DApp supporting a personal network that served as the system prototype. Two instances, one for Hyperledger Fabric and Ethereum networks, were recommended. Every node in the network has an RFID scanner. A DApp that is a component of the system has an interface as well as a front end. There are some more assumptions included in the prototype's design that could influence how it is put into practice. It is impossible to verify the system's authenticity. The only drug distribution actions that may be traced are those that adhere to the established protocols accepted by the regulatory body.

The study in Ref. [17] worked on improving drug traceability with the aid of Blockchain. The researchers used questionnaires and interviews to collect data.

According to the study, Blockchain, which is employed by browser-based Ethereum DApps, enables decentralized data storage. There was no real-world testing or application of the technology.

In Ref. [18], Haq and Esuka looked at how Blockchain technology could be used in the pharmaceutical sector to stop the sale of counterfeit drugs. The objective was to track medications using the system from producer to client delivery. A database will be created to store the patient's responses to each medicine for further reference. Only trustworthy parties are allowed to push data into the network's permissioned Blockchain, used to keep transactions. The item had a QR code with a certain number printed on it. The unique number was not generated at random, and smartphone owners are the only ones who can track and trace narcotics.

The primary focus of the investigation in Ref. [19] is the legal application of the technology known as Blockchain in the pharmacy industry. The authors offered advice on how to look into the possibilities of Blockchain technology to safeguard the rights of patients to high-quality medications. The approach is a natural synthesis of philosophical viewpoint, broad scientific theory, and specific legal research methodologies. Only the patient's right to high-quality pharmaceuticals was addressed in the study. There is no system in place to detect fake drugs.

The majority of current relevant studies are mainly theoretical analyses. The majority of Blockchain-based plans did not offer channels for user feedback or complaints (through which issues might be directed directly to reputable government health institutions or drug manufacturers). It was also observed that most authors tended to ignore the differences between the physical movement of the drug and web storage as well as the fact that allowing customers to authenticate is different from addressing issues that arise in the supply chain alone (SCM), where everyone involved, including the patient or customer, can check the products' origins online without authentication. Some of the associated works also have significant computational overheads and scalability issues.

It was discovered that clients using Blockchain technology solutions now in use lack the ability to give feedback or file complaints with the government or the company that made the product. Instead of complaining to the store where it was purchased, a consumer or patient who receives a counterfeit product may contact the manufacturer in order to take swift legal action and identify the source of the drugs. It is clear that customer involvement in this process is crucial to combatting drug counterfeiting and drug authentication in order to eliminate or decrease the use of illegal medicines.

19.2.2 Causes of substandard/falsified drugs

Several points can be inferred as the reasons for the increase in incidences of counterfeiting in drugs.

In actuality, the drugs regulatory body, with the power to authorize producers and as well register drugs, can take action against dishonest or negligent makers, which is one difference between fabricated and inferior medications. When the manufacturer is misrepresented, there is no such remedy. Only the producer's anonymity may be confirmed by the regulator, who will then refer the case to police enforcement. There is typically little to no proof linking the market-available fake drug to the offender, making it difficult for the police or security agents who inherit these criminal cases to compile enough evidence for a prosecution [20].

Substandard pharmaceuticals are a result of poor production procedures being disregarded. Small and medium-sized businesses and businesses in Africa struggle to get business improvement loans. These businesses may end up creating subpar medications [2].

Manufacturers are aware of the necessity to utilize high-quality ingredients and procedures because wealthy nations enforce strict quality standards for pharmaceuticals. Manufacturers are aware that these requirements are less likely to be upheld in low- and middle-income nations. As a result, some producers create pharmaceuticals of lower quality for less demanding and less affluent consumers (a process known as parallel or tiered production).

Fake or inferior pharmaceuticals may become more prevalent as a result of poor procurement methods. The companies that provide the lowest pricing do so by purchasing unclean substances and making shoddy formulations. Although it is best practice to reject the lowest-priced bids if they are of questionable quality, it can be challenging to resist the pull of the dollar sign. By taking the necessary precautions while buying pharmaceuticals, low-quality items can be kept out of the market. Controlling corruption and fostering openness are highly prioritized in effective procurement. The measures required for effective and transparent purchase of the highest-quality medications are outlined in the WHO's Model Quality Assurance System for purchase Agencies [4].

False pharmaceutical production and trafficking are lucrative industries managed by criminals. These crimes are typically opportunistic and arise in areas with lax regulatory frameworks. The security personnel of multinational, innovative pharmaceutical businesses compiles evidence to support convictions when criminals target their products. Additionally, police are looking into more drug-related offenses, but they often only conduct quick raids. Given the urgent need to investigate homicides and other violent crimes, it is challenging for security agencies to maintain consistency in prosecuting this dubious crime.

Similar to how subpar medications are frequently both fabricated and subpar, some potentiating circumstances encourage both types of issues. The trade in both fake and inferior medications is facilitated by factors like strong demand for drugs, an unpredictable supply, lax regulatory frameworks, and uneven public awareness.

Medicines are what economists refer to as inelastic goods, meaning that changes in the unit price have a relatively small impact on demand. The high relative price of medicines, along with price inelasticity, makes them a significant out-of-pocket expense for patients everywhere. The medication market is unstable; both supply and price change over time. Drug shortages increase drug costs and lure customers to unregulated marketplaces [3].

Drug shortage could be avoided by lowering the price and making medications more readily available. A supply of high-quality generic medications must be available on the market for the WHO-recommended generic substitution strategy to work. Costs associated with establishing bioequivalence and putting together a manufacturer's dossier for regulatory assessment might make entering the market unaffordable for generic manufacturers, which often operate on thin profit margins. The requirements of various regulatory authorities vary, frequently greatly. Many tiny regulatory agencies are unable to examine the bioequivalence data that generics firms submit, which furthers the issue [21].

The establishment of a robust generics business in underdeveloped nations is hampered by the high cost of market authorization. The scarcity of drugs as well as increases in price that drive the selling of low-quality products might be avoided with the support of a stronger generic drug industry. Regulatory agencies can seek to more effectively coordinate their processes, which will increase their effectiveness and lower entry bottlenecks for producers of high-quality generic drugs. Having more convergent regulatory frameworks also benefits regulators indirectly without requiring them to engage in time-consuming mutual recognition negotiations.

19.2.3 Reasons why detection of counterfeit drugs is important

In low- and middle-income nations with inadequate pharmacovigilance and drug regulation regimes, the economic effects of counterfeit and subpar medications are substantial. Antimicrobial resistance, unpleasant effects, higher healthcare expenditures, and a decline in public trust in healthcare systems are all consequences of using subpar drugs. Although fake medications may include hazardous components, due to their challenging identification, clinicians frequently overlook disease progression. High mortality in low- and middle-income nations is a result of inadequate life-saving medications. These nations' counterfeit and subpar antimicrobial medications develop drug resistance, endangering the general public's health. Poor antimicrobials may have low dosages or be diluted, exposing organisms to concentrations below what is considered therapeutic. Drugs of inferior quality exacerbate drug-resistant TB and staphylococcus infections and jeopardize efforts to eradicate malaria globally due to antimalarial resistance.

19.2.4 The socio-economic effects of fake medicines

Medications that are counterfeit and of low quality are more expensive for patients and health systems. Due to the high cost of medications, both individuals and governments waste money on ineffective medications. Long-lasting diseases reduce productivity, resulting in employees skipping work and spending more on medical care. Illegal drugs shorten a drug's useful life by fostering antimicrobial resistance. Drug development comes at a societal price, one that rises as medications get more complicated.

The public's trust in the healthcare system and all public institutions is damaged by substandard and counterfeit medications. Criminal cartels frequently engage in the trade in fake drugs. Their sale supplies money for other criminal activities, buys arms and weapons, and gives corrupt individuals access to power. Most victims of tainted and subpar pharmaceuticals are unaware that they are victims, depriving them of their entitlement to compensation. The trade in illegal medications contributes to a dangerous and evil cycle of crime as well as poverty, by further eroding the already fragile governmental infrastructure that permits their circulation [4,6].

19.2.5 The enormity of the problem

The prevalence of counterfeit and poor-quality medications in the community is difficult to estimate. Drug quality issues are monitored by governments and industry, although this data is often private. Data from the Pharmaceutical Security Institute, which is a network comprising the security sections of 25 significant pharmaceutical corporations, show that unlawful manufacture as well as distribution of medications is a widespread issue. In 2011, it had an impact on at least 124 nations, and the developing world bore a disproportionate share of the damage.

Pills and tablets are the most often contaminated products that the NAFDAC and FDA Office of Criminal Investigations investigate, and they are typically made by lone criminals rather than careless enterprises. Since 2008, 11 operations against illegal drugs have been carried out by Interpol, an international organization that promotes police cooperation. Tons of suspicious goods were seized by police participating in Interpol raids, sparking hundreds of inquiries and arrests.

Case studies—reports from doctors who find subpar or fake pharmaceuticals in the course of their regular work—make up a large portion of the scholarly literature on drug quality. This kind of study gives background on when/how various types of medications are harmed; it can also set off epidemiological studies. Convenience or nonprobability sampling is the most popular approach for examining drug quality. Such findings point to significant issues with antibiotics in developing nations and antimalarial medications in Southeast Asia and Sub-Saharan Africa.

Systematic random samples taken from a representative cross-section of drug suppliers by patient actors provide the most accurate estimation of the prevalence of illegal drugs. These studies are scarce and logistically challenging. The problem would be better understood and tracked if more studies were conducted in compliance with the most recent criteria for reporting medicine quality assessment results.

Uncertainty about the size of the market for counterfeit and subpar pharmaceuticals prevents coordinated international action. A system for the universal detection as well as monitoring of counterfeit and subpar medications is being developed by WHO. Continuous use of such a system, ultimately connecting it to the country-wide pharmaco-vigilance systems, would enhance global action and provide a more nuanced picture of the kinds of falsified, subpar, and un-registered drugs in use as well as the scope of the business.

Due to insufficient or absent active ingredients, the medication may not be effective. Because the medication includes too much of the active substance or other unidentified hazardous chemicals, it may be dangerous.

It's possible that the medication was created or stored in an unregulated setting without the necessary safeguards to guarantee its effectiveness and safety.

The risks or repercussions of using fake medications generally consist of treatment failure (or death), damage to end organs (such as the kidney, heart, or liver), toxicity (adverse effects/therapeutic failures), false vital signs, loss of confidence, and even financial losses [3]. An efficient or effective method to stop the dreadful threat of drug counterfeiting is desperately needed.

Recently, it has been observed that the adoption of Blockchain in the medical and healthcare sectors is expanding quickly. Various health industries, including data access management across medical institutions, secure exchange of electronic health records, medicine security and traceability, clinical trials, etc., have utilized Blockchain due to its secure attributes and nature. Since the data is dispersed and kept in blocks, there is no single point of failure when using Blockchain technology. Blockchain technology aids in resolving healthcare security issues. With digital signatures and smart contracts, Blockchain technology's secure, reliable, auditable, and immutable transactions make it ideal for the detection of fake drugs in drug information. The following characteristics [22] make Blockchain trustworthy for use in preventing the sale of fake drugs:

a) Peer-to-Peer Transmission: Instead of using a centralized node, communications occur straight among the peers or nodes.
b) Distributed Database: The entire database along with its complete history can be accessed by each entity or participant on the Blockchain. All the transactions taking place between two entities are recorded efficiently and in a secure way by the distributed ledger [23].
c) Computational Logic: The use of a digital ledger makes it possible to be computational logic with the transactions in a Blockchain.
d) Transparency with Pseudonymity: Each entity in a Blockchain assigned with a unique address. Every transaction in a Blockchain occurs between these addresses. It is up to the users whether they want to give proof of their identity or they want to remain hidden or unidentified to other entities.
e) Irreversibility of Records: The records cannot be altered once the transaction information is stored on the Blockchain [7,24].

Blockchain, according to several academics, is the ideal option in situations when data security and privacy protection are top priorities [25–27].

In light of the rising frequency of cyberattacks, the uses of Blockchain technology and/or the Internet of Things in healthcare research are presently of significant focus and are being investigated [28–31]. Its potential to offer a reliable platform where parties can provide and use a variety of services, such as electronic voting [32], secure data storage [33–37], and others [38], is also being investigated by other areas beyond the health care industry. This current study tests the possibility of using the technology as well as its principles (together with QR codes scanning) in a pharmaceutical surveillance system, toward combating the deadly crime of drug counterfeiting.

19.3 The proposed fake drug detection system

The functionality of the proposed detection system is majorly hinged on the fact that its web-based capability and the fact that it also uses Multi-Media Messaging as well as Short Messaging (MMS/SMS). The system gives drug detection and traceability facilities and collects requests from different drug information seekers. The system maintains a distributed data store (distributed system), here, approved participant on the Blockchain network will have copies of the data since it is a distributed ledger system that can be maintained and accessed from different areas by a considerable number of approved participants on the network. In this proposed counterfeit drug detection system, user-desired services will be readily available online and users from different areas can access it at all time.

The proposed system of counterfeit drug detection using Blockchain technology will be obtainable or accessible at all times, from any location, and show traceability of drugs, authenticity, as well as drug information.

The proposed system is a web and MMS/SMS platform that provides comprehensive and authentic information on drugs, with a view to enhancing the rational use of those drugs. Additionally, as users interact with the proposed system, they are permitted to post requests for drug-related queries on fake drugs detected, to the manufacturers directly (report criminal activities). The proposed system has a participant page to manage major system functionalities that embrace view, add, push drug, and manage additional task and manufacturer alone interact with the customer. The proposed system is accessible to only authorized entities including wholesaler, distributor, person authorized, or entitled to supply pharmaceutical. This is made even possible via its easy interface that makes search/ authentication by the customers quite easy.

The proposed system architecture calls for developing a mechanism for detecting fake drugs based on Blockchain and QR codes. The suggested system's architecture is shown in Figure 19.1.

Private/permissioned Ethereum Blockchain technology is suggested by this study. Each participant on the network is given a set of certain activities to perform using the cryptographically secure key pairs of the Blockchain. The network will be able to identify each participant by their own key pair (private and public). The transaction is signed using a private key that must be kept private.

The entire network receives the transactions that have been digitally signed. A digital signature, which is more secure than a handwritten one, is the secret. The signature phase and the verification phase are the two key stages that make up the suggested system. To send a message to a certain Distributor, for instance, a Manufacturer signs the message with his own private key, adds the produced signature, and then delivers the message to the Distributor. The Distributor (receiver), using the Manufacturer's public key, then confirms the legitimacy of the received signature.

The Distributor can then quickly determine whether the info has been altered or not. All of these can be expressed in full as follows:

Any sender is required to provide her public key() so that anyone wishing to validate her signatures may do so. She chooses a hash function and uses it to derive the digest document (m) that needs to be signed, as shown in (19.1).

$$h(m) = \breve{m} \tag{19.1}$$

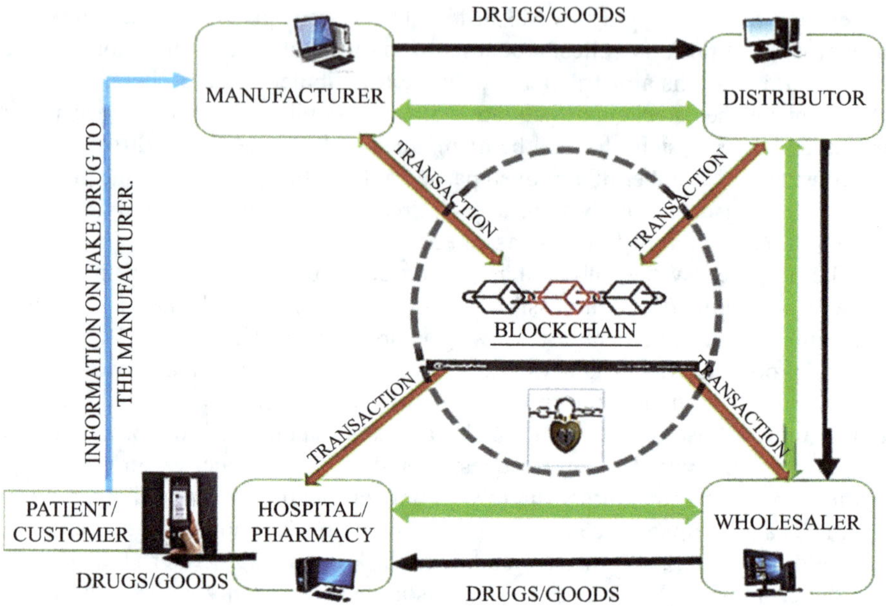

Figure 19.1 The proposed system architecture

The sender must then use (19.1)'s message hash to encrypt the message using her private key (a) and encryption algorithm (E). For that message, this results in her distinctive signature, as illustrated in (19.2):

$$\mathrm{E}A(\check{m}) = \c{S} \tag{19.2}$$

The message's calculated signature is then forwarded to the target recipient along with the associated signature ($\check{m}$) by the sender.

The recipient checks the validity of the sender's signature on the message at the next stage, known as verification. By using a combination of the decryption function and the public key of the sender, on the signature of the sender as shown in equation (19.3), the receiver must correctly adhere to the signature verification process;

$$DA(\c{S}) = DA\{\mathrm{E}a(\check{m})\} \tag{19.3}$$

$$DA(\c{S}) = M \tag{19.4}$$

The Elliptic Curve Digital Signature Algorithm (ECDSA) was used in this Blockchain-based system. The drug is regarded as a digital asset on the Ethereum Blockchain, with each one having a distinct hash (Unique ID). In the form of SnapTags, the special hash (Unique ID) will be affixed to the drug/tablet. Customers/clients must log onto the website of the manufacturer and choose their preferred button or tab choice (either the SMS or the scanning option) in order to access the authenticity of the medicine. The customer is required to enter his full name, phone number, location, and ultimately a scanned code from the integrated Snap-Tag App to the Ethereum network, in a new dialog box that appears after selecting one of the two possibilities. The customer can also photograph the Snap Tag of the manufacturer/company. These Snap Tag images can then be sent by SMS or a camera phone with picture messaging features. The suggested system will provide users with very intuitive and user-friendly web-based and short messaging interaction interfaces. Customers would be able to send drug-related questions, particularly if there is a suspicion of counterfeiting. Additionally, this system would enable communication between all authorized entities or stakeholders (e.g., the distributors, manufacturers, and even the wholesalers). The installed system would be able to provide accurate information on toxicity and toxicology caused by counterfeit and subpar medications.

Additionally, only authorized parties are able to read from and make updates to the content of the Blockchain and have access to the proposed system. In fact, the proposed method is anticipated to give authorized users the ability to encrypt their private data before storing it or sending it to the Blockchain. Any form of decryption would only be possible for the authorized recipient.

The proposed system permits manufacturers to store pertinent information about the unique identifiers of their chain partners, the product's coding scheme, its generic name, as well as the manufacturer's name and location, the location and name of the person who holds the marketing authorization, and a record of duly registered wholesalers who are permitted to keep as well as distribute medicines. Additionally, anti-tampering technologies for spotting instances of content replacement by dishonest people are anticipated to be included in the medicine packaging. Additionally, the newly developed Blockchain-based system for detecting falsified medications will show the legitimacy and traceability of drugs and drug information and be accessible at anytime, anywhere.

The proposed system was implemented using technologies such as Solidity-Etherum, JavaScript, CSS, HTML, and Cascading Style Sheets (CSS).

Four major subsystems make up the proposed system. For high coherence, the system is divided into components based on the specialized function it performs. Because there is only data exchange between interactions between subsystems, there is a very high level of coupling. Due to the client–server nature of the proposed architecture, the system will run on the server while having its output sent to the server. Therefore, a web browser that can decipher fundamental HTML tags can be employed on the client side. The system and database will be located on one side of the smart contract that is part of the Ethereum network. This study got contributions from scientific publication review, acquire data/information from private, public medical and paramedical professionals and their clients in the University of Teaching Hospital Akure, Nigeria as well as NAFDAC office, Federal Secretariat, Igbatoro Road, Akure, Nigeria.

19.3.1 Proposed system implementation

- This system was implemented using Blockchain, PHP, and Elliptic Curve Cryptography with curve pre-set secp256k1(Keccak 256 SHA3 Family), which involves the following processes:

- Blockchain Ethereum Encrypting: A private key and Ethereum address is obtained from Ethereum Blockchain, the system uses Secp256k1 to generate a sign signature from Ethereum address and save the signature Hex Signature Serializer. The saved signature can be used for generating the public key.
- Blockchain Ethereum Decrypting: The developed system uses the private key and address generated to develop sign signature, save the signature, and validate it, if the signed signature is on the Ethereum network. The network generates a public key from the address, private key and use it to verify if the authentication code provided the drug unique code or information is on the Ethereum network.
- When creating drug on the system an authentication key is generated and pushed to the Ethereum network.
- After saving a signed copy of the authentication to the network, a QR code is generated with the authentication code.
- After scanning the QR code, the system verifies if the scan authentication is on the network and displays information about the drug and if not, it allows the user to send message to manufacturer about a fake drug detected.
- QR code and SMS information is use as a medium of getting information of the drug on Ethereum network.

A few of the modules included in this include the home or landing page, login, as well as the registration pages, dashboard, management panel for inputting info, and drug information discipline panel. Here is a quick explanation of each module:

(a) The homepage
When a person logs into the website, the page is shown on their browser. All other website pages are linked to it. It had links to sales, confirmations, and other things (Figure 19.2).

Figure 19.2 The homepage

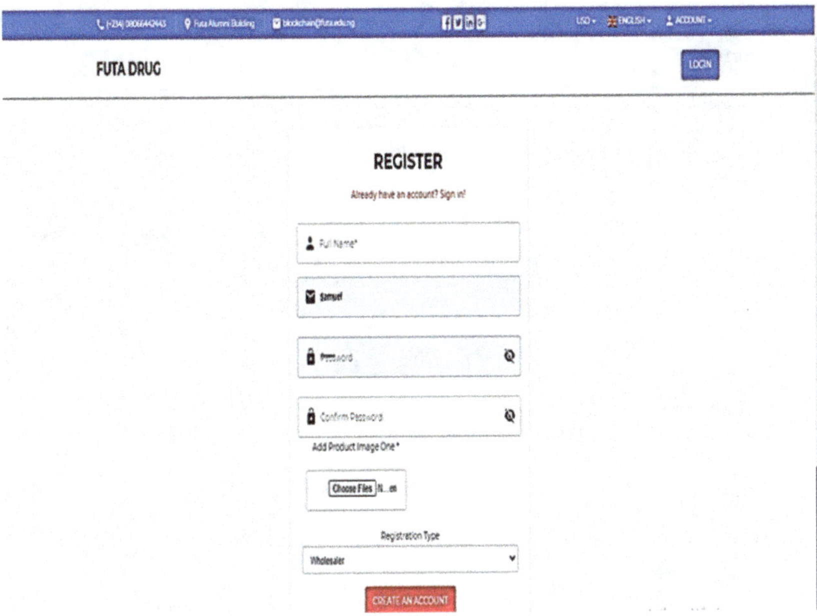

Figure 19.3 Registration page

On the Encrypted Ethereum System's registration page: Pharmacies, wholesalers, hospitals, and distributors can register an account with the medicine manufacturer using the registration page shown in Figure 19.3.

(b) The user login panel
Direct access to the login page is provided. Participants are able to log in to their accounts created with the medicine manufacturer. To cater for new member sign-up or existing member login, the developed system stores both their user name and the password. If the user forgets either, they can restore it by clicking the forget user name tab. Figure 19.4 shows the login page.

(c) The clients' dashboard
Figure 19.5 shows the dashboard of the client that intends to buy Product from the organization, Client can track their product and also check information about the drug they have purchased.

(d) The manufacturers' interface
Figure 19.6 shows the dashboard of the manufacturer with the link that allows the manufacturer to create drug and transfer drug to client.

(e) Drugs created
Figure 19.7 shows the snapshot of drug created with the QR code representation under the Ethereum network.

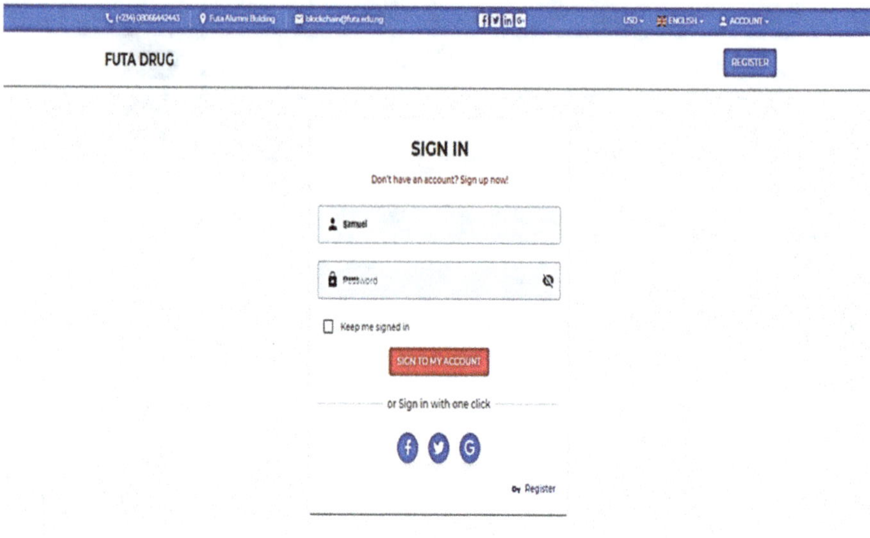

Figure 19.4 Login page

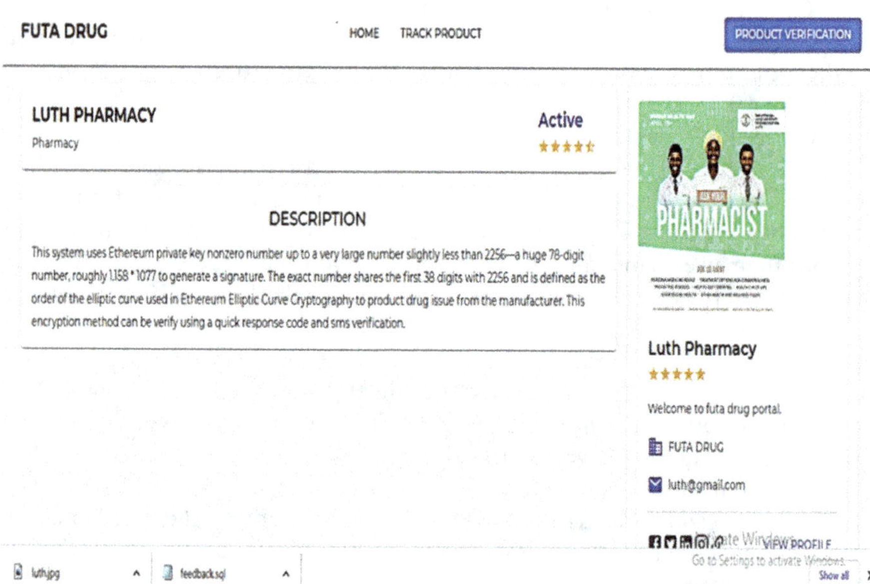

Figure 19.5 Pharmacy, hospital, wholesaler dashboard

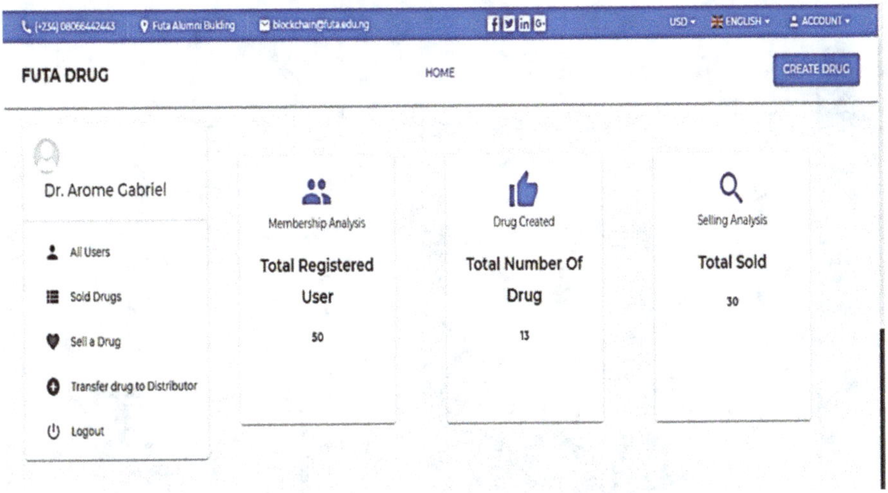

Figure 19.6 Manufacturer dashboard

19.3.2 The proposed system evaluation

A of the developed system's performance was carried out using standard metrics as discussed below;

a) *True-Positive (TP):* the overall of cases properly recognized to be true.
b) *False-Positive (FP):* the overall number of cases erroneously branded as true.
c) *True-negative (TN):* the overall number of cases properly recognized as false.
d) *False-Negative (FN):* the sum of cases that were incorrectly identified as false.
e) *Precision* (*P*): this information depicts the proportion of positively accurate forecasts. Equation 19.5 should be used to calculate precision.

$$P = \frac{TP}{TP + FP} \tag{19.5}$$

f) *Recall* (*R*): this is the proportion of all positive samples properly classed as positive. Equation 19.6 is used to determine Recall.

$$R = \frac{TP}{TP + FN} \tag{19.6}$$

g) *Specificity* (*S*): this stands for the proportion of every single negative samples properly classed as negative. Equation 19.7 can be utilized for determining specificity.

$$S = \frac{TN}{TN + FP} \tag{19.7}$$

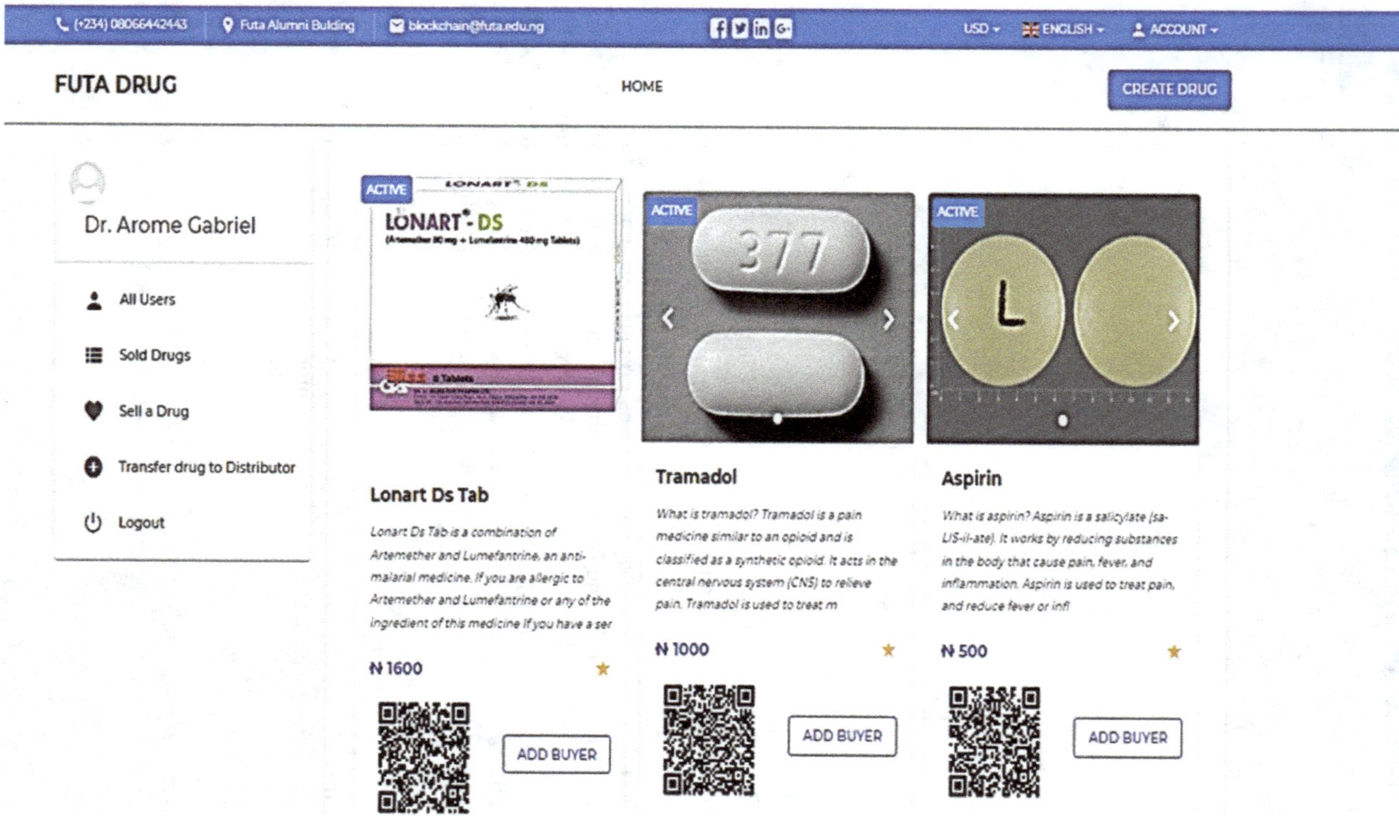

Figure 19.7 Drug created by the manufacturer

h) *F1-score* ($F1$): this puts together the recall as well as the precision as shown in equation 19.8:

$$F1 = \frac{2(P \times R)}{P + R} \tag{19.8}$$

i) *Accuracy* (A): refers to the model's gross accuracy, or the proportion of all samples properly classed. Equation 19.9 is used for computing accuracy.

$$A = \frac{TP + TN}{TP + TN + FP + FN} \tag{19.9}$$

Table 19.1 shows the evaluation of 500 users, so as to determine the Precision, Specificity, Balance Accuracy, $F1$ Score, Recall, and $F1$ Score of the proposed approach.

The summary of the system performance as regards to the performance metrics used, which are precision, recall, $F1$ score, Specificity and Balance accuracy, as computed using (19.5–19.9), is presented in Figure 19.8.

Figure 19.9 shows the results of other related works compared to the newly developed system. This comparative analysis is done in terms of standard metrics as highlighted in Figure 19.9.

A brief comparison of this current research with some other methodologies or approaches proposed in existing related works reveals that this project outperforms other existing related works. Our proposed approach is based on smart contract, with Ethereum as the network type. The newly developed system offers higher efficiency than some existing systems, like those reported in [11] as well as in [14]. Furthermore, this current study seems to be one of the few related works that went beyond system design to its actual implementation.

An admin is required to be in charge of the system, especially to manage the system and especially for maintenance and periodic updating. The new system can run on any Operating System platform and most common browsers.

Table 19.1 Evaluation matrix of 500 feedback from users

Metrics	Prospective users	Prospective users	Prospective users
Number of users	100	200	200
Precision (%)	89.6	92.2	95.2
Recall (%)	96.8	99.2	99.4
***F1* score (%)**	93.0	95.9	97.3
Specificity,TNR(%)	81.6	85	93
Balance accuracy (%)	89.2	94	96

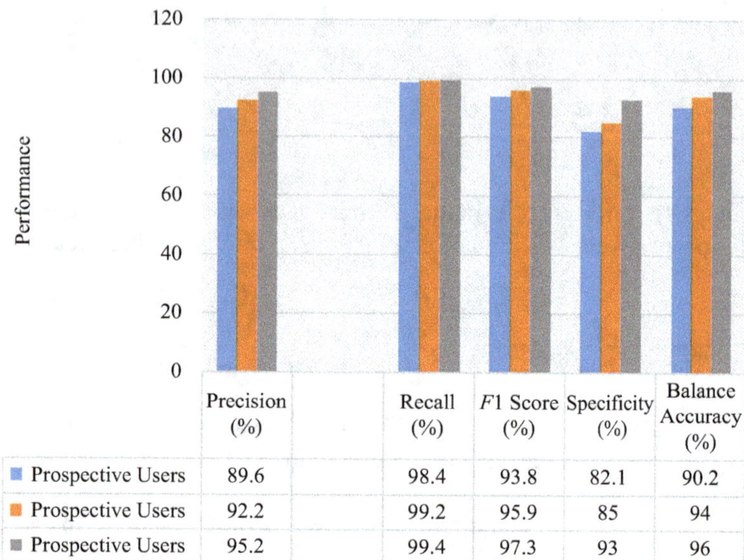

Figure 19.8 Evaluation Bar Chart of 500 feedback from users

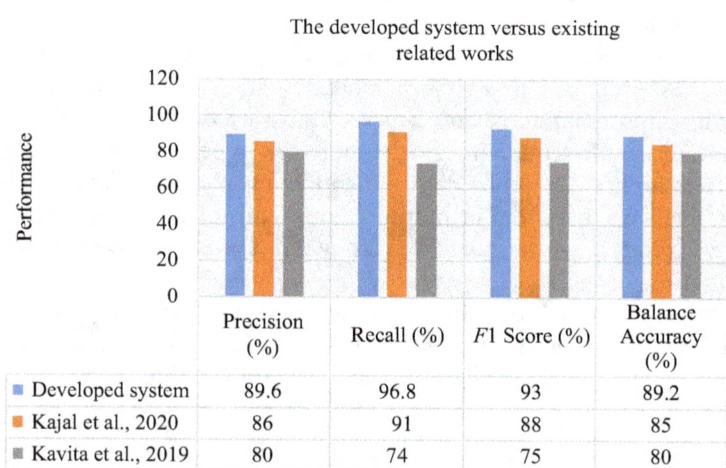

Figure 19.9 Evaluation of the developed system with other existing works

19.4 Conclusions and futures scope

Blockchain technology offers the ability to develop systems that allow various users to conduct transactions in a verifiable manner and lessen the need for trust between system participants. This study focused on examining the features of Blockchain technology and how they may be applied to combat phony drugs and goods. To do this, several Blockchain deployment methods and technologies were examined and debated, as well as the effects and issues with counterfeiting. Different strategies were devised and investigated, and it was discussed how and which Blockchain technology would be appropriate to utilize for various use cases. It became clear that while Blockchain technologies can be applied to prevent counterfeiting, they cannot stand alone as a solution. Blockchain can only be viewed as a component of a comprehensive strategy for resolving the problem, which must be situation specific and differ from case to case. The construction of a Counterfeit Drug Detection System was explicitly covered in this chapter. It offers web-based drug authentication with features from the Blockchain as well as smart contracts, as well as public accessibility, safety, and ease of use. The new system is designed such that after a fake drug is found, the user is able to interact with it by making requests or comments to the manufacturer in addition to false drug detection. The created Counterfeit Drug Detection System includes built-in features for independent administration. which makes it easier for the system administrator to manage all drug data, participants, drug categories, and user requests. The designed solution can operate on mobile devices and ought to function with all kinds of browsers. The system is also accessible at all times. Initiatives like this suggested technique should be investigated by the National Agency for Food and Drug Administration and Control (NAFDAC) of Nigeria and other food and drug regulatory agencies across the world in order to lessen the various risks associated with drug and product counterfeiting. This study has added to the body of knowledge by developing a system for accurately identifying fake medications utilizing the Blockchain and QR code/SnapTag technology. Future work can focus on exploring the possibility of using security schemes that are resistant to both classical and non-classical information security threats.

Acknowledgment

The Federal University of Technology, Akure, Nigeria, provided the workspace for the study.

References

[1] Food and Drug Administration Philippines. FDA. (2017). "FDA Warns vs Fake Products" URL: http://www.fda.gov.ph/announcement/474982-fda-warns-vs-fake-products.

[2] A. Bichell, (2017). "Fake Drugs are a Major Global Problem", *WHO Reports,* URL: https://www.npr.org/sections/goatsandsoda/2017/11/29/567229552/bad-drugs-are-a-major-global-problem-who-reports.

[3] Interpol (2018). "The Dangers of Counterfeit Medical Products. *INTERPOL.* 2018". Retrieved from: https://www.interpol.int/Crime-areas/Pharmaceutical-crime/The-dangers. Archived at: http://www.webcitation.org/6wahlZ6hX.

[4] World Health Organization (2017). "A Study on the Public Health and Socioeconomic Impact of Substandard and Falsified Medical Products". Geneva: World Health Organization; 2017. Licence: CC BY-NC-SA 3.0 IGO. Retrieved from http://www.who.int/medicines/regulation/ssffc/publications/se-study-sf/en.

[5] J. Tucker, T. Fischer, and L. Upjohn, (2018). "Unapproved Pharmaceutical Ingredients Included in Dietary Supplements Associated with US Food and Drug Administration Warnings". *JAMA Network Open*, 1(6), e183337–e183337.

[6] Bagozzi and Lindmeier (2017). "1 in 10 Medical Products in Developing Countries is Substandard or Falsified: WHO Urges Governments to Take Action". World Health Organization Media Center. Retrieved from http://www.who.int/mediacentre/news/releases/2017/substandard-falsified-products/en. Archived at: http://www.webcitation.org/6wagBrWKS

[7] G. Gnegel, C. Hauk, R. Neci, *et al.*, (2020). "Identification of Falsified Chloroquine Tablets in Africa at the Time of the COVID-19 Pandemic". *Am J Trop Med Hyg*. 2020; 103(1): 73–76. Published online 2020 May 12. DOI:10.4269/ajtmh.20-0363

[8] A. Thompson, A. Abayomi, and A. J. Gabriel, (2022). "Multifactor IoT Authentication System for Smart Homes Using Visual Cryptography, DigitalMemory, and Blockchain Technologies". In: S. Misra and A. Kumar Tyagi, (eds) *"Blockchain Applications in the Smart Era". EAI/Springer Innovations in Communication and Computing.* Springer, Cham. DOI:10.1007/978-3-030-89546-4_14

[9] O. J. Fayemi, A. F. Thompson, and O. A. Ayeni, (2022). Design and Implementation of Electronic Voting Using KECCAK256 Algorithm on Ethereum Network. In: A. Khanna, D. Gupta, S. Bhattacharyya, A. E. Hassanien, S. Anand, and A. Jaiswal, (eds) *International Conference on Innovative Computing and Communications. Advances in Intelligent Systems and Computing, vol 1394*. Springer, Singapore. DOI:10.1007/978-981-16-3071-2_35

[10] A. Thompson, H. Odekunle, and B. Alese, (2023). "A Secure Decentralized Privacy-Preserving Healthcare System Using Blockchain". In: K. Daimi, I. Dionysiou, and N. El Madhoun, (eds) *"Principles and Practice of Blockchains"*. Springer, Cham. DOI:10.1007/978-3-031-10507-4_9

[11] A. A. Sanghi and A. Katakwar, (2022). "Detection of Counterfeit Drugs in Medical Supply Chain Using Blockchain Technology". In *Advances in Manufacturing Technology and Management: Proceedings of 6th International Conference on Advanced Production and Industrial Engineering (ICAPIE)—2021* (pp. 651–659). Singapore: Springer Nature Singapore.

[12] M. Arumugam, S. Deepa, G. R. Sreekanth, G. Arun, and S. Nilesh, (2021). "Counterfeit Drugs Prevention Using Block Chain Techniques". In *IOP Conference Series: Materials Science and Engineering* (Vol. 1055, No. 1, p. 012109). IOP Publishing.

[13] Y. Huang, J. Wu, and C. Long, (2018). "Drugledger: A Practical Blockchain System for Drug Traceability and Regulation". In *2018 IEEE International Conference on Internet of Things (iThings) and IEEE Green Computing and Communications (GreenCom) and IEEE Cyber, Physical and Social Computing (CPSCom) and IEEE Smart Data (SmartData)* (pp. 1137–1144). IEEE.

[14] J. D. Evans, (2018). "Improving the Transparency of the Pharmaceutical Supply Chain Through the Adoption of Quick Response (QR) Code, Internet of Things (IOT), and Blockchain Technology: One Result: Ending the Opioid Crisis". *Pitt. J. Tech. L. and Pol'y*, 19, 35.

[15] K. Kumari, and K. Saini, (2019). "CFDD (Counterfeit Drug Detection) Using Blockchain in the Pharmaceutical Industry". *Int J Eng Res Technol (IJERT)*, 8, 1–4.

[16] P. Sylim, F. Liu, A. Marcelo, and P. Fontelo, (2018). "Blockchain Technology for Detecting Falsified and Substandard Drugs in Distribution: Pharmaceutical Supply Chain Intervention". *JMIR Research Protocols*, 7(9), e10163.

[17] M. Mohana, G. Ong, and T. Ern, (2019). "Implementation of Pharmaceutical Drug Traceability Using Blockchain Technology". *Inti Journal*, 2019(35).

[18] I. Haq, and O. M. Esuka, (2018). "Blockchain Technology in Pharmaceutical Industry to Prevent Counterfeit Drugs". *International Journal of Computer Applications*, 180(25), 8–12.

[19] V. Pashkov, and O. Soloviov, (2019). "Legal Implementation of Blockchain Technology in Pharmacy". In *SHS Web of Conferences,* Vol. 68, p. 01027. EDP Sciences.

[20] Y. Yun, (2020). "The Influence of Blockchain Technology on Fraud and Fake Protection". NSF grant DGE-1723635. Volume 7 Special Issue: *Interdisciplinary Cybersecurity Research*, Article 8. Available at: https://digitalcommons.odu.edu/ourj/vol7/iss1/8.

[21] M. J. Labaran and M. Haman-Adama, (2021). The Nigerian Pharmaceutical Supply Chain: Blockchain Adoption, Counterfeit Drugs and Successful Deployment of COVID-19 Vaccine in Nigeria". *Journal of Scientific Research and Reports*, 27(2): 20–36.

[22] R. H. Hasan, K. Salah, R. Jayaraman, *et al.*, (2020). "A Blockchain-Based Approach for the Creation of Digital Twins", *IEEE Access*. DOI:10.1109/ACESS.2020.2974810.

[23] X. Liu, S. S. Sun, and G. Huang, (2020), "Decentralized Services Computing Paradigm for Blockchain-Based Data Governance: Programmability, Interoperability, and Intelligence" *IEEE Transactions on Services Computing*, 13(2), pp. 343–355, 2020.

[24] M. Alsumidaie (2018). "Blockchain Concepts Emerge in Clinical Trials", *Applied Clinical Trials*, May 8, 2018. Available online: http://www.appliedclinicaltrialsonline.com/blockchain-concepts-emerge-clinical-trials (accessed on 3 October 2021).

[25] M. J. M. Chowdhury, K. Biswas M. S. Ferdous, and N. Chowdhury, (2019). "A Comparative Analysis of Distributed Ledger Technology Platforms". *IEEE Access* 2019, 7, 167930–167943.

[26] R. Bettin-Diaz, A. E. Rojas, and C. Mejia-Moncayo, (2018). Methodological approach to the definition of a Blockchain system for the food industry supply chain traceability. In: *Intl. Conf. on Computational Science and Its Applications*. pp. 19–33. Springer.

[27] L. Bell, J. W. Buchanan, J. Cameron, and O. Lo (2018). "Applications of Blockchain Within Healthcare", *Blockchain in Healthcare Today*, vol. 1, 2018.

[28] Imoize, Agbotiname Lucky, Irabor, Daisy Osarugue, Gbadega, Peter Anuoluwapo, and Chakraborty, Chinmay. "Blockchain Technology for Secure COVID-19 Pandemic Data Handling" (Healthcare Technologies, 2022), 'Smart Health Technologies for the COVID-19 Pandemic: *Internet of Medical Things Perspectives*', Chap. 6, pp. 141–179, DOI:10.1049/PBHE042E_ch6.

[29] A. L. Imoize, P. A. Gbadega, H. I. Obakhena, D. O. Irabor, K. V. N. Kavitha, and C. Chakraborty, (2022). "Artificial Intelligence-Enabled Internet of Medical Things for COVID-19 Pandemic Data Management". *Explainable Artificial Intelligence in Medical Decision Support Systems*, 357–380.

[30] A. L. Imoize, J. Hemanth, D. T. Do, and S. N. Sur, (Eds.). (2023). "Explainable Artificial Intelligence in Medical Decision Support Systems". *IET*.

[31] A. J. Gabriel, B. K. Alese, A. O. Adetunmbi, O. S., and O. A. Sarumi, (2019). "Post-Quantum Crystography System for Secure Electronic Voting". *Open Computer Science*, 9(1), 292–298. https://doi.org/10.1515/comp-2019-0018.

[32] A. J. Gabriel, (2021). "Secure Storage and Sharing of COVID-19 Data in Health Facilities Using AES-Cryptography and Audio Steganography". *Journal of Internet Technology and Secured Transactions (JITST)*, 9, 1. pp. 735–740.

[33] A. J. Gabriel, A. Darwsih, and A. E. Hassanien, (2021). Cyber Security in the Age of COVID-19. In: A. E. Hassanien and A. Darwish, (eds) "Digital Transformation and Emerging Technologies for Fighting COVID-19 Pandemic: Innovative Approaches". Studies in Systems, Decision and Control, vol. 322. Springer, Cham. DOI:10.1007/978-3-030-63307-3_18.

[34] H. C. Ukwuoma, A. J. Gabriel, A. F. Thompson, and B. K. Alese, (2022). "Optimised Privacy Model for Cloud Data," *2021 16th International Conference on Computer Science and Education (ICCSE)*, Lancaster, United Kingdom, 2021, pp. 267–269, DOI: 10.1109/ICCSE51940.2021.9569395.

[35] H. C. Ukwuoma, A. J. Gabriel, A. F. Thompson, and B. K. Alese, (2022). "Quantum Attack-Resistant Security System for Cloud Computing using Lattice Cryptography". *International Journal for Information Security Research (IJISR)*, 12, 1, Infonomics Society, pp:1053–1061, DOI: 10.20533/ijisr.2042.4639.2022.0119.

[36] O. Alabi, A. J. Gabriel, A. F. Thompson, and B. K. Alese, (2022). "Privacy and Trust Models for Cloud-Based EHRs Using Multilevel Cryptography and Artificial Intelligence". In: S. Misra, A. Kumar Tyagi, V. Piuri, L. Garg, (eds) *Artificial Intelligence for Cloud and Edge Computing. Internet of Things*. Springer, Cham. DOI:10.1007/978-3-030-80821-1_5

[37] H. Ukwuoma, A. J. Gabriel, A. F. Thompson, and B. K. Alese, (2022). "Post-Quantum Cryptography-Driven Security Framework for Cloud Computing". *Open Computer Science*, 12(1), 142–153. DOI:10.1515/comp-2022-0235

[38] T. Kumar V. Ramani I. Ahmad and A. Braeken (2018). "Blockchain Utilization in Healthcare: Key Requirements and Challenges," in *IEEE 20th International Conference on e-Health Networking, Applications and Services*, pp. 1–7, Czech Republic, 2018.

Chapter 20

Cybersecurity in centralized healthcare systems: overview, design framework, challenges, and research trends

Joseph Bamidele Awotunde[1], Abidemi Emmanuel Adeniyi[2], Peace Busola Falola[3], Matthew Olusegun Adigun[4], Femi Emmanuel Ayo[5], Agbotiname Lucky Imoize[6] and Demóstenes Zegarra Rodríguez[7]

Cybersecurity is an essential element of any healthcare system to protect patient data and ensure that information is used only for its intended purpose. Centralized healthcare systems are becoming increasingly interconnected and reliance on technology is increasing. Therefore, it is essential to have a comprehensive and robust cybersecurity framework in place to protect the system and its users. This chapter presents a summary of the present situation of cybersecurity in centralized healthcare systems, a framework for the design of such systems, and the challenges and research trends in this area. Using real-world examples, the chapter gives an in-depth evaluation of the role of cybersecurity in modern healthcare systems. It highlights the importance of designing and implementing effective cybersecurity measures, as well as the need for ongoing research to address the ever-evolving threats posed by malicious actors. Cybersecurity is an essential element of any healthcare system to protect patient data and ensure that information is used only for its intended purpose. This chapter primary focus is on a framework for designing such systems, as well as the difficulties and

[1]Department of Computer Science, Faculty of Information and Communication Sciences, University of Ilorin, Nigeria
[2]Department of Computer Science, College of Computing and Communication Studies, Bowen University, Nigeria
[3]Department of Computer Sciences, Faculty of Pure and Applied Sciences, Precious Cornerstone University, Nigeria
[4]Department of Computer Science, University of Zululand, South Africa
[5]Department of Mathematical Sciences, Olabisi Onabanjo University, Nigeria
[6]Department of Electrical and Electronics Engineering, Faculty of Engineering, University of Lagos, Nigeria
[7]Department of Computer Science, Federal University of Lavras, Lavras, Brazil

current research directions in this field. Using real-world examples, it highlights the importance of designing and implementing effective cybersecurity measures.

20.1 Introduction

An increasing hazard to the healthcare sector is health security breaches, assaults on medical devices and infrastructure, and loss of information and theft of funds [1]. Just one organization might face expenditures of up to US $7 million due to consequences, litigation, and image loss, especially in the case of hospital compromise of information safety [2]. Medical sector's overall effect of data leaks is estimated to be around US $6 billion [3]. Organizations in the healthcare sector are forced to invest a lot of money and effort in securing their systems since the healthcare sector lags behind other industries in data protection [4]. The intricacy of healthcare organizations make this, however, easier said than done. Hospitals are incredibly complicated organizations with a number of standard organizational traits turned up or down to extremities [5] like

- A technologically advanced platform: comparable to other businesses, they contend to control a variety of gadgets, from interconnected healthcare devices to antiquated information technology (IT); they have a vastly greater number of them than other organizations, ad hoc purchases made by doctors or free gifts provided by medical device manufacturers, rather than by a single IT department [6,7].
- Internal politics: they face the same issues as other sizable companies, but they are made more challenging by the organization's complex internal functions: similar to other organizations in terms of finances, information technology, and human resources-wise; unlike other enterprises, along with other specialties, they must also help pediatrics, cardiology, and radiology [5]. High levels of specialization are present. Each department has varied equipment requirements, patient care demands, and processes and employs highly skilled workers who undergo extensive training.
- Regulatory requirements: They must adhere to the rules set down by the state and federal governments, just like other organizations; however, healthcare information is seen as being especially delicate in the United States and is consequently safeguarded by additional particular data protection legislation [8].
- Patient-centered care: the ability of hospitals to earn significant net revenue is important to them, as it is to other American businesses. However, in contrast to other organizations, even for-profit ones have patient care as their top priority [9].

It is intriguing to think about how these traits might affect a particular hospital's capacity to withstand cyberattacks on a systemic level. But next think about the variety of potential distinctions between these organizations. For instance, a large, metropolitan research hospital has quite different interests than a rural community hospital. In terms of IT, smaller or more remote hospitals are more likely to outsource services, the most frequent role being transcription services

[10]. The choice of outsourcing overlaps with the preference for making modest investments in IT safety at these institutions [11].

The price of delivering healthcare is high and rising everywhere. In 2020, the United States alone spent $4.1 trillion, or astonishing 19.7% of GDP [12]. Notwithstanding substantial spending on healthcare, the majority of countries deal with ineffective medical infrastructures. Administrations are routinely held accountable for poor emergency response, delayed identification of urgent situations, insufficient surveillance of chronic patients, readmissions, and, most importantly, a high rate of avoidable mistakes. The fact that avoidable negligence is the main cause of fatalities in the United States will surprise some readers [13].

In order to improve treatment results via rapid and precise diagnosis and, at the same time, decrease the growing cost of medical care on government agencies, modern healthcare is becoming more and more dependent on technology. The utilization of Internet of Things (IoT) devices and multi-cloud computing for storage and analytics are becoming more common, according to trends. By 2022, a market intelligence group called International Data Corporation predicts that a startling 90% of medium and huge-sized enterprises will have adopted the cloud, incorporating hybrid and multiple clouds [14]. Multi-cloud growth in the healthcare industry is predicted to be 37% in 2021 compared to 19% in 2019 [15]. With these advancements, important patients who are hospitalized or in route by ambulance could receive timely diagnosis and care. In other words, they could significantly raise the likelihood that patients would live and recover from their illness.

The unintended consequence of the introduction of new technologies is the increased exposure of patients and hospitals to devastating nefarious assaults [16,17]. In total, 90% of healthcare businesses have experienced at least one cyberattack in the past two years [18]. In total, there will be 71% more breaches or occurrences in 2020 than there were in 2019 [19]. The healthcare industry accounted for the greatest proportion of ransomware-related insurance claims across all significant economic sectors between 2015 and 2019 [15]. Patients who are being diagnosed, treated, or transported in an ambulance pose serious risks from any attack on sensitive patient data going through a complexly organized healthcare system.

Cybersecurity threats in medical care platforms have been an increasing worry in recent years. The healthcare industry has become increasingly reliant on technology and electronic health records (EHRs), making it an attractive target for cybercriminals. Safeguarding computer systems, connections, and data against illegal entry, harm, theft, or interruption is the practice of cybersecurity [20]. It involves a set of measures, technologies, and processes designed to safeguard IT infrastructure, digital assets, and sensitive information from cyber threats and attacks. Given that cyberthreats are always evolving and becoming more advanced, cybersecurity is a continuous effort [21]. Organizations must stay updated on the latest security trends, adopt advanced technologies, and foster a security-first culture to protect their digital assets and sensitive information effectively. Collaboration and information sharing among cybersecurity professionals and organizations also play a vital role in building a more secure cyberspace [22,23].

The Internet has made the globe smaller in many respects, but it has also opened our eyes to external factors that have never been more varied and challenging. Safety and espionage both saw rapid evolution. Regarding cyber security, there are two points of view. One is that since companies who provide cloud computing only do a portion of what they do, they are well secured by the most innovative, state-of-the-art encryption technology. Protecting systems and data from major online attacks is a part of cybersecurity activities. There are several risks right now. Therefore, maintaining cyber security operations and strategy may be challenging, particularly in government and commercial networks where, in their most creative forms, cyberattacks typically strike the delicate political and military resources of a country or its population [20].

Due to the increasing expansion of biological data and healthcare ecosystems, smart healthcare technological advances have emerged as one of the most significant research areas. The fusion of cloud computing and IoT principles has encouraged the development of smart medical systems that are capable of diagnosis, monitoring, and gathering enormous volumes of health data and providing trustworthy analytical tools for analysis [24,25]. For the purpose of protecting and avoiding user data in the healthcare industry, the cybersecurity community has worked hard to build advanced security techniques [26,27]. Healthcare is one field where cybersecurity intelligence has had a significant impact. Several academics are working on innovative methods to improve the safety of healthcare systems. In addition, artificial intelligence (AI) has emerged as a major technology in recent years that can be used to make current approaches smarter.

Instances from the past few years include the ransomware assault that occurred in 2016 on the Hollywood Presbyterian Medical Center in Los Angeles and WannaCry, a non-targeted ransomware attack that hit more than 150 countries worldwide and briefly made parts of the UK's National Health Service unusable [28]. There is a need to create techniques that enable professionals to more accurately assess the real impact of such episodes on all specific patients and medical systems in general. The attacks involve millions of dollars in revenue losses and fines, as well as significant reputational loss. Despite the United States' healthcare and government sectors integrating robust emergency response and preparedness systems, the constantly changing cybersecurity risk toward medical institutions surpasses the present preventative measures and challenges in the "all-hazards" catastrophe readiness paradigm [28]. More epidemiologic research on clinical cybersecurity intrusions and their effects on the treatment of patients and medical results is needed to prevent and prevent such assaults.

20.1.1 Key contributions of the chapter

The following are the primary chapter contributions:

i. The chapter highlights the current cybersecurity practices in centralized healthcare systems.
ii. The chapter presents the current cybersecurity threats in centralized healthcare systems.
iii. The chapter presents the design framework and security mechanisms necessary for effective cybersecurity protection.

iv. The challenges and threats posed to modern healthcare systems are explored, along with current research trends in the field.

20.1.2 Chapter organization

Section 20.2 presents an overview of cybersecurity in centralized healthcare systems. Section 20.3 discusses the design framework for cybersecurity in centralized healthcare systems. Section 20.4 presents the research trends for cybersecurity in centralized healthcare systems. Section 20.5 discusses the critical lessons learned in this chapter, and finally, Section 20.6 concludes the chapter.

20.2 Overview of cybersecurity in centralized healthcare systems

In the context of computer-based technology, cybersecurity refers to the safeguarding against intentional or unintentional disruption caused by altering foundational software, hardware, or networked interconnections. Regardless of the fact that the subject and its methods have received significant focus in the technology, financial, industrial infrastructure, and national security sectors, healthcare cybersecurity is in a state of crisis, according to a 2017 report authorized by the Department of Health and Human Services (HHS). The following factors are a serious reason for worry, the research claims: (1) there is a severe lack of information safety experts, (2) the extensive use of old legacy technology, (3) innovation technologies that are too connected, and (4) the careless existence of software flaws in widely used devices.

On May 12, 2017, a noteworthy instance of the danger that cybersecurity flaws pose to public health took place, with the introduction and quick dissemination of the software virus WannaCry. Ransomware is an illustration of a subset of malevolent malware infections. Utilizing a bug in the Windows operating system's previous iterations, WannaCry was able to infect vulnerable machines [28]. The information previously saved on the computer was then encrypted by the virus, preventing the owner from accessing the data except a tribute in the sort of a digital coin that cannot be tracked was offered.

In the end, the ransomware infected thousands of machines across more than 150 nations. However, it might be argued that the infection of the NHS in Britain was where WannaCry had its greatest impact [29]. Over 80 hospitals had a 4-day interruption in their regular operations as a result. It was necessary to postpone tens of thousands of surgeries and clinical visits between May 12 and May 19; complicated medical devices, such as magnetic resonance imaging scanners, were momentarily turned off; and in other locations, ambulances had to be sent to clinics that were untouched, which caused disruptions in patient care [30]. At that moment, the NHS did not consistently gather particular data that would have made it possible to gauge how this might affect healthcare (i.e., the number of diversions, disease-specific morbidity, and mortality). As a result, it is impossible to accurately assess the impact on public health [31]. Using general mortality statistics and missed appointments, in Ref. [32] the authors tried to evaluate the medical impact of WannaCry. There was however no rise in mortality altogether; however, earlier studies have demonstrated implications on difficult death due to waits brought on by closures of roads during

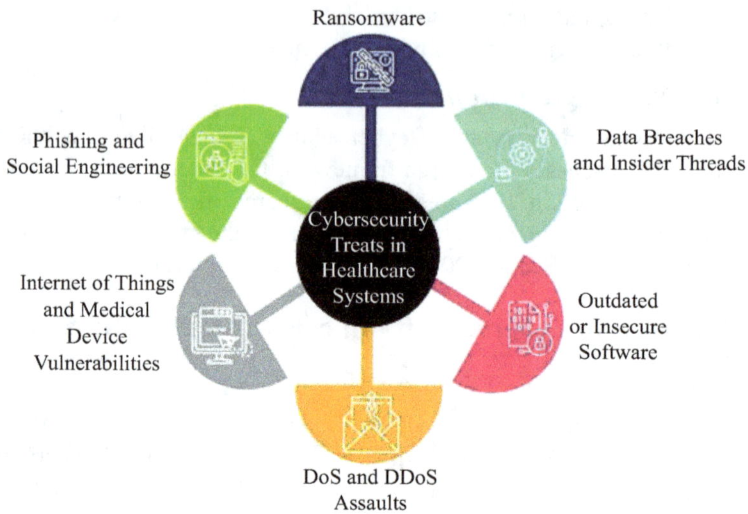

Figure 20.1 Common cybersecurity issues in healthcare systems

races. There were probably considerable unobserved repercussions [33]. From a monetary perspective, but the NHS unequivocally calculates that the WannaCry assault would cost at least £92 million an equivalent of US$115 million [34]. Figure 20.1 shows the common security treats in healthcare system.

While the majority of American Healthcare IT infrastructures were spared from WannaCry infestation, other ransomware assaults have impacted a number of institutions. Most significantly, a ransomware hacks with comparable unfavorable results happened at Hollywood Presbyterian Hospital in California in 2016 [35]. Unlike the WannaCry assault, but when the incident happened, Presbyterian Hospital opted not to alert the authorities. On the contrary, the hospital's data was seized captive for ten days before it finally paid the criminals a $17,000 bitcoin compensation [36]. This event's entire monetary and psychological consequences have not been assessed. However, other data security violations have cost hospitals up to $7 million in financing costs, legal expenses, and image damage [37]. Following the Presbyterian incident, the same ransomware was used in a large rise in attempted attacks in the neighboring city of Palo Alto [38].

The rise of digitalization and connectivity in healthcare systems has led to a pressing need for reliable cybersecurity protection. In many countries, the healthcare sector is highly centralized, with most healthcare data and services being stored on single networks. This necessitates the use of strong cybersecurity mechanisms to protect patient data and ensure safe and efficient operations within healthcare systems. Cybercrime emerged in the late 1970s when the computer IT industry started to gain form [39]. Over time, what began as spam evolved into viruses and other types of malware. The advanced capabilities and synergy of technology are increasing. The medical field is a well-liked target for hackers due to the fact that medical data includes critical private and monetary information.

In an effort to prevent the breach of medical data, the Health Insurance Portability and Accountability Act of 1996 (HIPAA) established structural and technological safeguards to guarantee critical information is safeguarded from hackers [40]. Physical precautions include things like controls over facility availability, media and device limits, and workstation use and security. Practical safeguards include things like an individual login number, a backup access mechanism, auto logoff, encoding, and decoding [41,42]. However, thieves are developing ways to circumvent these security measures. Medical technology deployment is a time-consuming process that needs extensive planning and implementation. Once installed, the software has to be upgraded often to remain abreast of the latest advances and safety holes that hackers have found. While spending a lot of money to become more integrated, organizations do not devote enough time or resources to maintaining software [43].

20.2.1 Cybersecurity threats in healthcare systems

If not from personal experience, then at least from a constant stream of news reports, the most of us are aware of cyber risks. According to reports, during the 2013 holiday shopping season, the private monetary information of tens of millions of people was taken from banks, credit card firms, and their favorite merchants. The Food and Drug Administration (FDA) was successfully breached via cyberspace, and foreign nations stole the designs of significant US military weapon systems [44]. Infrastructure and data related to healthcare are at least as susceptible as the majority of monetary and armed forces data [45]. Even more serious dangers to the architecture of the healthcare system and patient safety exist in addition to the financial, legal, and reputational issues related to data and identity theft.

An astounding 94% of healthcare organizations reported being the target of cyberattacks in recent research [46]. Information loss, theft of funds, assaults on medical technology, and infrastructure assaults have so far been the four main manifestations of cybercrime against the healthcare industry [47]. While some online criminals want financial gain, others aim to acquire intellectual property or client data, harm the reputation of an institution, or engage in “hacktivism” to make a political statement. Understanding of the need of protecting individual medical data has grown thanks to the HIPAA, which also provided a structure for regulation to encourage adherence, but security does not always follow from adherence [48]. The reality is that the majority of current HIPAA protection procedures depend on common technological techniques for isolating crucial data, but according to one latest study, many attackers are getting around these kinds of defenses without the need for stealthy methods. The technological domain and the regulatory compliance domain both have significant knowledge and focus gaps that need to be filled.

Despite the growing need for reliable cybersecurity, healthcare systems remain vulnerable to cyber threats. There are several reasons for this, including the lack of a centralized security strategy, outdated software, and insufficient detection and response measures. One of the most serious threats facing healthcare systems is data theft, which can result in the loss of private patient data. Other threats include ransomware attacks, malicious insiders, and distributed denial-of-service (DDoS) attacks (Figure 20.2).

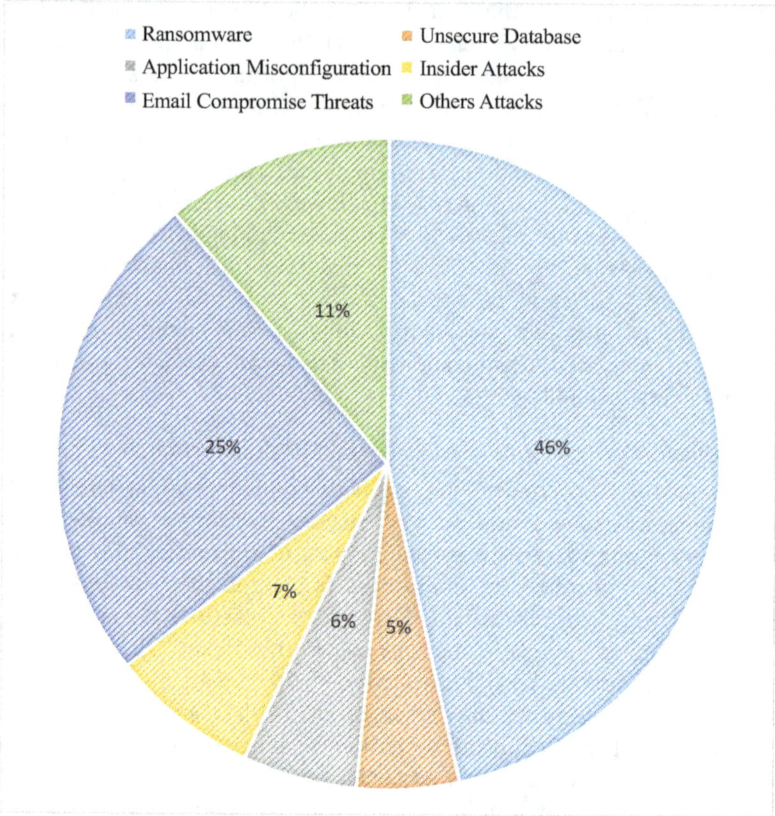

Figure 20.2 Data breach threats of report cases by types

The amount and type of data they collect and maintain, as well as their risk profile, healthcare institutions are especially at risk financially from data theft [49]. Of the 16 industries studied, healthcare had the highest per-record price whenever a loss of information took place, incurring approximately $233, according to the Ponemon Institute, a research organization specializing in privacy and data security [50], and the examination of information security policies. The retail sector incurred the lowest costs per record, at $78 on average across all industries [51]. Costs for victims' additional credit protection services and recovery efforts as well as expenditures in security-control measures are included. In the event that the WellPoint data breach of 2009–2010 incurred these projected expenses, more than 600,000 health plan members' personal and health information was made publicly available due to security issues [52]. In comparison to the $2 million in HIPAA fines that WellPoint was compelled to pay, the ultimate price would be in the billions. Hospitals, clinics, big group practices, and other institutions of the same nature within the medical field have become the focus of 72% of current illicit congestion, malware, and other assaults. Pharmaceutical companies, health insurance, provider connections, and other organizations will get the remaining 28%. In other words, the method of providing healthcare is under constant and unwavering assault.

Cybersecurity threats in healthcare systems have been a growing concern. Healthcare organizations, including hospitals, clinics, and medical facilities, manage enormous volumes of personal patient information and rely heavily on digital technologies for patient care and administrative purposes. Unfortunately, this increased reliance on technology has made healthcare systems attractive targets for cybercriminals [53]. Here are some of the common cybersecurity threats faced by healthcare systems:

20.2.1.1 Ransomware attacks in healthcare system

A form of virus known as ransomware encodes the information belonging to the victim and renders it unavailable unless an amount of money is paid. Healthcare systems often fall victim to such attacks because the loss of patient data can severely impact patient care, and the urgency of restoring access may lead organizations to consider paying the ransom [54]. Ransomware is malicious software that encrypts data on a healthcare system's network, making it inaccessible to authorized users [55]. Following that, the perpetrators request an amount of money in return for the decoding key. Ransomware attacks can disrupt medical services and potentially compromise patient safety if essential systems are affected [56].

In the medical sector, incidents involving ransomware have become a growing concern and a significant cybersecurity threat. Ransomware is a form of virus that encodes a victim's data, rendering it unusable till the perpetrators receive a ransom, who then provide the decryption key. Because they handle delicate and vital data, such as patient records and medical information, healthcare companies are prime targets for ransomware attacks [57,58]. These attacks can disrupt medical services, compromise patient safety, and result in significant financial losses.

Here are some key points to consider about ransomware attacks in healthcare:

Increased Targeting: Over time, ransomware assaults have increased in the medical sector. Attackers view hospitals, clinics, and other healthcare facilities as lucrative targets because they often rely heavily on digital systems and may have limited resources dedicated to cybersecurity.

Impact on Patient Care: Ransomware attacks can have severe consequences on patient care. Hospitals and clinics may lose access to patient records, medical imaging, and critical systems, leading to treatment delays and potential patient harm.

Financial Losses: Recovering from a ransomware attack can be costly. Healthcare organizations may face ransom demands, but even if they choose not to pay, they may still incur expenses related to incident response, data recovery, legal fees, and reputation damage.

Regulatory Compliance: Strong privacy regulations, like the Health Insurance Portability and Accountability Act (HIPAA) in the United States, apply to healthcare providers. A ransomware attack that compromises patient data can lead to regulatory penalties and legal repercussions.

Sophistication of Attacks: Ransomware attacks have become more sophisticated, employing various tactics to infiltrate networks, such as phishing emails, exploiting software vulnerabilities, or gaining access through third-party vendors.

Preventive Measures: Healthcare organizations must prioritize cybersecurity to protect against ransomware attacks. This includes regular data backups, system updates, employee training on recognizing phishing attempts, network segmentation, and the use of robust security solutions.

20.2.1.2 Collaboration and information sharing in healthcare systems

Healthcare organizations, government agencies, and cybersecurity experts need to collaborate and share information about emerging threats and best practices to strengthen the industry's overall security posture. Keep in mind that the situation regarding ransomware attacks is continually evolving, and it's essential to consult up-to-date sources for the latest information on this topic. To better comprehend how ransomware attacks are now affecting the healthcare industry, I recommend checking recent news articles, official reports from cybersecurity organizations, and government advisories related to cybersecurity threats in the healthcare sector.

20.2.1.3 Data breaches in healthcare system

Unapproved access to or exploitation of victim's information is one of the biggest concerns facing the healthcare industry [59]. This data can include personal information, medical history, test results, and billing details. Cybercriminals often sell these statistics on the gloomy web or use them for identity theft and financial fraud. Healthcare organizations store large volumes of personal and sensitive data, including patient medical records, financial information, and insurance details. Data breaches can occur due to vulnerabilities in systems, insider threats, or external hacking attempts [60]. Stolen medical records can be sold on the dark web or used for various forms of identity theft and fraud. Data breaches in healthcare systems are a significant concern because the information concerned is sensitive [61]. Numerous personal and medical details, such as names, locations, social security numbers, histories of illness, and more, are kept in great quantities by healthcare institutions. When these data are exposed or accessed by unauthorized individuals, it can lead to severe consequences for both patients and healthcare providers [62].

Common reasons for data breaches in healthcare systems include:

1. *Cyberattacks:* Cybercriminals and hackers attack healthcare systems in an effort to get patient data without authorization. They may exploit vulnerabilities in the organization's network or use phishing techniques to trick employees into revealing login credentials.
2. *Insider Threats:* Data breaches can also occur due to the actions of employees or insiders with access to sensitive information. These individuals might

intentionally or unintentionally disclose patient data, either for personal gain or due to negligence.

3. *Weak Security Measures:* Inadequate cybersecurity practices and outdated security software can make healthcare systems open to intrusions and data theft.
4. *Third-Party Risks:* For a variety of services, healthcare institutions frequently deal with outside contractors. If these companies don't put strong safety precautions in place, they can wind up serving as ports of admission for hackers to the healthcare system.

Consequences of healthcare data breaches include:

Identity Theft: When patient information is compromised, it can be utilized for crime and identity fraud. Monetary losses may result for those who are impacted by this.

Medical Fraud: Stolen medical information may be used to obtain medical services or prescriptions fraudulently, leading to incorrect treatments in the affected individual's medical record.

Damage to Reputation: Healthcare organizations that experience data breaches often suffer reputational damage, resulting in a decline in patient and investor trust.

Legal and Regulatory Penalties: Healthcare organizations that fail to protect patient data may face legal actions and regulatory fines for non-compliance with data protection laws.

The following steps should be put into practice by companies to lessen the likelihood of data leaks in healthcare systems:

Strong Cybersecurity Protocols: Implement robust cybersecurity measures, including encryption, breach detection systems, multi-factor authorization, and periodic safety audits.

Employee Training: Employees should get frequent training on data safety guidelines, including how to spot phishing scams and how to handle sensitive information properly.

Regular Audits and Assessments: To find system flaws and shortcomings, perform routine inspections and risk evaluations.

Third-Party Security: Verify that all collaborators and third-party providers have suitable safety procedures set up to safeguard data.

Incident Response Plan: Create and test a crisis management strategy to quickly address data breaches and limit the damage.

Data breaches in healthcare systems are complex and ever-evolving issues, requiring constant vigilance and investment in security measures to protect sensitive patient information.

20.2.1.4 Phishing and social engineering in healthcare systems

Social engineering tactics and phishing emails are frequently used by cybercriminals to deceive employees into disclosing critical data or clicking on malicious links [63]. A successful phishing attack can provide attackers with access credentials or other critical information. Fake emails, texts, or telephone calls are used by cybercriminals to deceive healthcare workers into disclosing sensitive data, including login passwords or patient information [64,65]. Social engineering attacks exploit human vulnerabilities rather than technical weaknesses. Phishing and social engineering are serious cybersecurity threats that can pose significant risks to any system, including healthcare systems [66,67]. Let's discuss how these threats can impact healthcare systems and some measures to mitigate them.

1. *Phishing:* Phishing is a type of cyberattack in which perpetrators use phony emails, messages, or Internet pages to coerce victims into disclosing confidential data like login passwords, financial information, or private details.

   Potential Impact on Healthcare Systems

   Unauthorized access: Attackers may gain access to sensitive patient records, medical data, or financial information, leading to potential data breaches.

   Ransomware: Phishing emails can deliver malicious attachments or links that, when opened, can infect the healthcare system with ransomware, locking users' data unless a ransom fee is paid

   Disruption of services: A successful phishing attack on healthcare staff could disrupt operations, leading to lags in medical care that might endanger the health of the patient.

   Mitigation Measures:

   Education and training: Healthcare staff should receive regular training on identifying phishing attempts and be educated about the consequences of falling victim to such attacks.

   Email filtering: Use effective email screening programs to identify and stop fraudulent emails before they are received by users.

   Multi-factor authentication (MFA): Accessing critical platforms or data should require MFA, which adds an additional layer of protection even if the credentials are stolen.

   Incident response plan: To swiftly identify, react to, and recuperate from a phishing assault, have a well-defined incident response strategy in place.

2. *Social Engineering:* Social engineering is the practice of persuading people to provide sensitive information or take security-compromising acts.

   Potential Impact on Healthcare Systems:

   Unauthorized access: Social engineering tactics can trick healthcare staff into revealing passwords or granting access to sensitive information.

   Impersonation: Attackers may pose as legitimate personnel to gain trust and access to restricted areas or information.

   Information leakage: Attacks using social engineering may result in the unintended exposure of private data to unknown parties.

Mitigation Measures:
Access control: Put in place reliable access control measures to guarantee that only those with the proper authorization may access sensitive information and locations.
Verification protocols: Establish strict procedures for verifying the identity of individuals before sharing sensitive information.
Limited disclosure: Encourage employees to follow the principle of "need-to-know" when sharing information, even within the organization.
Vigilance and skepticism: Train staff to be vigilant and skeptical of unsolicited requests for information, especially if they seem unusual or urgent.

Overall, cybersecurity in healthcare systems is crucial, given the sensitive nature of patient data. Combining technical measures and protecting against phishing and social engineering attacks may be achieved through staff education and clearly established rules and procedures. It's crucial to remain current with the latest cybersecurity practices and continuously improve the system's defenses to adapt to evolving threats.

20.2.1.5 Internet of things and medical device vulnerabilities

The increasing use of IoT devices and interconnected medical devices presents new attack vectors. These gadgets have flaws that can be used to alter medical equipment or obtain illegal entry into healthcare networks [68,69]. The adoption of wearable technology and medical gadgets that are online connected opens up new attack vectors. IoT devices that are out-of-date or insecurely configured can be used to access the healthcare network. The IoT has brought numerous advancements and conveniences to various industries, including healthcare [70]. IoT implies a network of networked medical equipment and systems that gather, transmit, and evaluate patient data in order to enhance patient care and boost healthcare productivity [71,72]. While IoT has the ability to change the medical sector, it also introduces certain vulnerabilities, particularly when it comes to medical devices. The safety and design faults of medical equipment linked to the Internet are known as medical device flaws in the IoT environment. Malicious actors may take advantage of these flaws for a variety of reasons, including patient injury, illegal access to patient data, interference with medical equipment, and data breaches [73]. Here are some common vulnerabilities associated with IoT medical devices:

1. *Weak Authentication and Authorization:* Some medical devices may have weak or default login credentials, making them susceptible to unauthorized access. If not properly secured, attackers can gain access to the device and manipulate its functions or steal sensitive patient data.
2. *Lack of Encryption:* Insufficient data encryption during transmission can expose patient data to interception and eavesdropping. This is particularly concerning when sensitive health information is being sent between devices or to a centralized system.
3. *Outdated Software and Firmware:* Manufacturers may not consistently provide software updates or patches for their medical devices. This leaves devices

running outdated software, which can have known vulnerabilities that attackers can exploit.

4. *Inadequate Security Testing:* Medical device manufacturers might not conduct thorough security testing during the development process, leaving vulnerabilities undiscovered until they are exploited in the real world.
5. *Physical Access Exploitation:* If physical access to the medical device is possible, attackers could potentially compromise the device directly, altering its functionality or extracting data.
6. *Insecure Communication Protocols:* Some devices use insecure communication protocols that are susceptible to interception or data manipulation.
7. *Data Privacy Concerns:* Significant privacy issues are raised by the enormous volume of sensitive patient data that medical IoT devices capture and communicate. This information can be misused to commit insurance fraud, identity theft, or even blackmail.
8. *Denial-of-Service (DoS) Attacks:* Attackers may carry out DoS assaults to overwhelm medical devices or the systems they connect to, causing disruptions in patient care or data processing.
9. *Interoperability Issues:* When medical devices from different manufacturers are integrated into a hospital or healthcare system, compatibility and security issues may arise, leaving gaps that attackers could exploit.

Addressing these vulnerabilities is important to ensuring the safety and security of IoT medical gadgets. To mitigate risks, healthcare organizations and device manufacturers should take several steps:

Implement reliable entry management and verification systems. Use strong encryption to keep data during transmission and storage. Regularly update software and firmware with security patches. Conduct thorough security testing, including penetration testing, during the development phase.

Physically secure medical devices to prevent unauthorized access. Choose secure communication protocols for data transmission. Follow data privacy laws, like the GDPR (General Data Protection Regulation) in the European Union or HIPAA (Health Insurance Portability and Accountability Act) in the United States.

Foster collaboration between device manufacturers, healthcare professionals, and cybersecurity professionals will exchange expertise and best practices. These actions are being made by healthcare groups and can significantly reduce the risk of IoT medical device vulnerabilities and ensure the safety and privacy of their patients.

20.2.1.6 Insider threats in healthcare system

Healthcare systems may be seriously jeopardized by the conduct of dishonest or careless staff, contractors, or other insiders [74,75]. Employees with access to sensitive data may intentionally or inadvertently leak information or compromise security. Insider threats in the healthcare system are security hazards brought on by employees who are permitted to access certain areas of the company to sensitive information or resources and exploit that access for malicious purposes. These individuals may include employees, contractors, volunteers, or any other personnel associated with the healthcare facility. Insider threats pose a significant risk to patient data, financial resources, and the overall integrity of the healthcare system.

Types of Insider Threats in Healthcare:

Data Theft: Insiders with access to patient records and sensitive medical information may steal this data for various reasons, such as selling it on the black market or using it to commit identity theft and fraud.

Sabotage: Disgruntled employees or individuals may intentionally disrupt healthcare operations, compromise patient care, or damage critical systems.

Fraud: Insiders can exploit their positions to manipulate financial records, insurance claims, or billing systems for personal gain or to benefit others.

Espionage: Competing healthcare organizations or external entities may attempt to infiltrate a healthcare facility by planting insiders who gather confidential information for competitive advantage or other malicious purposes.

Phishing and Social Engineering: Insiders can fall victim to phishing attacks or social engineering tactics, where external actors deceive them into divulging sensitive information or granting unauthorized access.

Medical Identity Theft: Insiders may misuse patient identities or healthcare provider credentials to access medical services, prescription medications, or medical equipment fraudulently.

Unauthorized Disclosure: Insiders might unintentionally or intentionally disclose sensitive information to unauthorized parties, violating patient privacy and confidentiality.

Unintentional Errors: Negligence or lack of proper training may lead to accidental data breaches or system vulnerabilities.

Prevention and Mitigation Strategies:

Access Control and Monitoring: Put in place strong access restrictions to make sure that workers are given only permission to use the systems and data they need to perform their jobs. Monitor access logs for unusual or suspicious activities.

Employee Training and Awareness: Inform staff members on a regular basis on safe online behavior, possible hazards, and how to spot and report them.

Employee Screening: Conduct thorough background checks before hiring new personnel, particularly for positions involving sensitive data or critical systems.

Security Policies and Procedures: Establish comprehensive security policies that address insider threats and ensure that all employees understand and adhere to them.

Encryption and Data Protection: To prevent unwanted access, encode private information during motion and at rest.

Whistleblower Protection: Create a culture that encourages reporting of suspicious activities, and protect whistleblowers from retaliation.

Behavioral Analytics: Utilize advanced monitoring tools that can detect anomalies in employee behavior, helping identify potential insider threats.

Two-Factor Authentication (2FA): Use 2FA to increase safety while accessing important devices and data.

Regular Auditing: Conduct periodic security audits to assess vulnerabilities and address potential risks proactively.

Incident Response Plan: To successfully address insider threats and other safety issues, create a thorough incident response strategy.

Healthcare insider threats necessitate a multi-layered security strategy that incorporates technology, rules, and staff education. It's crucial to maintain vigilance and regularly adjust safety precautions to counteract changing dangers in the healthcare sector.

20.2.1.7 Denial-of-service (DoS) and distributed denial-of-service (DDoS) attacks in healthcare system

The DoS and DDoS assaults seek to overwhelm the networks of healthcare systems, rendering them inaccessible to authorized users [23]. Such assaults can impair medical procedures and cause life-threatening delays in patient treatment. The DoS and DDoS attacks are serious cybersecurity threats that can significantly impact healthcare systems [76,77]. In a healthcare context, these assaults can result in negative outcomes. for patient care, data security, and overall system stability. Here's an overview of how these attacks can affect healthcare systems:

Denial-of-Service (DoS) Attacks: By bombarding a target system or network with an excessive quantity of traffic, requests, or resource usage, a DoS attack seeks to reduce its availability [78,79]. In the healthcare sector, this could mean the targeted disruption of critical services, medical devices, or infrastructure. Some ways in which DoS attacks can impact healthcare systems include:

Service Disruption: Attackers may overwhelm the servers or network of the healthcare system with a large number of traffic, which would make services sluggish to nonexistent. Slowdowns in patient care and possibly fatal circumstances can result from this.

Medical Device Malfunction: For management and tracking, a number of medical equipment, including infusion pumps and patient monitors, are connected to the network. A DoS attack on the network could prevent these devices from functioning correctly, endangering patient safety.

Electronic Health Record (EHR) Inaccessibility: Doctors and healthcare staff heavily rely on EHRs to access patient information. A DoS attack on EHR servers could render medical records inaccessible, hampering medical decision-making and continuity of care.

Distributed Denial-of-Service (DDoS) Attacks: DDoS attacks are a more sophisticated variant of DoS attacks. A DDoS assault involves the planned utilization of several hacked devices—often botnet members—to saturate the intended system with traffic. Due to their dispersed nature, DDoS assaults are more effective than standard DoS attempts. In a healthcare environment, DDoS attacks can cause the following problems:

Scalability and Complexity: DDoS attacks can target multiple points within the healthcare network simultaneously, making them harder to mitigate compared to single-source DoS attacks.

Network Congestion: With multiple attack sources, the incoming traffic can congest the network, affecting not only the target but also other connected systems, leading to a domino effect of disruptions.

Evasion of Defenses: DDoS attacks can attempt to evade mitigation efforts by varying attack patterns and source IP addresses, making it difficult to block the malicious traffic effectively.

Mitigation Measures: To protect healthcare systems from DoS and DDoS attacks, organizations can implement the following security measures:

1. *Network Monitoring:* Keep an eye on system performance and network traffic all the time to spot possible DoS and DDoS assaults early.
2. *DDoS Protection Services:* Use external DDoS defense services that are experienced in mitigating these assaults and have the capacity to efficiently manage large-scale attacks.
3. *Redundancy and Load Balancing:* Reduce the effect of an assault on a single point by using redundancy and load balancing to disperse traffic over several servers and data centers.
4. *Rate Limiting and Traffic Filtering:* Implement rate limiting and traffic filtering rules to block suspicious or excessive traffic from known attack sources.
5. *Intrusion Detection and Prevention Systems (IDPS):* Use IDPS tools to instantly identify and stop illicit traffic.
6. *Regular Security Audits:* Conduct routine safety inspections and susceptibility evaluations to find and fix any possible infrastructure flaws in the healthcare system.
7. *Employee Training:* Inform healthcare personnel on social engineering, cybersecurity guidelines, and how to spot and report possible security risks.

By taking proactive steps and staying vigilant, healthcare organizations can better protect their systems and patient data from the devastating effects of DoS and DDoS attacks.

20.2.1.8 Outdated or insecure software in healthcare systems

Healthcare systems may become exposed to known vulnerabilities and malware if security patches and upgrades are not applied in a timely manner [80]. Using outdated or insecure software in healthcare systems can pose significant risks to patient data, overall system integrity, and patient safety [81]. Healthcare organizations are often the primary objectives for cyberattacks due to the delicate and valuable information they store, making it crucial to maintain robust security measures and up-to-date software.

Here are some potential issues that can arise from using outdated or insecure software in healthcare systems:

Data Breaches: Hackers may use known weaknesses in outdated software to obtain patient data without authorization. Sensitive medical records, financial data, and other personally identifiable information (PII) may be exposed as a result of breaches.

Patient Safety Concerns: Insecure software could compromise patient safety directly if it is used in medical devices or equipment. Cyberattacks on critical medical devices, such as infusion pumps or pacemakers, could have life-threatening consequences for patients.

Regulatory Non-Compliance: Numerous healthcare institutions are governed by stringent data privacy laws, such as the General Data Privacy Regulation (GDPR) in the European Union and the Health Insurance Portability and Accountability Act (HIPAA) in the United States. Using insecure software may lead to non-compliance and result in legal consequences and financial penalties.

Loss of Trust: Data breaches and security incidents can erode patient trust in healthcare providers. Patients may be less likely to share sensitive information or seek medical treatment if they fear their data is at risk.

Disruption of Services: Cyberattacks or security breaches can disrupt healthcare services, leading to downtime in critical systems and hindering medical professionals from accessing essential patient information.

To mitigate these risks, healthcare organizations should adopt the following best practices:

Regular Software Updates: For quick application of security fixes and for resolving known vulnerabilities, keeping software current is essential.

Security Audits and Risk Assessments: Risk evaluations and safety audits on a regular basis can assist in finding possible vulnerabilities and rank security measures.

Strong Access Controls: Only authorized workers will be able to access patient data thanks to the implementation of strong access restrictions.

Data Encryption: Information may be protected even in the event of illegal access by encoding private data while it is at repose and in motion.

Employee Training: By regularly educating employees on cybersecurity best guidelines, security breaches can be prevented due to individual mistakes.

Vendor Management: Healthcare organizations should carefully vet software vendors to ensure their products meet security and compliance standards.

Incident Response Planning: Organizations may react to safety issues and lessen their effects by creating an extensive incident-handling strategy.

By prioritizing security and staying vigilant against potential threats, healthcare organizations can protect patient data and ensure the integrity and safety of their systems.

20.2.1.9 Unsecured mobile devices in healthcare systems

The use of portable gadgets like smartphones and tablets is growing in healthcare settings, but they can become points of vulnerability if not properly secured [82,83]. Lost or stolen devices may provide unauthorized access to patient data. Unsecured mobile devices in healthcare systems may pose substantial hazards to the security of patient data, system reliability, and privacy. With the increasing use of smartphones, tablets, and other mobile devices in the healthcare industry, it's crucial to understand and address the potential vulnerabilities they introduce. Here are some key issues and risks associated with unsecured mobile devices in healthcare:

1. *Data Breaches:* Mobile devices may store or access sensitive patient information, including medical records, test results, and personal details. If these devices are unsecured, they become susceptible to data breaches. Unauthorized access or loss of a mobile device potentially result in the disclosure of patient information, serious confidentiality breaches, and possibly legal repercussions.
2. *Malware and Viruses:* Unsecured mobile devices can be infected with malware and viruses. This malicious software can compromise the device's functionality, steal data, or grant unauthorized access to sensitive information. Malware can be introduced through various means, such as downloading untrusted apps or accessing compromised networks.
3. *Phishing Attacks:* Healthcare professionals using mobile devices may receive phishing emails or messages containing malicious links or attachments. If users fall victim to these attacks and unknowingly provide sensitive information or credentials, it can lead to unauthorized access to healthcare systems.
4. *Unauthorized Access:* When healthcare providers use unsecured mobile devices to access patient data or healthcare systems, it makes illegal access more likely. If the device is not adequately protected with passwords or other authentication measures, anyone who gains physical access to the device could potentially access patient information.
5. *Lack of Encryption:* Without proper encryption, data stored on or transmitted from mobile devices can be intercepted and read by unauthorized individuals. Encryption is essential to protect sensitive patient information and prevent it from being accessed if the device is compromised.
6. *Device Loss or Theft:* Mobile devices are easily misplaced, lost, or stolen. If healthcare professionals store sensitive patient data on these devices without proper security measures, it could lead to significant breaches and potential harm to patients.
7. *Regulatory Non-Compliance:* In many countries, healthcare providers are subject to rigorous laws, such as the Health Insurance Portability and Accountability Act (HIPAA) in the United States, that must be followed. Failure to secure mobile devices adequately could lead to non-compliance with these regulations, resulting in penalties and legal consequences.

Organizations should put the following procedures into place to reduce the dangers linked to using unprotected mobile devices in healthcare systems:

Device Management Policies: Establish comprehensive policies for the use and management of mobile devices in healthcare settings. This should include guidelines on data access, storage, encryption, and authentication protocols.

Mobile Device Security Software: Deploy safety software to defend against malware, viruses, and other cybersecurity dangers on mobile devices.

Encryption: To prevent unwanted access, make sure that all critical data saved on mobile devices is encoded.

Access Controls: To guarantee that only approved workers can see patient data on mobile devices, put robust authentication methods in place, such as biometric authentication or two-factor verification.

Remote Wiping and Tracking: Make mobile devices' remote cleaning and monitoring features available so that if they are lost or stolen, the data can be erased remotely, preventing unauthorized access.

Regular Training: Provide training to healthcare professionals on mobile device security best practices, including how to recognize and avoid phishing attacks.

Mobile Device Inventory: Keep a detailed inventory of all mobile devices used within the healthcare system to track their use and ensure appropriate security measures to be in place.

These actions will help healthcare institutions lower the dangers posed by unprotected cellphones and better safeguard patient information and privacy.

20.2.1.10 Weak authentication and access controls in healthcare systems

1. Inadequate security measures, such as using inadequate access controls or insecure passwords, can lead to unauthorized access to patient data and other critical systems [84]. Weak authentication and access controls in healthcare systems pose significant security risks and can lead to serious consequences for both patients and healthcare organizations [85,86]. Let's explore the potential issues associated with these weaknesses:
2. *Unauthorized Access:* Weak authentication mechanisms may allow unauthorized individuals to obtain access to delicate patient information, medical records, and other confidential data. This can result in data breaches, privacy violations, and identity theft.
3. *Data Breaches:* Cybercriminals frequently attack healthcare institutions because of the high value of patient information on the black market. Weak access controls increase the likelihood of successful cyberattacks, leading to data breaches and exposing patients' personal and medical information.
4. *Medical Identity Theft:* Insufficient authentication measures can enable criminals to impersonate patients and fraudulently access healthcare services, prescription medications, or insurance benefits. Medical identity theft can have severe implications for patient safety and financial wellbeing.
5. *Tampering with Medical Records:* Inadequate access controls may allow unauthorized individuals to modify or tamper with medical records. This puts

the health and safety of the patient at risk by resulting in inaccurate diagnoses, treatments, or prescriptions.

6. *Compliance Violations:* Various laws and standards, such as the Health Insurance Portability and Accountability Act (HIPAA) in the United States, apply to healthcare businesses. Non-compliance and possibly legal repercussions might emerge from lax authentication and access constraints.
7. *Disruption of Services:* In some cases, attackers may exploit weak access controls to disrupt healthcare services, leading to patient inconvenience and potential risks in critical situations.
8. *Patient Safety Risks:* If unauthorized individuals can access medical devices or systems controlling patient care, there is a risk of intentional or unintentional harm to patients.

Strong safety mechanisms should be implemented by healthcare systems to overcome these vulnerabilities:

Strong Authentication: Enforce strong passwords, multi-factor authentication (MFA), or biometric verification to guarantee that only authorized individuals have access to sensitive data.

Role-Based Access Control (RBAC): Implement RBAC to grant access privileges depending on the user's position and duties within the healthcare organization.

Regular Auditing and Monitoring: Conduct regular audits of access logs and monitor to look for suspicious behavior or illegal access attempts through user activity.

Encryption: To prevent unwanted possession of patient information, encode information both at repose and while it is being transmitted.

Employee Training: Inform healthcare personnel on the value of secure passwords, how to spot phishing scams, and how to follow security procedures.

Policies and Procedures: Develop and enforce clear security policies and procedures, ensuring all employees understand their roles in maintaining data security.

Penetration Testing and Vulnerability Assessments: To detect and proactively resolve any weaknesses, conduct frequent security assessments.

Continuous Updates and Patching: To reduce known weaknesses, keep software, apps, and systems updated with the most recent security updates.

Physical Security: Ensure physical access to critical systems and data centers is tightly controlled and monitored.

By implementing these procedures, healthcare businesses may drastically lower the risks connected to lax verification and access restrictions, protecting confidential patient information, and guaranteeing regulatory compliance.

20.2.1.11 Lack of cybersecurity awareness and training in healthcare systems

Security vulnerabilities frequently include a large amount of human mistakes. Employees who lack cybersecurity knowledge and instruction may unintentionally breach security. Healthcare systems' lack of cybersecurity education and awareness raises serious questions and has plagued the sector for a while. Healthcare institutions manage enormous quantities of private and sensitive information, which makes them desirable targets for hackers. Several factors contribute to the challenge of cybersecurity in healthcare:

1. *Limited Resources:* Healthcare institutions often have limited budgets and resources dedicated to cybersecurity. This can lead to outdated or insufficient security measures and a lack of investment in training staff on cybersecurity best practices.
2. *Complexity of Healthcare Systems:* With numerous integrated equipment, networks, and applications, healthcare systems are complicated. This intricacy makes it difficult to implement comprehensive security measures and increases the potential attack surface for cyber threats.
3. *Insider Threats:* Healthcare systems may face threats from insiders, such as disgruntled employees or unintentional mistakes by staff members who may not be adequately trained to recognize and respond to security risks.
4. *High Staff Turnover:* The healthcare industry experiences a relatively high turnover rate among employees, including IT staff. Frequent turnover can lead to knowledge gaps and a lack of consistent cybersecurity practices.
5. *Lack of Regulatory Pressure:* Although there are regulations in place (e.g., Health Insurance Portability and Accountability Act—HIPAA in the United States), enforcement and penalties for non-compliance have not always been stringent enough to drive organizations to prioritize cybersecurity.
6. *Rapid Adoption of Technology:* The rapid integration of new technologies in healthcare, such as IoT devices and telemedicine platforms, may outpace the implementation of appropriate security measures.
7. *Social Engineering Attacks:* Healthcare employees can be vulnerable to social engineering attacks, such as phishing emails or phone calls, due to the urgent nature of their work and their focus on patient care.

Addressing the lack of cybersecurity awareness and training in healthcare systems requires a multi-faceted approach:

Investment in Cybersecurity: Healthcare organizations must allocate sufficient resources to build and maintain robust cybersecurity infrastructures. This includes hiring skilled IT professionals, implementing up-to-date security technologies, and conducting regular security audits.

Employee Training and Awareness: All staff members, from doctors and nurses to administrative personnel, should receive regular training on cybersecurity best practices, recognizing potential threats, and the proper handling of sensitive data.

Strong Leadership and Governance: Leadership within healthcare organizations should prioritize cybersecurity and establish a culture of security from the top-down. This involves appointing Chief Information Security Officers (CISOs) and forming dedicated security teams.

Compliance and Regulation: Healthcare regulatory bodies should continuously update and enforce cybersecurity standards to ensure organizations adhere to best practices and face consequences for non-compliance.

Collaboration and Information Sharing: Healthcare organizations should collaborate with each other, sharing information about emerging threats and effective cybersecurity measures.

Data Encryption and Access Controls: Implementing encryption and strict access controls for patient data can help protect sensitive information even in the event of a breach.

Continuous Monitoring and Incident Response Plans: Healthcare systems need to have systems in place to continuously monitor for potential security breaches and establish well-defined incident response plans to handle and mitigate any attacks that occur.

Third-Party Vendor Assessment: Healthcare organizations should evaluate the cybersecurity procedures of partners and external providers to make sure that their systems don't pose additional risks.

By addressing these challenges and implementing comprehensive cybersecurity strategies, healthcare systems can better protect patient data, maintain the trust of their patients, and reduce the risk of costly data breaches and cyberattacks.

20.2.1.12 Third-party vendor risks in healthcare systems

Healthcare systems often work with external vendors for several services, and any vulnerabilities in these vendor systems can affect the overall security of the healthcare network. Third-party vendor risks in healthcare systems refer to the potential dangers and vulnerabilities that arise when healthcare organizations engage external vendors or third-party service providers to handle various aspects of their operations. These vendors could include software and technology providers, medical device manufacturers, cloud service providers, billing and claims processors, and many others.

While engaging with third-party vendors can offer several benefits, such as cost savings, expertise, and improved efficiency, it also introduces certain risks that can impact patient safety, data security, regulatory compliance, and overall business continuity. Some of the key risks associated with third-party vendors in healthcare systems are as follows:

1. *Data Breaches and Security Incidents:* Healthcare organizations deal with sensitive patient information, making them attractive targets for cybercriminals. If a third-party vendor handling patient data experiences a breach or security incident, it could lead to the exposure of protected health information (PHI) or other sensitive data.
2. *Regulatory Compliance:* Healthcare institutions are required to abide by a number of laws, including the Health Insurance Portability and Accountability Act (HIPAA) in the United States. The healthcare institution may face judicial and monetary repercussions if a third-party vendor doesn't comply with certain regulatory criteria.

3. *Service Disruptions:* Reliance on third-party vendors for critical services, such as EHR or cloud hosting, means that any service disruptions or outages experienced by the vendor can directly affect the healthcare organization's ability to deliver patient care or maintain operations.
4. *Inadequate Business Continuity Planning:* If a third-party vendor does not have robust business continuity and disaster recovery plans in place, it can leave the healthcare organization vulnerable to prolonged service disruptions during emergencies or disasters.
5. *Vendor Dependency:* Over-reliance on a single vendor for a particular service can create dependency issues. If the vendor faces financial difficulties, goes out of business, or is acquired by another company, it may lead to service disruptions and migration challenges for the healthcare organization.
6. *Lack of Vendor Oversight:* Inadequate vendor management and oversight can result in misunderstandings, miscommunications, and a lack of accountability in fulfilling contractual obligations, leading to subpar service delivery.
7. *Unsecure Software and Devices:* Third-party software or medical devices may have security flaws or vulnerabilities that could be exploited, potentially leading to patient safety risks or data breaches.
8. *Lack of Interoperability:* In healthcare, seamless integration and interoperability between systems are crucial. If a third-party solution lacks compatibility with existing systems, it can hinder the exchange of patient information and data flow.

To mitigate these risks, healthcare organizations should implement robust vendor management practices:

Due Diligence: Conduct thorough assessments of potential vendors before entering into contracts to ensure they meet security, compliance, and performance standards.

Contractual Agreements: Create precise contractual agreements that include obligations for data protection, service level agreements (SLAs), security precautions, and compliance standards.

Ongoing Monitoring: Continuously monitor the vendor's performance, security practices, and adherence to contractual obligations throughout the business relationship.

Security Assessments: Regularly assess the vendor's security measures, to find and fix potential flaws, including penetration testing and susceptibility assessments.

Business Continuity and Disaster Recovery Planning: Ensure that the vendor has robust plans in place to maintain service continuity during emergencies or disruptions.

Diversification: Avoid over-reliance on a single vendor by diversifying vendors for critical services where possible.

By being proactive in managing third-party vendor risks, healthcare organizations can better protect patient information and uphold ethical adherence and ensure the continuity of critical services. Addressing these cybersecurity threats requires a comprehensive approach involving robust security measures, regular security audits, employee training, and constant vigilance. Healthcare institutions should put cybersecurity first in order to safeguard patient information, uphold trust, and guarantee the continuity of essential medical services. Keep in mind that the threat landscape is continuously evolving, so it's essential for healthcare systems to continually update with the latest security practices and technologies.

20.3 Design framework for cybersecurity in centralized healthcare systems (FCCHS)

The requirement for information security and privacy has long presented difficulties for healthcare institutions. Organizations must implement sufficient measures to protect sensitive data, as well as show compliance with several state, federal, and industry regulations. Organizations have a strong desire for a framework that gives them a technique for implementing information security with the goal of delivering commercial benefits while attending to the necessary legal and regulatory obligations. Organizations from a variety of industries have used a variety of security frameworks over time to handle the difficulties of information protection. To solve their security concerns and give their customers comfort, healthcare businesses have long depended on some of the standards utilized in other industries (Figure 20.3).

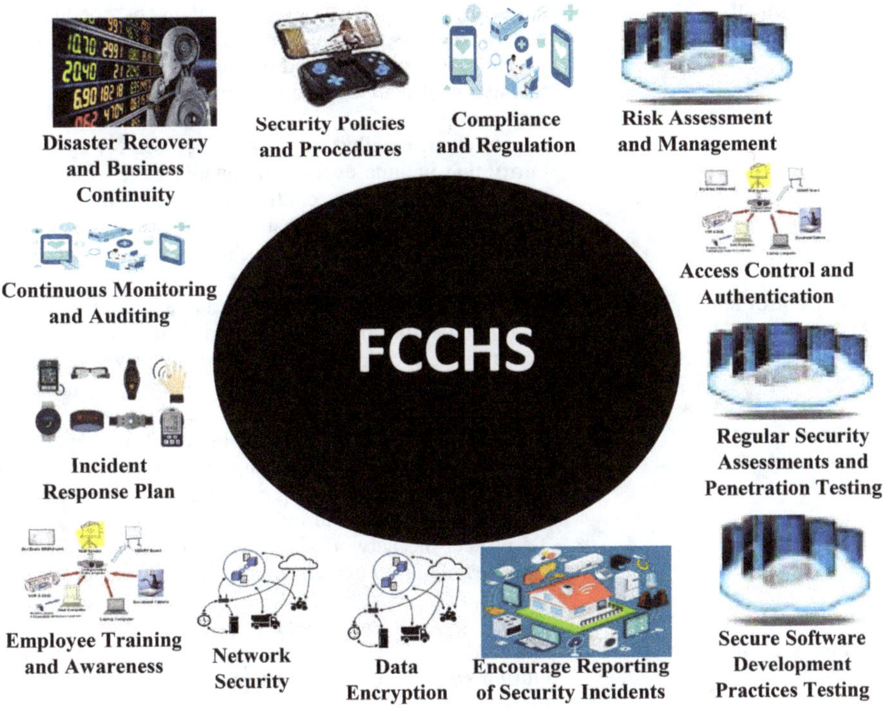

Figure 20.3 Framework for cybersecurity in centralized healthcare systems

The design of effective cybersecurity for healthcare systems requires a multi-layered approach, from the physical infrastructure to the operating system. At the lowest level, proper care must be taken to ensure the physical security of the system, such as through the use of access control systems. Other measures taken include regular patching and software updates, antivirus and malware protection, and the implementation of secure protocols. Access control and authentication should also be used to restrict user access to critical parts of the system. At higher levels, additional security measures should be incorporated into the system design. This includes data encryption, network segmentation, and data loss prevention. Advanced analytics and machine learning may also be utilized to identify possible cyber risks and take appropriate action. To safeguard critical patient data, centralized healthcare systems must be built with a strong cybersecurity foundation, maintain the integrity of medical records, and ensure the smooth functioning of healthcare services. Table 20.1 shows the framework to help establish a strong cybersecurity posture for centralized healthcare systems.

Table 20.1 Framework for cybersecurity in centralized healthcare systems

Cybersecurity posture	Description
Risk Assessment and Management	To find systemic weaknesses and dangers, conduct routine risk assessments. Prioritize risks based on their impact on patient care and data security. Develop a risk management plan that includes mitigation strategies and response protocols.
Security Policies and Procedures	Create clear, detailed rules and processes for cybersecurity that include every component of the healthcare system, such as access control, data processing, incident response, etc. Ascertain that these rules are understood by and taught to all personnel, independent contractors, and third-party providers.
Access Control and Authentication	Limit access to critical patient data and system resources by implementing tight access restrictions, such as multi-factor authentication. Using the lowest privilege principle, assign roles and privileges, only allowing users access to the data required for doing their jobs.
Data Encryption	To prevent unwanted access or interception of patient information, encode data during motion and at rest. Use key administration techniques and encoding methods that are accepted in the industry.
Network Security	To protect the network from inner and outside threats, use firewalls, intrusion detection and prevention systems (IDPS), and secure network segmentation. Keep a close eye on network traffic for any unusual activity.
Endpoint Security	On all devices linked to the hospital network, install cutting-edge endpoint security software, such as anti-malware and endpoint detection and response (EDR)

(Continues)

Table 20.1 (Continued)

Cybersecurity posture	Description
	programs. Update all endpoints, including medical equipment, with the most recent firmware and security fixes.
Incident Response Plan	Create a thorough incident response strategy that specifies what should be done in the case of a cybersecurity issue, such as a data leak or ransomware attack. Regularly do exercises and simulations to gauge how well the reaction strategy is working.
Continuous Monitoring and Auditing	Utilize technologies for ongoing surveillance to identify dangers quickly and take action. Conduct routine security audits to evaluate adherence to security policies and locate possible vulnerabilities.
Vendor Management	Examine the safety procedures followed by vendors and outside vendors who have access to medical data. Include security requirements in vendor contracts and monitor their compliance.
Employee Training and Awareness	All staff should attend periodic cybersecurity training sessions to learn about possible risks and effective security procedures. Encourage a culture of security and make employees an integral part of the cybersecurity defense. Employee training and awareness in healthcare systems are crucial components in order to guarantee the provision of excellent care for patients, rules must be followed and standards, and the protection of sensitive patient information. By investing in comprehensive and ongoing training and awareness programs, healthcare systems can provide their staff with expertise and abilities necessary to provide excellent patient care and maintain a safe and compliant environment.
Disaster Recovery (DR) and Business Continuity (BC)	Create a strong disaster recovery strategy to make sure that in the case of a significant cybersecurity incident, vital systems and services will be quickly restored. Regularly test the disaster recovery plan to verify its effectiveness. The DR and BC are important aspects of healthcare systems to ensure the uninterrupted delivery of essential services, patient care, and the preservation of sensitive data in the face of unforeseen events. In the context of healthcare, disasters can include natural disasters like earthquakes, hurricanes, and floods, as well as human-made disasters such as cyber-attacks, power outages, or pandemics. The DR and BC are essential components of healthcare systems to safeguard patient care and sensitive data during unforeseen events. Implementing comprehensive plans and conducting regular drills will better prepare healthcare organizations to respond effectively and minimize the impact of disasters.

(Continues)

Table 20.1 (Continued)

Cybersecurity posture	Description
Compliance and Regulation	Stay updated with healthcare industry regulations and comply with data protection laws (e.g., HIPAA in the United States). Appoint a dedicated compliance officer to ensure adherence to all relevant standards. Compliance and regulation are critical aspects of healthcare systems to ensure patient safety, data security, and ethical practices. Various rules and regulations must be followed by healthcare companies and standards to maintain the quality of care and protect both patients and healthcare providers. Failure to abide with healthcare rules can have serious repercussions, such as penalties and loss of authorization, legal actions, and damage to the organization's reputation. Therefore, healthcare organizations typically have compliance officers or teams responsible for overseeing adherence to relevant regulations and implementing necessary policies and procedures to maintain compliance
Regular Security Assessments and Penetration Testing	To proactively find systemic flaws and vulnerabilities, conduct routine security audits and penetration tests. A strong cybersecurity plan for enterprises must include regular security evaluations and penetration testing. These procedures aid in locating holes and flaws in their infrastructure, networks, applications, and information systems. A complete cybersecurity plan must include regular security evaluations and penetration testing. They assist businesses in identifying areas for improvement, strengthening existing security protocols, and lowering the likelihood of successful cyberattacks.
Secure Software Development Practices	Employ secure coding practices and conduct thorough security reviews during the development of healthcare applications and systems. Secure software development practices are essential for creating robust and resilient software that protects against various cyber threats and vulnerabilities.
Encourage Reporting of Security Incidents	Establish a process for employees and users to report any potential security incidents without fear of retribution. Reporting security incidents is a crucial and responsible action that can significantly improve the overall cybersecurity posture of individuals, organizations, and even society as a whole. It's essential to create an environment where reporting security incidents is not punished but encouraged. Organizations ought to have transparent rules and practices in place to handle incident reporting, ensuring that those who report incidents are supported and not subject to retaliation. By promoting a culture of openness and accountability, we can collectively enhance cybersecurity and protect against potential threats.

Remember that cybersecurity is an ongoing process, and the healthcare system's security measures must continuously evolve to stay ahead of new threats and vulnerabilities. Healthcare firms may dramatically improve their cybersecurity stance and successfully secure patient data and vital systems by putting in place an extensive architecture like this.

20.4 Research trends

Currently, there is a great deal of research being conducted in the field of healthcare cybersecurity. Much of this research focuses on developing novel technologies and techniques for protecting healthcare systems from cyber threats. For example, researchers are exploring the use of blockchain technology for secure data sharing, AI for malware detection, and machine learning for predictive analytics. In addition, research is being done on ways to improve user authentication, automated patching of software, and data encryption. Here are some research trends in cybersecurity for healthcare systems up till date:

1. **Regulatory Compliance and Standards:** Researchers have been focusing on understanding and implementing various cybersecurity standards and frameworks tailored specifically for the healthcare industry [87]. Compliance with regulations such as HIPAA (Health Insurance Portability and Accountability Act) and GDPR (General Data Protection Regulation) is critical to safeguarding patient data [88,89].
2. **Ransomware Mitigation and Recovery:** In ransomware attacks, cybercriminals encode confidential patient data and focus on healthcare companies, demanding payment to decrypt it. Researchers were focused on finding robust ways to prevent, detect, and respond to such attacks to protect patient information and ensure the continuity of healthcare services [90]. Ransomware attacks have been a significant concern in healthcare [91]. Research efforts have been directed toward developing better ransomware prevention strategies and effective recovery plans to minimize the impact of such attacks on patient care and data loss [91,92].
3. **Medical IoT Security and Vulnerabilities:** The proliferation of IoT devices in the medical sector, such as medical devices and wearables, presented new security challenges [70,93]. Researchers were investigating potential vulnerabilities in these devices and working on securing them to prevent unauthorized access or tampering. The IoT devices in healthcare, such as connected medical devices and wearables, have introduced new vulnerabilities. Researchers have been exploring ways to secure these devices, including encryption, authentication, and intrusion detection systems, to stop unauthorized access and potential manipulation of patient data [94,95].
4. **Vulnerability Assessment and Penetration Testing:** Continuous evaluation of healthcare systems for vulnerabilities and conducting penetration testing helps identify weaknesses before malicious actors exploit them. Researchers have been working on automating and improving these assessment techniques.

5. **Mobile Health (mHealth) Security:** The rise of mobile health apps and devices has presented new security challenges [96]. Researchers have been investigating methods to secure mobile health applications, protect data transmission, and secure user authentication [97]. mHealth Security refers to the measures and practices put in place to safeguard the privacy, accessibility, and reliability of health-related data and services transmitted and accessed through mobile devices and wireless technologies. As the use of mobile devices and apps for healthcare purposes continues to grow, ensuring the security of these platforms becomes crucial to maintain patient privacy and prevent illegal access to confidential data. The complexity of mHealth security requires collaboration between healthcare providers, app developers, mobile device manufacturers, and security experts to establish a safe ecosystem that ensures patient safety and data protection [98]. To find weaknesses and enhance the overall safety stance of mHealth apps and systems, periodic security audits and risk assessments are essential.
6. **Medical Device Security:** Connected medical devices and implantable technologies pose significant risks if compromised. Researchers were studying the security flaws in these devices and proposing solutions to safeguard them from potential cyber threats [99,100].
7. **Healthcare Data Privacy and Compliance:** With the growing volume of patient data being collected and stored, ensuring data privacy and compliance with regulations like HIPAA (Health Insurance Portability and Accountability Act) was crucial [101]. Research efforts were directed at developing frameworks and technologies to safeguard patient information and uphold adherence [102,103].
8. **Machine Learning for Threat Detection:** Machine learning and AI were being explored as tools to detect anomalies and potential threats in healthcare systems [104,105]. Researchers were working on developing algorithms capable of identifying suspicious patterns in real time to respond quickly to cyberattacks.
9. **AI and ML-based models for Security:** AI and machine learning algorithms have been applied to identify anomalies and patterns in network traffic, helping healthcare institutions detect and respond to potential cyber threats more effectively. These technologies can also improve malware detection and prediction of cyberattacks [106].
10. **Blockchain in Healthcare Security and Data Integrity:** Blockchain technology offers potential benefits in securing healthcare data by providing a decentralized and tamper-resistant platform [107,108]. Researchers were investigating how blockchain could be applied to improve data integrity and enhance cybersecurity in healthcare. A potential remedy has been investigated using blockchain technology to enhance the security and privacy of EHRs [109]. By creating a decentralized and immutable ledger, blockchain can protect patient data from unauthorized changes and ensure data integrity.
11. **Insider Threat Mitigation:** Insider threats, intentional or accidental, remained a significant concern for healthcare organizations. Research aimed

at identifying insider threat indicators and implementing measures to prevent and mitigate such risks [74,110].

12. **Cloud Security for Healthcare Data:** As healthcare providers increasingly adopted cloud services for data storage and management, researchers were focusing on addressing the specific security challenges associated with cloud-based healthcare systems [111,112]. As more healthcare providers adopt cloud-based services for data storage and processing, researchers have been working on improving cloud security measures. This includes secure data encryption, access control, and vulnerability assessments to protect sensitive patient information stored in the cloud [113].
13. **Cyber Threat Intelligence Sharing:** Cooperation and information exchange between healthcare institutions and other stakeholders were becoming more popular as a successful strategy for tackling cyber risks all at once [114,115]. Researchers were exploring ways to facilitate secure data-sharing platforms for sharing threat intelligence. Healthcare organizations have started collaborating and sharing cyber threat intelligence to enhance their group's capacity to detect and react to threats. Information sharing among different stakeholders can help mitigate potential attacks across the industry.
14. **Human Factors in Cybersecurity:** Recognizing that human error is a significant factor in cyber incidents, research has been conducted to better understand and address human-related vulnerabilities [116,117]. This includes training healthcare staff on cybersecurity best practices, promoting awareness of phishing attacks, and implementing access control measures.
15. **Cybersecurity Awareness and Training:** Healthcare employees and professionals' ignorance of cybersecurity has been identified as a weakness [118,119]. Research efforts were devoted to developing effective training programs to educate healthcare personnel about potential risks and best security practices [120–122].

Healthcare cybersecurity has been a crucial area of focus due to the increasing reliance on technology and digital systems within the healthcare industry. With the rapidly evolving landscape of cybersecurity threats and the healthcare industry becoming a focus for cyberattacks, several research trends have emerged to strengthen safety mechanisms and protect sensitive patient data. The field of cybersecurity in healthcare systems is already experiencing several notable trends. However, keep in mind that the landscape is continuously evolving, and new developments will still emerge in the nearest future.

20.5 Critical lessons learned

Studying cybersecurity in centralized healthcare systems has revealed several critical lessons that are vital for safeguarding private patient information and preserving the quality of medical services. The study of cybersecurity in centralized healthcare systems is crucial due to the increasing reliance on digital technologies in the healthcare industry. Centralized healthcare systems store sensitive patient data and are vulnerable to cyber threats, making them attractive targets for hackers. To ensure the security and integrity of patient information, it is essential to understand the critical lessons learned in this field. Here are some of the key lessons learned:

Challenges: Several challenges are encountered when dealing with cybersecurity in centralized healthcare systems:

1. *Data Breaches:* Cyberattacks that result in the loss or exploitation of patient data can have serious repercussions on the healthcare organization's finances and image.
2. *Insider Threats:* The safety of the system may be seriously compromised by employees who have evil intentions or who lack appropriate security knowledge.
3. *Legacy Systems:* Older and unsupported systems may lack the necessary security updates, making them susceptible to attacks.
4. *Interoperability:* Integrating various healthcare systems and devices can create vulnerabilities if not adequately secured.
5. *Compliance:* Healthcare systems must abide by a number of data protection and privacy laws, including HIPAA (Health Insurance Portability and Accountability Act) in the United States, which complicates cybersecurity measures.

Design Framework: A robust cybersecurity design framework for centralized healthcare systems should encompass the following key components:

1. *Access Control:* Restrict the accessibility of sensitive data to authorized individuals only by using robust authentication and permission processes.
2. *Data Encryption:* Utilize encoding mechanisms to safeguard data at repose and in motion, protecting patient information from unauthorized access.
3. *Network Security:* To track and defend the network from online threats, use firewalls, intrusion detection systems, and intrusion protection systems.
4. *Patch Management:* Upgrade software and firmware often to fix security flaws and lower the chance of exploitation.
5. *Employee Training:* Train healthcare staff on cybersecurity best practices to minimize human errors and prevent data breaches.
6. *Incident Response Plan:* Create a thorough incident response strategy to quickly identify, include, and mitigate cyber problems.

Research Trends: To address the evolving cyber threats in centralized healthcare systems, research in cybersecurity focuses on several trends:

1. *AI and Machine Learning:* Implementing AI and machine learning algorithms to detect anomalies and patterns in data traffic, facilitating early identification of cyber threats.
2. *Blockchain:* Exploring the use of blockchain technology to improve data safety, privacy, and integrity in healthcare systems.
3. *Zero Trust Architecture:* Adopting a zero-trust approach, where no user or device is inherently trusted, to strengthen access control and data protection.

4. *Cloud Security:* Developing robust security measures for cloud-based healthcare systems to guarantee the privacy and accessibility of patient information.
5. *Cybersecurity Regulations:* Studying the impact of existing and emerging regulations on healthcare cybersecurity practices and compliance.

Safeguarding centralized healthcare systems against cyber threats demands a multifaceted strategy that integrates people, procedures, and technology. By learning from past incidents and implementing robust cybersecurity measures, medical businesses may better safeguard patient information while upholding the confidence of their partners and clients. Therefore, the study of cybersecurity in centralized healthcare systems is a vital area of research and implementation. By understanding the overview, design framework, challenges, and research trends, In the midst of constantly developing cyber threats, stakeholders can better safeguard patient data and preserve the reliability of medical systems.

20.6 Conclusion

This chapter has presented an overview of cybersecurity in centralized healthcare systems. The design framework and security mechanisms necessary for effective protection have been outlined, along with the challenges and threats posed to modern healthcare systems. Additionally, current research trends have been highlighted. It is clear that cybersecurity in healthcare must be taken seriously and that further research in the field is required in order to keep patients and their data safe. Cybersecurity is an essential element of any healthcare system to protect patient data and ensure that information is used only for its intended purpose. This chapter provides a summary of the condition of cybersecurity today in centralized healthcare systems, a framework for the design of such systems, and the challenges and research trends in this area. In conclusion, cybersecurity is a critical concern in centralized healthcare systems because cyberattacks are becoming more frequent and sophisticated. Healthcare organizations and various actors in the healthcare industry have a shared responsibility to protect IT infrastructures, ensure the availability of health services, preserve safety and privacy of patient data, and prevent and respond to cyber-attacks. The COVID-19 pandemic has further emphasized the need for robust cybersecurity measures in telehealth services. Usability management frameworks and secure software development methodologies are essential to make sure medical information systems are secure and easy to use.

References

[1] Perakslis, E. D. (2014). Cybersecurity in health care. *N Engl J Med*, *371*(5), 395–397.

[2] Claunch, D., & McMillan, M. (2013). Determining the right level for your IT security investment: A rural medical center facing threats of data breaches discovered that hospital IT security investments go beyond just dollars and cents. *Healthcare Financial Management*, *67*(5), 100–104.

[3] Ponemon, I. (2016). Sixth annual benchmark study on privacy & security of healthcare data. *Technical Report.*

[4] Kruse, C. S., Frederick, B., Jacobson, T., & Monticone, D. K. (2017). Cybersecurity in healthcare: A systematic review of modern threats and trends. *Technology and Health Care*, *25*(1), 1–10.

[5] Smet, M. (2002). Cost characteristics of hospitals. *Social Science & Medicine*, *55*(6), 895–906.

[6] Islam, S. R., Kwak, D., Kabir, M. H., Hossain, M., & Kwak, K. S. (2015). The internet of things for health care: a comprehensive survey. *IEEE Access*, *3*, 678–708.

[7] Oyebiyi, O. G., Abayomi-Alli, A., Arogundade, O. T., Qazi, A., Imoize, A. L., & Awotunde, J. B. (2023). A systematic literature review on human ear biometrics: Approaches, algorithms, and trend in the last decade. *Information*, *14*(3), 192.

[8] Brookman, J. (2015). Protecting privacy in an era of weakening regulation. *Harv. L. & Pol'y Rev.*, *9*, 355.

[9] Cheng, T. L., Unaka, N. I., & Nichols, D. (2023). Crossing the quality chasm and the ignored pillar of health care equity. *Pediatric Clinics.*

[10] Menachemi, N., Burke, D., Diana, M., & Brooks, R. (2005). Characteristics of hospitals that outsource information system functions. *Journal of Healthcare Information Management: JHIM*, *19*(1), 63–69.

[11] Angst, C. M., Block, E. S., D'Arcy, J., & Kelley, K. (2017). When do IT security investments matter? Accounting for the influence of institutional factors in the context of healthcare data breaches. *MIS Quarterly*, *41*(3), 893–A8.

[12] Mandal, P. (2023). Healthcare costs vis-à-vis economic growth in pandemic crisis with technology adoption. *International Journal of Technology Management & Sustainable Development*, *22*(1), 7–20.

[13] Rodziewicz, T. L., Houseman, B., & Hipskind, J. E. (2021). Medical error reduction and prevention. 2021. StatPearls [Internet]. Treasure Island (FL): StatPearls Publishing.

[14] Expects, I. D. C. (2021). To Be the year of multi-cloud as global COVID-19 pandemic reaffirms critical need for business agility. URL: https://www. idc. com/getdoc. jsp.

[15] Gupta, L., Salman, T., Ghubaish, A., Unal, D., Al-Ali, A. K., & Jain, R. (2022). Cybersecurity of multi-cloud healthcare systems: A hierarchical deep learning approach. *Applied Soft Computing*, *118*, 108439.

[16] Abikoye, O. C., Oladipupo, E. T., Imoize, A. L., Awotunde, J. B., Lee, C. C., & Li, C. T. (2023). Securing critical user information over the internet of medical things platforms using a hybrid cryptography scheme. *Future Internet*, *15*(3), 99.

[17] Cooper, P. W. (2014). Global State of Information Security® Survey 2015. *Annual State of Information Security Survey.*

[18] Awotunde, J. B., Misra, S., Ajagbe, S. A., Ayo, F. E., & Gurjar, R. (May 2023). An IoT machine learning model-based real-time diagnostic and

monitoring system. In *Machine Intelligence Techniques for Data Analysis and Signal Processing: Proceedings of the 4th International Conference MISP 2022*, Volume 1 (pp. 789–799). Singapore: Springer Nature Singapore.

[19] Almulihi, A. H., Alassery, F., Khan, A. I., Shukla, S., Gupta, B. K., & Kumar, R. (2022). Analyzing the implications of healthcare data breaches through computational technique. *Intelligent Automation & Soft Computing, 32*(3).

[20] Seemma, P. S., Nandhini, S., & Sowmiya, M. (2018). Overview of cyber security. *International Journal of Advanced Research in Computer and Communication Engineering*, *7*(11), 125–128.

[21] Mijwil, M., Filali, Y., Aljanabi, M., Bounabi, M., & Al-Shahwani, H. (2023). The purpose of cybersecurity governance in the digital transformation of public services and protecting the digital Environment. *Mesopotamian Journal of Cybersecurity*, *2023*, 1–6.

[22] Nizich, M. (2023). Preparing the cybersecurity workforce of tomorrow. In *The Cybersecurity Workforce of Tomorrow* (pp. 117–146). Emerald Group Publishing Limited.

[23] Awotunde, J. B., Ayo, F. E., Panigrahi, R., Garg, A., Bhoi, A. K., & Barsocchi, P. (2023). A multi-level random forest model-based intrusion detection using fuzzy inference system for Internet of things networks. *International Journal of Computational Intelligence Systems*, *16*(1), 31.

[24] Chakraborty, C., Nagarajan, S. M., Devarajan, G. G., Ramana, T. V., & Mohanty, R. (2023). Intelligent AI-based healthcare cyber security system using multi-source transfer learning method. *ACM Transactions on Sensor Networks*.

[25] Ayo, F. E., Awotunde, J. B., Folorunso, S. O., Adigun, M. O., & Ajagbe, S. A. (2023). A genomic rule-based KNN model for fast flux botnet detection. *Egyptian Informatics Journal*, *24*(2), 313–325.

[26] Ferreira, L., Silva, D. C., & Itzazelaia, M. U. (2023). Recommender systems in cybersecurity. *Knowledge and Information Systems*, 1–37.

[27] Nizich, M. (2023). An introduction to the field of cybersecurity and the current workforce gap. In *The Cybersecurity Workforce of Tomorrow* (pp. 1–35). Emerald Group Publishing Limited.

[28] Tully, J., Selzer, J., Phillips, J. P., O'Connor, P., & Dameff, C. (2020). Healthcare challenges in the era of cybersecurity. *Health Security*, *18*(3), 228–231.

[29] Kumar, R. L., Wang, Y., Poongodi, T., & Imoize, A. L. (Eds.). (2021). *Internet of Things, Artificial Intelligence and Blockchain Technology*. Cham: Springer.

[30] Paulsen, J. E., Hazelett, M. B., & Schwartz, S. B. (2018). CIED cybersecurity risks in an increasingly connected world. *Circulation*, *138*(12), 1181–1183.

[31] Smart, W. (2018). Lessons learned review of the WannaCry ransomware cyber attack. *Department of Health and Social Care: London, UK*, *1*, 10–1038.

[32] Ghafur, S., Kristensen, S., Honeyford, K., Martin, G., Darzi, A., & Aylin, P. (2019). A retrospective impact analysis of the WannaCry cyberattack on the NHS. *NPJ Digital Medicine*, *2*(1), 98.

[33] Choi, S. J., & Johnson, M. E. (2019). Do hospital data breaches reduce patient care quality?. *arXiv preprint arXiv:1904.02058*.

[34] Martin, G., Ghafur, S., Kinross, J., Hankin, C., & Darzi, A. (2018). WannaCry—a year on. *BMJ*, 361.

[35] Winton, R. (2016). Hollywood hospital pays $17,000 in bitcoin to hackers; FBI investigating. *Los Angeles Times*, 18.

[36] Slayton, T. B. (2018). Ransomware: The virus attacking the healthcare industry. *Journal of Legal Medicine*, *38*(2), 287–311.

[37] Jalali, M. S., & Kaiser, J. P. (2018). Cybersecurity in hospitals: A systematic, organizational perspective. *Journal of medical Internet research*, *20*(5), e10059.

[38] Hammill, A. (2017). *The Rise and Wrath of Ransomware and What It Means for Society* (Doctoral dissertation, Utica College).

[39] Wall*, D. S. (2008). Cybercrime, media and insecurity: The shaping of public perceptions of cybercrime. *International Review of Law, Computers & Technology*, *22*(1–2), 45–63.

[40] Mia, M. R., Shahriar, H., Valero, M., *et al.* (2022). A comparative study on hipaa technical safeguards assessment of android mhealth applications. *Smart Health*, *26*, 100349.

[41] Parker, S., Wu, Z., & Christofides, P. D. (2023). Cybersecurity in process control, operations, and supply chain. *Computers & Chemical Engineering*, 108169.

[42] Kavitha, K. V. N., Ashok, S., Imoize, A. L., *et al.* (2022). On the use of wavelet domain and machine learning for the analysis of epileptic seizure detection from EEG signals. *Journal of Healthcare Engineering, 2022*.

[43] Hyder, A., Uddin, B., Siddiqui, H., Naeem, M., & Waheed, A. (2023). Mediation of reverse logistics in sustainable resources and organizational performance: Sustainable resources and organizational performance. *South Asian Journal of Operations and Logistics (ISSN: 2958-2504)*, *2*(1), 11–27.

[44] Dorn, T. M. (2023). *US Critical Infrastructure: Its Importance and Vulnerabilities to Cyber and Unmanned Systems*. Page Publishing Inc.

[45] Cao, L. (2023). AI and data science for smart emergency, crisis and disaster resilience. *International Journal of Data Science and Analytics*, *15*(3), 231–246.

[46] Bhuyan, S. S., Kabir, U. Y., Escareno, J. M., *et al.* (2020). Transforming healthcare cybersecurity from reactive to proactive: current status and future recommendations. *Journal of Medical Systems*, *44*, 1–9.

[47] Alsuwaidi, A., Hassan, A., Alkhatri, F., Ali, H., Mohammad, Q. H., & Alrabaee, S. (April 2020). Security vulnerabilities detected in medical devices. In *2020 12th Annual Undergraduate Research Conference on Applied Computing (URC)* (pp. 1–6). IEEE.

[48] Flaumenhaft, Y., & Ben-Assuli, O. (2018). Personal health records, global policy and regulation review. *Health Policy*, *122*(8), 815–826.

[49] Frik, A., Nurgalieva, L., Bernd, J., Lee, J., Schaub, F., & Egelman, S. (2019). Privacy and security threat models and mitigation strategies of older adults. In *Fifteenth Symposium on Usable Privacy and Security (SOUPS 2019)* (pp. 21–40).

[50] Meglio, M. (2020). Embracing insecurity: Harm reduction through a no-fault approach to consumer data breach litigation. *BCL Rev.*, *61*, 1223.

[51] Ponemon, L. (2013). Cost of data breach study: Global analysis. *Poneomon Institute Sponsored by Symantec*, 205–2.

[52] Austin, D. A., & Hungerford, T. L. (September 2009). The market structure of the health insurance industry. Congressional Research Service, Library of Congress.

[53] Awotunde, J. B., Folorunso, S. O., Imoize, A. L., *et al.* (2023). An ensemble tree-based model for intrusion detection in industrial Internet of things networks. *Applied Sciences*, *13*(4), 2479.

[54] Ogundokun, R. O., Awotunde, J. B., Misra, S., Abikoye, O. C., & Folarin, O. (2021). Application of machine learning for ransomware detection in IoT devices. In *Artificial Intelligence for Cyber Security: Methods, Issues and Possible Horizons or Opportunities* (pp. 393–420). Cham: Springer International Publishing.

[55] Vehabovic, A., Ghani, N., Bou-Harb, E., Crichigno, J., & Yayimli, A. (2022, June). Ransomware detection and classification strategies. In *2022 IEEE International Black Sea Conference on Communications and Networking (BlackSeaCom)* (pp. 316–324). IEEE.

[56] Moore, G., Khurshid, Z., McDonnell, T., Rogers, L., & Healy, O. (2023). A resilient workforce: patient safety and the workforce response to a cyber-attack on the ICT systems of the national health service in Ireland.

[57] Sadiku, M. N., Chukwu, U. C., & Sadiku, J. O. (2023). Cybersecurity in healthcare. *European Journal of Modern Medicine and Practice*, *3*(6), 22–29.

[58] Argyridou, E., Nifakos, S., Laoudias, C., *et al.* (2023). Cyber hygiene methodology for raising cybersecurity and data privacy awareness in health care organizations: Concept study. *Journal of Medical Internet Research*, *25*, e41294.

[59] Abiodun, M. K., Awotunde, J. B., Ogundokun, R. O., Adeniyi, E. A., & Arowolo, M. O. (2021). Security and information assurance for IoT-based big data. In *Artificial Intelligence for Cyber Security: Methods, Issues and Possible Horizons or Opportunities* (pp. 189–211). Cham: Springer International Publishing.

[60] Chou, T. S. (2013). Security threats on cloud computing vulnerabilities. *International Journal of Computer Science & Information Technology*, *5*(3), 79.

[61] Chernyshev, M., Zeadally, S., & Baig, Z. (2019). Healthcare data breaches: Implications for digital forensic readiness. *Journal of Medical Systems*, *43*, 1–12.

[62] Ronquillo, J. G., Erik Winterholler, J., Cwikla, K., Szymanski, R., & Levy, C. (2018). Health IT, hacking, and cybersecurity: National trends in data breaches of protected health information. *JAMIA Open*, *1*(1), 15–19.

[63] Muthuswamy, V. V. (2023). Cyber security challenges faced by employees in the digital workplace of Saudi Arabia's digital nature organization. *International Journal of Cyber Criminology*, *17*(1), 40–53.

[64] Kalla, D., Samaah, F., Kuraku, S., & Smith, N. (2023). Phishing detection implementation using databricks and artificial intelligence. *International Journal of Computer Applications*, *185*(11), 1–11.

[65] Awotunde, J. B., Adeniyi, A. E., Ogundokun, R. O., Ajamu, G. J., & Adebayo, P. O. (2021). MIoT-based big data analytics architecture, opportunities and challenges for enhanced telemedicine systems. *Enhanced telemedicine and e-health: advanced IoT enabled soft computing framework*, 199–220.

[66] Mashtalyar, N., Ntaganzwa, U. N., Santos, T., Hakak, S., & Ray, S. (2021, July). Social engineering attacks: Recent advances and challenges. In International Conference on Human-Computer Interaction (pp. 417–431). Cham: Springer International Publishing.

[67] Aldawood, H., & Skinner, G. (2019). Reviewing cyber security social engineering training and awareness programs—Pitfalls and ongoing issues. *Future Internet*, *11*(3), 73.

[68] Lopatina, K., Dokuchaev, V. A., & Maklachkova, V. V. (October 2021). Data Risks Identification in Healthcare Sensor Networks. In *2021 International Conference on Engineering Management of Communication and Technology (EMCTECH)* (pp. 1–7). IEEE.

[69] Awotunde, J. B., Ameen, A. O., Oladipo, I. D., Tomori, A. R., & Abdulraheem, M. (2016). Evaluation of four encryption algorithms for viability, reliability and performance estimation. *Nigerian Journal of Technological Development*, *13*(2), 74–82.

[70] Paul, M., Maglaras, L., Ferrag, M. A., & AlMomani, I. (2023). Digitization of healthcare sector: A study on privacy and security concerns. *ICT Express*.

[71] AbdulRaheem, M., Awotunde, J. B., Chakraborty, C., Adeniyi, E. A., Oladipo, I. D., & Bhoi, A. K. (2023). Security and privacy concerns in smart healthcare system. In *Implementation of Smart Healthcare Systems using AI, IoT, and Blockchain* (pp. 243–273). Academic Press.

[72] Adeniyi, E. A., Ogundokun, R. O., Misra, S., Awotunde, J. B., & Abiodun, K. M. (2022). Enhanced security and privacy issue in multi-tenant environment of green computing using blockchain technology. In *Blockchain Applications in the Smart Era* (pp. 65–83). Cham: Springer International Publishing.

[73] Awotunde, J. B., Jimoh, R. G., Folorunso, S. O., Adeniyi, E. A., Abiodun, K. M., & Banjo, O. O. (2021). Privacy and security concerns in IoT-based healthcare systems. In *The Fusion of Internet of Things, Artificial Intelligence, and Cloud Computing in Health Care* (pp. 105–134). Cham: Springer International Publishing.

[74] Yeo, L. H. (2023). *Unintentional Insider Threat Assessment Framework: Examining the Human Security Indicators in Healthcare Cybersecurity* (Doctoral dissertation, Eastern Michigan University).

[75] Usmani, M. A., Usmani, K. A., Kaleem, A., & Samiuddin, M. (2023). Cyber threat migration: Perpetuating in the healthcare sector and agriculture and food industries. In *Advances in Cyberology and the Advent of the Next-Gen Information Revolution* (pp. 62–85). IGI Global.

[76] Tuscano, A., & Joshi, S. (2023, March). Significance of cyber security of IoT devices in the healthcare sector. In *2023 Somaiya International Conference on Technology and Information Management (SICTIM)* (pp. 12–16). IEEE.

[77] Al-Qarni, E. A. (2023). Cybersecurity in healthcare: A review of recent attacks and mitigation strategies. *International Journal of Advanced Computer Science and Applications*, *14*(5).

[78] Mammadova, K., & Aslanov, R. (2023). Installation of integrated intellectual information security systems in open corporate networks–DDoS attack. *Scientific Collection «InterConf+»*, *32*(151), 643–651.

[79] Ortega-Fernandez, I., & Liberati, F. (2023). A review of denial of service attack and mitigation in the smart grid using reinforcement learning. *Energies*, *16*(2), 635.

[80] Mahmood, M., Khan, M. I., Hussain, H., *et al.* (2023). Improving security architecture of Internet of medical things: A systematic literature review. *IEEE Access*.

[81] Lehto, M., Neittaanmäki, P., Pöyhönen, J., & Hummelholm, A. (2022). Cyber security in healthcare systems. In *Cyber Security: Critical Infrastructure Protection* (pp. 183–215). Cham: Springer International Publishing.

[82] Ali, A., Somroo, N. A., Farooq, U., Asif, M., Akour, I., & Mansoor, W. (October 2022). Smartphone security hardening: Threats to organizational security and risk mitigation. In *2022 International Conference on Cyber Resilience (ICCR)* (pp. 1–12). IEEE.

[83] Njuguna, D., & Kanyi, W. (2023). An evaluation of BYOD integration cybersecurity concerns: A case study. *Int. J. Recent Res. Math. Comput. Sci. Inf. Technol*, *9*, 80–91.

[84] Bandari, V. (2023). Enterprise data security measures: A comparative review of effectiveness and risks across different industries and organization types. *International Journal of Business Intelligence and Big Data Analytics*, *6*(1), 1–11.

[85] Hasan, M. K., Ghazal, T. M., Saeed, R. A., *et al.* (2022). A review on security threats, vulnerabilities, and counter measures of 5G enabled Internet-of-Medical-Things. *IET Communications*, *16*(5), 421–432.

[86] Roobini, S., Kavitha, M., Sujaritha, M., & Kumar, D. R. (2022). Cybersecurity threats to IoMT-enabled healthcare systems. In *Cognitive Computing for Internet of Medical Things* (pp. 105–130). Chapman and Hall/CRC.

[87] Abraham, C., Chatterjee, D., & Sims, R. R. (2019). Muddling through cybersecurity: Insights from the US healthcare industry. *Business Horizons*, *62*(4), 539–548.

[88] Bradford, L., Aboy, M., & Liddell, K. (2020). COVID-19 contact tracing apps: A stress test for privacy, the GDPR, and data protection regimes. *Journal of Law and the Biosciences*, *7*(1), lsaa034.

[89] Sokol, A. J. (2017). Clinical research and data: HIPAA, the common rule, the general data protection regulation, and data repositories. *Merrill Series on the Research Mission of Public Universities*, 47–62.

[90] Albahri, A. S., Zaidan, A. A., Albahri, O. S., Zaidan, B. B., & Alsalem, M. A. (2018). Real-time fault-tolerant mHealth system: Comprehensive review of healthcare services, opens issues, challenges and methodological aspects. *Journal of Medical Systems*, *42*, 1–56.

[91] Thamer, N., & Alubady, R. (2021, April). A survey of ransomware attacks for healthcare systems: Risks, challenges, solutions and opportunity of research. In *2021 1st Babylon International Conference on Information Technology and Science (BICITS)* (pp. 210–216). IEEE.

[92] Blatchly, J. (2023). *The Impact of Ransomware–A Comparison of Worldwide Governmental Policies and Recommendations for Future Directives* (Doctoral dissertation, Utica University).

[93] Adeniyi, A. E., Abiodun, K. M., Awotunde, J. B., Olagunju, M., Ojo, O. S., & Edet, N. P. (2023). Implementation of a block cipher algorithm for medical information security on cloud environment: Using modified advanced encryption standard approach. *Multimedia Tools and Applications*, 1–15.

[94] Alalhareth, M., & Hong, S. C. (2023). An improved mutual information feature selection technique for intrusion detection systems in the Internet of medical things. *Sensors*, *23*(10), 4971.

[95] Ayo, F. E., Awotunde, J. B., Olalekan, O. A., Imoize, A. L., Li, C. T., & Lee, C. C. (2023). CBFISKD: A combinatorial-based fuzzy inference system for keylogger detection. *Mathematics*, *11*(8), 1899.

[96] Galetsi, P., Katsaliaki, K., & Kumar, S. (2023). Exploring benefits and ethical challenges in the rise of mHealth (mobile healthcare) technology for the common good: An analysis of mobile applications for health specialists. *Technovation*, *121*, 102598.

[97] Lin, W., Xu, M., He, J., & Zhang, W. (2023). Privacy, security and resilience in mobile healthcare applications. *Enterprise Information Systems*, *17*(3), 1939896.

[98] Iwaya, L. H., Nordin, A., Fritsch, L., *et al.* (2023). Early labour app: Developing a practice-based mobile health application for digital early labour support. *International Journal of Medical Informatics*, 105139.

[99] Jmal, R., Ghabri, W., Guesmi, R., Alshammari, B. M., Alshammari, A. S., & Alsaif, H. (2023). Distributed blockchain-SDN secure IoT system based on ANN to mitigate DDoS attacks. *Applied Sciences*, *13*(8), 4953.

[100] Tariq, U., Ahmed, I., Bashir, A. K., & Shaukat, K. (2023). A critical cybersecurity analysis and future research directions for the Internet of things: A comprehensive review. *Sensors*, *23*(8), 4117.

[101] Thantilage, R. D., Le-Khac, N. A., & Kechadi, M. T. (2023). Healthcare data security and privacy in data warehouse architectures. *Informatics in Medicine Unlocked*, 101270.

[102] Iguenane, B. (2023). Impact of information security on online operations: The mediating role of risk management. *International Journal of Computations, Information and Manufacturing (IJCIM)*, *3*(1), 27–34.

[103] Akanbi, M.B., Jimoh, R.G., Imoize, A.L., *et al.* (2023). Enhanced template protection algorithms based on fuzzy vault and cuckoo hashing for fingerprint biometrics. *Fusion: Practice and Applications*, 10(2), pp. 08–24.

[104] Yagi, M., Yamanouchi, K., Fujita, N., Funao, H., & Ebata, S. (2023). Revolutionizing spinal care: Current applications and future directions of artificial intelligence and machine learning. *Journal of Clinical Medicine*, *12*(13), 4188.

[105] Javed, A. R., Saadia, A., Mughal, H., *et al.* (2023). Artificial intelligence for cognitive health assessment: State-of-the-art, open challenges and future directions. *Cognitive Computation*, 1–46.

[106] Adeniyi, E.A., Imoize, A.L., Awotunde, J.B., *et al.* (2023). Performance analysis of two famous cryptographic algorithms on mixed data. *Journal of Computer Science*, 2023, 19(6), pp. 694–706.

[107] Khatri, S., Agarwal, A., Kumar, R., & Khan, R. A. (2023). Use cases of smart contracts in decentralized health infrastructure. In *Advances in Information Communication Technology and Computing: Proceedings of AICTC 2022* (pp. 497–509). Singapore: Springer Nature Singapore.

[108] Adeniyi, J. K., Adeniyi, T. T., Awotunde, J. B., Abiodun, M. K., & Atanda, O. G. (2023, April). Agrolend: A blockchain implementation approach of smart contract farming platform. In *2023 International Conference on Science, Engineering and Business for Sustainable Development Goals (SEB-SDG)* (Vol. 1, pp. 1–7). IEEE.

[109] Reegu, F. A., Abas, H., Gulzar, Y., *et al.* (2023). Blockchain-based framework for interoperable electronic health records for an improved healthcare system. *Sustainability*, *15*(8), 6337.

[110] Abiodun, M. K., Adeniyi, A. E., Victor, A. O., Awotunde, J. B., Atanda, O. G., & Adeniyi, J. K. (2023, April). Detection and prevention of data leakage in transit using LSTM recurrent neural network with encryption algorithm. In *2023 International Conference on Science, Engineering and Business for Sustainable Development Goals (SEB-SDG)* (Vol. 1, pp. 01–09). IEEE.

[111] Adams, A. (2023). *A Qualitative Inquiry into the Security Concerns Affecting Cloud Adoption Rates of Healthcare Organizations* (Doctoral dissertation, Colorado Technical University).

[112] Kumar, M., Kumar, A., Verma, S., *et al.* (2023). Healthcare Internet of things (H-IoT): Current trends, future prospects, applications, challenges, and security issues. *Electronics*, *12*(9), 2050.

[113] Vijarania, M., Gupta, S., Agrawal, A., Adigun, M. O., Ajagbe, S. A., & Awotunde, J. B. (2023). Energy efficient load-balancing mechanism in integrated IoT–fog–cloud environment. *Electronics*, *12*(11), 2543.

[114] Kuntal, D. (2023). *SHSP: A Scalable Framework for Healthcare System using Polygon Blockchain* (Doctoral dissertation).

[115] Esmaeilzadeh, P. (2023). Evolution of health information sharing between health care organizations: Potential of nonfungible tokens. *Interactive Journal of Medical Research*, *12*(1), e42685.

[116] Alhasan, I. Y. (2023). *Human Factors in Cybersecurity: A Cross-Cultural Study on Trust* (Doctoral dissertation, Purdue University Graduate School).

[117] Mwim, E. N., Mtsweni, J., & Chimbo, B. (2023, March). Conceptual mapping of the cybersecurity culture to human factor domain framework. In *Future of Information and Communication Conference* (pp. 729–742). Cham: Springer Nature Switzerland.

[118] Klein, G., & Zwilling, M. (2023). The weakest link: Employee cyber-defense behaviors while working from home. *Journal of Computer Information Systems*, 1–15.

[119] Kioskli, K., Fotis, T., Nifakos, S., & Mouratidis, H. (2023). The importance of conceptualising the human-centric approach in maintaining and promoting cybersecurity-hygiene in Healthcare 4.0. *Applied Sciences*, *13*(6), 3410.

[120] Kubale, V., Lobnikar, T., Gabrovec, B., & Dvojmoč, M. (May 2023). Ensuring corporate security and its strategic communication in healthcare institutions in Slovenia. In *Healthcare* (Vol. 11, No. 11, p. 1578). MDPI.

[121] Wisnubroto, D. S., Khairul, K., Basuki, F., & Kristuti, E. (2023). Preventing and countering insider threats and radicalism in an Indonesian research reactor: Development of a human reliability program (HRP). *Heliyon*, *9*(5).

[122] Stenzinger, A., Moltzen, E. K., Winkler, E., *et al.* (2023). Implementation of precision medicine in healthcare–a European perspective. *Journal of Internal Medicine*.

Chapter 21

Artificial intelligence and blockchain for robust healthcare delivery: from the perspective of security and confidentiality

Joseph Bamidele Awotunde[1], Abidemi Emmanuel Adeniyi[2], Peace Busola Falola[3], Agbotiname Lucky Imoize[4], Anjan Bandyopadhyay[5], Akash Kumar Bhoi[6,7] and Demóstenes Zegarra Rodríguez[8]

Blockchain technology and artificial intelligence (AI) have recently enabled the medical industry to undergo a transformation with regard to information protection and privacy. This chapter explores the opportunities to apply these innovative technologies in healthcare, addressing the implications for security and privacy from both a technical and regulatory perspective. In the first section of this chapter, both AI and blockchain technologies are briefly introduced and the current trends in their application in healthcare. It also explains the characteristics of the healthcare sector that make it particularly suitable for employing AI and blockchain solutions. The second part examines the technical safety and confidential benefits of employing AI and blockchain technology and the security and privacy implications of their adoption in healthcare. It also considers the regulatory implications associated with their implementation, and the need for robust regulatory frameworks to ascertain the safety and confidential of patient and healthcare data. Finally, the chapter explores the potential practical applications of AI and blockchain in healthcare and the current

[1]Department of Computer Science, Faculty of Information and Communication Sciences, University of Ilorin, Nigeria
[2]Department of Computer Science, College of Computing and Communication Studies, Bowen University, Nigeria
[3]Department of Computer Sciences, Faculty of Pure and Applied Sciences, Precious Cornerstone University, Nigeria
[4]Department of Electrical and Electronics Engineering, Faculty of Engineering, University of Lagos, Nigeria
[5]Kalinga Institute of Industrial Technology, KIIT Deemed to be University, India
[6]KIET Group of Institutions, India
[7]AB-Tech eResearch (ABTeR), India
[8]Department of Computer Science, Federal University of Lavras, Brazil

challenges in their implementation. It concludes by offering recommendations on how to ascertain the secure and private use of AI and blockchain in healthcare. Overall, this chapter demonstrates that AI and blockchain can be powerful tools for ensuring the safety and confidential of healthcare data. However, further research and development are needed to ensure their successful implementation and to ensure the implementation of robust security and regulatory frameworks.

21.1 Introduction

Over the years, big data has streamlined and facilitated our routine duties in the clinical and health care fields; however, the approach taken to get there requires comprehension of how to arrange and evaluate the data so as to accomplish the ultimate objective, which is to enhance the medical system in relation to expenses and advantages, individuals standard of life, and outcomes [1]. Beyond a requirement for central power, a dispersed, decentralized environment is now conceivable thanks to blockchain technology. Due to the employment of cryptographic principles, transactions are safe and trustworthy [2]. In the last few years, blockchain technology has taken over a number of sectors, partly due to the popularity of cryptocurrencies.

Blockchain technology has immense promise in the medical field since it can link disparate systems, enhance the precision of health data, and adopt a more patient-focused strategy for medical systems. Blockchain enables inter-entity transactions between parties without the use of a middleman. It relies on validators, who are typically miners, to accomplish decentralized transaction validation by acting as intermediaries. Distributed consensus, the ability of several parties that lack confidence in each other to reach an agreement, is used to achieve this. The spending twice issue facing the global community of cryptocurrencies is related to this computation challenge because it concerns how to ensure that a particular amount of an electronic coin hasn't been previously spent without the consent of an unbiased third group (usually a financial institution), which records every transaction and people's balances [3].

Artificial intelligence (AI) describes a system or process that adapts its behavior in response to environmental inputs in order to improve a measure of outputs [4,5]. There are two reasons for the current rise of AI in healthcare: (a) Open-source AI architectures' general-purpose accessibility enables non-AI experts to use sophisticated AI models without having to complete special AI training, and (b) the capacity to synthesize disparate information to build large databases and study challenging health management issues [4].

The phrase "machine learning," which is an aspect of AI, refers to a system's capacity to identify trends in databases using statistical and mathematical techniques, as well as to learn from errors through experience with previously developed algorithms. The main distinction between a conventional database and a blockchain is how the data is structured. Blockchain technology ensures that data is decentralized legitimate and safe. In contrast to how data is organized in databases as tables, information is organized in blockchains as chains of blocks. As Chen *et al.*, [6] work termed "LearningChain" and the author's most recent work, "CrowdSFL," [7], both indicate that combining machine learning (ML) with the security and dependability of blockchain systems can produce incredibly precise results. Examples of how blockchain and ML are linked are CloudBurst [8] and ExplorerChain [9].

By parallelizing the short-read mapping process and enhancing the flexibility of processing extensive genomic data, the CloudBurst computing paradigm accelerates the process of genome mapping to a rate that is 24 times quicker than that of traditional computing paradigms [8]. ExplorerChain integrates AI and blockchain technologies via distributed networks in medical care/genomic datasets to provide a number of enhancements, like authority over the use of computing assets, an unalterable audit path, the avoidance of single points of breakdown, and improved security. ExplorerChain was shown to have comparable discrimination power but a little longer running time than the central server-based method [9].

Blockchain and AI-based technology are novel breakthroughs in the healthcare sector. Several governing authorities use data from Internet investigations to build healthcare benchmarks. To create health indices, data from Google polls conducted by numerous federal regulators is used. Blockchain technology makes it easier to store the encrypted data that AI demands [10]. Blockchain allows medical professionals to examine patient health records (PHRs), and AI will employ a variety of suggested algorithms, decision-making abilities, and vast amounts of data [11]. Therefore, the healthcare system will evolve to be more cost-effective and efficient while also democratizing healthcare by adopting the most recent innovations [12]. The ability to process massive data sets in real time has also improved thanks to cutting-edge technology, allowing for faster illness detection that facilitates openness and interaction between patients and medical providers.

In order to reuse commercial medications and investigate the efficacy of prescription compositions and dosage control, clinical trials can be tracked using quantitative drug design techniques and AI [13,14]. Governments must choose the best methods for leveraging resources and accelerating transformation while maintaining the necessary consistency and compliance in light of this rapidly changing environment. Blockchain technology makes it possible to create and maintain content blocks known as ledgers and to analyze data in a safe and automated manner [3]. Blockchain helps in the analysis and forecasting of health data. Technology helps in many different ways, according to research, including evaluating medical supply files, coming across computational learning with pharmacological warnings, successfully implementing medical and therapy zones, and the possibility of rebuilding. Medical experts, healthcare professionals, and payers receive fast updates thanks to the collected medical data. The integration of AI and blockchain further improves this. Machines can now discern health trends and patterns thanks to AI. Furthermore, the industry for self-driving cars has shown that it can effectively use AI to create autonomous vehicles. However, some companies are creating strategies for using ML to identify financial risks and detect fraud.

AI contributes to predictive value and makes it easier to evaluate medical data. Studies have shown that AI helps in an efficient way, for instance by comparing medical supply files, encountering computerized instructions with pharmaceutical warnings, properly incorporating wellness and cure areas, and the possibility of reassembling. To take into account the aforementioned aspects, researchers have employed a variety of strategies built on blockchain and AI technologies. These methods enable the medical sector to examining data at extraordinary speeds while ensuring integrity and data safety, and they give specific professionals temporary access to their data. The main motivation of this chapter is to draw attention to the work that researchers have done to inform us about the function and significance of using blockchain-AI in healthcare systems especially in the area of safety and confidentiality perspective.

21.1.1 Key contributions of the chapter

The following are the major chapter contributions:

i. The chapter highlights how the combination of AI enabled with blockchain can boost the safety and confidentiality of medical system. The blockchain is known to be an immutable and transparent when it comes to data accessibility. AI-based models reduce and enhance the chance of data theft by helping to detect and stop unauthorized entry.
ii. The chapter presents recent research in the areas of AI-based algorithms enabled with Blockchain technology in medical systems for safety and confidential issues.
iii. The chapter discusses cutting-edge case studies of AI-based algorithms and Blockchain for safety and confidential medical sectors.
iv. This chapter offers a full understanding of the practical uses of blockchain and AI in healthcare systems, particularly in the areas of safety and confidentiality of patient data. The following are the major chapter contributions: This chapter greatly advances knowledge and encourages further research and development in the field of safe and effective healthcare systems.

21.1.2 Chapter organization

Section 21.2 presents the applicability of blockchain in Healthcare System. Section 21.3 discusses the applicability of AI algorithms in Healthcare Systems. Section 21.4 presents AI-based algorithms for security and privacy for Healthcare System. Section 21.5 discusses the Integration of AI and Blockchain in Healthcare Systems, Section 21.6 presents open issues and future research directions. Section 21.7 discusses the critical lessons learned in the chapter, and finally, Section 21.8 concludes the chapter.

21.2 Applicability of blockchain in healthcare systems

Effective access control models for medical systems must take security and privacy into account. More significantly, the internet has an impact on how people live their lives and communicate, including how they work and interact with others. The application of small sensor-based gadgets to connect the real and virtual worlds is known as the Internet of Things (IoT) [14,15]. The use of blockchain-based frameworks offers more decentralized and tamper-proof communication between nodes. A distributed and immutable ledger is another name for blockchain [16]. As a result, it provides performance, management, applications, and access whenever needed [17]. However, networking devices and other suggestions and implementations are still expanding. As a result, the majority of sectors are moving toward IoT and adopting blockchain technology [18,19].

Furthermore, blockchain-based models have serious confidentiality and safety problems, especially when healthcare institutions are involved. For IoT-based systems, security issues including denial-of-service (DoS), SQL injection, tampering listening in, and replay assaults are a problem. These dangers affect the confidentiality, genuineness, and authorization of safety applications. In order to offer protection for IoT gadgets that use blockchain-based applications, it is imperative to solve these issues and provide an innovative framework. It goes without saying that a node with inadequate safety might permit accessibility to patient information. It is believed that an electronic health record (EHR) is the most crucial and delicate type of data since it includes a great deal of private data about patients and diagnoses. However, as digital healthcare systems develop and evolve, EHR data are becoming more susceptible to security breaches [20]; therefore, security and privacy must be taken seriously in the scenario of confidence and decentralization [21].

IoT may offer additional security and functionality to a variety of consumers, according to a crucial component [22,23]. The growth of linked devices at an exponential rate worldwide led to billions documented in 2020 because of the increased accessibility in getting to the web and the rise in intelligent interaction among individuals, objects, data, and processes [24]. As a result, the fundamental conditions for addressing such difficulties are with IoT apps' security. As a result, there has been an increase in their complexity, as highly sophisticated devices offer less security when performing access control. Supervision for entry is the fundamental safety measure for EHR data from any source. As a result, EHR and PHR access control policies must be created [25]. The creation of PHR systems uses a blockchain-based digital healthcare infrastructure known as Hyperledger Fabric. PHRs are influenced globally by security, privacy, and cross-domain authorization. Based on the safety vulnerability level index [26], millions of data are hacked digitally on a daily basis. Researchers must look into these difficulties in order to assess the safety and confidentiality concerns with relation to the usage of ledger technology in PHR.

A cross-domain organization method in a digital medical system can give clinicians and patients access to data that is dispersed across several domains. However, accessing data via a cross-domain organization necessitates greater security and adaptable permission rules. A policy lays up guidelines and stringent requirements for participant and data properties. Additionally, data can be protected using encryption techniques [27]. The circle identities and cluster identities from the literature form the foundation for the researchers' encryption techniques [15,28].

Blockchain is an innovative and groundbreaking innovation that is mostly employed in situations where privacy is crucial and centralization is inappropriate [29–31]. Health data are of special relevance to blockchain [32–34], with a focus on sharing, dissemination, and encryption. The core ideas behind a blockchain are decentralization and cryptographic hashing. Blockchain databases and information are reachable by everybody on the network. Every member of the network has access to the blockchain contents thanks to the network's creation of a distributed, decentralized chain. Consensus is a process that safeguards the network's security. An agreement system uses a collection of principles and is fault-tolerant to help all participants reach the necessary consensus regarding the condition of the blockchain ledger. The three main parts of a blockchain are blocks, nodes, and miners. In this context, a block is analogous to a page in a record book that stores a few or all of the most current transaction data that was not previously saved in a block.

The blockchain advances to the following block whenever a block is finished or mined. Each block, starting with the genesis block, contains information, its own special nonce, and a hash value that connects to the prior block via a hash label, forming a series of blocks and eliminating any possibility of alteration [35]. A blockchain network's nodes ensure that the given data is kept in the decentralized database and are in charge of maintaining the network's functionality. The blockchain is replicated on each node, and any node that contributes adds fresh blocks to the chain receives incentives. In order to prevent security vulnerabilities like double-spending attacks, the consensus process grants equal access to the distributed ledger to all network users and shields the chain from outside parties [36].

Only a few of the consensus approaches that are available include proof-of-work (PoW), Byzantine faulty tolerant (BFT), zero-knowledge proof (ZKP), and proof-of-stake (PoS) [37]. Additionally, smart contracts use blockchain technology to make it possible to create immutable contracts that are accessible, helping to increase honesty and confidence between two parties. A blockchain network's participants each have an alphanumeric identity which is a special code that keeps track of their deals. As a result, the distributed ledger's users may easily track and see every action. The smart contract's secure transactions aid in preventing intervention from consolidated systems. Platforms such as Ethereum Virtual Machine or Solidity might be utilized to create smart contracts for automating auditing procedures, permitting time-limited access to distributed patient information, and enhancing pharmaceutical product supply chain administration [38]. The amount of data in the medical sector has multiplied, and blockchain technology can assist stakeholders in successfully managing this enormous volume of data. Blockchain also creates secure and private data exchange protocols in the medical industry. Blockchain technology has shown exciting prospects in the medical sector due to its irreversible and decentralized state through implementations including safe data management [39,40], open clinical record keeping [41], and medical information confidentiality [42–44]. A summary of blockchain technology capabilities in the healthcare industry is given in Figure 21.1.

Blockchain is a fairly young and evolving technology that has found adoption in the medical field and provides innovative applications. Among all the renowned

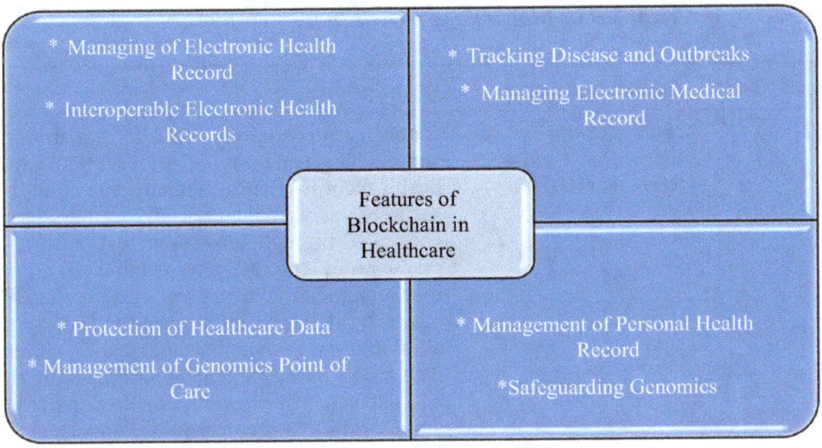

Figure 21.1 Blockchain technology capabilities in the healthcare industry

network members and medical professionals, efficient, productive information exchange and distribution is essential to the creation of inexpensive therapies and innovative cures for a variety of ailments. This will speed up the expansion of the medical industry during the next years. Possibilities for blockchain technology in the logistics industry that were recently revealed emphasize the advantages for the medical industry. The technological advance improves and progresses in this initial phase since it quickly impacts living standards. Additionally, gaining prominence is blockchain technology, notably in the finance and medical sectors. It offers the medical sector a lot of major and spectacular potential, from research and logistics to interactions between physicians and patients [29,45,46]. The medical sector might gain greatly from and be improved by blockchain technology. By solving important issues like safety of information, connectivity, and openness, blockchain technology offers the capacity to completely transform the healthcare industry. The following are some crucial areas in which blockchain can be used in healthcare. The important uses of blockchain in healthcare are covered in Table 1.

While blockchain offers several benefits, there are also challenges and considerations to address. These include scalability issues, regulatory compliance, standardization of data formats, and the need for collaboration among various stakeholders to adopt the technology. Implementing blockchain technology demands considerable preparation and attention in the healthcare industry of regulatory compliance, interoperability, and adoption challenges. While it holds great promise, the successful integration of blockchain into the healthcare system will depend on collaboration between stakeholders, robust infrastructure, and addressing potential privacy concerns. Overall, blockchain technology has the capacity to completely transform the healthcare industry by improving the safety of data, connectivity, and productivity while giving patients greater control over their medical records. We may anticipate additional cutting-edge scenarios and implementations in the medical field as the innovation grows to develop and become more widely used.

Table 21.1 Applications of blockchain in healthcare systems

Authors	Applications area	Description
[47–51]	**Interoperability of Electronic Health Records (EHRs)**	Blockchain technology can offer a distributed and unchangeable way of preserving electronic health records (EHRs). Patient data could be securely encrypted, and access to it could be controlled through smart contracts, ensuring privacy and data integrity. Additionally, blockchain can help in creating interoperability between different healthcare providers' systems, allowing seamless and secure sharing of patient data. Blockchain can enable seamless sharing and exchange of electronic medical records among different medical professionals and institutions. Patients can have control over their data and grant access to specific healthcare professionals when needed, streamlining the process and reducing duplication of tests and procedures. Healthcare systems frequently have issues with connectivity, making it challenging to share data securely and efficiently. Blockchain can serve as a standardized platform for data exchange, enabling different healthcare providers and institutions to access patient records seamlessly, ensuring consistency and security throughout the process.
[52–57]	**Clinical Trials and Research**	Blockchain's capacity to provide data with openness, tracking, and inviolability helps simplify the medical trial procedure. Researchers can securely share trial data, and the results can be verified independently. This can help in reducing fraud and speeding up the research process. By capturing data, blockchain can improve the reliability and openness of clinical trials in all stages of the trial, from data collection to results. This helps prevent data manipulation and ensures the authenticity of trial data, leading to more reliable research outcomes.
[57–61]	**Supply Chain Management**	Blockchain can be utilized by the pharmaceutical sector to trace the complete supply chain, from medicine manufacturers to patients. This can help in preventing counterfeit drugs, ensuring the authenticity of medications, and improving drug safety. Pharmaceuticals may be tracked using blockchain throughout the supply chain, from manufacturers to distributors to pharmacies. This improves transparency and helps identify and eliminate counterfeit drugs from the market, ensuring patient safety. Beyond patient data, blockchain can enhance security

(Continues)

Table 21.1 (*Continued*)

Authors	Applications area	Description
		and traceability in pharmaceutical supply chains. Every stage of the supply chain is documented on the blockchain, from manufacturer to distributor to patient, it becomes harder for counterfeit drugs to infiltrate the system.
[54,62–65]	**Medical Credentialing and Licensing**	Blockchain can facilitate a more efficient and trustworthy medical credentialing process. Healthcare professionals' credentials and licenses can be stored on the blockchain, enabling easy verification by healthcare organizations and authorities.
[59,66–69]	**Healthcare Payments and Billing**	Blockchain can simplify healthcare payments and billing processes by creating a decentralized ledger for tracking transactions between insurers, providers, and patients. This can reduce administrative costs and prevent fraudulent billing. Blockchain can simplify and secure healthcare payments by reducing the number of middlemen employed in the process. Smart contracts can automate payment agreements between insurers, healthcare providers, and patients, reducing administrative costs and ensuring prompt payment.
[70–76]	**Telemedicine and Remote Patient Monitoring**	Blockchain can enhance the security and privacy of telemedicine services and remote patient monitoring. It can enable secure communication between patients and healthcare providers while safeguarding sensitive medical data. Blockchain can facilitate secure communication and data exchange between patients and remote healthcare providers. This enables remote patient monitoring and telemedicine services while maintaining data privacy and security.
[77–81]	**Health Data Analytics and AI**	With the consent of patients, healthcare information kept on the blockchain can be used for research purposes and training AI models. Blockchain data integrity ascertains that the information used for analysis is reliable and tamper-proof. Blockchain can facilitate secure and privacy-preserving health data analytics. Researchers can access anonymized data stored on the blockchain without compromising the identities of individual patients, thus encouraging data sharing for medical research while protecting privacy.
[42,54,82–85]	**Public Health Surveillance**	Blockchain can aid in tracking disease outbreaks, public health data, and vaccination records, ensuring accurate and information that

(Continues)

Table 21.1 (*Continued*)

Authors	Applications area	Description
		is current for public health officials. Additionally, blockchain technology has the capacity to enhance disease surveillance networks in situations where breakouts of illness cause local and international health catastrophes. Blockchain can be utilized in these situations to pinpoint potential health security issues, evaluate and take precautionary action and make decisions more quickly. Although it has flaws, blockchain-based research and applications have shown promise.
[66,86–89]	**Data Security and Privacy**	Blockchain's decentralized and immutable nature makes it the best solution for securing sensitive patient data. Medical records and personal information can be kept in encrypted blocks on the blockchain, reducing the risk of data breaches and unauthorized access. Blockchain can facilitate patient-controlled access to their health records. Instead of relying on a central authority to store and manage data, patients may provide particular healthcare professionals or researchers access to their medical information through cryptographic keys. This approach gives patients greater control over their data and enhances privacy.
[62,90,91]	**Medical Credentialing and Licensing**	Blockchain can streamline the verification and sharing of medical credentials and licenses for healthcare professionals, making the process more efficient and secure. To make sure they have the proper licenses to practice medicine, professionals must confirm their identities. Additionally, they must knowingly divulge their individual data in order to validate submitting their credentials to the medical institution where they seek to continue further education or the hospital where they plan to practice medicine both of which are insufficiently secure and where the greatest risk of identity theft exists. A system that can quickly and easily verify the digital credentials of a healthcare professional disclosure is needed to solve these two primary issues.
[92–97]	**Healthcare Research Data Sharing**	Researchers can securely share and access large datasets for scientific research without compromising patient privacy. Blockchain distributed nature allows for collaborative research while maintaining data integrity and privacy. The exchange of healthcare data will

(Continues)

Table 21.1 (Continued)

Authors	Applications area	Description
		increase research development in this field. Patients who share their medical information, however, must deal with significant privacy and security issues. This study suggests a blockchain-based system architectural design to demonstrate what blockchain technology can do to support (i) sharing of health data that is secure and transparent and (ii) processing of access permissions to healthcare data.
[98–101]	**Healthcare IoT Devices**	The safety of data produced by Internet of Things (IoT) sensors in the medical industry can be improved via blockchain. By doing this, wearable device-generated patient data is protected and other IoT sensors remain tamper-proof and trustworthy. In the Blockchain-powered system, a unique ID will be given to a person and connected to the Blockchain. He may decide who gets access to the information collected from his intelligent gadgets. When there are many IoT gadgets, he may also choose which ones, if any, should communicate information with the medical provider. According to the report, blockchain technology is mostly utilized to improve information safety, including data honesty, access control, and safeguarding privacy, for managing information jobs in healthcare and IoT.
[102–105]	**Healthcare Insurance Claims Processing**	Blockchain can simplify the insurance claims process by providing a transparent and auditable trail of claim transactions. This reduces fraud and speeds up claims processing for both insurers and patients. Blockchain technology and AI can do a lot of solving the issues handling health insurance applications. Some of the applications of these innovations can be helpful include utilizing blockchain openness by granting access to a larger dataset and using AI techniques, which may improve the precision of AI models. to examine data stored on the blockchain for fraud detection.
[106–109]	**Data Integrity and Immutability**	In healthcare, maintaining the integrity of patient data is crucial. Data cannot be removed or changed after it has been recorded because to the decentralized and unchangeable nature of blockchain technology. This feature helps prevent data tampering and unauthorized access, which enhances security. This enables the

(Continues)

Table 21.1 (*Continued*)

Authors	Applications area	Description
		production of a transaction record that is secure, transparent, and impervious to alteration. Blockchains are frequently connected to cryptocurrencies like Bitcoin, but the technology has a wide range of other potential applications, such as the secure and open tracking of data in the supply chain, the development of secure and unchangeable voting systems, and the facilitation of secure and open record-keeping for a variety of industries.
[110–115]	**Consent and Identity Management**	Blockchain smart contract capabilities can be leveraged to manage patient consent effectively. Patients can define specific terms and conditions for data usage, and these conditions can be automatically enforced through smart contracts. This approach ensures that data is only used for authorized purposes, minimizing privacy risks. Blockchain-based identity management systems can enable more secure patient identification and authentication processes. This helps prevent medical identity theft and fraud, guaranteeing that only people with permission can access private medical information. The hash of the block before it is enclosed in each subsequent block, ensures the ledger's immutability. Without a single point of trust, blockchain technologies offer serializability, immutability, and cryptographic verifiability.
[53,113,116,117]	**Secure Health Information Exchange**	Blockchain can streamline health information exchange between different entities, such as medical facilities, drugstores, and insurance firms while maintaining data integrity and privacy. Each transaction is securely recorded on the blockchain, ensuring transparency and reducing the risk of data breaches.

Blockchain technology has the potential to significantly enhance safety and confidentiality in the healthcare system. Despite these advantages, it's important to acknowledge that implementing blockchain in healthcare comes with its challenges, such as scalability, adherence to regulations, and compatibility with current systems. Additionally, while blockchain can enhance data security, it does not solve all healthcare privacy and security concerns on its own. Complementary measures, such as strong encryption, access controls, and cybersecurity best practices, should also be in place to ensure a comprehensive security and privacy framework in the healthcare system.

21.3 Applicability of artificial intelligence algorithms in healthcare systems

AI-based models are everywhere in technology and are increasingly integrated into daily life. Additionally, Accenture researchers [118] forecasted that between 2014 and 2021, the market for AI applications in healthcare is likely to grow from $600 million to $6.6 billion. Recent research demonstrates that ML and DL models powered by AI are used to address coronavirus-related problems [119]. Medical imagery offers a great deal of potential for using ML to identify trends and anomalies. In order to help healthcare professionals make decisions more automatically, it then matches such data into learning models [120]. For instance, AI may be used in a framework that automatically recognizes faces and measures body heat in order to protect those with coronavirus infections [121]. Healthcare is using AI more and more. The growth of AI in healthcare calls for research and discussion of AI-related ethical issues.

Applications of AI-based technologies in the medical sector offer fresh possibilities [122]. Several hospitals are using AI-enabled systems in the context of decision-support systems (DSSs) for health personnel in the perspective of detection and cure [123]. AI technologies also affect how treatment is delivered organizationally, improving the efficiency of different operations including nursing and administration activities in hospitals [124]. With the deployment of AI, there are ethics that have to be acknowledged and resolved in an effective, evidence-based manner. AI in the healthcare industry involves a variety of complex ethical issues. An additional careful strategy for the use of AI in healthcare has been recommended in recent analyses of the effects of AI on community wellness, even if more research is being done to assure ethical AI design and deployment. AI may still have the power to enhance people's health and help keep healthcare systems resilient and sustainable [125]. Figure 21.2 shows the applicability of AI in healthcare system.

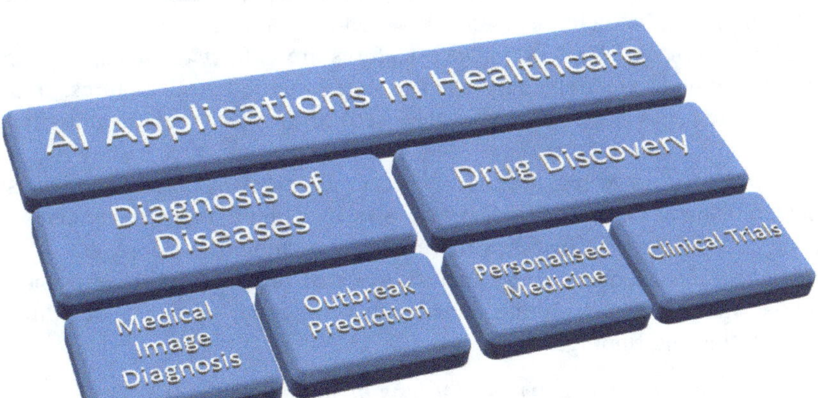

Figure 21.2 The applicability of AI-based algorithms in healthcare system

AI algorithms have found numerous applications in the healthcare system, transforming how medical professionals diagnose, treat, and manage patient care. Algorithms have tremendous applicability in healthcare platforms and have the capacity to revolutionize patient care, diagnosis, treatment, and administrative processes. Among the most significant uses of AI in healthcare is:

Medical Image Analysis: X-rays, ultrasounds, magnetic resonance imaging (MRIs), computed tomography (CT) scans, positron emission tomography (PET), and pathology slides are just a few examples of the medical pictures that AI algorithms may examine to aid in the detection and diagnosis of diseases such as cancer, fractures, and neurological disorders [126]. AI models can often identify abnormalities with high accuracy, potentially reducing human error and improving diagnostic efficiency. They can spot patterns and irregularities that the human eye would find challenging to spot, resulting in quicker and more accurate diagnoses. Medical Image Analysis is a field of study within medical imaging that includes the interpretation and extraction of useful data from medical pictures using computer algorithms and methodologies [127,128]. The main objective of medical imaging analysis is to aid healthcare professionals in diagnosing diseases, monitoring treatment progress, and conducting medical research. Here are some of the key aspects of medical image analysis:

1. *Image Preprocessing:* Medical images often contain noise, artifacts, and non-relevant information that can hinder accurate analysis. To increase the resolution and conformity of the pictures, preprocessing methods such as noise decrease, picture improvement, and picture registration are used.
2. *Segmentation:* Segmentation involves dividing the medical image into meaningful regions of interest, such as organs, tumors, blood vessels, or other anatomical structures. Segmentation is crucial for quantitative analysis and targeted interventions.
3. *Feature Extraction:* After segmentation, relevant features are extracted from the regions of interest. These features may include shape, texture, intensity, or other characteristics that help distinguish between normal and abnormal tissues.
4. *Classification and Detection:* Once features are extracted, ML and computer vision methods are frequently used to categorize medical pictures. into different categories (e.g., healthy vs. diseased) or to detect specific abnormalities (e.g., tumors and fractures).
5. *Registration:* Image registration is used to align several pictures of the same person taken at various periods or using various photographic techniques. This is crucial for tracking disease progression or treatment response.
6. *Visualization:* Medical image analysis systems provide visual representations of the analysis results, aiding healthcare professionals in understanding and interpreting the findings.

Applications of Medical Image Analysis include:

Disease Diagnosis: Detection and diagnosis of various conditions, such as cancer, neurological disorders, cardiovascular diseases, etc.

Treatment Planning: Assisting in treatment planning for surgeries, radiation therapy, or other interventions.

Image-Guided Interventions: Providing real-time guidance during minimally invasive procedures.

Drug Development and Research: Supporting medical research by quantifying changes in tissues or evaluating treatment outcomes in clinical trials.

Medical Image Analysis is an interdisciplinary field that combines principles from computer science, image processing, ML, and medicine. It plays a vital role in modern healthcare, aiding clinicians in making accurate and timely diagnoses while improving patient care and outcomes.

Personalized Medicine and Treatment Plans: To create individualized treatment recommendations, AI may assess patient data comprising medical records, genes, and lifestyle variables [129]. This can lead to more effective treatments tailored to individual patients, improving outcomes and reducing adverse reactions. Utilizing information about a patient's genetic composition and way of life, AI can assist in customizing therapies for specific individuals, and health history, improving treatment outcomes, and minimizing adverse effects [130]. Precision medicine, sometimes referred to as personalized medicine, is a method of providing medical that particularly tailors medical choices and treatments to each patient by taking into consideration their individual genetic composition, way of life, surroundings, and other characteristics. By tailoring therapies to the unique needs of each patient, personalized medicine aims to increase the efficacy, safety, and efficiency of healthcare [131].

Key elements of personalized medicine and treatment plans include:

1. *Genetic Testing:* Genetic tests analyze a person's DNA to identify specific genetic variations or mutations that may influence their response to certain medications or their risk of developing certain diseases. By understanding a patient's genetic profile, healthcare providers can select drugs that are more likely to be effective and avoid those that might cause adverse reactions.
2. *Biomarker Identification:* Biomarkers are measurable indicators that can provide information about a patient's health status or response to treatment. In personalized medicine, biomarkers are used to recognize individuals who are probably to benefit from a particular therapy or who may require alternative treatments.
3. *Tailored Treatment Selection:* Based on the genetic and biomarker information, healthcare providers can choose methods that are likely to be the most successful for a specific individual. This approach minimizes the trial-and-error process in finding the right treatment for a patient.
4. *Dosing Optimization:* Personalized medicine can also help determine the most appropriate dosage of medication for an individual, considering factors such as metabolism and potential drug interactions.
5. *Prevention and Early Detection:* Personalized medicine is not only about treating diseases but also about identifying individuals who are at higher risk of developing certain conditions. This proactive approach enables early detection and preventive measures to reduce the impact of diseases.

6. *Monitoring and Follow-up:* Continuous monitoring and analysis of a patient's health data allow healthcare providers to adjust treatment plans as needed, ensuring that the chosen therapies remain effective and safe over time.
7. *Integration of Lifestyle Factors:* Personalized treatment plans also consider lifestyle factors such as diet, exercise, and stress management. These factors can significantly impact a patient's response to treatment and overall health outcomes.
8. *Data Privacy and Ethics:* Given that the gathering and evaluation of individual health data is a key component of customized therapy, it's essential to prioritize patient privacy and maintain ethical standards in handling this sensitive information.

Personalized medicine holds great promise for revolutionizing healthcare by switching to a more flexible strategy rather than a one-size-fits-all tailored and effective form of treatment. As technology and research continue to advance, we can expect further advancements in this field, leading to improved health outcomes for patients worldwide.

Drug Discovery and Development: AI algorithms can analyze vast datasets to identify potential drug candidates for various diseases [132]. AI-driven drug discovery can significantly speed up the research process, potentially leading to the creation of novel therapies and the repurposing of existing drugs for different conditions. By analyzing massive databases of genetic and molecular data, finding new drug candidates, and other tasks, AI may dramatically speed up the drug development process and simulate their interactions with biological systems [133]. Drug development is a difficult and drawn-out procedure aimed at identifying, designing, testing, and bringing new medications to market to treat various diseases and conditions. It involves numerous scientific disciplines, regulatory approvals, and significant investments of time and resources [134]. Here's a summary of the key stages involved in the drug research and development process:

Target Identification and Validation

The process begins with locating a particular biological target like a protein or enzyme that has a role in a disorder or illness. Scientists study the target's role in the disease and assess its potential as a therapeutic target.

Hit Discovery

Researchers search for "hits"–molecules or compounds that engage the target in some way that could potentially lead to a therapeutic effect. High-throughput screening and computational methods are commonly used to identify initial hits from large libraries of compounds.

Lead Optimization

The most promising hits are further optimized to enhance their potency, selectivity, and safety profile. Medicinal chemists modify the lead compounds' chemical composition to enhance their drug-like characteristics.

Preclinical Research: Before testing the drug in humans, to evaluate the safety of a medicine, preclinical research is carried out utilizing cell cultures and animal models, efficacy, and pharmacokinetics (absorption, distribution, metabolism, and excretion).

Investigational New Drug (IND) Application: If the preclinical studies show promising results and safety, researchers file an Investigational New Drug application with regulatory authorities (such as the FDA in the United States) to request permission to begin human clinical trials.

Clinical Trials

To assess the drug's efficacy, safety, and best dose in human subjects, clinical studies are carried out in stages.

Phase I: Small-scale trials to assess safety and dosing.

Phase II: Larger trials to evaluate efficacy and further assess safety.

Phase III: Even larger trials to confirm efficacy, monitor adverse reactions, and compare the drug to standard treatments.

Phase IV: Post-marketing studies conducted after regulatory approval to gather additional information about the security of the medication and effectiveness in real-world use.

New Drug Application (NDA)

After successful completion of clinical trials, researchers submit an NDA to the regulatory agency, providing comprehensive data from preclinical and clinical studies. The agency reviews the data to determine whether the drug is safe and effective for its intended use.

Regulatory Approval: If the regulatory agency is satisfied with the data, they approve the drug for marketing and commercial use.

Post-Marketing Surveillance: After approval, the drug is continuously monitored for any adverse effects or long-term safety issues.

The entire drug discovery and development process can take over a decade and involves collaboration among scientists, researchers, clinicians, pharmaceutical companies, and regulatory authorities. It also requires substantial financial investment to fund research, development, and clinical trials. Only a small percentage of drug candidates that enter the pipeline ultimately make it to market as a result of the high failure rates at various stages of the process.

Virtual Health Assistants (VHAs): AI-powered VHAs can interact with patients, providing basic medical advice, scheduling appointments, and answering general health-related questions. These applications can lighten the load on healthcare providers and enhance patient engagement [135]. AI-powered chatbots and VHAs can interact with patients, answer their questions, provide health information, and even offer basic medical advice, enhancing patient engagement and access to healthcare [136]. VHAs are AI-powered applications or software designed to provide healthcare-related services and support to users [137]. These assistants leverage natural language processing and ML algorithms to interact with individuals, understand their health-related inquiries, and provide relevant information, advice, or assistance. Key features and functionalities of VHAs may include:

1. *Health Information:* VHAs can access vast databases of medical knowledge and provide information about symptoms, diseases, treatments, medications, and preventive measures.

2. *Symptom Assessment:* They can ask users questions about their symptoms to offer potential diagnoses or recommend whether professional medical attention is necessary.
3. *Medication Reminders:* VHAs can serve as a reminder for users to take their prescriptions on time and provide information about dosage and potential interactions.
4. *Health Monitoring:* Some VHAs can connect with wearable devices or health-tracking apps to monitor a user's health metrics, such as heart rate, activity levels, and sleep patterns.
5. *Appointment Scheduling:* Users can use VHAs to book appointments with healthcare providers or specialists.
6. *Virtual Consultations:* In some cases, VHAs may facilitate virtual consultations with healthcare professionals through video conferencing.
7. *Mental Health Support:* VHAs can offer emotional support, relaxation techniques, and coping strategies for managing stress and anxiety.
8. *Health Tips:* VHAs can deliver personalized health tips and recommendations based on a user's health profile and preferences.
9. *Diet and Nutrition:* They can provide information about healthy eating habits, dietary restrictions, and personalized meal plans.
10. *Chronic Disease Management:* VHAs can help individuals manage chronic conditions by offering reminders, monitoring progress, and providing educational resources.

Benefits of Virtual Health Assistants:

Accessibility: VHAs can be accessed from any location with an internet connection, increasing healthcare accessibility, especially for people in remote or underserved areas.

Time Efficiency: VHAs can quickly respond to queries, reducing how long it requires for someone to find relevant health information.

24/7 Availability: VHAs can be available around the clock, offering support and guidance at any time.

Personalization: Advanced AI algorithms enable VHAs to tailor responses and recommendations to each user's specific health needs and preferences.

Empowerment: VHAs can empower people to take control of their well-being by providing education and resources for self-care.

Despite the many advantages, it's crucial to remember that VHAs have certain drawbacks. They are not a replacement for qualified medical guidance, diagnosis, or care. While they can give a general description and support, users should always consult healthcare professionals for specific medical concerns and advice. Additionally, privacy and security concerns must be carefully addressed when implementing VHAs to safeguard sensitive health data.

Predictive Analytics: AI algorithms may examine patient information to forecast the likelihood of disease occurrence, readmissions, and complications [138]. This enables early intervention and proactive management of patients at high risk, enhancing patient outcomes and cutting back on healthcare expenses. In order to forecast the probability of particular health events, such as medical hospitalizations, disease advancement, or consequences, AI systems can examine vast amounts of patient data [139]. This can help in early intervention and preventive care.

Administrative Support and Efficiency: AI can streamline administrative tasks such as billing, coding, and scheduling, improving the overall efficiency of healthcare organizations and allowing healthcare professionals to focus more on patient care. AI algorithms can optimize hospital workflows, resource allocation, and scheduling, leading to better resource management and reduced waiting times for patients.

Remote Patient Monitoring (RPM): AI-powered devices and wearables can continuously monitor patients' important signs and health metrics in real time. This data can be examined to detect early signs of deterioration or potential health issues, allowing for timely intervention and reducing hospital readmissions. AI-powered wearables and remote monitoring devices can continuously collect and analyze patient data, enabling early detection of health issues and better management of chronic conditions [2,35]. RPM is a healthcare practice that utilizes technology to monitor patients' health remotely. It enables healthcare professionals to collect and track medical data from patients outside of traditional healthcare settings, such as hospitals or clinics. RPM enables ongoing observation of a patient's health, vital signs, symptoms, and other relevant health information without the need for frequent in-person visits.

Key components of Remote Patient Monitoring may include:

1. *Sensors and Devices:* Patients use various wearable or non-invasive devices equipped with sensors that gather information about bodily functions including heart rate, blood pressure, glucose levels, oxygen saturation, temperature, and more. These devices can be integrated with smartphones or other monitoring systems.
2. *Telecommunication Infrastructure:* RPM relies on a secure and reliable telecommunication network to transmit data from the patient's devices to the healthcare provider or a central monitoring system.
3. *Data Management and Analysis:* The collected data is stored and managed in a secure database or cloud-based platform. Healthcare professionals can access and analyze the data to identify trends, deviations, or abnormalities in a patient's health condition.
4. *Alerts and Notifications:* The RPM system can be designed to generate alerts or notifications when certain health parameters go beyond predetermined thresholds. This helps healthcare providers respond promptly to any critical changes in the patient's condition.
5. *Patient Portals and Mobile Apps:* Patients often have access to their data through web-based portals or mobile applications. This empowers them to take an active role in managing their health and staying informed about their health status.

Benefits of Remote Patient Monitoring include:

Improved Patient Outcomes: RPM enables early health concern discovery enabling healthcare professionals to take action before conditions worsen, leading to better outcomes and reducing hospital readmissions.

Enhanced Patient Engagement: Patients are more involved in their health management, as they can see real-time data, set goals, and track progress, which can improve adherence to treatment plans.

Cost Savings: RPM can lead to cost savings for both patients and healthcare providers by reducing hospital visits, unnecessary tests, and hospital readmissions.

Access to Remote or Underserved Areas: RPM helps extend medical care to remote or underserved regions where healthcare facilities may be limited.

Chronic Disease Management: RPM is especially advantageous for people with chronic illnesses like diabetes and hypertension, or heart diseases, as it allows for continuous monitoring and timely intervention.

It's important to note that while RPM has shown great promise in transforming healthcare, it is not meant to replace all in-person visits or emergency care. Rather, it complements traditional care and enhances the overall patient experience by providing continuous and personalized monitoring.

Robot-Assisted Surgery: Robots with AI can help surgeons with difficult operations, offering enhanced accuracy and lowering the invasiveness of certain surgeries [140]. This can lead to quicker recovery times and improved patient outcomes. Robotic surgery, commonly referred to as robot-assisted surgery, is a kind of less-invasive surgical method that makes use of robotic equipment to support surgeons during operations [141]. The goal of robot-assisted surgery is to enhance surgical precision, flexibility, and control, while also providing potential benefits for patients, such as reduced pain, faster recovery, and smaller incisions.

Key components of robot-assisted surgery:

1. *Robotic System:* The core of robot-assisted surgery is the robotic system, which includes a console where the surgeon sits and controls the instruments, and a patient-side cart with robotic arms equipped with surgical instruments. The surgeon operates the robotic system through the console, and the robotic arms mimic the surgeon's movements with enhanced precision and range of motion.
2. *Surgical Instruments:* Specialized surgical tools are mounted on the robotic arms such as scalpels, scissors, forceps, and cameras. These instruments can be smaller and more maneuverable than traditional surgical tools, allowing for more precise movements in confined spaces.
3. *3D Visualization:* Robot-assisted surgery typically incorporates a 3D high-definition camera system that provides the surgeon with a magnified and detailed view of the surgical site. This enhanced visualization helps the surgeon make precise decisions during the procedure.
4. *Computer Assistance:* The robotic system often includes computer software that can interpret the surgeon's movements and translate them into precise

actions by the robotic arms. The system can also assist in reducing hand tremors and other minor inconsistencies in the surgeon's motions.

Advantages of robot-assisted surgery:

Enhanced Precision: The robotic system allows for more precise movements and greater dexterity than traditional laparoscopic or open surgeries, potentially leading to better surgical outcomes.

Reduced Trauma: Robot-assisted surgery typically involves smaller incisions, resulting in less tissue damage, reduced scarring, and faster recovery times for patients.

Improved Visualization: The 3D camera system provides a clearer and more detailed view of the surgical site, helping the surgeon perform intricate procedures with greater accuracy.

Greater Flexibility: The robotic arms can access hard-to-reach areas within the body, enabling surgeons to perform complex surgeries that may be challenging or impossible with conventional techniques.

Less Blood Loss: The precise movements of the robotic instruments may lead to reduced blood loss during surgery.

Shorter Hospital Stays: Due to the minimally invasive nature of the procedure, patients may experience shorter hospital stays and quicker overall recovery times.

It's important to note that robot-assisted surgery is not suitable for all types of procedures, and its implementation may depend on the surgeon's expertise and the specific requirements of the patient's condition. As with any surgical technique, there are potential risks and limitations associated with robot-assisted surgery, and patients should discuss these aspects with their healthcare providers before making decisions about their treatment.

Disease Detection and Outbreak Prediction: To identify disease outbreaks, AI systems may scan enormous volumes of data from several sources monitor public health trends, and predict potential epidemics. This information can help public health authorities prevent and limit the spread of infections by being proactive. Disease detection and outbreak prediction are essential components of public health surveillance systems aimed at monitoring the prevention of infectious illness transmission. With advances in technology and data analysis, several approaches have been created to improve disease detection and outbreak prediction. Some of these approaches include:

Syndromic Surveillance: Monitoring certain symptoms or syndromes is known as symptomatic surveillance.

rather than confirmed diagnoses. By analyzing data from sources such as trips to emergency rooms, over-the-counter medication sales, and Internet search trends, public health officials can detect unusual patterns that may indicate the early stages of an outbreak.

1. *Digital Disease Detection:* With the widespread use of digital technologies, social media, and Internet-connected devices, data can be mined for signals of

potential disease outbreaks. This approach involves using natural language processing and ML algorithms to analyze online content and identify relevant keywords and phrases related to diseases and symptoms.

2. *Early Warning Systems:* These systems use data from various sources, including health facilities, meteorological data, and environmental monitoring, to identify early warning signs of an outbreak. By combining multiple data streams, these systems can provide more accurate predictions and early alerts to health authorities.
3. *Genomic Surveillance:* Genomic sequencing of pathogens can provide crucial insights into the origin and spread of infectious diseases. Tracking the genetic changes of pathogens over time allows scientists to understand how diseases are evolving and potentially predict their future behavior.
4. *One Health Approach:* The One Health philosophy acknowledges the interdependence of environmental, animal, and people health. By monitoring diseases in both humans and animals, public health officials can identify potential zoonotic diseases (those transmitted between animals and humans) and take early preventive measures.
5. *Machine Learning and AI:* Big data sets may be analyzed by ML algorithms to find trends that human analysts would miss. By training models on historical disease data, AI can assist in predicting disease outbreaks with higher accuracy and speed.
6. *Real-time Data Sharing and Collaboration:* Timely data sharing and collaboration between different health agencies and countries are crucial for early detection and containment of outbreaks that may have cross-border implications. Organizations like the World Health Organization (WHO) facilitate such information sharing and coordination.

It is crucial to understand that despite these approaches can significantly improve disease detection and outbreak prediction, they are not perfect, and challenges like data quality, privacy concerns, and resource limitations must be considered. Additionally, public health efforts are still essential for effective disease control, including vaccination campaigns, contact tracing, and implementing appropriate preventive measures.

Natural Language Processing (NLP) for Medical Records: AI-powered NLP can extract relevant information from medical records, making it simpler for medical professionals to obtain and understand patient data efficiently. NLP algorithms can extract valuable insights from unstructured clinical notes, research papers, and patient records, aiding in medical research and knowledge discovery.

Diagnostics and Decision Support: AI can assist healthcare professionals in diagnosing diseases by analyzing patient data, symptoms, and medical history. AI-based decision support systems can provide personalized treatment recommendations based on the individual patient's characteristics and historical data. It is important to note despite the fact that AI has the ability to transform medical care, it must be implemented and regulated carefully to ensure patient safety, privacy, and ethical considerations are taken into account. Additionally, the usage of AI should be as a supplementary tool for healthcare professionals rather than a replacement for human expertise and judgment.

As it provides cutting-edge and improved functionality in the smart healthcare system, a smart gadget contains a significant amount of sensitive patient data. The delivery of healthcare services to individuals will change significantly as a result of the interconnection of healthcare system components via the Internet [142]. A smart healthcare system's effectiveness is hampered by serious dangers and vulnerabilities that have arisen as a result of simple access to healthcare applications and services. Considering that a substantial number of heterogeneous devices create data that is different in size and kind, it is also challenging to manage the data in the healthcare database and safeguard it from intruders who wish to profit from the data. Thus, network intrusions, system-level attacks, hardware- and software-based attacks, as well as other security problems that might threaten patient lives, could have an impact on smart healthcare systems [142]. An examination of the literature revealed a research vacuum since most security research on the medical care ecosystem concentrated on security risks rather than integrating modern technologies to address them. We thus conduct a full study of the numerous current security issues and remedies in the setting of intelligent healthcare in this chapter.

An efficient way to combat the rising tide of cyberattacks plaguing the healthcare ecosystem is to implement AI technology in intelligent medical care systems [143]. In order to provide an endogenous security solution, the AI contributes a significant role in analyzing the malevolent behavior of the attacker. The utilization of AI in the smart healthcare system has been suggested by several researchers as a reliable and practical security solution. AI systems, however, are unable to counteract data integrity assaults, in which a perpetrator intercepts a transmission in order to obtain and insert harmful code into lawful data. The attacker also listens covertly and passively to network traffic in order to gather sensitive data about healthcare resources, such as how many people are in serious situations, the limits of implantable devices, and login information for patient information systems [144]. This information is crucial from a security perspective because, in the event that it gets into the wrong hands, major privacy-related issues might put the sophisticated healthcare system in jeopardy. The implementation of blockchain technology, which is characterized by decentralization, immutability, openness, and safety, is therefore required [145,146].

21.4 Artificial intelligence security and privacy for healthcare system

Data Protection: AI algorithms require large datasets for training. Ensuring patient data privacy and protection is crucial. Anonymization, encryption, and differential privacy techniques can be employed to safeguard sensitive information.

Model Security: Protecting AI models from adversarial attacks is essential. These attacks involve manipulating input data to mislead AI systems. Robust model training, using techniques like adversarial training, can help improve model resilience.

AI Bias: AI systems that were educated on skewed data can reinforce current healthcare prejudices. Addressing this issue involves careful curation of training data, regular auditing of models, and transparency in algorithm design.

Explainability and Interpretability: In healthcare, it's critical to understand the decision-making process of AI models. Black-box AI systems can be concerning. Employing explainable AI techniques can make AI more transparent and trustworthy.

21.4.1 Artificial intelligence (AI) in healthcare security

AI can be used to strengthen security in healthcare in various ways:

Anomaly Detection: Large volumes of data from EHRs, medical devices, and other sources to detect unusual patterns or behaviors that may indicate a security breach or unauthorized access may be analyzed by AI algorithms.

Predictive Analytics: AI can predict potential security threats based on historical data, enabling healthcare organizations to proactively take measures to prevent or mitigate such threats.

Behavioral Biometrics: AI-powered systems can use behavioral biometrics (e.g., typing patterns, voice recognition) to validate the identity of healthcare professionals and patients, reducing the risk of unauthorized access.

Natural Language Processing (NLP): NLP algorithms can automatically scan and analyze text-based data, such as medical records and emails, to identify sensitive information and flag potential privacy breaches.

Cybersecurity Automation: AI can automate routine security tasks, such as system monitoring, threat hunting, and incident response, improving efficiency and accuracy.

Anomaly Detection: AI algorithms can monitor network activities, user behaviors, and data access patterns to identify unusual or suspicious activities. This helps in detecting potential security threats or unauthorized access attempts.

Intrusion Detection and Prevention: AI-powered intrusion detection systems can continuously analyze network traffic and system logs to identify and block malicious activities or cyberattacks in real time.

Predictive Security: AI can analyze historical security data and patterns to predict future threats, enabling proactive measures to prevent potential attacks.

User Authentication: AI can improve user authentication mechanisms by using biometric data, voice recognition, or facial recognition to ensure the identity of users accessing sensitive data.

Data Encryption and Decryption: AI can enhance encryption and decryption processes, making it more secure and less susceptible to traditional brute-force attacks.

21.4.2 Artificial intelligence (AI) for privacy in healthcare

AI can help protect patient privacy and maintain confidentiality in healthcare systems through various techniques:

De-identification: AI can automatically de-identify or anonymize patient data before it's used for research or analysis, ensuring that individuals' identities are not exposed.

Privacy-Preserving Machine Learning: AI methods such as federated learning or differential privacy allow for collaborative model training without sharing raw patient data, thus protecting sensitive information.

Access Control and Data Governance: AI-driven access control mechanisms can ensure that only allowed personnel can access specific patient data, lowering the possibility of data breaches.

Natural Language Processing (NLP) for Privacy Policy Compliance: AI-powered NLP can analyze privacy policies and consent forms to ensure that they adhere to relevant regulations and standards, such as GDPR and HIPAA.

21.4.3 Blockchain for security and privacy in healthcare system

Blockchain is a distributed and immutable ledger technology that can contribute to healthcare safety and confidentiality in the following ways:

Data Integrity: Blockchain strength lies in its immutable ledger. However, ascertaining the accuracy and honesty of medical data before it enters the blockchain is crucial. Garbage in, garbage out (GIGO) still applies. Blockchain ensures the integrity of healthcare data by creating a tamper-resistant record of all transactions and changes to patient records. Because of the immutability of blockchain technology, data that has been stored cannot be changed or erased without the network's users' consent. This feature helps maintain the integrity of patient records and prevents unauthorized modifications.

Access Control: Blockchain decentralized nature can make access control more challenging. Implementing robust access control mechanisms is essential to prevent unauthorized access to patient data.

Consensus Mechanisms: Different blockchain consensus mechanisms (e.g., Proof of Work, Proof of Stake) have their security trade-offs. Ensuring the chosen mechanism aligns with security and privacy requirements is vital.

Smart Contract Vulnerabilities: Smart contracts, while powerful, are susceptible to bugs and vulnerabilities. Thorough testing and code audits are essential to prevent exploitable weaknesses.

Consent Management: Blockchain can facilitate patient-controlled consent management, allowing individuals to grant or revoke access to their medical data for specific entities.

Interoperability: Blockchain reduces the danger of data silos and improves cooperation by enabling safe data exchange and connectivity between various healthcare providers and systems.

Identity Management: Identity management systems built on blockchain technology can be more safe and distributed, lowering the chance of theft and identity fraud.

Clinical Trials and Research: Blockchain can simplify the handling of clinical trial data while maintaining patient confidentiality and assuring openness and traceability.

21.4.3.1 Blockchain in healthcare privacy

Blockchain technology can significantly enhance privacy in the healthcare system:

Decentralization: Patient information is frequently kept in consolidated databases by conventional healthcare institutions, making them vulnerable to single points of failure and security breaches. Blockchain decentralized architecture distributes data across a network of nodes, making it more resistant to attacks.

Patient Consent Management: Blockchain can facilitate secure and transparent patient consent management systems, allowing patients to limit who has exposure to their medical information and how it is used.

Interoperability: Blockchain enables seamless and secure data sharing across different healthcare providers while maintaining strict access controls. This can improve collaboration and patient care without compromising data security.

Auditing and Compliance: Blockchain transparent and auditable nature simplifies regulatory compliance, ensuring that healthcare organizations adhere to data privacy laws and guidelines.

21.5 Integration of artificial intelligence and blockchain in healthcare systems

The convergence of AI and blockchain in healthcare can create even more robust security and privacy solutions. For example:

Private and Decentralized Health Data AI Models: AI algorithms can be trained on decentralized data kept on the blockchain, ascertaining that sensitive information remains private while enabling collaborative research and development of AI models.

Federated Learning: Blockchain can facilitate federated learning approaches, where AI models are trained across multiple healthcare organizations' data without sharing raw data, preserving privacy.

Smart Contracts for Data Access Control: Smart contracts on the blockchain can manage fine-grained access controls to health data, allowing patients to grant permission to specific AI applications or researchers while retaining full control over their data.

Data Off-Chain vs. On-Chain: Deciding which data is stored on-chain (immutable but slower) and which data is processed off-chain (faster but mutable) requires careful consideration of security and privacy requirements.

Decentralization vs. Centralization: Determining the level of decentralization in the system impacts security. Fully decentralized systems may lack a central authority to address security issues effectively.

Regulatory Compliance: HIPAA and GDPR: Healthcare systems dealing with patient data must comply with relevant regulations like the Health Insurance Portability and Accountability Act (HIPAA) and the General Data Protection Regulation (GDPR).

Interoperability: Ensuring compatibility between different AI systems and blockchain networks is crucial to maintain data integrity and prevent security breaches.

Regular Audits and Assessments: It is important to conduct regular safety audits and risk assessments in order to find vulnerabilities and make the required corrections.

The healthcare sector might undergo a change thanks to AI and blockchain technology, which will increase data safety, openness, and productivity. However, safety and confidentiality concerns raised by their execution also demand due attention. Blockchain and AI are two cutting-edge technologies that might significantly improve safety and confidentiality in the healthcare industry. Blockchain and AI are two game-changing technologies that have the potential to have a substantial influence on the safety and confidentiality features of the healthcare system. Some of the most important safety and confidentiality factors from both angles include:

21.6 Open issues and future research directions

Access to cutting-edge technologies in the healthcare system: As a result of the development of innovative medical systems, medical professionals and staff must now manage cutting-edge technology to operate medical equipment for the virtual surveillance of patients. However, not all medical providers have the necessary expertise and experience to address a patient's health symptoms using cutting-edge technologies. Despite the fact that doing so might be expensive for hospitals, the administration of the hospital should educate its medical professionals or staff about these technologies [147].

Scalability: One of the main issues that must be handled during the wireless communication between the patient and the doctor in the remote treatment setup is scalability. Healthcare providers may need a variety of medical tools and implantable sensors depending on the patient's health symptoms in order to collect patient health information and decide on further therapy. A person's health issue might worsen, cause mortality, or leave them in a very terrible condition if interaction among users and health practitioners is delayed due to insufficient scalability. Network bandwidth in intelligent healthcare platforms needs to be maximized for the rapid and dependable therapy of patients [148].

Security standardization in smart healthcare is insufficient: Present health and security regulations are out-of-date and overly traditional. They are not strong enough to withstand contemporary security threats either. Standardization is necessary, especially in the healthcare industry, to reduce error risk, boost patient safety, and significantly improve patient experience. Furthermore, security concerns that arise as a result of patients being monitored remotely may harm their health and make them less likely to take medication from that particular healthcare practitioner. As a result, it may harm the hospital management standing, which may impact overall income [149].

Smart healthcare systems are vulnerable to modern security assaults: In addition to common assaults like DDoS, MITM, and ransomware, attackers have found novel ways to attack a system. The most recent attacks involve software supply chain attacks, in which criminals exploit a healthcare institution's supplier network and weakness. Assaults on the IoT, currently, a huge range of remote connections to the Internet are made by endpoint devices. The malware evaluates the system's modifications and affects the signals it receives to perform harmful actions [150].

Access control at the physical layer is not available: The physical security layer serves as the foundation for all security measures. Only the application layer is subject to the access control limits imposed by the current security measures. The emerging security dangers target wireless communication since it is not safeguarded in the physical layer. The smart healthcare system is often entirely exposed when physical security is lost. Furthermore, a hacker can easily change the data from inserted medical devices, such as pacemakers, fabricated ligaments, and heart attaches, attached to the patient's body, which poses security risks in wireless communication among patients and medical care experts during online care [151].

21.7 Critical lessons learned

Based on a safety and confidentiality standpoint, investigating AI and blockchain in the context of healthcare has revealed key insights that may steer the responsible development and use of these technologies. Investigating the convergence of AI and blockchain for Healthcare Systems has yielded useful insights into the possible advantages and problems of using these technologies in the healthcare business. Examining the use of AI and blockchain in healthcare has revealed some important insights in terms of security and privacy. As these innovations advance, it is critical to address the problems and hazards connected with their application in healthcare. Learning about the convergence of AI and blockchain-based systems for healthcare from the standpoints of safety and confidentiality has highlighted important lessons. new lectures emphasize the difficulties, possibilities, and best practices to guarantee the safe and accountable implementation of novel innovations in the medical sector. Here are some key findings from this research:

1. *Data Privacy and Confidentiality are Paramount:* Medical data is extremely delicate and must be treated with extreme caution. Data security and confidentiality ought to be prioritized in AI and blockchain applications in medical services, ensuring that only authorized persons have access to patient information.
2. *Data Privacy and Ownership:* Healthcare data is extremely sensitive and subject to stringent privacy restrictions (e.g., HIPAA in the United States). It is critical to establish explicit data ownership rights and guarantee that patient consent and privacy are honored throughout the data lifecycle when employing AI and Blockchain in healthcare.
3. *Data Privacy and Consent:* Highly susceptible and private information is contained in healthcare data. When using AI and Blockchain technologies, it is critical to ensure patient privacy and gain informed permission for data usage. To secure patient information, consent management systems and comprehensive data anonymity mechanisms must be deployed.
4. *Research and Collaboration:* AI and blockchain advancement in healthcare is strongly reliant on collaboration among multiple stakeholders, including technological builders, medical professionals, scholars, and regulatory agencies. This collaboration promotes the exchange of information and best practices, as well as the progress of the field.
5. *Decentralization and Consensus Mechanisms:* The decentralized structure of blockchain and its consensus procedures improve security by removing single points of failure and lowering the possibility of data tampering. However, in order to guarantee privacy, the consensus model must be carefully designed, as some consensus algorithms may disclose sensitive data. Decentralization and immutability are two key characteristics of blockchain technology. While these traits improve data security and integrity, they also offer GDPR compliance issues, since the right to erasure becomes problematic in an immutable ledger. It is critical to include methods to manage data change requests while maintaining the chain's integrity. Understanding the various consensus processes used in healthcare blockchains (e.g., Proof of Work and Proof of Stake) is critical. Each mechanism has trade-offs with respect to safety, capacity, and energy consumption, and selecting the proper one for the specific healthcare use case is crucial.
6. *Decentralization and Data Security:* The decentralized structure of blockchain provides advantages in terms of data security by decreasing single points of failure and possible breaches. However, it complicates administering access limits and preserving data integrity inside the decentralized network.
7. *Immutable Records are not always Appropriate:* While blockchain's immutability is a beneficial trait, it might be problematic in the context of healthcare. Medical records may require updates or revisions, and sensitive information, such as a patient's right to be forgotten, should be erasable.
8. *Interoperability Challenges:* Because of interoperability difficulties, integrating AI and blockchain solutions with current healthcare infrastructure

might be difficult. It is critical to provide seamless communication and data flow between different systems while preserving security. It is difficult to provide smooth data interchange and communication across multiple healthcare systems, both AI and blockchain. Standardization initiatives are required to enable interoperability, which allows diverse systems to function efficiently together.

9. *Smart Contracts and Auditing:* Smart contracts in healthcare can help automate operations, but they must be extensively examined for security flaws. Smart contract flaws can have serious ramifications, especially when dealing with sensitive patient data. Because smart contracts on a Blockchain network may perform automatic tasks, they are appealing for healthcare applications like insurance claims processing and prescription administration. However, it is critical to ensure the security and validity of smart contracts in order to avoid vulnerabilities and potential exploitation. Thorough auditing and testing are essential when deploying smart contracts in healthcare to minimize vulnerabilities or unforeseen outcomes that might jeopardize patient safety or data privacy.
10. *Smart Contracts for Healthcare Transactions:* Smart contracts on the blockchain can help simplify administrative operations like insurance claims, billing, and supply chain management. These self-executing contracts have the potential to minimize administrative expenses while also increasing transparency.
11. *Trust and Transparency:* AI and blockchain technology are both seen as sophisticated and difficult to grasp. Transparent communication of these systems' methods and operations to patients, healthcare professionals, and stakeholders is critical for obtaining confidence and acceptance.
12. *Cybersecurity Risks:* Artificial intelligence and distributed ledger systems are vulnerable to cyberattacks. To guard against data breaches, ransomware attacks, and other security threats, healthcare businesses must deploy effective cybersecurity procedures.
13. *Regulatory Compliance:* Healthcare is a highly regulated business, and deploying AI and blockchain technologies necessitates adherence to current data protection and privacy laws. To prevent any legal complications, it is critical to understand the legal and regulatory ramifications.
14. *Bias and Fairness in AI Algorithms:* To avoid biases and assure justice, AI systems used in healthcare must be properly built and evaluated. Biased AI algorithms may provide discriminating results, affecting patient care and treatment decisions.
15. *Training AI Models with Privacy-preserving Techniques:* To train AI models while keeping patient data secure and private, medical professionals and AI developers must use privacy-preserving strategies such as federated learning or differential privacy.
16. *Regulatory Compliance:* Healthcare rules and compliance procedures must be followed at all times. AI and Blockchain applications should be designed with compliance in mind, taking into account regional and worldwide legislation that regulates the use of health data.

17. *Informed Consent and Data Ownership:* Patients should have access to their data and be aware of how it will be utilized. To get express authorization for data exchange and analysis, informed consent protocols should be in place.
18. *Data Quality and Integrity:* The "garbage in, garbage out" idea of blockchain also applies to healthcare. It is critical for trustworthy analysis and decision making to ensure the correctness and integrity of data that enters the blockchain.
19. *Scalability and Performance:* AI and blockchain technology may both be computationally demanding. It is critical to provide scalability and performance while retaining security, especially in high-throughput healthcare situations. Scalability difficulties plague blockchain networks, particularly public ones like Bitcoin and Ethereum. To manage massive volumes of healthcare data, technologies like permissioned blockchains or off-chain protocols must be investigated.
20. *Education and Training:* It is vital to provide proper education and training to healthcare professionals and workers who will be using these technologies. They must comprehend how AI and blockchain systems operate, as well as the possible hazards and best practices for maintaining security and privacy. Because AI and blockchain deployment in healthcare necessitates specific expertise, there is a need for continual education and training programs for healthcare professionals and technology specialists. This guarantees that the potential advantages are fully achieved while minimizing the hazards.
21. *Real-World Testing and Validation:* Real-world testing and validation in controlled conditions are critical for fully understanding the impact and usefulness of AI and blockchain in healthcare. Pilot studies and clinical trials can assist in identifying issues and refining technology for wider use.
22. *Data Validation and Provenance:* The immutability of blockchain provides an ideal framework for protecting data integrity and provenance. Using this functionality, healthcare systems may track the origin and modification history of data, lowering the risk of false or erroneous data.
23. *Hybrid Approaches:* In certain circumstances, combining traditional centralized databases with blockchain technology might provide a more practical solution by balancing the benefits of both worlds.
24. *Ethical Considerations:* As AI applications become more capable and autonomous, the importance of ethical frameworks grows. It is critical to ensure that AI algorithms and blockchain systems do not propagate prejudice or discrimination in healthcare choices.
25. *User Education and Awareness:* Healthcare professionals, patients, and other stakeholders must be informed about the advantages, disadvantages, and limits of AI and Blockchain in healthcare. Raising awareness can aid in the development of trust and appropriate usage of these technologies.
26. *Collaboration and Industry Standards:* Collaboration among healthcare providers, technology professionals, researchers, and politicians is critical for developing industry standards that safeguard the security and privacy of AI and Blockchain applications for healthcare.

By adopting the aforementioned lessons in the invention and deployment of AI and Blockchain approaches, healthcare companies may optimize the potential advantages while protecting patient data and privacy, resulting in better healthcare results. These important insights may be used in the development and implementation of AI and blockchain technologies in the healthcare business. We can build a more secure, private, and responsible environment that benefits patients, medical professionals, and all stakeholders.

21.8 Conclusion and future scope

By combining AI and blockchain technologies, healthcare systems can significantly enhance security and privacy, which are critical aspects in an industry dealing with sensitive patient information. However, it's essential to consider regulatory compliance and ethical implications while implementing these technologies to strike the right balance between innovation and the protection of patients' rights. Despite the potential benefits, it's important to address challenges related to scalability, interoperability, regulatory compliance, and data governance when implementing AI and blockchain in healthcare. Additionally, it's crucial to prioritize the ethical use of AI and ensure that patient privacy remains a top priority throughout the implementation process. In summary, leveraging AI and blockchain in healthcare offers immense potential but must be approached with careful attention to security and privacy concerns. Collaborations between AI experts, blockchain developers, and healthcare professionals can help design robust and secure systems to drive innovation while protecting patient data. Additionally, adherence to relevant regulations and industry standards is essential for successful and ethical implementation.

References

[1] Pablo, R. G. J., Roberto, D. P., Victor, S. U., Isabel, G. R., Paul, C., & Elizabeth, O. R. (2021). Big data in the healthcare system: A synergy with artificial intelligence and blockchain technology. *Journal of Integrative Bioinformatics*, *19*(1), 20200035.

[2] Awotunde, J. B., Chakraborty, C., & Folorunso, S. O. (2022). A secured transaction based on blockchain architecture in mobile banking platform. *International Journal of Internet Technology and Secured Transactions*, *12*(4), 287–303.

[3] Hölbl, M., Kompara, M., Kamišalić, A., & Nemec Zlatolas, L. (2018). A systematic review of the use of blockchain in healthcare. *Symmetry*, *10*(10), 470.

[4] Abidi, S. S. R., & Abidi, S. R. (July 2019). Intelligent health data analytics: A convergence of artificial intelligence and big data. In *Healthcare Management Forum* (Vol. 32, No. 4, pp. 178–182). Sage CA: Los Angeles, CA: SAGE Publications.

[5] Benke, K., & Benke, G. (2018). Artificial intelligence and big data in public health. *International Journal of Environmental Research and Public Health, 15*(12), 2796.

[6] Chen, X., Ji, J., Luo, C., Liao, W., & Li, P. (December 2018). When machine learning meets blockchain: A decentralized, privacy-preserving and secure design. In *2018 IEEE International Conference on Big Data (Big Data)* (pp. 1178–1187). IEEE.

[7] Li, Z., Liu, J., Hao, J., Wang, H., & Xian, M. (2020). CrowdSFL: A secure crowd computing framework based on blockchain and federated learning. *Electronics*, *9*(5), 773.

[8] Schatz, M. C. (2009). CloudBurst: Highly sensitive read mapping with MapReduce. *Bioinformatics*, *25*(11), 1363–1369.

[9] Kavitha, K. V. N., Ashok, S., Imoize, A. L., *et al.* (2022). On the use of wavelet domain and machine learning for the analysis of epileptic seizure detection from EEG signals. *Journal of Healthcare Engineering, 2022.*

[10] Vyas, S., Shabaz, M., Pandit, P., Parvathy, L. R., & Ofori, I. (2022). Integration of artificial intelligence and blockchain technology in healthcare and agriculture. *Journal of Food Quality*, 2022.

[11] Awotunde, J. B., Misra, S., & Pham, Q. T. (November 2022). A secure framework for internet of medical things security based system using lightweight cryptography enabled blockchain. In *International Conference on Future Data and Security Engineering* (pp. 258–272). Singapore: Springer Nature Singapore.

[12] Gorkhali, A., Li, L., & Shrestha, A. (2020). Blockchain: A literature review. *Journal of Management Analytics*, *7*(3), 321–343.

[13] Cha, S. C., Chen, J. F., Su, C., & Yeh, K. H. (2018). A blockchain connected gateway for BLE-based devices in the internet of things. *IEEE Access*, *6*, 24639–24649.

[14] Awotunde, J. B., Misra, S., Ajagbe, S. A., Ayo, F. E., & Gurjar, R. (May 2023). An IoT machine learning model-based real-time diagnostic and monitoring system. In *Machine Intelligence Techniques for Data Analysis and Signal Processing: Proceedings of the 4th International Conference MISP* 2022, Volume 1 (pp. 789–799). Singapore: Springer Nature Singapore.

[15] Ali, A., Rahim, H. A., Pasha, M. F. *et al.* (2021). Security, privacy, and reliability in digital healthcare systems using blockchain. *Electronics*, *10* (16), 2034.

[16] Ali, A., Naveed, M., Mehboob, M., Irshad, H., & Anwar, P. (April 2017). An interference aware multi-channel MAC protocol for WASN. In *2017 International Conference on Innovations in Electrical Engineering and Computational Technologies (ICIEECT)* (pp. 1–9). IEEE.

[17] Adeniyi, J. K., Adeniyi, T. T., Awotunde, J. B., Abiodun, M. K., & Atanda, O. G. (April 2023). Agrolend: A blockchain implementation approach of smart contract farming platform. In 2023 *International Conference on Science, Engineering and Business for Sustainable Development Goals (SEB-SDG)* (Vol. 1, pp. 1–7). IEEE.

[18] Abiodun, M. K., Adeniyi, A. E., Victor, A. O., Awotunde, J. B., Atanda, O. G., & Adeniyi, J. K. (April 2023). Detection and prevention of data leakage in transit using LSTM recurrent neural network with encryption algorithm. In *2023 International Conference on Science, Engineering and Business for Sustainable Development Goals (SEB-SDG)* (Vol. 1, pp. 01–09). IEEE.

[19] Singh, P., Masud, M., Hossain, M. S., & Kaur, A. (2021). Cross-domain secure data sharing using blockchain for industrial IoT. *Journal of Parallel and Distributed Computing, 156*, 176–184.

[20] Idrees, S. M., Nowostawski, M., Jameel, R., & Mourya, A. K. (2021). Security aspects of blockchain technology intended for industrial applications. *Electronics, 10*(8), 951.

[21] Sharma, A., Sarishma, Tomar, R., Chilamkurti, N., & Kim, B. G. (2020). Blockchain based smart contracts for internet of medical things in e-healthcare. *Electronics, 9*(10), 1609.

[22] Hameed, K., Ali, A., Naqvi, M. H., Jabbar, M., Junaid, M., & Haider, A. (August 2016). Resource management in operating systems-a survey of scheduling algorithms. In *Proceedings of the International Conference on Innovative Computing (ICIC), Lanzhou, China* (pp. 2–5).

[23] Vijarania, M., Gupta, S., Agrawal, A., Adigun, M. O., Ajagbe, S. A., & Awotunde, J. B. (2023). Energy efficient load-balancing mechanism in integrated IoT–fog–cloud environment. *Electronics, 12*(11), 2543.

[24] Hasnain, M., Pasha, M. F., Ghani, I., Mehboob, B., Imran, M., & Ali, A. (2020). Benchmark dataset selection of web services technologies: A factor analysis. *IEEE Access, 8*, 53649–53665.

[25] Liu, J., Li, X., Ye, L., Zhang, H., Du, X., & Guizani, M. (December 2018). BPDS: A blockchain based privacy-preserving data sharing for electronic medical records. In *2018 IEEE Global Communications Conference (GLOBECOM)* (pp. 1–6). IEEE.

[26] Khan, F. A., Asif, M., Ahmad, A., Alharbi, M., & Aljuaid, H. (2020). Blockchain technology, improvement suggestions, security challenges on smart grid and its application in healthcare for sustainable development. *Sustainable Cities and Society, 55*, 102018.

[27] Awotunde, J. B., Misra, S., Ayoade, O. B., Ogundokun, R. O., & Abiodun, M. K. (2022). Blockchain-based framework for secure medical information in internet of things system. In *Blockchain Applications in the Smart Era* (pp. 147–169). Cham: Springer International Publishing.

[28] Ogundokun, R. O., Arowolo, M. O., Misra, S., & Awotunde, J. B. (2022). Machine learning, IoT, and blockchain integration for improving process management application security. In *Blockchain Applications in the Smart Era* (pp. 237–252). Cham: Springer International Publishing.

[29] Griggs, K. N., Ossipova, O., Kohlios, C. P., Baccarini, A. N., Howson, E. A., & Hayajneh, T. (2018). Healthcare blockchain system using smart contracts for secure automated remote patient monitoring. *Journal of medical systems, 42*, 1–7.

[30] Zhao, J. L., Fan, S., & Yan, J. (2016). Overview of business innovations and research opportunities in blockchain and introduction to the special issue. *Financial Innovation*, *2*(1), 1–7.

[31] Clohessy, T., Treiblmaier, H., Acton, T., & Rogers, N. (2020). Antecedents of blockchain adoption: An integrative framework. *Strategic Change*, *29*(5), 501–515.

[32] Kaushik, K., & Kumar, A. (2023). Demystifying quantum blockchain for healthcare. *Security and Privacy*, *6*(3), e284.

[33] Adeniyi, E. A., Ogundokun, R. O., Misra, S., Awotunde, J. B., & Abiodun, K. M. (2022). Enhanced security and privacy issue in multi-tenant environment of green computing using blockchain technology. In *Blockchain Applications in the Smart Era* (pp. 65–83). Cham: Springer International Publishing.

[34] Dong, Y., Mun, S. K., & Wang, Y. (2023). A blockchain-enabled sharing platform for personal health records. *Heliyon*..

[35] Awotunde, J. B., Chakraborty, C., & Folorunso, S. O. (2022). A secured smart healthcare monitoring systems using blockchain technology. In *Intelligent Internet of Things for Healthcare and Industry* (pp. 127–143). Cham: Springer International Publishing.

[36] Rawal, B. S., Manogaran, G., & Hamdi, M. (2021). Multi-tier stack of block chain with proxy re-encryption method scheme on the internet of things platform. *ACM Transactions on Internet Technology (TOIT)*, *22*(2), 1–20.

[37] Barhanpure, A., Belandor, P., & Das, B. (2019). Proof of stack consensus for blockchain networks. In *Security in Computing and Communications: 6th International Symposium*, SSCC 2018, Bangalore, India, September 19–22, 2018, Revised Selected Papers 6 (pp. 104–116). Springer Singapore.

[38] Rathore, H., Mohamed, A., & Guizani, M. (2020). A survey of blockchain enabled cyber-physical systems. *Sensors*, *20*(1), 282.

[39] Bacorn, K. (2020). *GreenBlocks: A New Green Building Rating System Created on the Blockchain* (Doctoral dissertation, Harvard University).

[40] Massaro, M. (2021). Digital transformation in the healthcare sector through blockchain technology. Insights from academic research and business developments. *Technovation*, 102386.

[41] Xie, Y., Zhang, J., Wang, H., *et al.* (2021). Applications of blockchain in the medical field: Narrative review. *Journal of Medical Internet Research*, *23* (10), e28613.

[42] Bhattacharya, S., Singh, A., & Hossain, M. M. (2019). Strengthening public health surveillance through blockchain technology. *AIMS public health*, *6* (3), 326.

[43] Deshpande, K. V., Patil, T., Nagare, S., Sarode, R., & Dhanke, A. (June 2023). MedNcrypt: A blockchain based decentralised health record storage system using IPFS. In *2023 International Conference on Sustainable Computing and Smart Systems (ICSCSS)* (pp. 1579–1587). IEEE.

[44] Anjelin, D. P., & Kumar, S. G. (2023). Blockchain technology to improve security in healthcare data breaches. *International Journal of Intelligent Systems and Applications in Engineering*, *11*(7s), 332–339.

[45] Fu, J., Wang, N., & Cai, Y. (2020). Privacy-preserving in healthcare blockchain systems based on lightweight message sharing. *Sensors*, *20*(7), 1898.

[46] Satamraju, K. P. (2020). Proof of concept of scalable integration of internet of things and blockchain in healthcare. *Sensors*, *20*(5), 1389.

[47] Dagher, G. G., Mohler, J., Milojkovic, M., & Marella, P. B. (2018). Ancile: Privacy-preserving framework for access control and interoperability of electronic health records using blockchain technology. *Sustainable cities and society*, *39*, 283–297.

[48] Abikoye, O. C., Oladipupo, E. T., Imoize, A. L., Awotunde, J. B., Lee, C. C., & Li, C. T. (2023). Securing critical user information over the internet of medical things platforms using a hybrid cryptography scheme. *Future Internet*, *15*(3), 99.

[49] Schmeelk, S., Kanabar, M., Peterson, K., & Pathak, J. (2022). Electronic health records and blockchain interoperability requirements: A scoping review. *JAMIA open*, *5*(3), *ooac*068.

[50] Reegu, F. A., Abas, H., Gulzar, Y., *et al.* (2023). Blockchain-based framework for interoperable electronic health records for an improved healthcare system. *Sustainability*, *15*(8), 6337.

[51] Puneeth, R. P., & Parthasarathy, G. (2023). A survey on security and interoperability of electronic health records sharing using blockchain technology. *Acta Informatica Pragensia*, *12*(1), 160–178.

[52] Andrew, J., Isravel, D. P., Sagayam, K. M., Bhushan, B., Sei, Y., & Eunice, J. (2023). Blockchain for healthcare systems: Architecture, security challenges, trends and future directions. *Journal of Network and Computer Applications*, 103633.

[53] Kumar, M., Raj, H., Chaurasia, N., & Gill, S. S. (2023). Blockchain inspired secure and reliable data exchange architecture for cyber-physical healthcare system 4.0. *Internet of Things and Cyber-Physical Systems*.

[54] Sharma, P., Namasudra, S., Chilamkurti, N., Kim, B. G., & Gonzalez Crespo, R. (2023). Blockchain-based privacy preservation for IoT-enabled healthcare system. *ACM Transactions on Sensor Networks*, *19*(3), 1–17.

[55] Joshi, S., & Sharma, M. (2023). Assessment of implementation barriers of blockchain technology in public healthcare: Evidences from developing countries. *Health Systems*, *12*(2), 223–242.

[56] Raj, A., & Prakash, S. (2023). Privacy preservation of the internet of medical things using blockchain. *Health Services and Outcomes Research Methodology*, 1–28.

[57] Emmanuel, A. A., Awokola, J. A., Alam, S. *et al.* (2023). A hybrid framework of blockchain and IoT technology in the pharmaceutical industry: A comprehensive study. *Mobile Information Systems*, *2023*.

[58] Hu, H., Xu, J., Liu, M., & Lim, M. K. (2023). Vaccine supply chain management: An intelligent system utilizing blockchain, IoT and machine learning. *Journal of business research*, *156*, 113480.

[59] Nanda, S. K., Panda, S. K., & Dash, M. (2023). Medical supply chain integrated with blockchain and IoT to track the logistics of medical products. *Multimedia Tools and Applications*, 1–23.

[60] Aljabhan, B., & Obaidat, M. A. (2023). Privacy-preserving blockchain framework for supply chain management: Perceptive craving game search optimization (PCGSO). *Sustainability*, *15*(8), 6905.

[61] Srivastava, P. R., Zhang, J. Z., & Eachempati, P. (2023). Blockchain technology and its applications in agriculture and supply chain management: A retrospective overview and analysis. *Enterprise Information Systems*, *17*(5), 1995783.

[62] Saha, S., Nova, S. N., & Iqbal, M. I. (May 2023). Healthcare professionals credential verification model using blockchain-based self-sovereign identity. In *Proceedings of the Fourth International Conference on Trends in Computational and Cognitive Engineering: TCCE* 2022 (pp. 381–392). Singapore: Springer Nature Singapore.

[63] Purwono, P., Nisa, K., Wibisono, S. K., & Dewa, B. P. (2023). Private blockchain in the field of health services. *Journal of Advanced Health Informatics Research*, *1*(1), 10–15.

[64] Aldamaeen, O., Rashideh, W., & Obidallah, W. J. (2023). Toward Patient-centric healthcare systems: Key requirements and framework for personal health records based on blockchain technology. *Applied Sciences*, *13*(13), 7697.

[65] Babu, E. S., Yadav, B. R. N., Nikhath, A. K., Nayak, S. R., & Alnumay, W. (2023). MediBlocks: Secure exchanging of electronic health records (EHRs) using trust-based blockchain network with privacy concerns. *Cluster Computing*, *26*(4), 2217–2244.

[66] Singh, P., Sinha, P., & Raghav, A. (2023). A Blockchain IoT hybrid framework for security and privacy in a healthcare database network. In *Dynamics of Swarm Intelligence Health Analysis for the Next Generation* (pp. 210–225). IGI Global.

[67] Shobana, M., Mukeshkumar, A., Vaishnavi, S., & Prasad, C. G. (January 2023). Relating the DT framework in securing the healthcare data using blockchain. In *2023 International Conference on Computer Communication and Informatics (ICCCI)* (pp. 1–4). IEEE.

[68] Tanniru, M. R., Woo, C., & Dutta, K. (2023). A conceptual model to share resources and align goals: Building blockchain application to support care continuity outside a hospital. *Journal of Risk and Financial Management*, *16*(4), 247.

[69] Zhang, G., Yang, Z., & Liu, W. (2022). Blockchain-based privacy preserving e-health system for healthcare data in cloud. *Computer Networks*, *203*, 108586.

[70] Bawany, N. Z., Qamar, T., Tariq, H., & Adnan, S. (2022). Integrating healthcare services using blockchain-based telehealth framework. *IEEE Access*, *10*, 36505–36517.

[71] Kumar, R. L., Wang, Y., Poongodi, T., & Imoize, A. L. (Eds.). (2021). *Internet of Things, Artificial Intelligence and Blockchain Technology*. Cham: Springer.

[72] Cheikhrouhou, O., Mershad, K., Jamil, F., Mahmud, R., Koubaa, A., & Moosavi, S. R. (2023). A lightweight blockchain and fog-enabled secure remote patient monitoring system. *Internet of Things*, *22*, 100691.

[73] Upadrista, V., Nazir, S., & Tianfield, H. (2023). Secure data sharing with blockchain for remote health monitoring applications: A review. *Journal of Reliable Intelligent Environments*, 1–20.

[74] Albassam, A., Almutairi, F., Majoun, N. *et al.* (2023). Integration of blockchain and cloud computing in telemedicine and healthcare. *IJCSNS*, *23*(6), 17.

[75] Faruk, M. J. H., Shahriar, H., Valero, M., Sneha, S., Ahamed, S. I., & Rahman, M. (September 2021). Towards blockchain-based secure data management for remote patient monitoring. In *2021 IEEE International Conference on Digital Health (ICDH)* (pp. 299–308). IEEE.

[76] Zaabar, B., Cheikhrouhou, O., Ammi, M., Awad, A. I., & Abid, M. (October 2021). Secure and privacy-aware blockchain-based remote patient monitoring system for internet of healthcare things. In *2021 17th International Conference on Wireless and Mobile Computing, Networking and Communications (WiMob)* (pp. 200–205). IEEE.

[77] Mistry, C., Thakker, U., Gupta, R. *et al.* (June 2021). MedBlock: An AI-enabled and blockchain-driven medical healthcare system for COVID-19. In *ICC 2021-IEEE International Conference on Communications* (pp. 1–6). IEEE.

[78] Hannan, S. A. (2023). Challenges of blockchain technology using artificial intelligence in healthcare system. *International Journal of Innovative Research in Science, Engineering and Technology (IJIRSET)*, *12*(01), 64–74.

[79] Bibhu, V., Das, L., Rana, A., Sharma, S., & Salagrama, S. (2023). AI model for blockchain based industrial application in healthcare IoT. In *AI Models for Blockchain-Based Intelligent Networks in IoT Systems: Concepts, Methodologies, Tools, and Applications* (pp. 163–184). Cham: Springer International Publishing.

[80] Tyagi, P., & Bargavi, S. M. (2023). Using federated artificial intelligence system of intrusion detection for IOT healthcare system based on Blockchain. *International Journal of Data Informatics and Intelligent Computing*, *2*(1), 1–10.

[81] Selvarajan, S., & Mouratidis, H. (2023). A quantum trust and consultative transaction-based blockchain cybersecurity model for healthcare systems. *Scientific Reports*, *13*(1), 7107.

[82] Kamal, R., Hemdan, E. E. D., & El-Fishway, N. (2023). Care4U: Integrated healthcare systems based on blockchain. *Blockchain: Research and Applications*, 100151.

[83] Sharma, P., Namasudra, S., Crespo, R. G., Parra-Fuente, J., & Trivedi, M. C. (2023). EHDHE: Enhancing security of healthcare documents in IoT-enabled digital healthcare ecosystems using blockchain. *Information Sciences*, *629*, 703–718.

[84] Zhao, H., Bai, P., Peng, Y., & Xu, R. (2018). Efficient key management scheme for health blockchain. *CAAI Transactions on Intelligence Technology*, *3*(2), 114–118.

[85] Mallick, S. R., Lenka, R. K., Goswami, V. *et al.* (2023). BCGeo: Blockchain-assisted geospatial web service for smart healthcare system. *IEEE Access*.

[86] Kiania, K., Jameii, S. M., & Rahmani, A. M. (2023). Blockchain-based privacy and security preserving in electronic health: A systematic review. *Multimedia Tools and Applications*, 1–27.

[87] Kumar, A., Bhushan, B., Shristi, S., Kalita, S., Chaganti, R., & Obaid, A. J. (2023). Blockchain embedded security and privacy preserving in healthcare systems. In *Blockchain Technology Solutions for the Security of Iot-Based Healthcare Systems* (pp. 241–261). Academic Press.

[88] Wen, B., Wang, Y., Ding, Y., Zheng, H., Qin, B., & Yang, C. (2023). Security and privacy protection technologies in securing blockchain applications. *Information Sciences*, 119322.

[89] Alsuqaih, H. N., Hamdan, W., Elmessiry, H., & Abulkasim, H. (2023). An efficient privacy-preserving control mechanism based on blockchain for E-health applications. *Alexandria Engineering Journal*, *73*, 159–172.

[90] Gropper, A. (August 2016). Powering the physician-patient relationship with HIE of one blockchain health IT. In *ONC/NIST use of Blockchain for Healthcare and Research Workshop. Gaithersburg, Maryland, United States: ONC/NIST* (Vol. 212).

[91] Rahman, M. S., Alabdulatif, A., & Khalil, I. (2022). Privacy aware internet of medical things data certification framework on healthcare blockchain of 5G edge. *Computer Communications*, *192*, 373–381.

[92] Theodouli, A., Arakliotis, S., Moschou, K., Votis, K., & Tzovaras, D. (August 2018). On the design of a blockchain-based system to facilitate healthcare data sharing. In *2018 17th IEEE International Conference on Trust, Security and Privacy in Computing and Communications/12th IEEE International Conference on Big Data Science and Engineering (TrustCom/BigDataSE)* (pp. 1374–1379). IEEE.

[93] Shen, B., Guo, J., & Yang, Y. (2019). MedChain: Efficient healthcare data sharing via blockchain. *Applied Sciences*, *9*(6), 1207.

[94] Cyran, M. A. (2018). Blockchain as a foundation for sharing healthcare data. *Blockchain in Healthcare Today*.

[95] Jaiman, V., & Urovi, V. (2020). A consent model for blockchain-based health data sharing platforms. *IEEE Access*, *8*, 143734–143745.

[96] Zhang, P., White, J., Schmidt, D. C., Lenz, G., & Rosenbloom, S. T. (2018). FHIRChain: Applying blockchain to securely and scalably share clinical data. *Computational and Structural Biotechnology Journal*, *16*, 267–278.

[97] Zheng, X., Mukkamala, R. R., Vatrapu, R., & Ordieres-Mere, J. (September 2018). Blockchain-based personal health data sharing system using cloud storage. In *2018 IEEE 20th International Conference on E-health Networking, Applications and Services (Healthcom)* (pp. 1–6). IEEE.

[98] Srivastava, G., Parizi, R. M., & Dehghantanha, A. (2020). The future of blockchain technology in healthcare internet of things security. *Blockchain Cybersecurity, Trust and Privacy*, 161–184.

[99] Rajawat, A. S., Rawat, R., Barhanpurkar, K., Shaw, R. N., & Ghosh, A. (2021). Blockchain-based model for expanding IoT device data security. *Advances in Applications of Data-Driven Computing*, 61–71.

[100] Abou-Nassar, E. M., Iliyasu, A. M., El-Kafrawy, P. M., Song, O. Y., Bashir, A. K., & Abd El-Latif, A. A. (2020). DITrust chain: Towards blockchain-based trust models for sustainable healthcare IoT systems. *IEEE Access*, *8*, 111223–111238.

[101] Baucas, M. J., Spachos, P., & Plataniotis, K. N. (2023). Federated learning and blockchain-enabled fog-IoT platform for wearables in predictive healthcare. *IEEE Transactions on Computational Social Systems.*

[102] Hawayek, J. (2023). Problems with medical claims that artificial intelligence (AI) and blockchain can fix. *Blockchain in Healthcare Today*, *6*(2).

[103] Khatun, M., Islam, R. A., & Islam, S. (2023). B-SAHIC: A blockchain based secured and automated health insurance claim processing system. *Journal of Intelligent & Fuzzy Systems, (Preprint)*, 1–22.

[104] Ananna, T. N., Saifuzzaman, M., Chowdhury, M. J. M., & Ferdous, M. S. (2023). Managing health insurance using blockchain technology. *arXiv preprint arXiv:2306.10329*.

[105] Molnár, B., Pisoni, G., Kherbouche, M., & Zghal, Y. (2023). Blockchain-based business process management (BPM) for finance: The case of credit and claim requests. *Smart Cities*, *6*(3), 1254–1278.

[106] Naveed, N., Sultan, A., Khan, F., & Tahir, S. (March 2023). Efficient, immutable and privacy preserving e-healthcare systems using blockchain. In *2023 International Conference on Communication Technologies (ComTech)* (pp. 140–145). IEEE.

[107] Islam, M. S., Ameedeen, M. A. B., Rahman, M. A., Ajra, H., & Ismail, Z. B. (2023). Healthcare-chain: blockchain-enabled decentralized trustworthy system in healthcare management Industry 4.0 with cyber safeguard. *Computers*, *12*(2), 46.

[108] Isong, B., Vhahangwele, T., & Abu-Mahfouz, A. M. (2023). Blockchain-enabled vaccination registration and verification system in healthcare management. *Journal of Information Systems and Informatics*, *5*(2), 719–741.

[109] Pinto, R. P., Silva, B. M., & Inacio, P. R. (2022). A system for the promotion of traceability and ownership of health data using blockchain. *IEEE Access*, *10*, 92760–92773.

[110] Harrell, D. T., Usman, M., Hanson, L. *et al.* (2022). Technical design and development of a self-sovereign identity management platform for patient-centric health care using blockchain technology. *Blockchain in Healthcare Today*, *5*.

[111] Oyebiyi, O. G., Abayomi-Alli, A., Arogundade, O. T., Qazi, A., Imoize, A. L., & Awotunde, J. B. (2023). A systematic literature review on human ear biometrics: Approaches, algorithms, and trend in the last decade. *Information*, *14*(3), 192.

[112] Venkatraman, S., & Parvin, S. (2022). Developing an IoT identity management system using blockchain. *Systems*, *10*(2), 39.

[113] Anderson, C., Carvalho, A., Kaul, M., & Merhout, J. W. (2023). Blockchain innovation for consent self-management in health information exchanges. *Decision Support Systems*, 114021.

[114] Zhuang, Y., Shyu, C. R., Hong, S., Li, P., & Zhang, L. (2023). Self-sovereign identity empowered non-fungible patient tokenization for health information exchange using blockchain technology. *Computers in Biology and Medicine*, *157*, 106778.

[115] Peyrone, N., & Wichadakul, D. (2023). A formal model for blockchain-based consent management in data sharing. *Journal of Logical and Algebraic Methods in Programming*, *134*, 100886.

[116] Li, C., Huang, Y., Wu, Y. *et al.* (2023). Intelligent data sharing strategy supported by artificial intelligence and blockchain technology: Based on medical data. *Annals of Operations Research*, 1–25.

[117] Colace, F., De Santo, M., Marongiu, F., Santaniello, D., & Troiano, A. (2022). Secure medical data sharing through blockchain and decentralized models. In *Robotics and AI for Cybersecurity and Critical Infrastructure in Smart Cities* (pp. 249–262). Cham: Springer International Publishing.

[118] Awotunde, J. B., Ajagbe, S. A., & Florez, H. (October 2022). Internet of things with wearable devices and artificial intelligence for elderly uninterrupted healthcare monitoring systems. In *International Conference on Applied Informatics* (pp. 278–291). Cham: Springer International Publishing.

[119] Nguyen, D. C., Ding, M., Pathirana, P. N., & Seneviratne, A. (2021). Blockchain and AI-based solutions to combat coronavirus (COVID-19)-like epidemics: A survey. *Ieee Access*, *9*, 95730–95753.

[120] Wysocki, O., Davies, J. K., Vigo, M. *et al.* (2023). Assessing the communication gap between AI models and healthcare professionals: Explainability, utility and trust in AI-driven clinical decision-making. *Artificial Intelligence*, *316*, 103839.

[121] Chakraborty, S., Raut, R. D., Rofin, T. M., & Chakraborty, S. (2023). A comprehensive and systematic review of multi-criteria decision-making methods and applications in healthcare. *Healthcare Analytics*, 100232.

[122] Khan, B., Fatima, H., Qureshi, A. *et al.* (2023). Drawbacks of artificial intelligence and their potential solutions in the healthcare sector. *Biomedical Materials & Devices*, 1–8.

[123] Awotunde, J. B., Babatope, O., Ayoade, P. R., Garg, A., & Bhoi, A. K. (2022). Explainable artificial intelligence-based framework for medical decision support systems. *Explainable Artificial Intelligence in Medical Decision Support Systems*, 91.

[124] Ayoade, O. B., Oladele, T. O., Imoize, A. L. *et al.* (2022). *Explainable Artificial Intelligence (XAI) in Medical Decision Systems (MDSSs): Healthcare Systems Perspective*. The Institute of Engineering Technology (IET).

[125] Vishwakarma, L. P., Singh, R. K., Mishra, R., & Kumari, A. (2023). Application of artificial intelligence for resilient and sustainable healthcare

system: Systematic literature review and future research directions. *International Journal of Production Research*, 1–23.

[126] Koul, A., Bawa, R. K., & Kumar, Y. (2022). Artificial intelligence in medical image processing for airway diseases. In *Connected e-Health: Integrated IoT and Cloud Computing* (pp. 217–254). Cham: Springer International Publishing.

[127] Gupta, P., & Sahoo, P. K. (2022). Applications of artificial intelligence in medical images analysis. In *Biomedical Signal and Image Processing with Artificial Intelligence* (pp. 287–308). Cham: Springer International Publishing.

[128] Awotunde, J. B., Ajagbe, S. A., Oladipupo, M. A. *et al.* (October 2021). An improved machine learnings diagnosis technique for COVID-19 pandemic using chest X-ray images. In *International Conference on Applied Informatics* (pp. 319–330). Cham: Springer International Publishing.

[129] Hasanzad, M., Patrinos, G., Sarhangi, N., Sarrami, B., & Larijani, B. (2023). *Using ChatGPT to Predict the Future of Personalized Medicine.*

[130] Patil, S., & Shankar, H. (2023). Transforming healthcare: Harnessing the power of AI in the modern era. *International Journal of Multidisciplinary Sciences and Arts*, *2*(1), 60–70.

[131] Alkhodari, M., Xiong, Z., Khandoker, A. H., Hadjileontiadis, L. J., Leeson, P., & Lapidaire, W. (2023). The role of artificial intelligence in hypertensive disorders of pregnancy: Towards personalized healthcare. *Expert Review of Cardiovascular Therapy*, (just-accepted).

[132] Floresta, G., Zagni, C., Patamia, V., & Rescifina, A. (2023). How can artificial intelligence be utilized for de novo drug design against COVID-19 (SARS-CoV-2)?. *Expert Opinion on Drug Discovery*, 1–4.

[133] Vora, L. K., Gholap, A. D., Jetha, K., Thakur, R. R. S., Solanki, H. K., & Chavda, V. P. (2023). Artificial intelligence in pharmaceutical technology and drug delivery design. *Pharmaceutics*, *15*(7), 1916.

[134] Ravali, R. S., Chellathurai, A., Auguskani, J. P. L., Reddy, L. K. V., Narapureddy, B. R., & Mavaluru, D. (2023). Transforming healthcare innovations: Integrating AI in drug discovery, development, and nursing practice. *Latin American Journal of Pharmacy*, *42*(2), 673–681.

[135] Harry, A. (2023). The future of medicine: Harnessing the power of AI for revolutionizing healthcare. *International Journal of Multidisciplinary Sciences and Arts*, *2*(1), 36–47.

[136] Kaur, M., Sharma, R., & Bansal, N. (2023). 24/7 healthcare services with AI-powered virtual assistants: An update. *Journal of Advanced Research in Embedded System*, *10*(1), 6–9.

[137] KS, N. P., Sudhanva, S., Tarun, T. N., Yuvraaj, Y., & Vishal, D. A. (May 2023). Conversational chatbot builder–smarter virtual assistance with domain specific AI. In *2023 4th International Conference for Emerging Technology (INCET)* (pp. 1–4). IEEE.

[138] Arowolo, M. O., Akubor, V. A., Misra, S., Garg, L., Adebiyi, M. O., & Awotunde, J. B. (December 2021). Development of a chi-square approach for classifying ischemic stroke prediction. In *International Conference on*

Information Systems and Management Science (pp. 268–279). Cham: Springer International Publishing.

[139] Ajagbe, S. A., Awotunde, J. B., Oladipupo, M. A., & Oye, O. E. (2022). Prediction and forecasting of coronavirus cases using artificial intelligence algorithm. In *Machine Learning for Critical Internet of Medical Things: Applications and Use Cases* (pp. 31–54). Cham: Springer International Publishing.

[140] Ahmad, A., Tariq, A., Hussain, H. K., & Gill, A. Y. (2023). Equity and artificial intelligence in surgical care: A comprehensive review of current challenges and promising solutions. *BULLET: Jurnal Multidisiplin Ilmu, 2* (2), 443–455.

[141] Tariq, A., Gill, A. Y., & Hussain, H. K. (2023). Evaluating the potential of artificial intelligence in orthopedic surgery for value-based healthcare. *International Journal of Multidisciplinary Sciences and Arts*, *2*(1), 27–35.

[142] Alabdulatif, A., Khalil, I., & Saidur Rahman, M. (2022). Security of blockchain and ai-empowered smart healthcare: Application-based analysis. *Applied Sciences*, *12*(21), 11039.

[143] Awotunde, J. B., Ayo, F. E., Panigrahi, R., Garg, A., Bhoi, A. K., & Barsocchi, P. (2023). A multi-level random forest model-based intrusion detection using fuzzy inference system for Internet of things networks. *International Journal of Computational Intelligence Systems*, *16*(1), 31.

[144] Li, C., Raghunathan, A., & Jha, N. K. (June 2011). Hijacking an insulin pump: Security attacks and defenses for a diabetes therapy system. In *2011 IEEE 13th International Conference on E-Health Networking, Applications and Services* (pp. 150–156). IEEE.

[145] Ayo, F. E., Awotunde, J. B., Folorunso, S. O., Adigun, M. O., & Ajagbe, S. A. (2023). A genomic rule-based KNN model for fast flux botnet detection. *Egyptian Informatics Journal*, *24*(2), 313–325.

[146] Aggarwal, S., Kumar, N., & Tanwar, S. (2020). Blockchain-envisioned UAV communication using 6G networks: Open issues, use cases, and future directions. *IEEE Internet of Things Journal*, *8*(7), 5416–5441.

[147] Navaz, A. N., Serhani, M. A., El Kassabi, H. T., Al-Qirim, N., & Ismail, H. (2021). Trends, technologies, and key challenges in smart and connected healthcare. *IEEE Access*, *9*, 74044–74067.

[148] Jasim, A. M., & Al-Raweshidy, H. (2023). Optimal intelligent edge-servers placement in the healthcare field. *IET Networks*.

[149] Ahad, A., Ali, Z., Mateen, A., *et al.* (2023). A comprehensive review on 5G-based smart healthcare network security: Taxonomy, issues, solutions and future research directions. *Array*, 100290.

[150] Abdulhamid, A., Kabir, S., Ghafir, I., & Lei, C. (2023). An overview of safety and security analysis frameworks for the internet of things. *Electronics*, *12*(14), 3086.

[151] Imoize, A. L., Udeji, F., Isabona, J., & Lee, C. C. (2023). Optimizing the quality of service of mobile broadband networks for a dense urban environment. *Future Internet*, *15*(5), 181.

Index

www.ingramcontent.com/pod-product-compliance
Lightning Source LLC
LaVergne TN
LVHW011537200926
848484LV00001B/273

* 9 7 8 1 8 3 9 5 3 8 6 3 6 *